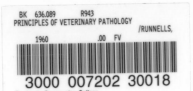

# Principles of
# VETERINARY PATHOLOGY

*Principles of Veterinary Pathology* has been developed as the successor to the former five editions of *Animal Pathology* under single authorship of Russell A. Runnells.

# Principles of

# VETERINARY PATHOLOGY

**RUSSELL A. RUNNELLS,** M.S., D.V.M.
Consultant, The Upjohn Company
Formerly head,
Department of Veterinary Pathology
Michigan State University

**WILLIAM S. MONLUX,** D.V.M., Ph.D.
Iowa Veterinary Diagnostic Laboratory
Iowa State University

**ANDREW W. MONLUX,** D.V.M., M.S., Ph.D.
Head, Department of Veterinary Pathology
Oklahoma State University

**The Iowa State University Press,** *Ames,* **Iowa, U.S.A.**

Previous copyrights under the title *Animal Pathology*:

First edition, 1938
Second edition, 1941
Third edition, 1944
Fourth edition, 1946
Fifth edition, 1954

Present volume, 1960

Library of Congress Catalog Card Number: 60-7254

# Preface

THE PUBLICATION of *Principles of Veterinary Pathology* marks the end of an era for *Animal Pathology*. The era began in the early 1930's with the lithoprinting of the forerunner of the present text and continued through five editions. The project was a venture by a single individual in a field not yet represented by a textbook in America. The era closes with that author being joined by two of his former students, William S. Monlux and Andrew W. Monlux, as co-authors. Following this edition the project will be solely theirs.

From the beginning, *Animal Pathology* was written particularly for veterinary students in the beginning courses in pathology. To emphasize the continuance of that policy the title of the text has been changed to *Principles of Veterinary Pathology*.

Upon retiring from authorship the senior author wishes there were some way for him to convey his gratitude adequately to scores of individuals who in one way or another helped to make *Animal Pathology* possible. He is mindful of the assistance given in various ways by colleagues and students with whom he has been associated. He is aware of the debt he owes to investigators in the United States and other countries whose researches formed the basis for the text. He hopes that all who contributed illustrations can derive some satisfaction in realizing that students gained some of their knowledge of pathology by viewing them.

An author is always most grateful to librarians for facilities and assistance in searching the literature. In this connection the senior author is indebted to the librarians at the universities of Michigan, Colorado, Georgia, and Florida, and of the state universities of Michigan, Iowa, and Colorado. He cannot forget the pleasant associations and fine cooperation of the staff of the Iowa State University Press, especially Marshall Townsend, Kathryn Lapp, and Raymond Fassel.

In preparing the manuscript for *Principles of Veterinary Pathology* the senior author is particularly indebted to Dr. D. A. Sanders, Dr. W. R. Pritchard, and Mr. Fred Bryant at the University of Florida, and the librarians at the Upjohn Company in Kalamazoo for special facilities for library work. And lastly he is exceedingly grateful for the helpful, friendly criticisms and suggestions of his close colleague, Dr. E. A. Benbrook, throughout the years.

RUSSELL A. RUNNELLS

# Contents

## Part 4—SPECIAL PATHOLOGY OF THE SYSTEMS

# PART I

# Introduction and History

CHAPTER 1 | # Introduction

The past, *today,* and the future concern the thoughts of all of us in veterinary medicine. Naturally, our primary interest lies in today. In the practice of veterinary medicine, whether it involves the pathologist, anatomist, pharmacologist, or clinician, the urgent problems are the current ones — the problems of today.

The knowledge of today is built on the knowledge of yesterday, and likewise, the knowledge of the future is based upon what we are doing today. To understand and appreciate the evolution of the veterinary art it is necessary to study the history of veterinary medicine. Since this text is concerned with pathology, it is especially important to study the history of pathology.

Throughout history, one single bit of information, at times seemingly insignificant, has resulted in an entire revolution of medicine or perhaps has added that cementing substance necessary for a workable understanding of the accumulated knowledge. These milestones of medical progress stand out quite clearly as we delve into the past.

The printing press was a singular advancement because it allowed medical compilers to disseminate the available knowledge throughout the world. The introduction of dissection of the cadaver in university classrooms by Ptolemy was another milestone in medicine. Then, for the first time, alterations in the body as the result of disease could be observed, determined, and appreciated. The circulation of the blood, described by William Harvey, was one of the most important single contributions to medicine because it explained how nutrients and oxygen are carried to distant parts of the body. It explained hyperemia, hemorrhage, thrombosis, embolism, and many of the other alterations observed in pathology. The work of van Leeuwenhoek, Bichat, and Mueller opened the field of histopathology. When the value of the microscope in the study of medicine was made clear, Virchow demonstrated the importance of the microscopic examination of tissue in a book on cellular pathology. The study of bacteria by Pasteur, Koch, and Klebs emphasized the fact that these minute organisms were the cause of disease. Cohnheim and Metchnikoff depicted the vascular and cellular changes that occurred in inflammation, thus clearing the field for a thorough understanding of this interesting subject.

The emphasis in medicine and in pathology is now being placed upon cytochemistry and upon chemical, clinical, and physiological pathology rather than on the anatomical pathology in which the pioneering work was done.

Today we have a working knowledge of both the macroscopic and microscopic alterations that occur in tissue as the result of disease. We know that these alterations are comparatively few and that one alteration can be produced by many etiological factors. Like an alphabet, the use of terms associated with these lesions builds the language of medicine so that individuals who have mastered the basic terminology can communicate freely with their colleagues.

Great advances are being made in the field of etiology in the recognition and study of new viruses, pleuropneumonia-like organisms, rickettsiae, and bacteriophages. These discoveries are revealing the reasons why certain diseases have appeared in the general population. They also explain why confusion has existed in the past when the course and epidemiology of certain diseases were obscured due to the presence of diseases simulating each other.

Today, advances are being made in the study of the many industrial products sold to the public. Many of them are extremely toxic to animals.

The advent of the atom bomb, the presence of ionizing substances in our midst, and the treatment of both infectious and neoplastic diseases with radioactive isotopes have opened entirely new fields to which only our imaginations can give us a clue for the future.

The future is not of great concern to any of us. We can philosophically examine the future and speculate as to the type of medicine and the types of diseases that populations will be subject to in years to come; but in the busy life of today there is little time to worry about the problems of future veterinarians and future man. Rightly so, because we do not know which discovery today may revolutionize the entire field of medicine or even the entire civilization. So, other than from a speculative point of view, we are not too concerned with the future.

This book will be concerned primarily with the problems of today. As new diseases are described and new developments are made, this book will change to keep the student abreast of current knowledge.

The study of animal diseases has resulted in the compilation of a large amount of data. This information has been collected, classified, and organized until veterinary medicine is a highly specialized art. Veterinary medicine was once practiced by the blacksmiths, horse traders, and those handy men in the community who seemed to have a gift for the medication of domestic animals. It was part of the duty of the apprentice in the blacksmith shop to learn something of the veterinary art.

The need for specialized training became apparent during the nineteenth century, when courses in veterinary medicine began to be listed in the college catalogues of public and private institutions. At first the courses were six weeks in length, later they became three months, soon they advanced to two years, then three years, finally four years, then five years, and now all schools in this country require six years of study — two years of preveterinary study and four years in veterinary subjects. In this way veterinary medicine has progressed from the blacksmith shop and the livery stable to the university. It has now advanced to the graduate school level, and for those few individuals who continue their study in veterinary medicine, a considerably longer period of time is required to receive the Master of Science or Doctor of Philosophy degrees.

Since there are many applicants for admission into our colleges of veterinary medicine, the colleges now have admission committees whose function is to select the most desirable candidates. This rigid selection has resulted in a much better type of student and veterinarian.

Until the sophomore year in the veterinary curriculum, the student studies certain basic sciences (chemistry, physics, English, mathematics, anatomy, histology, embryology, and animal sciences of various types). At this point he is finally in possession of the basic information necessary for the study of disease. With this in mind, pathology comes to occupy the fulcrum position in the study of veterinary medicine.

*The object of the study of pathology is to acquaint the student with the changes occurring in tissues as the result of disease.* The mastery of pathology will make the study of veterinary medicine much easier during the years of clinical study. By studying pathology diligently, the student will learn to apply the basic sciences he has mastered, and as he progresses to his junior and senior years (the clinical years), he will have a better understanding of the changes that take place within an animal as the result of disease. He will be able to visualize tissue changes and appreciate why the symptoms he observes have appeared. Pathology becomes that correlating study by which the pre-pathology courses are coordinated so that a better understanding of the clinical subjects will be possible. At the time of graduation the student will have received a well-rounded presentation of the subject of veterinary medicine.

# CHAPTER 2

# History of Pathology

To appreciate veterinary medicine and to understand how it has developed through the past centuries, some attention must be given to its history. Through the ages it has been closely allied with human medicine just as it is today. The diseases of animals are often the diseases of man, and therefore their histories are closely intertwined.

## PREHISTORIC AND STONE AGE MEDICINE

We know that the art of healing was practiced in one form or another far back into the Stone Age. Just when the art of medicine appeared in prehistoric periods is not known, and there is no way of determining the exact time. We know diseases have existed for centuries, and probably man and animals have been afflicted with various diseases since the beginning of their time on earth. It is difficult to determine the exact nature of the diseases present during prehistoric times, but archeological studies have indicated some of the lesions. The fossil remains, the skeletons, and the mummies that are discovered today are very carefully studied for lesions that will give some indication of the diseases afflicting these early people. Consequently, some excellent reports are available on the diseases of early man. The Egyptian mummies have been carefully examined and much valuable information has been obtained. The an-cient Egyptians had much the same types of diseases that afflict us today.

Man probably began his practice of medicine by licking his wounds much as dogs, cats, and other animals do. Since he was endowed with greater intelligence than his animal associates, man soon discovered that certain plants, herbs, oils, and protective devices aided in the healing of wounds and in the treatment of his diseases. Gradually, over the expanse of centuries, the art of medicine evolved. The medical practices carried out by savage tribes can be observed today, probably in much the same form as they have existed for centuries, in the cultures of the Bushman of Australia and New Guinea, the inhabitants of the South Sea Islands, and the American Indians.

The knowledge of ancient medicine was controlled by the witch doctor, who used secret herbs, vegetable and animal concoctions, noise, and hideous dress to drive away evil spirits. How much good he did is questionable, but certainly some of the medicaments used were beneficial since we still use a few of the same drugs (quinine, podophyllum, and cocaine).

## RECORDED HISTORY

Recorded history reveals that medical practice existed in all of the more advanced ancient civilizations. Babylon, Persia, Egypt, India, China, Greece, and

Rome all had advanced medical practices and all had a well-developed medical science. It is interesting to observe that considerable skill was developed in certain phases of these medical arts, particularly in those that dealt with war.

If we examine museums and the ruins of these ancient civilizations, we find sculptured figures and designs in marble, granite, and terra cotta — figures that indicate the diseases of those ancient days. There are illustrations of individuals with varicose veins, tumors, dropsy, ulcers, and obesity. The artists of that time depicted the diseases present in the population, and we find they are identical with the diseases causing us so much misery and expense today.

## ASSYRIAN ERA

The Assyrian Empire under Hammurabi (2100 B.C.) is of particular interest to the student of veterinary medicine because at that time veterinary medicine was first mentioned in recorded history. Horses were of great importance in the Assyrian civilization and were used in war to great advantage. The Assyrian Empire obtained much of its strength and much of its prestige through the use of cavalry. The equestrian army found that special care was needed for their horses if they were to keep them in the field on long campaigns. For this reason alone veterinary medicine achieved a considerable degree of skill. In the *Laws of Hammurabi* rigid regulations were laid down as to the conduct of veterinary practitioners. History indicates that these rules and laws were enforced. Considerable space was devoted to the fee charged for services. Medical care was expensive just as it is today. It was found that certain regulations were necessary to control the charges for veterinary services to prevent the public from being exploited and to prevent unfair competitive practices. Even today, in the United States, somewhat similar controls are maintained by the state boards of veterinary examiners, the offices of the state veterinarians, and

by various legislative committees. Fortunately, regulations in the United States have dealt with who shall practice and with the conduct of the veterinarian and have not regulated the fees charged for services rendered.

Other peoples of that time (Hebrews, Babylonians, Carthaginians, and Greeks) contributed to a voluminous literature on veterinary medicine. Unfortunately, most of it was destroyed by the Crusades and by the invasions of the barbarians from the north just as were many other arts and sciences. Only a small amount of the veterinary literature of this period is still available, so our knowledge of early medicine has been acquired from a meager amount of information in our museums and libraries.

## EGYPTIAN ERA

The people of the Nile began to influence medicine about 4000 B.C. Some of these ancient people became very adept in certain phases of medicine, especially skull surgery. The museums of today contain numerous skulls with trephine openings or scars where openings had been made. The scars indicate that healing had taken place and reveal that at least some patients survived. Skull surgery probably developed because of the numerous fractures obtained during war. When compression fractures of the head occurred, it was discovered that by correcting these injuries (by removal of clotted blood and fragments of bone) some of the individuals would recover.

One of the remarkable arts in Egyptian culture was that of *embalming*. Even after several thousand years these mummies are still so well preserved that postmortem examinations can be made and the cause of death can, at times, be determined. The extensive studies made on these mummies indicate that these ancient people died with the same diseases we are afflicted with today. Embalming of thousands of bodies was carried out over a period of about fifty centuries. However, there is a noticeable gap in the recorded history of Egypt, for we find no information on lesions or diseases discovered during embalming. Apparently there was no association made between the changes in the internal organs of these individuals and the causes of death. Bodies were taken into the embalming temples and no one but the priests saw them. The theological cause of disease was stressed, and it is quite possible that the priests recognized changes in organs, and although they themselves knew that certain changes took place in the organs, they kept the information secret. They wished to retain the theory of the theological cause of disease — that illness was the result of Divine displeasure. By so doing they could maintain their theological hold on the people.

## HEBREW ERA

The *Mosaic Doctrine* on clean and unclean flesh must be set down as the first recorded evidence of *systematic meat inspection*. Since Moses lived in the fifteenth century B.C., it is now thirty-five centuries since the transmissibility of animal diseases to human beings was officially recognized. The Laws of Moses, described in detail in Exodus and Leviticus, are exact and nearly complete from the sanitary point of view, and actually little has been added or retracted from these laws during the past thirty-five centuries. The Laws specified that meat which had touched unclean things was unsuitable for human consumption. The clothing of individuals who handled unclean carcasses had to be washed before the wearer could resume his place among the people. The flesh of shellfish and crawling creatures in general was officially declared unfit for human use. Leviticus, Chapter 11, tells us:

3 Whatsoever parteth the hoof, and is clovenfooted, and cheweth the cud, among the beasts, that shall ye eat.

4 Nevertheless these shall ye not eat of them that chew the cud, or of them that divide the hoof: as the camel, because he cheweth the cud, but divideth not the hoof; he is unclean unto you.

6 And the hare, because he cheweth the cud, but divideth not the hoof; he is unclean unto you.

7 And the swine, though he divide the hoof, and be clovenfooted, yet he cheweth not the cud; he is unclean to you.

10 And all that have not fins and scales in the seas, and in the rivers, of all that move in the waters, and of any living thing which is in the waters, they shall be an abomination unto you.

These very exacting, good laws, so similar to those we have today, are well worth reading. The animals listed by Moses are the same that are of concern to the public health official today. These foods are not wholesome even today if the animals are raised and food is processed and stored under inadequate sanitary conditions. Modern canning and food handling procedures have made some of these products, formerly unsuitable for consumption, safe for human consumption today. We can understand why some of the Laws of Moses concerning food came about when we observe unsanitary swine husbandry. The pig is a scavenger, and in this role he is capable of becoming infected with a wide variety of diseases. In the hog, tapeworm cysts, trichinae, erysipelas, and paratyphoid are infectious for man. In a country where there was no refrigeration, it is little wonder that regulations concerning the use of pork were instituted. As to the laws against the consumption of shellfish, there is no better way of transmitting typhoid fever than by human consumption of oysters which have fed in water contaminated with human feces. Today we have very rigid regulations as to where and when oysters may be gathered, for the simple reason of avoiding the enteric complications sometimes associated with their consumption. Think of the centuries of misery that must have existed for ancient pastoral people afflicted with tapeworms, anthrax, trichinosis, salmonellosis, tuberculosis, and other diseases that ravaged animals and were capable of spreading to the masses. Think of the misery experienced by these people before they became aware of the importance of meat and meat products in the transmission of diseases. It is no wonder that intelligent and far-sighted Moses developed and laid down these Laws.

During the period when the Israelites were slaves of Pharaoh, the flocks and herds of the Egyptians were destroyed by a plague while those of the Israelites escaped. We see in Exodus, Chapter 9:

> 4 And the Lord shall sever between the cattle of Israel and the cattle of Egypt: and there shall nothing die of all that is the children's of Israel.
>
> 6 And the Lord did that thing on the morrow, and all the cattle of Egypt died: but of the cattle of the children of Israel died not one.

Divine displeasure against the enemy of a favored people is the Biblical explanation. The actual explanation of this historic tragedy is that Moses practiced simple laws of livestock sanitation, he understood hygiene, and he practiced and lived by those rules. Pharaoh and his people maintained a miserable livestock sanitary program as they had for centuries and did for centuries after the period of Moses. History indicates that this plague was probably anthrax. The reason for the high incidence of the disease in the cattle of Pharaoh and no losses in the cattle of the Israelites is that the cattle of Pharaoh were pastured in the river bottoms, in the swamps, and in the wet inundated areas along the river where the vegetation was lush — areas where anthrax is found. The Israelites, on the contrary, kept their flocks and their herds on the high ground away from the river, and for that reason their animals escaped the disease.

Although the Hebrews were great hygienists and were to be admired for their food sanitation (many of our modern laws have been based on their ancient laws), we cannot help but notice that they accepted the theological concept as the cause of disease just as did the Egyptians, Babylonians, and Assyrians. Although they were well ahead of these nations in hygiene and the control of disease, they still looked to the cause of disease as being the result of Divine displeasure. Did the leaders — intelligent men of the standard of Moses — recognize the cause of disease as being other than theological, but in order to hold the people, did they push the truth into the background and nourish mysticism and the theological concept of etiology?

## GREEK ERA

The contributions of the Greek physicians of the classical period did not deal with the nature of disease nor with the exact changes that occurred in the body as the result of disease, but they did elucidate the principles of exact and careful clinical observation. The Greeks crystallized these observations into a system of medicine. In this manner they became the first clinicians — individuals who met the general public, studied the symptoms of the patient, and by organizing these observations, arrived at a diagnosis. They were the *fathers*, or the originators, *of clinical medicine* as we know it today.

Undoubtedly the most outstanding individual in the history of Greek medicine was HIPPOCRATES (460–375 B.C.). In fact, he is one of the most notable physicians in history. His impact on medical science was so great that the physicians of today consider him as the *father of medicine*. In respect to this old gentleman, medical students of today, at the time of graduation, take the *Oath of Hippocrates*, concerning the practice and ethics of medicine.

The writings of Hippocrates are the basis for the *humoral theory of disease*. It is very questionable if all the documents credited to him were written by his own hand. Many of his writings and theories were not truly his but were rather the product of the School of Hippocrates and the work of his students. Hippocrates was very influential and persuasive, he had many students, he was a great teacher and no doubt implanted many ideas and thoughts in the minds of his followers. Although the result was not the immediate work of Hippocrates, it is just to give him credit for the thought since the seed had been planted in the minds of the students, grew there, and developed into something worthwhile. Today it matters little whether Hippocrates actually wrote the material credited to him or not, but the information was advanced, it was recorded, and fortunately some of it remains for us today even though much of the knowledge was lost during the Crusades and the invasion by the northern barbarians.

Some historians would have Hippocrates as the father of veterinary medicine, but most veterinarians do not agree. The writings of Hippocrates indicate that he never intended his oath to include veterinarians; in fact some of his contributions would suggest that he rather looked down on the "doctors of horses," perhaps even sneering at their efforts.

The humoral theory of disease was developed by the School of Hippocrates and followed the typical Greek philosophical approach. Greek philosophy was based on units of four. The *four elements* of Greek philosophy were *air, water, fire,* and *earth.* The *four qualities* were *moisture, cold, warmth,* and *dryness.* Since Hippocrates and his students were trained basically in philosophy and this governed their general outlook on life, it is natural that their concepts of disease would be divided into units of four. They decided the body consisted of *four humors* (four fluids): the *blood* that was warm and moist like the air, the *phlegm* that was cold and moist like the water, the *yellow* bile that was warm and dry like the fire, and the *black bile* that was cold and dry like the earth. The *origins* of these four humors were closely defined: The blood came from the heart, the phlegm originated in the brain, the yellow bile found its origin in the liver, and the black bile (the most serious of all) came from the spleen.

According to Hippocrates, *health* was believed to be due to a proper mixing or blending of these four humors. In contrast, *disease* was thought to be an improper blending or mixing of the humors.

The clinical explanation of disease according to the humoral theory is as follows: When the phlegm, that originates in the brain, begins to gravitate downward and appears at the nose, the individual has a cold. If it gravitates into the lungs, the patient has pneumonia. Should it continue to gravitate into the lungs for a long period of time, tuberculosis is the result. When the gravitation extends still lower and reaches the intestine, dysentery is the result. Finally, when the phlegm descends into the rectum, hemorrhoids occur.

Diseases of the black bile were considered to be the most serious. When the plagues swept through Europe and other portions of the world during the Middle Ages, they were attributed to disturbances of the black bile. In fact, disturbances of the black bile were so numerous that the period from Hippocrates through the Renaissance is often referred to as the *period of the black bile.*

Each of the four humors was most likely to cause illness during particular seasons of the year. Dyscrasias or disturbances of the phlegm were most commonly observed during the winter. This was the season when colds and pneumonia were present, and tuberculosis was more likely to appear in individuals with respiratory difficulties. Disturbances of the blood occurred in the spring when the blood was "hot" and the population became warlike and wanted to fight. The turmoil of love and war appeared when there was an improper blending or a cooking of the blood. Diseases of the yellow bile were most common during the summer. This was due to malaria and hepatic disease in which the individuals became icteric as the result of an excessive hemolysis of the erythrocytes or the interference with the elimination of bile by the liver. The period of the black bile occurred during the late summer and autumn. This was the period of the year for many of the plagues — diseases in which the spleen, the source of the black bile, became enlarged.

Hippocrates was of the opinion that a disease passed through three stages: a *preliminary stage,* a *ripening stage,* called by him the period of coction, or pepsis, in which there was a mixing, cooking, and boiling of the humors, and finally the *stage of crisis* in which the individual either recovered or died. Today similar stages in the pathogenesis of a disease are recognized: the period of incubation, the period during which the symptoms of the disease develop, and the stage of crisis followed by recovery or death.

The writers of the period of Hippocrates left many good descriptions of inflammation, wounds, rhinitis, pharyngitis, and puerperal sepsis. They knew that patients with suppurative diseases experienced chills and fever. They considered pus as merely transformed blood that was heated by the disease until it putrefied. They were very keen clinical observers, and by philosophical methods they attempted to explain the cause of disease and the alterations they observed. All of this work was done without the aid of the autopsy, and their entire medical science was based on the outward appearance of the individual.

Although the humoral theory of Hippocrates seems odd to us today, it served as the basis for medical practice for two thousand years. In fact, it was not until the end of the nineteenth century that its hold upon the medical world was finally broken when modern pathology, bacteriology, and physiology proved it to be wrong.

ARISTOTLE (384–323 B.C.), another Greek philosopher, was the *originator of modern anatomy and physiology.* This great scholar, although he contributed much to medicine, never dissected a human cadaver. Autopsy examinations were forbidden in Grecian times because of theological concepts. The Greeks usually cremated their dead, and, according to their religious rites, the body had to be intact at the ceremony of cremation. If the body were not intact and did not pass through the ceremony of cremation as dictated by the priests, the soul was condemned to wander aimlessly forever along the banks of the Styx (a mythical stream) searching for the lost parts. For that reason it is easy to understand why the family of the deceased would not allow the cadaver to be dissected.

Because of his excellent work, Aristotle had great influence on future anatomical studies in medicine. He dissected many animals, carried out experiments in physiology, and studied the growth and development of animal life. Because of this pioneering work, many consider him as the *father of zoology.*

Aristotle had a very outstanding royal student, PTOLEMY OF MACEDONIA (367–283 B.C.). In fact, Aristotle was his private tutor. Young Ptolemy was sent as a ruler to Alexandria, Egypt, by the ruler of Greece, Alexander of Macedonia. Ptolemy remembered the teachings of his famous tutor and continued with his study of anatomy. He went into the dissection rooms and there, together with other members of the royal family, dissected and examined the dead. With this royal sanction of dissection, the medical culture of Alexandria flourished. Ptolemy established the University of Alexandria, the Museum of Alexandria, and the great Alexandrian Library. Here, for the first time in medical history, anatomy and dissection of the cadaver took its rightful place in medicine. The culture of the University of Alexandria reigned for four hundred years until destroyed by Caesar when he invaded Egypt. Caesar destroyed the museum and burned the university, the library, and the literature. Only a few scholars and a few remnants of the writings of the period escaped the Roman torch.

## ROMAN ERA

The Romans embraced the medical thoughts of the Greeks and the humoral theory of Hippocrates. A few new ideas and theories dealing with medicine did appear but did not attract many followers and did not become established. The most important of these new ideas was the theory of ASCLEPIADES (128–56 B.C.), a Greek physician who lived in Rome. He believed in the atomic, or corpuscular, theory which placed blame for disease on an inharmonious motion of the corpuscles of the body. The object of his treatment was to restore harmony by use of diet, friction, bathing, and exercise.

CLAUDIUS GALEN (131–206 A.D.), a Greek physician practicing in Rome, was probably the greatest individual in medical history and had more influence on medicine than any other man. Galen was a staunch follower of Hippocrates. He preached the theories of Hippocrates, wrote profusely, was an excellent speaker, and so impressed the people and influenced Roman literature that the humoral theory of Hippocrates lived for two thousand years. Galen is also remembered for his views on meat inspection. He insisted that animals used for human food should be inspected prior to slaughter, and especially so if the meat from these animals was to be consumed by human beings who were ill.

Although Galen wrote a very large number of documents, much of his work was inaccurate. However, it was very convincing and attracted many students. Probably many of the errors in his publications and the inaccuracies in his teaching resulted because he was not able to perform a human autopsy. Dissection of the cadaver was forbidden by Roman law. Fortunately, Galen had been exposed to the information that had survived the destruction of the University of Alexandria. This information and the knowledge he acquired through the dissection of animals formed the basis for his writings.

Another important Roman of this era was CORNELIUS CELSUS (30 B.C.–38 A.D.). Celsus was not a physician. He was a Roman patrician, a man of leisure, who had a wide variety of interests and a taste for literature. Probably because of his nonprofessional position, his work was ignored and unknown by the medical profession of his day. In 1443 Pope Nicholas V, while looking through some ancient literature, came across eight volumes containing a rich storehouse of pathological observations written by Celsus. These writings described and discussed the "cardinal signs of inflammation" (redness, swelling, heat, and pain). These eight volumes can be considered as the *first special pathology.*

APSYRTUS flourished as a veterinary teacher and author in Constantinople during the middle of the fourth century A.D. He was an army officer and was engaged in the treatment and care of the cavalry mounts of Emperor Constantine. He described the principal diseases of horses and instructed the cavalrymen in equine medicine. His keen observations and excellent writings had great influence on the thoughts of veterinarians living in later years and particularly those of the Arab Era.

Another Roman veterinarian, RENATUS VEGETIUS (450–500 A.D.), is credited with being the first author of the Christian Era to write a textbook devoted exclusively to veterinary medicine. Not much is known about the background of this man. Some of his biographers claim he was a man of letters while others claim he was nothing more than a common horse dealer. Nevertheless, he was a keen observer, a good writer, and possessed a great amount of native intelligence. His concepts of the diseases of animals had great influence on his many students and on the animal industry of that time. He was among the first to urge people to disregard Divine displeasure as the cause of disease and to base their treatments and concepts of disease on a thorough knowledge of anatomy, surgery, and medicine. His ideas were a start in the right direction, but it required many years before the goal was realized. Far-sighted Vegetius can certainly be commended for his advanced thinking. Because of the book he wrote and the influence he had on veterinary medicine, he is considered as the *father of veterinary medicine.*

The literature of this period makes very interesting reading. We are sometimes amazed to note how little we have actually added to medical literature and how little we have improved upon the methods used by these ancient people. At times a comedy of errors is encountered in these old documents, but in spite of this they contain considerable sound advice. Unfortunately, much of the work of Vegetius, Apsyrtus, and others was destroyed, along with nearly all art and literature, when the barbarians from the north and the Crusaders invaded Asia Minor. Certainly this period became the Dark Ages as far as veterinary medicine was concerned.

## MEDIEVAL PERIOD

Leaving the Roman Empire and passing into the Middle Ages, or the Medieval Period, we find, in general, a lack of interest in literature, art, and medicine. A few men, notably Paracelsus and Fracastoro, tried to refute the dogma of Galen and Hippocrates. Fracastoro propounded an entirely sound theory on the contagiousness of disease, but like so many other theories in those days, his ideas were not noticed.

## ARAB ERA

The Arabs were quite active in medical circles during the Medieval Period. The Arab Era extended from the seventh to the twelfth century. It was during this time that the Prophet Mohammed introduced the Mohammedan religion. He and his followers attempted to conquer the known world. They invaded Asia Minor, Egypt, North Africa, Spain, and France.

Even today the Arab influence can be seen in the countries they invaded or conquered.

The invaders soon realized that to maintain their strength and to exploit the subjugated countries it was necessary to bring a certain amount of science into their culture, particularly in the fields of agriculture, animal industry, and veterinary medicine. The Arabs lacked a technical background of their own, having very little to draw upon as far as agriculture, animal industry, and veterinary medicine were concerned. They found it necessary to borrow from the cultures of that period. They employed Hebrew scholars to translate the information into the Arabic tongue. Once they had this information in their possession, they used it and added to it so that great progress was made in certain fields. Much of the information we have on early veterinary medicine survived from this work of the Arabs and the Hebrew translators.

As a result of the destructive Seljuk invasion of Asia Minor during the eleventh century, much of the literature of that period was destroyed. A work on agriculture and veterinary medicine by IBN-AL-AWAN is pointed out by all veterinary historians as an example of the excellent quality of the veterinary art of this period. Unfortunately, it represents only a small portion of the information that had been available.

## RENAISSANCE

During the Renaissance, human and veterinary medicine began to take form. This was the transition period in medicine when sacramental patterns and Divine displeasure as the cause of disease were gradually beginning to disappear and sensible people were beginning to resort to surgery, medicine, and common sense. The people were weary of tolerating the diseases that afflicted them and their livestock. Their flocks had been destroyed by anthrax, blackleg, rabies, tetanus, scabies, and wound infection. They demanded action. Pressure was placed upon the state, and little by little that pressure was felt. Gradually there was an elimination of superstition and fear. Medical and veterinary literature began to appear. Here and there a school of veterinary medicine made its appearance. With the advent of books and periodicals, the progress became more and more rapid.

## SIXTEENTH CENTURY

Before medicine could develop, flourish, and become the beneficial science it is today, certain monumental discoveries had to be made. These milestones in medicine began to appear in the sixteenth century.

In the sixteenth century, autopsies were becoming fairly common, and routine dissections were commonplace. The *printing press,* a Chinese discovery, had made its appearance. This single discovery had a great influence on medicine because men could write and record their findings, their thoughts could be printed, and this knowledge could be disseminated throughout the world. Compilers began to make their appearance, accumulating the protocols of others, adding some of their own, arranging them in book form, and publishing them. Many of these compilations were composed of the curiosities and rarities of medicine rather than complete well-balanced medical descriptions. Little by little, men with common sense began to see the fallacy of just recording curiosities and rarities and began to devote their attention to the accumulation of knowledge that would give medicine the sound, solid footing it needed.

## SEVENTEENTH CENTURY

The seventeenth century was a bewildering period when science and literature flourished with incredible vigor in spite of religious strife, the Thirty Years War, and the English Revolution. One of the outstanding individuals of this time was WILLIAM HARVEY (1578-1657). In 1628 he described the blood vascular system and the circulation of the blood through it. This single discovery had a tremendous impact upon medicine. Without a knowledge of the circulation of the blood, most of the tissue alterations studied in pathology could not be explained. Hyperemia, hemorrhage, edema, embolism, infarction, pyemia, miliary tuberculosis, and the metastasis of neoplasms — none of these common pathological conceptions could be explained unless the circulation of the blood was understood. *No single discovery has had a more far-reaching effect on pathology than the discovery of the circulation of the blood.*

The next major advance in medicine was made by ANTONY VAN LEEUWENHOEK (1632-1723). He cannot be given credit for the discovery of the microscope because others had demonstrated the magnification of lenses long before his time. We do, however, give him credit for being the *first to show that the microscope had practical importance* in the study of tissues and other minute objects. Without the microscope the study of histology would be impossible. By demonstrating the practical use of the microscope, Leeuwenhoek paved the way for the minute examination of tissues. With his simple, crude instrument which magnified about sixty times, Leeuwenhoek saw and described many things. A book, *Antony Van Leeuwenhoek and His "Little Animals,"* by Clifford Dobell, describes and illustrates the many objects he observed.

## ANATOMICAL PATHOLOGY

One of the first compilers of medical literature was a Frenchman by the name of JEAN FERNEL (1497-1558). He accumulated the information of his time and was the *first to attempt to codify the new knowledge of pathology.* He brought together the observations made by the dissections of that time and attempted to bring this information into a form that could be used by others in the study of disease. His text of pathology was the principal one used for many years.

Jean Fernel was followed by a famous Italian compiler, GIOVANNI BATTISTA MORGAGNI (1682-1771). Modern pathology began with Morgagni. His life is interesting in that he was unknown until he was seventy years of age, at which time he published five volumes entitled *The Seats and Causes of Disease.* In these volumes he systematically recorded 700 complete autopsies with comments on the relation of the structural changes to the signs shown by these individuals during life. *This was the first time that anyone had attempted to correlate pathological alterations in the dead individual with the symptoms shown by that individual during life.* This was an extremely important text in medicine. After Morgagni, pathology could never again be slipshod or superficial — the new standard was too high.

A young Frenchman by the name of MARIE-FRANCOIS XAVIER BICHAT (1771-1802) opened a new field in medical science. During his brief life span of 31 years he established the *foundation for the study of histology.* He presented a new concept of anatomy and showed that the body was composed of twenty-one tissues — vascular, muscular, osseous, cartilagenous, etc. An even more remarkable thing about this discovery is that Bichat's observations were made entirely by physical and chemical methods since he did not possess a microscope, and yet he is considered as the *father of histology.* With simple methods such as putrefaction, maceration, cooking, and chemical disintegration using acids and bases, he was able to divide the tissues of the body into these twenty-one groups. Later, users of microscopes were attracted by his findings and wondered what the difference might be in these tissues. With their microscopes they scrutinized the subdivisions that Bichat had pointed out, and in this manner they brought forth microscopic descriptions of the basic tissues of the body. Bichat's work was so brilliantly done that he is given a place in

the foundation of microscopic pathology. His observations formed the bridge between the systematic pathology of Morgagni and the cellular pathology of Virchow.

Modern veterinary medicine originated in France. French domination of veterinary medicine began with a man by the name of JACQUES LABESSIE DE SOLLEYSEL (1617-1680). In 1664 he published the first complete veterinary classic of this period. It was entitled *Le Parfait Marechal.* The publication of this work, with its influence upon veterinary medicine, was the outstanding event of the seventeenth century in veterinary medicine. In this publication Solleysel points out the lamentable situation created by allowing the veterinary art to fall so completely into the hands of the farrier. This was especially apparent in Paris. This book marks the beginning of the end of the horseshoer's regime and his control of veterinary medicine.

The second dominating veterinarian in France was CLAUDE BOURGELAT (1712-1779). Bourgelat was engaged in the practice of law but was vitally interested in horses. It soon became apparent that he was gifted in equine husbandry. In 1751 he wrote *Elements of Hippiartry and the New Knowledge of Equine Medicine.* His exceptional talents became obvious in this book. As a result he was asked to investigate the glanders outbreak in French cavalry mounts and was successful in eradicating the disease for the French army. Bourgelat was then requested to establish a veterinary school, and this he did in Lyon, France.

The *first modern veterinary school* was established in Lyon, France, on January 1, 1762. Bourgelat immediately utilized the facilities of this school to combat the epidemics prevalent in the area. From his success in this venture he built a prestige for veterinary medicine that has never been lost, and as a result veterinary education flourished in France.

Bourgelat was called to Paris in March,

1764. There, by royal decree, he established the school known as l'Ecole veterinaire nationale d'Alfort. This is one of the most outstanding veterinary schools, is in existence today, and retains the distinction of being one of the dominating centers of veterinary science in the world. It is located in Alfort, a suburb of Paris, on the banks of the Marne. The buildings, surrounded with a wall, are placed in a garden setting, and many of the historic documents and statues depicting early veterinary education can be found here.

The third prominent French veterinarian of this period was CHARLES VIAL DE SAINT-BEL (1753–1793). Saint-Bel was a graduate of Lyon. Following graduation he went to Paris and taught at Alfort. Later he became the director of this school. During the French Revolution he was forced to flee to England. After considerable difficulty he was able to establish the Veterinary College of London in April, 1791. This school is in existence today. Unfortunately this brilliant young man died two years later, in 1793, as the result of glanders, a disease he acquired from one of his equine patients.

Saint-Bel is of great interest to American veterinarians because of his influence on veterinary education in the United States. The early veterinarians that came to America were graduates of the Veterinary College of London or were students of men from there. So Saint-Bel, although he was never aware of it, had direct influence on modern veterinary education in this country.

The next major contribution to medicine was made by an Englishman, JOHN HUNTER (1728–1793). He is considered to be the *first experimental pathologist.* He was a man of great curiosity and was interested not only in medicine but in all phases of biology. He is best known for his extensive studies, *Blood and Inflammation, Gunshot Wounds,* and a treatise, *Venereal Disease.* His great zeal for experimental pathology led him to infect himself with syphilis in order to study this disease more closely. He developed a typical case of the disease, which was probably the cause of his death. A brother and nephew of John Hunter also contributed much to medical science, but their work is overshadowed by his.

The Germans soon came to dominate the field of pathology. This was probably because of CARL ROKITANSKY (1804–1878) who lived in Vienna. He is considered as the *supreme descriptive pathologist* of all time. It was he who firmly established the structural basis of disease. He wrote his first protocol in 1827 and by 1866 had written 30,000. At the termination of his career he had 70,000 protocols at his disposal. It was he who established necropsy technic — the systematic examination of every organ by methods that preserved organ continuity yet revealed the lesions they contained. Little change has been made in his necropsy technic. Although he was the ablest descriptive pathologist, he was not capable of controlling his imagination and dramatic instinct. It was a crushing blow when in his old age he saw his brilliant theories demolished and his air castles crumbled before the sound theories of cellular pathology as presented by Virchow.

## CELLULAR PATHOLOGY

As we look back into the middle of the last century we find pathology in an advanced but curiously helpless state. The major factors in gross pathology had been explained. The brilliant work of Rokitansky and others had described most of the changes encountered in tissues. Yet, in spite of this, there was no common cementing substance to bring all of these isolated ideas together, no principle to explain why these changes occurred or to explain the relation of one isolated fact to another. Many theories were advanced, but one by one they fell by the wayside, not being able to survive critical analysis. Even Rokitansky, in spite of his brilliance, could not formulate some common cementing substance to hold and bring all of these facts together.

The necessary cementing substance was *cellular pathology*. It began in Germany and resulted in a reformation of all pathology. The inspiration for this development came from a remarkable man, JOHANNES MUELLER (1801–1858), who lived in Bonn and Berlin. We might say he was the last of the philosophers whose learning comprehended all branches of science. From this time on, the development in the various phases of science became so great that one man could never command it all again. This man is considered as the greatest teacher of the nineteenth century as far as medicine is concerned. He was one of the first to use the microscope in the study of tissues. He remembered that Bichat had demonstrated the body to be composed of twenty-one tissues. He knew that Antony van Leeuwenhoek had shown the microscope to have practical importance in the examination of tissues. So Mueller brought all of this information together and impressed upon the world the necessity of examining tissues with the microscope in order to appreciate and understand the changes that were occurring. One of his works, *The Finer Structure and Form of Morbid Tumors*, probably had more influence on proving the necessity of microscopic study in pathology than any other piece of writing.

Mueller had many famous students. Among them were Theodore Schwann, Matthias Schleiden, Jacob Henle, and Rudolph Virchow. The greatest of these was RUDOLPH VIRCHOW (1821–1902). In 1847, when but twenty-six years old, Virchow began the publication of the journal known as *Virchow's Archives*. This journal has been in continuous publication for more than one hundred years. It is the most complete work of pathology in existence. Practically everything known in pathology is contained within its pages. Unfortunately it is written in German and is unavailable to many stu-dents because of the language barrier. Virchow's greatest work was the publication of his *Cellular Pathology*. This was a compilation of his lectures and was one of the first publications of this new period. Most of the terms (such as thrombosis and embolism) used in pathology are the coinage of Virchow. His discussion on embolism explains how tumors, bacteria, and other objects are transported from one part of an individual to another.

Cellular pathology was no mere replacement, no new system, of Virchow's own. Instead, it was the simple but early recognition of the principle to which all biologic teaching has to come — the study of cellular life. Biology, zoology, botany, entomology, medicine, etc., must be approached from the cellular point of view. Virchow made it evident for all time that one cell follows another just as surely as one animal follows another or as one plant follows another. He proceeded to rebuild pathology on the concept of the body as an organized cell state — a social system of continuous development in which each microscopic unit has a specific place and function. All areas of pathology were clarified with this concept, and in each of these areas Virchow led the way.

Today all pathologists are cellular pathologists. It is difficult to realize that a time existed when cellular pathologists were not in existence. In the field of degenerative pathology, Virchow was particularly prominent. Most of the terms used today (fatty degeneration, fatty infiltration, amyloidosis, etc.) were coined and explained by Virchow. He gave pathology the push it needed, and from then on its development was rapid.

Although SEMMELWEISS (1818–1865), a Hungarian, was not a pathologist, his contribution to medicine is a monumental reform in medical sanitation. Up until the time of Semmelweiss, the hospitals had such a high death rate that they were usually considered as places to go in order to die. Patients admitted to the hospitals were often placed in the large five- or seven-man beds that were common during this period. During the night one or more of the patients in the same bed might die. The new patient might be placed in a bed where an individual had glanders, another had anthrax, a third typhoid, a fourth scarlet fever, and a fifth a wound infection. He would have little chance of leaving that bed without acquiring at least one of these diseases. The medical men of that period would perform an autopsy and, without washing their hands or changing their clothes, would go into the surgery rooms to deliver babies, do leg amputations, and other surgery. The mortality was particularly severe for women during childbirth, and streptococcic septicemias following childbirth were common. The streptococci were carried from one individual to another by the attending physician.

Semmelweiss *instituted hospital sanitation* by requiring the attendants of the hospital to wash and clean themselves and to wear clean clothing. He insisted on the segregation of the ill and attempted to divide them into infectious and noninfectious groups. All of this was done without the knowledge of bacteriology, because at this time bacteria as a cause of disease were not known. The results of his efforts were remarkable, for soon his success became known and his methods spread to other hospitals.

The importance of infectious organisms in disease was demonstrated by LOUIS PASTEUR (1822-1895) in France. He was one of the originators of the new field of *bacteriology* and of the theory that bacteria were the cause of some diseases. Pasteur was a chemist who became interested in microorganisms while trying to solve some of the problems associated with the fermentation of beer, the souring of wine, and the death of silkworms. His studies carried him into the field of human and animal diseases (pasteurellosis, anthrax, rabies, etc.). He showed that individuals could be successfully immunized by vaccine prepared with organisms.

About the same time, in Germany, ROBERT KOCH (1843-1910), another etiologist, came into prominence. Like Pasteur, he was also a chemist who later became a bacteriologist. He isolated many microorganisms, showed that many bacteria caused diseases, and was the first to use artificial solid media in the attainment of pure cultures. It was he who established *Koch's Postulates*, a procedure necessary for proving a specific microorganism as the cause of a specific disease.

Although Robert Koch and Louis Pasteur did much to show that bacteria caused disease, it was EDWIN KLEBS (1834-1913) who demonstrated the importance of bacteria in pathology. Klebs was a student of Virchow. Most of Virchow's work was done before it was known that bacteria could cause disease, and it was over this point that Klebs differed with Virchow. Virchow never appreciated the importance of bacteria in disease.

Another Virchow student who attained great prominence was JULIUS COHNHEIM (1839-1884). Cohnheim revealed some of the errors in the teachings of the old master, Virchow, particularly in the field of inflammation. Cohnheim's methods of investigation were almost entirely experimental, and because of this he is credited as being the *originator of modern experimental pathology*. His most notable experiment concerned the vascular and cellular changes in the mesentery of the frog when acted upon by an irritant. He opened the abdomen of a frog and viewed the mesentery with a magnifying lens. When he placed a drop of acetic acid upon this mesentery, he noted that the vessels dilated. At first the rate of flow of the stream of blood through this vessel was quickened, then the current slowed and the red and white corpuscles previously indistinguishable in this swift stream became visible. Presently he observed an astonishing fact — the leukocytes passed through the capillary wall, migrated toward the site of injury, and accumulated where the obnoxious agent had been deposited. The conclusion was unequivocal: Pus cells found in the region of inflammation were blood leukocytes. It is readily understandable how important this discovery was in the explanation of cellular alterations in inflammation. This simple observation is the *basis for the pathology of inflammation.*

There were many other individuals who contributed to medical science during this period. One of the most outstanding was NEGRI. It was he who described the intracellular inclusion body — later called the Negri body — in the cytoplasm of the neurons of individuals having rabies.

## AMERICAN VETERINARY COLLEGES AND INSTITUTIONS

During the nineteenth century quite a number of private veterinary schools appeared in the United States. The early schools were very short-lived, but some of the later schools survived until the 1920's. Many practitioners graduated from these schools. Most of the men attending these schools for periods of six weeks to four years had considerable experience in animal industry before they enrolled. They received intensive training in clinical medicine. With their excellent knowledge of animals they were able to apply what they learned and, as a result, were excellent practitioners. In contrast, the modern veterinary student lacks basic animal training. All too often the reason for the downfall of some veterinarians is that they do not understand basic animal husbandry.

None of the private schools is in existence today. All of the colleges of veterinary medicine in this country today are state supported and are associated with various colleges and universities. When the state-supported schools of veterinary medicine first appeared on the campuses of our colleges and universities, they were the subject of much derision. The livestock industry and the older veterinarians could not imagine a veterinarian being a college graduate. It was not long before the private schools and the practitioners found it difficult to compete with the state-supported schools, and one by one the private schools were forced to close.

Rapid advances in veterinary education in America began about 1861. During the next ten to fifteen years a number of well-trained individuals from the British Isles, principally from the Royal Veterinary College of Edinburgh, came to this country. These men founded veterinary education in North America.

The first school of veterinary medicine in America to be associated with colleges and universities appeared in Canada. One of the first individuals to arrive was Andrew Smith who founded the school at Toronto. Later this school became known as the Ontario Veterinary College under the sponsorship of the Provincial Agricultural Society. This school is in existence today. It has been a very prominent school, and many excellent graduates have come from this exceptional educational institution.

Another pioneer was Duncan McEachran who founded the Montreal Veterinary College, which later became the Veterinary Department of McGill University.

At the time of the Civil War Ezra Cornell brought James Law to this country to teach courses in veterinary medicine at Cornell University where he founded a veterinary department. There the first courses in veterinary medicine on the campus of a college or university in the United States were offered. This veterinary department later became the New York State Veterinary College.

Although courses were first offered in veterinary medicine at Cornell University, the first veterinary school was established at Iowa State College in 1879. The most outstanding individual in veterinary medicine in Iowa history has been the late dean, Charles H. Stange, who was responsible for the present arrangement of buildings and course of study.

There are a number of other singular individuals in the history of veterinary medicine in the United States. Among these is Theobald Smith. He was a physician and a close friend of James Law. He was associated with Johns Hopkins, Harvard, and the Rockefeller Institute. One of his greatest contributions was the demonstration that arthropods were capable of transmitting protozoan diseases. He showed that Texas Fever, caused by a protozoan, *Babesia bigemina*, could be transmitted by a tick from one animal to another.

To control the diseases of animals and to enforce meat inspection, the Bureau of Animal Industry was established. Many of our outstanding veterinarians have been associated with this governmental agency. Daniel E. Salmon and John Mohler have been particularly active in this agency. Dorset, Niles, and McBride, prominent figures in swine research, showed that swine could be immunized against hog cholera. Maurice C. Hall, a parasitologist, was outstanding in the control of parasitic diseases.

## PATHOLOGY IN AMERICA

WILLIAM HENRY WELCH (1850–1934), a student of Cohnheim, is credited with bringing pathology to the United States. He was professor of pathology at Johns Hopkins University in Baltimore. He probably has had more influence on pathology and medicine in this country than any other individual. He was followed by a number of other prominent figures. Among these were Councilman, Mallory, Prudden, Hektoen, Ophuls, and Warthin — all German trained and all excellent students. These men formed the nucleus around which pathology was built in this country.

Veterinary pathology began with VON BRUCKMULLER, who, in 1869 in Vienna, published his *Textbook of Pathological Zoo-anatomy of Domestic Animals.* He was followed by another German pathologist, Theodore Kitt. Kitt wrote an excellent three-volume veterinary pathology text now translated into English. Although it is outdated, the basic principles of pathology are well described. In 1926 Ernst Joest, a prominent German pathologist, published a five-volume text on veterinary pathology. It is the most complete compilation of veterinary pathology in existence. Little has been added to his work except in the area of infectious diseases. In the 1930's Nieberle published an excellent veterinary pathology textbook that is well adapted to the needs of the student.

In the United States the first veterinary pathologist of prominence was Walter Crocker who taught at the University of Pennsylvania. Ohio State was fortunate in having Leonard Goss as a pathologist. This country has several well-trained working pathologists at the present time. One of the most distinguished of these is Peter Olafson, Cornell University, Ithaca, New York. He is a brilliant man and certainly a leader in the field of pathology. At Iowa State University Edward Benbrook has been the dominating figure in pathology since 1918. Herman Seibold has been particularly active in governmental agencies and is probably our best histopathologist. Charles Davis, Denver, Colorado, has been the dominating pathologist in federal meat inspection. He has probably seen more pathological tissue than any other pathologist in this country. Veterinary medicine in the United States is fortunate in having many younger men who are active in the field of pathology and who will contribute much to medicine. Of these younger men Donald Cordy has shown outstanding ability.

Since World War II, Albert Hjarre and Sven Rubarth, Stockholm, Sweden, have been the most prominent European pathologists. The excellent work produced by these two men and their students should be read by every student of veterinary medicine.

Sir Arnold Theiler has been responsible for the development of veterinary medicine in South Africa and for the building of the excellent research institute and school at Onderstepoort, South Africa. He was born in Switzerland and went to Africa as a young man. Nearly every disease known in Africa today was investigated by him. He exhibited unusual ability in determining the etiology and control of the African diseases. Probably no modern veterinarian contributed as much to veterinary medicine as this individual who was handicapped during his entire life by having only one arm.

## DEFINITIONS

Before engaging in the study of any subject, it is well to define some of the terms peculiar to that field so their meanings will be appreciated. There are a number of general terms used to designate the major areas of pathology and related subjects as indicated in the following paragraphs.

**Pathology** is the study of the anatomical, chemical, and physiological alterations in an organism as the result of disease. Pathology is subdivided into several fields or specialties:

1. *General pathology* is concerned with the basic alterations in tissues as the result of disease. It involves those changes common to all tissues or organs (thrombosis, embolism, fatty degeneration, fatty infiltration, amyloidosis, etc.).

2. *Special pathology* is the application of the basic alterations learned in general pathology to the various specific diseases that involve the individual as a whole. It consists of a systematic examination of the individual organ by organ and the recording of alterations resulting from infectious or parasitic diseases, malnutrition, trauma, etc.

3. *Experimental pathology* is concerned with the production of lesions by experimental methods. It is the type of pathology employed in research when certain etiologic agents are applied to an individual so that the resultant alterations in various organs may be studied.

4. *Macroscopic or gross pathology* is the examination of an individual by systematic dissection without the aid of a magnifying lens.

5. *Post-mortem pathology* is the examination of an individual after death. This is the basis for modern medicine.

6. *Microscopic pathology, histopathology, or cellular pathology* is the examination of tissue with the aid of a magnifying lens and usually implies the use of stained preparations mounted on glass slides.

7. *Clinical pathology* embraces certain laboratory methods used by clinicians to aid them in arriving at a diagnosis. It includes the examination of blood, urine, feces, exudates, skin scrapings, and biopsy material.

8. *Humoral pathology* is the study of the alterations in the antibodies (agglutinins, precipitins, lysins, opsins, antitoxins, etc.) that occur in an individual as the result of disease.

9. *Chemical pathology* is the study of the chemical alterations of the body fluids and tissues that result from disease. For example, in nephritis there is a retention of certain substances (nonprotein nitrogen, urea-nitrogen, creatinine, etc.) by the kidney that can be detected in the blood by chemical methods. By determining the amount of these retained substances as well as the fluctuations in amount from day to day, the clinician and pathologist are able to estimate the amount of damage occurring in the kidney.

10. *Physiological pathology* is concerned with the function of organs (motility, digestion, excretion, metabolism, etc.).

**Necropsy, post-mortem examination, or autopsy** is the examination of an individual after death by systematic dissection. The term necropsy is preferred in veterinary medicine. In human medicine the term autopsy is still preferred.

**Morbid changes** are those alterations in tissue found at necropsy examination that are the result of disease.

**Pathognomonic lesion** is an alteration that indicates without doubt the cause of a particular disease. For example, the Negri body is a pathognomonic lesion. When this inclusion body, having the correct tinctorial properties, is found in the cytoplasm of the neurons of the hippocampus, it indicates the animal had rabies.

**Biopsy** is the removal and examination of tissue obtained from the living animal.

**Health** is the state of an individual living in complete harmony with his environment. The individual has a feeling of well-being. However, he may be healthy and still show lesions at necropsy examination, but the tissue alterations are not great enough to prevent complete adaptation with his surroundings.

**Disease** is a condition in which an individual shows an anatomical, chemical, or physiological deviation from the normal. The terms health and disease are used every day, and yet little thought is given to the difficulty of determining whether an individual is healthy or whether he has a disease. The differentiation becomes very arbitrary, especially when it concerns the so-called physiological functions. If we hold strictly to the definition, is anyone in perfect health? If a necropsy examination is made, some minor alteration might be revealed; and if so, that individual would not be healthy. So, actually, health is a relative state.

Several common illustrations can be used to demonstrate how difficult it is to determine whether an individual is healthy or not. In the process of fattening cattle, consider the very fat beef animal fitted for the show. Is that animal healthy? Are we not producing a pathological individual with our feeding methods? Are we not creating an individual, considered to be ideal, that is actually a sick animal? Observe the fat beef animal. He moves with difficulty, perhaps even groans as he walks because of the effort associated with his movements. With any exertion or during warm weather he suffers from the heat; and if he is subjected to much exertion he may die merely because he is overfat. If the fat animal happens to be a cow, she will probably be sterile since fat animals often do not reproduce.

In France the fat livers of geese are a great delicacy. To produce these livers the geese are confined in a cage with only their heads and necks protruding. A mixture of grains is stuffed into the geese at intervals throughout the day. Arsenic and phosphorus are frequently added to the ration to produce hepatic injury and to increase the amount and rapidity of the deposition of fat in the liver. After a period of time the geese develop very large livers that are yellow in color and distended with fat. Is this health or disease?

Another example is the old, pampered family dog, so obese that he almost rolls down the sidewalk as he walks. It is an effort for him to move, and about the only movement he makes is to obtain more food. He suffers from the heat in warm weather. If he is required to exert himself, he may die. Where do we draw the line between obesity and the amount of fat necessary for health?

It is difficult to determine whether or not certain organs are present by observing the external appearance of an individual. One kidney may be absent or so injured that it does not function. The remaining kidney may be twice its normal size since it has assumed the function of the defective kidney. This is called compensatory hypertrophy, and if the change came about gradually, the individual might not be aware that anything had taken place. To all outward appearances that individual is normal.

**Scientific medicine** is based on sound anatomical, chemical, and physiological investigation. It is the basis of modern medicine.

**Empiric medicine** is not based on sound anatomical, chemical, and physiological investigation. It is the medicine practiced by the quack, charlatan, or empiric. There are all too many examples of this type of medicine. One of the common examples of empiric veterinary medicine is the mythical disease "hollow horn." When a cow becomes ill some livestock men drill a hole in the base of the horn, and if the horn is hollow the disease is diagnosed as "hollow horn." The fallacy of this method of investigation is that all horns are hollow. The individual has not dissected cattle to determine if all horns are hollow, and his curiosity is not great enough to question the advice some empiric has given him. Frequently the cure for this disease is the injection of one or two ounces of turpentine through this opening in the horn into the frontal sinus. The cow must experience excruciating pain when the turpentine comes in contact with the mucous membranes of the frontal sinus. To the empiric an indication of the beneficial results of this treatment is the pouring of exudate from the nose of the cow. The turpentine produces an inflammation of sufficient magnitude that exudate flows out of the sinuses, into the nasal passages, and is discharged through the external nares.

Another example of veterinary quackery is the condition known as "wolf in the tail." A cow is ill and for some unknown reason the diagnosis of "wolf in the tail" is made. To cure this disease several longitudinal incisions are made in the tail, salt is rubbed into the incisions, and the site is bandaged with a dirty rag. Still another example is the tying of a string around the base of the tail to cure diarrhea. Occasionally the string is drawn so tightly that circulation of blood in the tail is prevented and gangrene is the result.

## THE STUDY

The study of veterinary medicine and pathology is concerned with six important aspects.

**Etiology** is the study or the theory of the cause of disease. Etiology is divided into two categories.

1. *Intrinsic causes of disease,* or the predisposing factors, are those characteristics (genus, breed, sex, age, etc.) of an individual over which he himself has no control and which determine the type of disease present.
2. *Extrinsic causes of disease* are those environmental factors (mechanical, chemical, thermal, infectious, or parasitic) capable of producing disease in the individual.

**Pathogenesis** is the progressive development of a disease process from the time it is initiated to its final conclusion in recovery or death. Pneumonia is a very good illustration of pathogenesis. The individual is infected with bacteria that are capable of producing pneumonia. The irritation produced by these bacteria results in a stage of congestion in which there is an increased amount of blood and fluid in the lungs. Soon the stage of red hepatization appears, in which the plasma in the alveoli of the lung coagulates and the lung becomes solidified or hepatized. When leukocytes invade the hepatized tissue, the lung acquires a gray color. This is designated as the stage of gray hepatization. Finally there is the stage of resolution or recovery in which the leukocytes destroy the irritating substances and remove the exudate. This progression of events is known as pathogenesis.

**Lesion** is the macroscopic or microscopic alteration occurring in tissue as the result of an injury. An illustration of this is the fragmentation of bone that occurs when a fracture is produced.

**Pathologic biochemistry** is the study of the altered chemical composition of fluids and tissue during an illness. For example, in nephritis certain substances (nonprotein nitrogen, urea-nitrogen, creatinine, phosphorus, etc.) are retained by the kidney. By chemical means these substances can be detected in a sample of blood, and the course of the disease can be followed by fluctuations in the amount of these substances.

**Symptom** is a clinical sign (lameness, incoordination, baldness, swelling, fever, etc.) manifested by the *living* individual as the result of tissue changes.

**Result, or termination,** of a disease occurs in three ways:

1. *Recovery.* The animal has an illness, the damage produced by the disease is repaired, and after a short period of time there is no outward manifestation of injury.

2. *Invalidism.* The animal has an illness and tissue damage is great. The body is not able to completely repair the alteration and, although tissue damage is present, the extent of the injury is not so great that the individual is rendered incompatible with life.

3. *Death.* The body defenses are overcome and the tissue damage is so great that the basic functions required for life cannot be maintained and the individual dies.

PART II

# ETIOLOGY

# CHAPTER 3 | Intrinsic Cause of Disease

**Definition.** The intrinsic, or predisposing, causes of disease are those factors that determine the type of disease present within an individual and over which he himself has no control.

The intrinsic causes of disease are divided into seven major groups.

**1. Genus** is of extreme importance because certain diseases involve specific genera. Hog cholera is a disease of the hog. No other animal is naturally affected with this disease. It is true that by manipulation the virus can be transmitted to the rabbit, but it does not maintain itself in this animal. Canine distemper is primarily a disease of the dog. At times, mink and a few other animals are infected with the virus. It does not affect the horse, cow, sheep, or pig.

**2. Race and breed** also influence the type of disease present. Dairy cattle are much more susceptible to various diseases than are beef cattle. Dairy cattle have been bred for milk production. All too often they seem to have lost much of their resistance to disease and will not tolerate as much as the beef animal. Within the dairy breeds, the Jersey and Guernsey are less resistant to various diseases than is the Holstein. In the canine, the German shepherd, great Dane, and Saint Bernard are more severely af-

fected with bone disease and canine distemper than are the other breeds of dogs. They are larger than most other breeds, perhaps having greater nutritional requirements during the period of growth so that nutritional deficiencies are more serious. Brain tumors are common in the bulldog breeds. The boxer dog has a very high incidence of brain tumors as compared with other breeds, and every boxer brain should be examined for neoplasms at necropsy even though the animal showed no symptoms of a locomotor disturbance.

**3. Family** is of special importance to the livestock producer because it is from the family that the genetic characteristics of the individual are derived. Certain families of animals have various lethal genes or other undesirable characteristics that bring about the destruction of the individual. Some families possess unusual resistance to certain diseases. Families of chickens that have unusual resistance to leukosis can be produced in contrast to other families that have a very high mortality rate from this disease.

Hernias in swine may become a serious herd problem when defects are present in the abdominal wall as the result of a hereditary abnormality of growth. Herds of cattle are observed in which the calves have hydrocephalus (accumulation of fluid in the ventricles of the brain). The fluid presses upon the brain, destroys the brain, and results in death of the individual.

Susceptibility to many diseases may change quite rapidly. In a period as short as ten years, the entire situation may change due to an alteration in the breeding program. Intensive inbreeding tends to accentuate defects, and all too many of our livestock breeders have discovered that although they have achieved maximum milk production, maximum beef production, or some other desirable characteristic in their animals, they have also produced certain undesirable qualities. Frequently, the particular group of animals in which the defect appeared has had to be discarded.

4. **Age** is very important as a predisposing factor since certain diseases are found in definite age groups. Tumors are most frequently observed in older animals. Sarcomas are most likely to occur in younger individuals while carcinomas are usually encountered in old animals. By knowing the age of the individual, it is possible to arrive at some conclusion as to the probable type of tumor present. Canine distemper is a disease of young dogs. It is not a disease of old dogs because they either have had the disease or have an unusual amount of resistance to the infection. Strangles (a disease of the upper respiratory tract) in the horse is a disease of young horses rather than old horses. Nutritional anemia in swine occurs as the result of a deficiency of iron and copper in the milk. It is observed between the third and the sixth week of life, corresponding with a critical period in iron metabolism and hemoglobin formation. Prostatic hyperplasia (enlargement of the prostate) occurs in old dogs and is seldom observed in young dogs. The prostate may become so large that it causes a stenosis of the urethra, preventing the flow of urine. At times, the enlargement becomes so great as to compress the rectum and cause constipation. Cecal coccidiosis in the chicken is a disease of young birds. Through previous infection, older birds have become immunized against the disease.

5. **Sex** naturally exerts an influence on the type of disease because of the different types of organs found in the two sexes. Reproductive diseases are more common in the female than in the male. Certain diseases (metritis, mastitis, acetonemia, and milk fever) are confined to the female. Nephritis in the dog is two or three times more common in the male than in the female, but in the bovine, nephritis is more common in the female.

6. **Color** is extremely important in animal diseases. Melanosarcomas are very common in gray and white horses but are seldom observed in brown or black horses. Animals with non-pigmented skin, or only slightly pigmented skin, are much more susceptible to photodynamic diseases. When these animals consume various plants containing phytoporphyrins, a chemical reaction occurs following exposure of the cutaneous surface to sunlight, and injury to the skin is the result. If pigment is present in the skin, it protects the individual by preventing the sunlight from penetrating the skin, thus inhibiting the chemical reaction. Chester white hogs are easily injured by the sun, and blistering of the ears and back may interfere with the proper weight gains of these animals. White bulldogs are often deaf, and deafness is associated with the lack of pigment.

7. **Idiosyncrasy** is an unusual reaction to some substance and is of great importance to the veterinarian. Some animals exhibit an unusual reaction when a drug is administered. These individuals, even when a small portion of the recommended amount of the drug is administered, will die or show other serious manifestations of unusual toxicity.

# CHAPTER 4

# Extrinsic Cause of

# Diseases of A Nutritional Nature

No other factor is as important as a cause of disease as is food. Two-thirds of the body weight consists of water in which is suspended a heterogeneous mixture of proteins, carbohydrates, fats, minerals, and essential substances called vitamins. The balance between these substances fluctuates within rather narrow limits.

The body is essentially a large chemical laboratory in which there is a continuous fermentation process. This chemical process is known as **metabolism.** Metabolism consists of two opposing processes. The first is **catabolism,** a continuous fermentation process of deterioraton which, if allowed to continue, would eventually bring about the destruction of the body. To prevent the complete disintegration of an individual there is a second opposing process known as **anabolism,** which is a continuous reconstructive fermentation going on within an individual. In order that this anabolic process may continue, it is necessary that food substances be consumed, digested, and the products of digestion be absorbed and distributed throughout the body. The type of food ingested will vary greatly (corn, wheat, oats, forage crops, meat, etc.) but the basic constituents in the ration must fall within rather narrow limits. If there is too much variation in these essential substances and they do not meet the basic requirements,

it is not long before some nutritional disease will appear, possibly resulting in the death of the individual.

## EXCESS OF FOOD

Everyone has experienced discomfort from the extreme dilatation of the stomach that occurs after overeating. The glutton experiences pain and discomfort for several hours following engorgement. Most animals are gluttons. A good example is the dog suddenly confronted with more food than he has ever seen before. He apparently feels he must consume every bit of it, and after doing this he is in misery for several hours. His attitude and facial expressions indicate the pain he is experiencing.

Acute pancreatitis, especially in the human being, is associated with overeating. For that reason, the human physician frequently observes the disease in individuals who have just eaten a large meal. A few hours after consuming the repast, the individual experiences severe abdominal pain. The pathogenesis of the disease indicates there is a reverse peristalsis of the pancreatic duct. Some of the bile or ingesta from the intestinal tract is carried into the pancreas, and acute pancreatitis is the result.

Acute dilatation of the stomach is frequently associated in animals with the consumption of a large amount of dry feed. It is much the same situation that occurs when water is added to dried beans or rice. The dry feed swells as it becomes infiltrated with water. Gastric dilatation occurs in all animals and is particularly common in the horse. A horse may gain access to a granary and consume all of the dry feed (oats, corn, etc.) he can hold. The saliva and gastric secretions, in the process of digestion, add moisture to this mass. In addition, the horse may add more moisture by drinking water. The feed swells and finally there is no additional space for expansion in the stomach. The pyloric sphincter allows only partially digested food to pass. As the pain increases with gastric dilatation, there may be a spasm of the pyloric sphincter so that no ingesta can pass. The cardiac sphincter of the horse stomach will not allow regurgitation, and therefore no relief can be obtained by vomiting. The food swells, the stomach is distended, and finally ruptures, the contents being discharged into the peritoneal cavity. Death of the horse from peritonitis and septicemia usually results within six hours.

Human gluttons are much more prone to develop degeneration of the liver than are moderate eaters. They have a very high incidence of arteriosclerosis and are frequently afflicted with gout. Insurance companies are well aware of this fact and consider gluttons as poor insurance risks. Sometimes they refuse to insure these individuals, knowing they will probably die at an early age.

Extremely well-fed horses are much more susceptible to heatstroke and sunstroke. They also often experience a very serious necrosis of skeletal muscles. Horses that have been worked must be fed a reduced ration during vacation periods; otherwise muscle necrosis and death may occur. The disease, azoturia, is often referred to as Monday morning sickness because it is on Monday morning after a weekend of rest that many horses are afflicted with the disease. Within an hour or two after an animal is put to work following a holiday, he begins to experience cramps in the heavy muscles of the legs and back. Soon he is unable to move his legs because of the cramping muscles. Later he is unable to stand and may die. The urine is red because myoglobin, liberated when the muscle is destroyed, is being eliminated through the kidneys. If the animal recovers, he may be permanently lame or unsuitable for work because of the destruction of the skeletal muscles. The disease may be prevented by reducing the amount of feed and by exercising the horse during vacation periods.

Overeating disease in lambs is very common. Whenever the amount of feed consumed by the lamb each day is more than about a pound and a half, symptoms of overeating disease can be expected. The affected animal suddenly begins to stagger, throws his head back, goes into a convulsion, kicks a few times, and dies. It is the best lambs that are involved because they are consuming the most feed. The cause of death is associated with the large amount of feed consumed because this results in a change in the bacterial flora of the rumen and intestinal tract. Among the many organisms present are members of the *Clostridium* group that are capable of producing a powerful toxin. When this toxin is absorbed, death of the individual is the result. The same disease occurs in cattle that are on full feed.

Laminitis, a disturbance in cell metabolism in the sensitive laminae of the hoof, occurs in overfed horses. Usually there is a digestive disturbance followed by extreme soreness of the feet when alterations in the sensitive laminae of the hoofs occur. In severe cases the animals are unable to stand. This disease has become one of the major pony diseases because these pets are usually overfed or improperly fed.

## DEFICIENCY OF FOOD

The quantitative lack of food or starvation is the biggest problem of the world today. In some areas the problem is seasonal, while in other areas it is a problem throughout the entire year. Large areas of the world are continually faced with famine because of tremendous populations (China and India). Too little food is always a problem during periods of drought or in the late winter and early spring when food is no longer available. It is particularly serious in wildlife because they have no way of storing food. If there has been a dry summer followed by a severe winter, the death loss in wildlife during the late winter and early spring is tremendous. Many animals avoid this period of food shortage by being able to hibernate or migrate.

Starvation may also result from the inability to prehend, swallow, or digest food. This occurs when there are diseases of the teeth, foreign bodies of various types in the digestive tract, tumors involving the organs of digestion, or an increased motility of the digestive tract causing food to pass so rapidly through it that digestion and assimilation cannot occur.

Since man restricts the movement of his animals and feeds them what he wishes, the problem of starvation in domestic animals is the problem of the farmer. All too often starvation occurs because the owner is not intelligent enough to assume the responsibility of providing for the needs of his animals.

During a period of starvation the process of catabolism continues. To supply the substances required for anabolism and to maintain the vital functions, the reserve stores of nutrient contained within the individual are drawn upon. Glycogen, which is the most readily usable substance for energy, is the first to be utilized. The fat deposited in the various body fat depots (around the kidney, in the mesentery and omentum, and in the subcutaneous tissue) is used next. Then the fat contained within the parenchymatous organs is utilized. If starvation continues, the protein comprising the cytoplasm of the cells is used. Finally, a stage is reached when so much protein has been used that the cells of the body are no longer able to perform the functions necessary for maintaining life, and death is the result.

Man and carnivorous animals can survive starvation for a period of two to four weeks and recover. If they are starved for a longer period of time, tissue depletion is so great that recovery cannot occur. An abundance of water will prolong the period of survival. The survival time in many animals depends upon the ability to hibernate. Salamanders and turtles will survive a year or more, frogs for nine months, and snakes for six months; however, if water is entirely removed from their environment, death results much more rapidly.

The ability of animals to resist bacterial infection is greatly reduced when the body defenses are impaired as the result of starvation. It has been shown experimentally that if mice are completely deprived of food for 36 to 48 hours and then inoculated with staphylococci, they are less resistant to infection than those fed continuously on a ration containing minimal nutrient requirements. This may explain in part the prevalence of infectious diseases among farm animals following long-distance shipping during which their food is withheld.

If underfeeding is continued for a long period of time, the digestive tract loses its muscular tone and becomes smaller than normal, and the parenchymatous organs are reduced in volume. Along with the diminution in size, these organs also lose the ability to utilize fully the available food. Animals that have survived a period of starvation cannot be given all of the feed they wish when it is again available. The reason for this is that the digestive tract, as well as the other organs associated with digestion and assimilation, is not able to utilize the food. The amount of secretion they can produce is inadequate and the musculature of the organs is not able to move the food through the digestive tract. If the digestive tract is overloaded, the animal will die as the result of impaction, bloat, and injurious bacterial fermentations of the ingesta.

The bodies of starved animals become more angular because of the disappearance of the subcutaneous fat. For the same reason the outlines of the muscles become more prominent. Bony prominences become more conspicuous. The abdomen appears small and "tucked up" due to the emptiness of the gastrointestinal tract and the disappearance of the extra- and intra-abdominal fat. The eyes appear sunken because the orbital fat diminishes.

Post-mortem examination of an individual that has died from starvation reveals atrophy of the fat depots (perirenal region, omentum, mesentery, subcutaneous tissue, etc.). The organs of the body show a decrease in size and weight as compared to those of normal individuals. The heart and brain show the least loss of weight. The digestive tract is usually empty. Anemia is present, and all of the tissues throughout the body are extremely edematous. Microscopic examination reveals the cells are smaller than normal, and the intercellular spaces are filled with edematous fluid.

A qualitative deficiency of food is just as important as a quantitative lack of food. Even though an abundance of food is present, the ration may be deficient in proteins, carbohydrates, fats, minerals, vitamins, and other substances. The need for these various components of the ration varies with the species of animal and its work requirements. The cow may require more of one substance than the pig, or the dog may require more of this substance than the horse. Not only is there a species variation but there may also be a variation between individuals. Likewise, the need for these various ingredients varies from day to day depending upon the weather and the diseases to which the individual is exposed. It is extremely important that all veterinarians be aware of the variation in the daily requirements of the individual animal as well as variations that occur in the feed. It is imperative that deficiency diseases in a herd be studied very closely to determine why they are present.

The feed industry has become a major agricultural enterprise. The feed manufacturer is doing everything possible to produce a feed that meets the average requirements of an average individual under average conditions. The farmer is not buying a feed that will meet all of the nutritional requirements that may exist on his farm. Whenever animal husbandry practices are altered on the farm, when a disease appears, when antibiotics are added to the ration, or the feed is stored or is mixed with other types of feed, the nutritive requirements of that group of animals are changed. Then the feed purchased at the mill may no longer be adequate to meet the requirements of that particular group of individuals. Whenever a disease appears in a group of animals, there is no way of determining the individual nutritive needs. Requirements of certain ingredients, such as vitamins, may be increased two or three times, perhaps even ten or fifteen times. Under these conditions, if a nutritional deficiency is found, that farmer cannot hold the feed company responsible because he did not buy a feed that would supply the needs of all individuals under all conditions. Additional vitamin supplements are usually needed whenever animals are ill.

Malnutrition may bring about a decreased function or loss of function of organs or groups of organs. The organs of special function are the first to show this change. Disturbances in fertility and reproduction are frequently the first manifestations of a nutritional deficiency. This is observed in the corn belt in beef animals when farmers forget that breeding animals need a well-balanced ration. Sterility is frequently observed in herds where the ration consists of corn and a little roughage — the same ration he is giving to his feeder cattle. When a well-balanced ration is substituted, the sterility problem usually disappears. The eye is particularly sensitive to a deficiency of vitamin A, and when this deficiency is present in cattle they are unable to see at night.

## PROTEIN

Protein is a vital substance in the body and forms the basic constituent of protoplasm. In this basic protein structure the metabolic activities of the body, involving proteins, carbohydrates, fats, minerals, and other essential substances, take place. To maintain this basic protoplasmic structure, protein is necessary. In the young growing animal additional protein is needed for growth and development. When adequate protein, containing the essential amino acids, is not present, the anabolic activities cannot take place or are retarded, and the animal does not grow properly and is stunted.

### Excess of Protein

Good quality protein is not injurious in amounts far above that needed for body requirements. This protein must be in a form that can be utilized. Carnivora need nothing but meat of good quality in their ration. Hogs do very well on a ration consisting almost entirely of protein; in fact, it is very doubtful if the so-called protein poisoning in pigs ever occurs. Chickens can consume much more protein than it is economical to feed. Herbivorous animals can consume large amounts of protein but do need considerably more carbohydrate in the form of roughage than do other species of animals because their digestive tract is designed for cellulose digestion. When large amounts of protein are fed to the ruminant not adjusted to a high protein ration, a serious gastrointestinal disturbance will result. Horses or cattle will sometimes gorge themselves on tankage, and an extremely serious toxemia will occur because the rumen and intestinal microorganisms cannot digest the protein, the bacterial flora is altered, and toxic products from putrefaction of protein are absorbed by the animal.

### Deficiency of Protein

Under normal conditions of growth in both wild and farm animals, there is probably no protein deficiency. In modern agriculture where every effort is made to raise and fatten animals in the shortest possible time through the use of rapidly maturing animals, concentrate feeds, ad-

ditional vitamins, and growth stimulating substances (antibiotics and hormones), additional protein is needed. This is especially true in the pig and the chicken where the rate of growth is extremely rapid. If protein is not available in adequate amounts to meet the requirements of this accelerated rate of growth, maximum gains in weight and production will not be obtained.

Ruminants are less susceptible to critical deficiencies of individual amino acids in their food protein than are the rat, pig, and chicken. Rumen microorganisms contribute much to the supply of protein digested in the intestine. For this reason ruminants can obtain high quality microbial protein from nonprotein nitrogenous compounds such as urea.

An inadequate amount of protein is of considerable economic importance to livestock producers. The indications of a deficiency of protein are reduction in growth rate, slow rate of gain, hypogalactia, poor egg production, and a light fleece. The common causes of a protein deficiency are as follows:

1. When the ration contains inadequate protein or protein that cannot be utilized, a deficiency will result. This is commonly observed in young growing animals where the needs for protein are great. It is frequently observed in calves that are pail-fed a ration consisting entirely of milk for a much longer interval of time than the usual nursing period. It is observed in young nursing animals whose mothers are deficient in protein. This is most commonly observed in sows that are fed inadequate amounts of protein supplement and have been pushed for maximum production and maximum number of litters in the shortest possible period of time. Protein deficiency is observed in fattening pigs fed a ration consisting exclusively of corn without the addition of a protein supplement. Cows and sows in heavy milk production will suffer from a protein deficiency when inadequate amounts are present in the ration. Hens in full egg

production will become deficient in protein because so much is lost in the egg unless adequate protein is added to the ration. Protein deficiency is frequently observed in ewes, cattle, and horses wintered on poor quality roughages (cornstalks) without a supplemental ration of grain and hay that contains protein. Protein is very apt to be deficient in areas of drought or in semi-arid countries where plants are scarce and do not develop properly.

2. A deficiency of protein is seen in animals on a ration in which the more expensive protein is replaced by a cheaper protein or in which the amount of protein in the ration is drastically reduced. This protein deficiency is frequently observed in both man and animals during times of war, for example in Europe during the past two world wars. During these wars a national protein deficiency existed, and the protein in the ration was reduced to a minimum. Because the condition is associated with periods of conflict, the resulting disease is called war edema. In this disease the amount of blood protein becomes so low that the normal osmotic pressure of the blood can no longer be maintained. As a result, plasma constituents leave the blood stream and appear in the tissue spaces and body cavities. This accumulation of fluid is known as edema.

3. A protein deficiency may occur when an animal is ill and does not wish to eat or when diseases of the tongue, teeth, and esophagus prevent the ingestion of food.

4. A protein deficiency occurs when diseases of the stomach and intestine increase the motility of the organs and the food passes through them so rapidly that the food is not digested and absorbed. It will also occur when alterations in the wall of the intestine (paratuberculosis of cattle and necrotic enteritis of swine) do not allow the absorption of food.

5. A deficiency of plasma protein occurs when diseases of the liver cause so much damage that the synthesis of plasma protein is inadequate or is prevented.

6. A deficiency of plasma protein is observed in animals (especially lambs and calves) infected with gastrointestinal parasites (Hemonchus, Ostertagia, and Trichostrongylus species) because of the hemorrhage they produce.

7. Plasma protein may become deficient when renal disease is present. This is commonly observed in the human being but is of little importance in domestic animals because they seldom have a glomerulonephritis. The greatest amount of plasma protein is lost through the kidney when oak bud poisoning or amyloidosis is present. However, the protein lost in amyloidosis is never great enough to be of any concern.

The importance of an adequate supply of proteins in the rations of domestic animals can be appreciated when one considers how proteins function in helping to build the natural and acquired defenses of the body against the entrance of pathogenic microorganisms.

The epidermis is covered with an elastic, but very resistant, protein substance, keratin, whose function is to act as a barrier against the entrance of harmful microorganisms. It is aided by the enzyme, lysozyme, another protein, which causes the lysis of some, but not all, harmful bacteria (notably *Mycobacterium tuberculosis*). Lysozyme is present in high concentration in the lacrimal secretion and quite probably prevents the entrance of some bacteria into the conjunctivae, the tear ducts, and the anterior nares. The mucous membranes lining the tubular-shaped structures that communicate with the exterior of the body secrete mucus, a mucoprotein whose function is to enclose microorganisms and remove them in the flow of mucus discharged by the individual. With protein the bone marrow forms leukocytes, the indispensable phagocytes in inflammatory reactions.

When a foreign protein, such as an exotoxin, endotoxin, or a virus, enters the body, changes occur in the blood, principally in the gamma-globulin fraction of the plasma proteins. These changes can be demonstrated by serological tests which detect the presence of antibodies (agglutinins, antitoxins, lysins, opsonins, and precipitins). These protein substances are a very important part of the mechanisms which animals possess for their defense against infection.

When the plasma proteins become diminished (hypoproteinemia), the protein reserve is drawn upon. The reserve consists of the protein in the cells and organs. If dietary protein is not forthcoming after the reserve has been drawn upon, or even before, the animal's resistance to infection becomes lowered because there is a lack of globulin for antibody production.

Gamma-globulin is a complete protein and as such contains all of the nitrogenous compounds necessary for the body. It can be produced only when there is an abundant supply of amino acids available in the tissues and organs, or in the food. Not only must there be an adequate supply of amino acids but also energy for the synthesis of them into gamma-globulin in the liver. This energy must be furnished by the oxidation of carbohydrates and fats assisted by the activating influences of suitable enzymes and vitamins (particularly riboflavin).

It should be emphasized here that it requires a period of several weeks to deplete an animal's protein reserve, but it seems reasonable that any reduction in the amount of gamma-globulin would be serious during the incubation period of an infectious disease when the number of microorganisms is increasing rapidly and ever-increasing quantities of antibodies are needed to combine with them.

While it is not a part of the animal's mechanism for defense against infection, another blood protein, oxygen-carrying hemoglobin, must be mentioned here because its presence in the body in an adequate amount is imperative for existence. In protein deficiency the body gives preference to hemoglobin production over that of the plasma proteins, but even then, in hypoproteinemia, hemoglobin cannot be adequately supplied and anemia occurs.

The serum normally carries a small, but important, amount of iron in combination with a globulin fraction of the plasma proteins. This is probably iron on the way from the liver to the bone marrow. When the plasma proteins have become reduced in protein-deficient animals, there is also a proportional reduction in the iron-binding capacity of the serum so that a state of hypoferremia results. It appears that copper is also in combination with a protein in the plasma. In protein deficiency there is also a plasma-copper reduction (hypocupremia). A similar hypoferremia also occurs in acute and chronic infections. Realizing this, one can speculate on the seriousness of infection in a protein-deficient animal — an animal in which an already diminished plasma-iron level is further lowered by the effects of infection. In infection the iron accumulates in the spleen and liver.

## CARBOHYDRATE

The quality of ingested carbohydrate is probably not as critical as that of the fats and proteins. The important thing in carbohydrate metabolism is the availability of the carbohydrate according to the form in which it is presented. Carbohydrates may be present in abundance and yet the individual is unable to utilize them. Man and carnivorous animals have considerable difficulty in digesting certain crude carbohydrates because they do not possess cellulose-digesting chambers as do ruminants. Some carbohydrates may become suitable for man and carnivorous animals if the food is processed. Cooking of potatoes and other vegetables brings about a disintegration of the plant cells and alterations in the carbohydrate so the food may be utilized by a simple digestive tract.

An excellent example of the manipulation of the ration in a manner resulting in the utilization of relatively indigestible carbohydrate was demonstrated during World War II in the Scandinavian countries. A food shortage was one of the problems of these countries since they could not import certain necessary foods because of trade restrictions. The Swedish people had to rely on their own farms for all of the food they needed. Since the human population required a greater share of the available food, a shortage of feed for cattle and horses developed. This in turn resulted in a decreased amount of dairy products and equine labor. During this time, paper pulp could not be exported and was accumulating on the wharves and around the mills. It was discovered that this paper pulp could be utilized by the ruminant if the normal rumen bacterial flora could be maintained. The pulp, apparently palatable to the bovine, was reconstituted by soaking in water until it resembled a soft mash. To maintain a normal rumen flora that would digest the cellulose of the paper pulp, it was found that 100 grams of molasses per day per cow was needed. The readily available carbohydrate, in the form of molasses, supplied the nutritive requirements of the rumen flora. When this was provided, the rumen flora was able to digest the cellulose and convert it into carbohydrates and other substances needed by the ruminant. Thus, the food shortage was alleviated and dairy products became available.

### Excess of Carbohydrate

Excessive amounts of usable carbohydrate, over and above that needed for cell metabolism, heat, and energy, are converted into fat. This process is used in fattening animals.

### Deficiency of Carbohydrate

An inadequate amount of carbohydrate or an inability to digest the available carbohydrate is manifested by thinness, weakness, debility, and death. A number of diseases are associated with a deficiency of carbohydrate, and several of them will be discussed in the following paragraphs.

**Pregnancy disease** of ewes is associated with a deficiency of carbohydrates. It is also known as the toxemia of pregnancy,

preparturient paralysis, acidosis, and acetonemia. The susceptible animals are mature or aged ewes which are fed a rather non-nutritious roughage not supplemented with sufficient grain. Aged ewes with deficient dentition, when fed whole corn as a grain supplement, are easy victims of this condition. While a carbohydrate deficiency is the principal cause of pregnancy disease, it is associated with advanced pregnancy and lack of exercise.

The part advanced pregnancy plays in the etiology of this disease is usually dependent upon the number of fetuses a ewe carries. A ewe carrying a single fetus seldom has pregnancy disease unless the lamb is unusually large. Affected ewes usually carry twins or triplets. The lack-of-exercise factor is almost always directly related to inclement weather conditions such as sleet storms, heavy snow falls, and blizzards which restrict the activity of the animals.

When the feeding of a deficient carbohydrate ration, advanced twin or triplet pregnancy, and lack of exercise are combined, some ewes develop symptoms characterized by depression and coma. They usually die within a week.

The pathogenesis of the disease can be explained in the following manner: Ewes have an extremely low normal glucose blood level. They, like other animals, convert the glucose into glycogen in the liver where much of it is stored. The relative amount stored, however, is very small. The liver of a single lamb fetus contains three times as much glycogen as its mother's. Twins and triplets together store an amount that must be a considerable drain on the already inadequate amount for a well-nourished ewe. When the ration of such a ewe is deficient in carbohydrate or when she fails to eat, the liver glycogen content becomes diminished more rapidly than it can be replenished. Depot fat is then transported to the liver to replace the glycogen lost by the hepatic cells. In this instance the liver fat content is increased from 3 to 4 per cent of the fresh weight of the organ to as much as 35 per cent. In the oxidation of this hepatic fat, ketone bodies (acetoacetic acid and beta-hydroxybutyric acid) are formed in excess. In a normal animal the skeletal muscles utilize the ketone bodies for energy. In inactive ewes these substances accumulate in the blood (ketonemia) and large amounts are excreted in the urine (ketonuria). Two factors then are operating to cause a state of ketosis — increased production of ketone bodies in the liver and decreased utilization of them by the muscles. In the body's effort to excrete these two organic acids, the alkali reserve is depleted and the ewe dies in a state of acidosis.

In the post-mortem examination three things are outstanding: (1) advanced pregnancy with a single, large, well-developed fetus, or more often with twins or triplets, (2) an extreme fatty degeneration of the liver, and (3) the presence of ketone bodies in the urine.

**Macroscopic appearance.** The color of the liver is distinctly bright yellow. The surface is smooth and, because the organ is greatly enlarged, the borders are rounded. Even though the total weight of the liver is increased, small excised portions of it will float on water due to the high fat content. The cut surface is greasy.

**Microscopic appearance.** The liver cells contain droplets of fat. The droplets are large; in fact, a single droplet may nearly fill a cell. To accommodate the infiltrated fat, the cells become enlarged and rounded. They have the appearance of adipose tissue cells. The nuclei stain normally but are pushed to the periphery of the cells and are often converted from spheres into crescents. If the condition which causes the fatty infiltration subsides, the cells recover. Apparently the excessive infiltration of fat does not seriously interfere with the function of the liver in all cases.

**Acetonemia** is a serious disturbance of carbohydrate metabolism in high-producing dairy cattle. The sudden onset of heavy lactation at the end of pregnancy provides a combination of factors that completely upsets carbohydrate metabolism and causes ketosis. The cow normally has a lower blood glucose level (40 to 60 mg. per cent) than do other domestic animals (100 to 120 mg. per cent). This low blood glucose probably exerts some influence on the appearance of acetonemia.

The complete pathogenesis of ketosis has not been clarified. A very brief review of the salient points in this process makes it understandable why there is so much uncertainty about the real cause of ketosis. This review begins with digestion in the rumen where large numbers of microorganisms (bacteria and protozoa), by means of enzymes, digest carbohydrates. In the fermentation of digestion, volatile fatty acids (acetic, butyric, and propionic) are formed and absorbed. These acids eventually furnish energy for the cow. Acetic and butyric acids form ketone bodies. Propionic acid counteracts the formation of these bodies and is also used in the production of liver glycogen.

Acetic and butyric acids, that are ketogenic in effect, comprise almost 80 per cent of the fatty acids produced and absorbed by the rumen. Propionic acid, which counteracts their effects because it is utilized in glycogenesis, comprises about 20 per cent of the total. In health this appears to be the proper proportion of each that prevents clinical ketosis from occurring. Late in pregnancy when a cow is storing glycogen in the liver of her fetus and at parturition when she diverts it into her milk, the balance may not be maintained. This allows the effects of the ketogenic fatty acids to exceed those of the glycogenic propionic acid in the dam.

Ruminal bacteria also synthesize vitamin B and protein. Among the vitamins, $B_{12}$ is especially needed to stimulate the bacteria to increase the rate of cellulose digestion.

When a cow freshens, her milk production suddenly increases from nothing to ten or more gallons per day. To meet the demand for nutrient with which to make this volume of milk, digestion in the rumen must be accelerated. The efficiency and magnitude of rumen digestion are dependent upon the number and kinds of bacteria present. They cannot thrive unless the readily available nutrients they need are present in the rumen. Their requirements are proteins, carbohydrates, minerals (calcium, phosphorus, and cobalt), and sulfur for the synthesis of vitamin $B_{12}$ and other vitamins.

In carbohydrate metabolism in the cow vitamin $B_{12}$ is important because it is concerned with the formation of epinephrine in the adrenal cortex. Epinephrine has a variety of functions in carbohydrate metabolism which could have some bearing on the cause of ketosis. Important among the functions of epinephrine are: (1) It increases the quantity of blood sugar by releasing glycogen from the liver; (2) it transforms muscle glycogen into lactic acid that is utilized by the liver in the formation of glycogen; (3) it regulates the blood sugar level when the cow is subjected to stress (parturition and the onset of heavy lactation); and (4) it stimulates the pituitary gland to release the adrenocorticotrophic hormone (ACTH) which in turn causes the adrenal cortex to increase the production of cortisone. Cortisone stimulates the formation of glycogen by converting fat and protein to fatty acids and glycerol. Glycogen is produced by the liver from glycerol.

A high-producing dairy cow is very delicately balanced from the standpoint of carbohydrate metabolism. When the nutritive intake and requirements are in balance, the varied and complex processes just mentioned take place in proper sequence, and a state of health is maintained. The most critical time for maintaining this balance is during late pregnancy, parturition, and early lactation. This is the time of severe stress and the time when there is a sudden demand for an increase in nutritive requirements. However, this is often the period when feed is restricted to prevent congestion of the mammary gland. As parturition approaches, there is a gradual decrease in the blood sugar level. After parturition there is a more sudden decrease, designated as hypoglycemia, which persists for a period of time. During this period, ketone bodies (acetone, acetoacetic acid, and beta-hydroxybutyric acid) are present in the blood. The quantity of these bodies in a normal cow at this time varies from a trace to 5 or 6 mg. per cent in the blood and a trace to 15 or 16 mg. per cent in the urine. There are no symptoms of illness and a state of subclinical ketosis does not exist.

Clinical ketosis rarely occurs if the cow's appetite remains good and the ration is adequate. If either is lacking, ketone bodies accumulate in the blood (80 mg. per cent) and are excreted in the urine (550 mg. per cent). At the same time the blood sugar level decreases as much as 50 per cent (20 to 30 mg. per cent). Ketonemia, ketonuria, and hypoglycemia exist and the cow has clinical ketosis.

Signs of clinical ketosis are anorexia, hypogalactia, and rapid loss of weight with dehydration, listlessness, incoordination, and constipation. Ketone bodies are readily detected by the odor of the expired air and the voided urine.

Recovery from uncomplicated ketosis occurs when the glycogen content of the liver is high enough to prevent hypoglycemia and the excessive production of ketone bodies. ACTH, cortisone, and synthetic steroid hormones may accomplish this by causing glucogenesis (the conversion of protein and fat in the liver to glucose). Sodium propionate may accomplish this by being converted into glucose or glycogen in the liver. Intravenous administration of glucose gives temporary improvement by immediately increasing the blood sugar level. During the period of temporary improvement, a ration containing the essential substances mentioned early on this page, especially carbohydrates, must be provided if complete recovery is to be accomplished.

Secondary ketosis may occur when a high-producing cow develops anorexia due to metritis, traumatic gastritis, nephritis, or an acute infectious disease such as mastitis.

# FAT

Fat is utilized for energy when carbohydrate is not available. The fat ingested above that required for metabolism is converted into body fat. When carbohydrates are ingested in excess of the requirement, they are converted into fat and are stored in that form as a reserve source of energy.

The amount of fat consumed and required varies with the species of animal. The ruminants for the most part do not ingest fat as do other species of animals. Most of their body fat is derived from a conversion of carbohydrate into fat. The type of carbohydrate consumed exerts a decided effect on the consistency of the body fat. Barley and corn produce a very firm fat that makes a desirable meat carcass. This is of considerable importance in the feeding of livestock.

## Excess of Fat

When too much fat is consumed in the ration, the individual gains weight since the fat is stored in the fat depots of the body. The consistency of the body fat varies with the type of fat ingested. Dogs fed large amounts of mutton tallow will eventually have body fat resembling sheep fat in some of its physical and chemical characteristics. The ability of the ingested fat to alter the character of the body fat is of great importance in the feeding of livestock. The oil in soybeans and peanuts produces a very soft fat if it is fed in excessive amounts. It is difficult for the packer to produce a desirable product from hogs that have been fattened with these oils. These carcasses are discriminated against because the fat is so soft that oil will actually drip from them as they hang in the refrigerator.

Excessive fat or oil in the ration results in an increased motility of the intestinal tract and may result in diarrhea. This is especially apt to occur if the oil is of a non-digestible type such as mineral oil. If the oils are not digested, they will coat the food and interfere with the penetration of digestive enzymes. When the oils cause an increased rate of intestinal motility, the food passes through the intestinal tract so rapidly that it is only partially digested and malnutrition is the result.

The fat-soluble vitamins are removed from the food by excessive amounts of oil. If undigested oil passes through the intestinal tract, it will carry the fat-soluble vitamins with it and a vitamin deficiency will result. This is of considerable concern in poultry when too much cod-liver oil is placed in the ration. A vitamin D deficiency is prevented by the addition of fish oil to the ration, but vitamin E is extracted by the oil so that the chicks develop nutritional encephalomalacia. In calves, coagulation necrosis of the skeletal and cardiac muscles occurs when the ration contains so much fish oil as to extract the vitamin E.

When a diarrhea is present as the result of the excessive intake of oil, injury to the tail may occur. This is especially common in the rat. A mass of oily feces covers the tail, causes dermatitis, exerts external pressure on the vascular system of the tail, and the result is gangrene and sloughing of the tail.

## Deficiency of Fat

A certain amount of fat is needed in the ration for normal growth and development. The need is especially great if the amount of carbohydrate is limited and if large amounts of energy are required.

Fat apparently contains certain essential substances. As a whole, little attention has been paid to them, and the specific substances have not been isolated and identified. Human beings and dogs in the arctic require considerable fat in their ration. If it is lacking, central nervous disorders result. In the human being, insanity, locomotor disturbances, irritability, and other symptoms of degeneration of the central nervous system and the peripheral nerves are manifested. Sled dogs in the arctic on a low fat ration develop convulsions, fits, and a maniacal tendency to the extent that it is often confused with the central nervous form of canine distemper and rabies. Just how serious this is can be exemplified by the experience of Amundsen on his first polar expedition. When the time came for him to use his sled dogs in the trip to the North Pole, he found they were afflicted with arctic madness. As a result, the expedition was a failure because he did not have a means of transporting his supplies to the North Pole. On his second expedition he took large amounts of barreled salt pork along with him. An adequate amount of pork was fed daily, arctic madness was prevented, and he was able to reach the Pole because his dogs were healthy. This essential substance is most abundant in seal fat. Pork does not contain as much of this substance but it is still present in adequate amounts to prevent the disease.

Fat is essential for normal growth and development of experimental rats. If fat is not available, the growth rate is retarded, there is excessive scaliness of the skin along with a poor hair coat, and some of the rats may die.

## WATER

The functions of water depend upon its properties as a solvent and as a vehicle. In these capacities water aids the digestive fluids in the absorption of food, transports soluble substances in the blood and lymph, facilitates the excretion of soluble waste products, keeps the constituents of the cells and tissues in solution so that chemical reactions can take place, maintains the proper dilutions of salts in the tissues, helps to regulate the temperature of the body by removing excessive heat through the evaporation of water from the surface of the body, and acts as a lubricant on the serous surfaces.

### Excess of Water

When an individual consumes too much water, a condition known as water sickness appears. Water sickness is usually associated with warm weather and high humidity. Under these conditions, large amounts of water are drunk for the cooling effect and to replace the water lost through sweating and evaporation. This condition is frequently observed in farmers, men working in foundries or mills, and in those individuals engaged in the canning industry. It is especially common during the warm humid summer days. The condition is of considerable concern in troops required to maneuver in the tropics. Under these conditions, when large amounts of water are consumed and the loss of chlorides is not replaced with salt, a depletion of the chlorides will result.

Men afflicted with water sickness show vague digestive disturbances, headache, abdominal and muscular cramps, nausea, vomiting, diarrhea, incoordination, unconsciousness, and frequently the disease terminates in death.

Water sickness is also observed in swimmers who remain in water for long periods of time. Tremendous amounts of water are absorbed through the skin of the individual unless the skin is greased. The swimmer also, intentionally or inadvertently, swallows some water. As the result of the excessive intake of water, the swimmer experiences a dull, depressed, weak sensation that may persist for several hours.

Water sickness may be observed in hunting dogs, particularly in young nervous dogs that are hunting for the first time. The dogs run excessively, become extremely excited, frequently develop diarrhea, and begin to drink water at every pond and stream they encounter. As the result of the excessive intake of water, the chlorides in the body are depleted, and the dogs are unable to hunt because of exhaustion. Dogs usually do not die from this condition because they will not continue to work after they are ill as will horses.

The symptoms of water sickness are due to the elimination of chlorides in the form of sweat, the dilution of chlorides within the body as the result of the excessive water intake, and the loss of chlorides by vomiting. The latter occurs because the chloride ion in the hydrochloric acid of the gastric juice is derived from sodium chloride. When the chlorides are depleted, the normal osmotic pressure of the body fluids cannot be maintained. Then the exchange of nutrients and metabolites between the blood and the cells is no longer possible. Normal cell metabolism is suppressed or prevented, and this produces serious clinical symptoms and may cause death.

Treatment is directed toward replacing the chlorides. Salt solution may be given intravenously to bring about immediate relief, and then, when the patient shows improvement, additional salt is given by mouth.

Indirectly, too much water in a community is of concern to the livestock industry because certain diseases become prevalent when an abundance of moisture is present. When there is excessive rain, swamps, ponds, and mud holes appear. These serve as breeding sites for mosquitos and other insect vectors. The mosquito is capable of carrying many diseases (equine viral encephalomyelitis, equine infectious viral anemia, malaria, etc.). Muddy barnyards and especially the muddy hog wallow are ideal sites for the development of the intermediate stages of the life cycle of various parasites infectious for animals. The mud becomes contaminated with enteric bacteria capable of spreading to other animals and causing a serious endemic or epidemic.

Water is of concern to the cattle and sheep industry when animals are forced to stand in mud for long periods of time and their legs become macerated. A dermatitis of the legs, especially between the claws, results. The tissues are invaded with various types of bacteria, and the disease known as foot rot is the result.

Mud is a problem with horses when it becomes caked in the feather of the legs. The wet mud macerates the skin, acts as an irritant, and produces a dermatitis. The injured skin is invaded with bacteria and a serious suppurative inflammation of the skin is the result. This is one of the reasons why the Clydesdale and the Shire, breeds with much feather on the legs, were never very popular in areas where mud was present during the rainy season.

A serious condition known as lumpy wool disease occurs in sheep in areas where there is an abundance of rainfall. Constant rain washes the oil out of the wool, the wool becomes wet, and the wet wool on the backs of the sheep becomes a macerating blanket. Whenever skin is soaked in water for a long period of time, it loses its ability to resist bacterial invasion, and a dermatitis is the result. Exudate accumulates on the skin and mats the wool. The rotting wool, containing odoriferous exudate, attracts flies. The flies lay their eggs, maggots hatch from the eggs, and death of the animal may occur when the maggots invade the tissues.

### Deficiency of Water

Before considering what actually happens in the body during water depletion, one should recall that water is present in three so-called compartments or depots — vascular, interstitial, and cellular — or one may think of water distribution in the body as being extracellular (vascular and interstitial) and intracellular. The extracellular water (vascular and interstitial) is in close association with sodium chloride. The association is so close that in speaking of water depletion, salt must continually be brought into the discussion.

It is not difficult to understand what happens in water depletion. First, the extracellular fluid (vascular and interstitial) becomes hypertonic because water leaves the body by the lungs, the skin, and the kidneys, while salt is not lost to the same extent. Next, water is drawn out of the cells (cellular compartment) to maintain the extracellular fluid. The result is **dehydration** of all three compartments. Since the loss of salt is very slight in this type of dehydration, it is dangerous to administer saline solution intravenously in these cases. There is already an excessive amount of salt in proportion to water in the body, and the extra amount in saline solution "adds fuel to the fire." It is the rule in human medicine not to administer isotonic saline when it is not necessary because there is a tendency for patients receiving the solution to retain sodium and chlorine out of proportion to water.

An animal must excrete a certain minimum amount of water in order to rid the body of metabolites. If less than this minimum amount is excreted, the metabolites accumulate in the blood, and a severe intoxication called **uremia** results. If water is not supplied, death occurs probably as a result of uremia and hemoconcentration (as in shock).

Birds, by means of their uric acid metabolism, are able to conserve water much more efficiently than mammals. The uric acid is eliminated as urate, which is a semisolid substance that does not require the volume of water for excretion as does urine when excreted by the mammal. This method of water conservation is absolutely essential in the developing chicken embryo since an additional supply of water cannot be introduced into the egg during the period of incubation.

The effects of the deprivation or depletion of water occur more rapidly and more severely than those caused by starvation. The animals naturally are extremely thirsty. Thirsty animals refuse food. The amount of digestive fluids diminishes. The blood becomes more viscid (hemoconcentration). There is loss of weight and great emaciation. The skin appears to be too big for the animal, and consequently becomes wrinkled, dry, and scaly.

Two-thirds of the body consists of water. Normally the water intake exceeds the requirements of the animal and the surplus is excreted by the kidneys. When the intake ceases and losses of water continue by vaporization (skin and lungs) and by urination, the body loses water at the rate of about 2 per cent of the body weight daily. A 10 per cent loss of the water content of the body causes alarming disturbances, and a 20 per cent loss re-

sults in death. The survival time will vary considerably depending upon the humidity of the surroundings, temperature, and activity of the individual. In humid surroundings, there is profuse sweating and an abundance of water is lost in this way. In dry areas, loss of water by evaporation is great. The temperature of the surroundings is extremely important because the higher the temperature, the greater is the amount of sweating, the more rapid is the evaporation, and the shorter is the period of time the individual will survive. An individual that can remain quiet will survive without water much longer than one that is moving about, because the rate of metabolism is less in the resting individual. Three to four days is about as long as an animal can survive without water. If the temperature is low and the humidity is ideal, the animal may survive for a period of one to two weeks or until about 20 per cent of the body weight has been lost.

Water starvation is a world-wide problem when rain has been deficient and wells and streams become dry. Unless water can be brought into the community, death from water starvation will result. This is particularly serious in wild animals because they are unable to survive the period of time required to move to a new area where water is available when their water supply is gone.

In the Midwest, one of the most common causes of water starvation is the freezing of the water supply. The animals are unable to break the ice and reach the water underneath. For this reason it is absolutely imperative that water heaters be maintained in the watering system on the farm to prevent the freezing of water. The heaters are also needed to warm the water to a temperature at which the animals will consume it in amounts adequate for metabolism and proper gains in weight.

Water starvation is frequently observed in poultry and swine during the fall of the year when they are brought from the pasture or range into the houses. All too frequently the farmer neglects to bring watering facilities into the house. A serious water deficiency is present before the error is recognized.

In the search for various labor-saving devices, there is a tendency to rely too much on the automaticity of the mechanical drinking fountain. Defective mechanical appliances may result in water deficiency. For this reason, every drinking device should be checked at least once a day to determine if it is operating correctly. Frequently, in a milking line, one automatic drinking device will not be operating. A single cow may suffer from water starvation and may die before the cause of the disorder is recognized.

In desert countries obtaining water is always a serious problem. By training, both man and animals can go for much longer periods of time on a minimum amount of water than will the untrained individual. Water training is practiced in the armed services so that individuals in combat in desert areas or for survival at sea will learn to conserve the small amount of water that may be available. Even the camel must undergo periods of water training if he is to survive on the desert for considerable periods of time without water. The camel that is to be used on the desert is not allowed to have all of the water he will drink and is maintained on a constant water discipline. By training, the tissues and cells of the camel become adjusted to a minimum amount of water and, as a result, he can survive for astonishingly long periods of time with only a limited supply of water.

While our first thought in connection with water deficiency is relative to the lack of water for normal animals, there is another phase of the subject which is probably of much greater importance to veterinarians. It is the matter of water depletion in sick animals — surgical and medical cases that are too weak to drink, animals that are in a state of coma such as cows and sheep with ketosis and cows

with parturient paresis, and animals that cannot swallow (dysphagia), such as calves with diphtheria and horses with encephalomyelitis. Dehydration is a contributing factor in the death of many sick and weak animals.

## MINERALS

The most important minerals in the rations of domestic animals are sodium chloride, calcium, phosphorus, magnesium, iodine, iron, copper, cobalt, and manganese. Variations in the amounts of these result in various structural and functional changes in the body.

### Sodium Chloride

Sodium chloride aids in maintaining osmotic pressure in the blood, the interstitial tissue, and the cells; in fact, 65 per cent of the total osmotic pressure of the blood is due to sodium chloride. This pressure makes possible the exchange of cell nutrients for cell metabolites. Salt in the plasma decreases the viscosity of the blood. The source of the chlorine ion in the gastric hydrochloric acid is sodium chloride.

The same fluid depots (extracellular and intracellular) of the body that are so important in water metabolism are likewise of importance in salt metabolism. The movement of fluids through cell membranes, in the process of carrying nutrient material to the cells and metabolites away from the cells, is determined by the relative osmotic pressure of the area. The osmotic pressure is rather delicately balanced to maintain a state suitable for the diffusion of fluids in and out of the cells so that the essential substances will enter the cell and undesirable substances will leave. If the interstitial fluid becomes hypertonic, water will be drawn out of the cells (dehydration); if hypotonic, the cells will gorge themselves with water. The water balance between the cells and the interstitial tissue is maintained by the action of the electrolyte ions — sodium, chlorine, and bicarbonate ions in the interstitial fluid, and potassium and phosphate ions in the cells.

Sodium chloride is not only an important constituent of the extracellular fluid but also of the alimentary secretions and sweat. It has already been said that its principal function in the extracellular fluid is to supply osmotic pressure so that the intracellular fluid (protoplasm) is kept in an isotonic state. Salt also plays an important role in maintaining the acid-base balance of the extracellular fluid, which normally is slightly alkaline. It accomplishes this purpose by means of its sodium ions, which supply more than 90 per cent of the base, and its chlorine ions, which provide more than 70 per cent of the acid.

The maintenance of the isotonicity of the extracellular fluid is under the control of a very complicated mechanism. In England, Verney (1948) determined by experiment that the concentration of sodium chloride in the carotid arterial plasma (carotid osmotic pressure) stimulates receptors in the carotid body, and that impulses travel to the neurohypophysis (posterior lobe) which secretes an antidiuretic hormone. This hormone in turn regulates kidney function so that the extracellular fluid is maintained in an isotonic state.

### EXCESS OF SODIUM CHLORIDE

If animals have free access to salt, the intake exceeds the requirements of the body. The surplus is excreted primarily by the kidneys and a little is eliminated by the skin and alimentary tract. However, if renal disease is present so that the excretion of the chlorides is prevented, or if sufficient water is not available to dilute the chlorides and eliminate them through the kidneys, salt poisoning will occur. Salt poisoning frequently occurs when excessive amounts of physiological saline are administered to animals that are ill.

Salt poisoning is observed in animals on rations excessively high in salt content. In an effort to save labor, ranchers have devised a method of feeding cotton-seed meal. The cottonseed meal is necessary in range country during the winter to supply the protein, phosphorus, and other substances needed by animals forced to feed on the poor winter roughage of the range. Cattle are extremely fond of cottonseed meal and will gorge themselves upon it if allowed to have all they wish. If a large amount of salt is added to the meal, the animals will only consume a small amount of the meal each day because the salt renders it somewhat unpalatable. Therefore, ranchers can place large amounts of the cottonseed meal and salt mixture in bunkers or self-feeders once or twice a week and the animals will not eat excessively. This cottonseed meal and salt mixture may be fed if adequate amounts of water are available. The high salt content increases the amount of water needed by the animals because the excess salt must be diluted and eliminated in an aqueous solution. If the water supply is frozen and the animals consume a large amount of the cottonseed meal and salt mixture, salt poisoning is the result. These animals have a severe gastroenteritis, and the tubules of the kidneys are distended with white crystals of sodium chloride. Renal tubular degeneration and necrosis occur. Death is due to dehydration, gastroenteritis, and uremia.

Salt poisoning is commonly observed in pigs that consume large amounts of salt and do not have water available. The pig seems to be particularly susceptible to salt poisoning. It is the sodium ion rather than the chloride ion that produces the toxicity, since other sodium salts will produce the same symptoms and lesions. Salt poisoning is observed in pigs after they have consumed brine from vats used to pickle meat or fish, have drunk salt water contained within salt boxes or blocks following a rain, or have eaten a ration containing excessive salt. The pigs have a catarrhal gastroenteritis and an eosinophilic meningoencephalitis.

Salt poisoning is also observed in chicks

when the self-feeders or feeding troughs are not cleaned out regularly. The salt settles out of the ration to the bottom of the feeder or trough. When the chicks eat this feed containing a high concentration of sodium chloride, poisoning occurs. Chicks dying from salt poisoning show ascites. Adult poultry may also be poisoned with salt when they consume salted meat or fish, or the brine in which meat or fish has been pickled.

## DEFICIENCY OF SODIUM CHLORIDE

The amount of salt in the natural feeds of most species of animals is not sufficient. The need for additional salt in the ration depends upon (1) the species of animal, (2) the type of food consumed, (3) the amount of water in the ration, (4) the temperature, (5) the humidity, and (6) the work requirements of the individual. This is particularly true of animals that sweat while working or exercising.

Horses sweat profusely while at hard work during hot seasons and lose excessive amounts of sodium chloride. The resulting sodium chloride depletion of the body causes the symptoms associated with heat exhaustion. The disturbance of cell metabolism caused by the alteration in the osmotic pressure prevents the exchange of oxygen and nutrient for metabolites through the cell wall and explains the symptoms associated with heat exhaustion. The nervous manifestations shown by these animals are the result of alterations (cloudy swelling and lipoidal degeneration) in the neurones. Herbivora (horses, cattle, sheep, and goats) suffer from a deficiency of sodium chloride because plants are usually deficient in this salt. The predominating salts of plants are those of potassium, not sodium.

Carnivorous animals usually do not have a salt deficiency if they are fed a ration suitable for the carnivora, as there is a considerable amount of salt in meat. The modern house dog is frequently fed a ration low in salt, particularly when his food consists of cereal grains. During the heat of summer when the dog consumes large amounts of water, a salt deficiency may occur unless it is added to the ration. If swine and poultry receive milk and tankage, they are supplied with a sufficient amount of salt, but when these animals are fed solely on grain, symptoms of salt deficiency appear.

Salt deficiency is frequently observed in sows nursing large litters of pigs. Because of the fear of salt poisoning in pigs, many farmers feed rations that contain inadequate amounts of salt. Sows secrete a large amount of milk and, as a result, considerable salt is eliminated and salt depletion occurs. The sows show anorexia, constipation, hypogalactia, agalactia, and loss of weight. The animals recover quickly when salt is administered intravenously or is included in the ration.

When an animal does not receive sufficient sodium chloride, or for any reason loses the supply it normally should have in the body, the extracellular fluid ceases to be isotonic and becomes hypotonic due to the loss of electrolytes. Because of the alteration in osmotic pressure, the free flow of fluids through the cell wall (a semipermeable membrane) is suppressed, the exchange of nutrient and oxygen for metabolites does not occur, and metabolites accumulate within the cells. The volume of vascular fluid (plasma) diminishes because the kidneys excrete water in an attempt to keep the extracellular fluid in an isotonic state. The diminished volume of vascular fluid leaves the plasma proteins in a more concentrated form, increasing the colloidal osmotic pressure exerted by them and pulling water from the interstitial tissue. This state of water depletion of the extracellular compartments of the body is called **dehydration.**

In an experiment to determine the effects of salt deficiency conducted in Wisconsin several years ago, several dairy cows were deprived of salt for a year. Within two or three weeks after the beginning of the experiment, the animals showed a pronounced craving for salt, but no general impairment of health. Later, the cows began to show anorexia, hypogalactia, and general emaciation. Some of the animals died at the time of parturition or shortly thereafter. In an experiment in Iowa, in which ewes were deprived of salt, it was noted that they lost weight, gave birth to lambs of low vitality, and showed a decrease in wool production.

Inadequate intake of sodium chloride is not the only reason for salt depletion. Excessive sweating, vomiting, and diarrhea may cause excessive loss of salt which also may lead to dehydration. One-half of the body salt may be lost before death occurs. Salt depletion can be detected in these cases by examining the urine for sodium chloride by means of the Fantus test.

Salt is lost when vomiting and diarrhea occur because sodium chloride is present in the secretions of the gastrointestinal tract. Animals that vomit and scour persistently dehydrate rapidly. Loss of sodium chloride from vomiting and diarrhea also disturbs the acid-base balance in the body. The loss of chlorine ions in the gastric juice results in **alkalosis,** and loss of sodium ions in the intestinal secretions leads to **acidosis.** In treating dehydration resulting from sweating, vomiting, and diarrhea, one must remember that the salt lost must be replaced as well as the water. Water cannot be held in the body without salt. Six or seven grams of sodium chloride will retain one liter of water.

## Calcium

Calcium is found in the soil and is absorbed by vegetation. The leaves and stems of plants contain an abundance of calcium, but grains are deficient. Calcium is eliminated from the body in secretions and excretions, but the intestine and kidney remove most of the excess.

Calcium is essential for the ossification of bone, calcification of cartilage, regulation of skeletal and cardiac muscle tone, coagulation of blood, and maintainance of osmotic pressure and pH. Calcium metabolism is under the control of the parathyroid gland, and vitamin D is necessary for its deposition in cartilage and bone.

EXCESS OF CALCIUM

Calcium, as ingested by the individual, must be in a definite proportion to other minerals, particularly phosphorus, in the ration. The calcium-phosphorus ratio varies with the species of animal and the type of work (e.g. lactation and egg production) to which the animal is subjected. For most species of animals the ratio should be approximately two parts of calcium to one part of phosphorus (2:1) if normal bone metabolism is to be maintained. The ratio between calcium and phosphorus fluctuates constantly, being broader at times and narrower at other times, but if the variation from this rather basic ratio becomes excessive and persists for a long period of time, a disturbance in calcium metabolism will cause a bone disease.

When excessive amounts of calcium are administered to an individual along with excessive amounts of vitamin D, calcification of many tissues, other than bone, may occur throughout the body. This condition is observed in animals when a vitamin- and mineral-conscious owner administers excessive amounts of vitamin D and calcium to his animals. In northern latitudes where a fear of vitamin D deficiency exists and where fish scrap and fish oils are relatively cheap, excessive amounts of vitamin D in the form of fish oil are often given to calves. This oil extracts vitamin E from the ration and the deficiency of vitamin E results in coagulation necrosis of cardiac and skeletal muscle. Since there is an excessive amount of vitamin D and calcium, this mineral is deposited in the necrotic muscles.

Excessive amounts of calcium are present in the blood when tumors of the parathyroid gland occur. A tumor of the parathyroid gland produces an abundance of parathyroid hormone. The excess of hormone causes decalcification of the skeleton. When the amount of calcium in the blood exceeds 12 mg. per cent, precipitation of the calcium occurs in organs, especially muscles, where it is not normally found. The individual is said to have become petrified.

Parakeratosis in swine occurs when there are excessive amounts of calcium in the ration. Excessive calcium interferes with the metabolism of zinc which is necessary for the normal growth of skin (see Chapter 22).

## DEFICIENCY OF CALCIUM

The amount of calcium in the blood stream fluctuates between 10 and 11 mg. per cent depending upon the species of animal. Although the amount of calcium varies constantly, it cannot depart very much from the basic normal figure for the species or alarming symptoms of a calcium deficiency will appear. The calcium in the blood is maintained in a supersaturated solution. This supersaturation is necessary if adequate amounts of calcium are to be available when sudden requirements for it appear. If the calcium content of the blood exceeds 12 mg. per cent, the supersaturation can no longer be maintained and precipitation occurs in various tissues of the body. If the blood calcium decreases to 8 mg. per cent, symptoms (tetany and incoordination) of calcium deficiency appear, and if the calcium content of the blood reaches 6 mg. per cent or lower, tetany, paralysis, coma, and death occur.

A reserve supply of calcium is contained within the skeleton. It is deposited in the osteoid tissue along with phosphorus and other minerals, and this mineralization converts the osteoid tissue into osseous tissue. Normally, a rather definite balance exists between the calcium in the blood and in the bones. This balance is under the direct control of the parathyroid gland and is closely associated with vitamin D. Since calcium is being brought into the body constantly and calcium is being used at varying rates by the body, the calcium content of the bones is in a state of constant fluctuation during both physiological and pathological conditions. The calcium content of the ration may be adequate for

normal body metabolism, but our domestic animals are subject to a number of stresses or functions that require additional calcium. If adequate amounts of calcium are not contained within the ration, the reserve supply in the bones is withdrawn. This depletion of calcium from the bones and the resulting softening is called osteomalacia.

One of the physiological functions requiring large amounts of calcium is pregnancy. Throughout the gestation period the plasma calcium content of the mother falls slightly below the normal amount while that of the fetus becomes higher than that of the mother. When the blood calcium of the mother decreases in amount, it is replaced by a mobilization of calcium from the storehouse in the skeleton. As a result, the bones become softer and softer as calcium is removed. When gestation terminates and the period of lactation begins, large amounts of calcium are eliminated in the milk. Again calcium is removed from the skeleton to supply the necessary amount of calcium in the milk. Throughout the lactation period, tremendous amounts of calcium are being eliminated constantly from the body through the milk. If adequate stores of calcium have not been built up in the bones, and if the owner of the animal does not supply additional calcium in the ration, a serious bone disease occurs. Multiple fractures of the skeleton occur, and, in addition, there may be serious distortion of the skeleton when the decalcified bones can no longer support the weight of the individual or resist constant tension by the muscles. As a result, locomotor disturbances, bowing of the legs, abnormal curvatures of the back, and distortions of the pelvis occur.

The rapid depletion of calcium from the blood at the beginning of lactation may result in symptoms of tetany, incoordination, muscular spasms, unconsciousness, and death. When the calcium content of the blood is reduced from its normal 10 to 11 mg. per cent to 8 mg. per cent, muscular spasms and irritability are observed. When the calcium content of the blood is reduced to 6 mg. per cent, tetany, incoordination, paralysis, inability to stand, and unconsciousness are observed. By the time the level of calcium falls to 3 mg. per cent, death occurs. This disturbance of calcium metabolism is known as postparturient paresis, milk fever, hypocalcemia, or eclampsia. It is most frequently observed in the cow, dog, and sow.

The treatment of hypocalcemia consists of the administration of various calcium salts intravenously. Calcium gluconate is the most desirable chemical. The response to the intravenous administration of calcium is a startling reaction. As soon as the calcium content of the blood has been restored to a near normal level, the symptoms of eclampsia disappear. Often, before the entire amount of drug has been given, the animal will stand up, move about, and begin to graze.

A number of years ago veterinarians used to inflate the mammary gland with air. The insertion of air into the mammary gland prevented the flow of milk, and this, in turn, prevented the elimination of calcium. As a result, depletion of blood calcium did not occur and tetany was prevented. It is believed that hypocalcemia, in some cows, is due to an extremely low parathyroid activity. The parathyroid in this type of cow cannot compensate physiologically for the sudden heavy demand for calcium in the colostrum and milk. Apparently parathyroid development, in this case, has not kept pace with the development of the mammary gland and its ability to produce larger and larger quantities of milk.

The bones of the laying hen are also depleted as the period of egg production advances. The fluctuations in the calcium content of the bones are easily demonstrated in poultry by sawing the long bones of a non-laying hen lengthwise and comparing these bones with the sawed bones of other hens in various stages of egg production. The hen that is not laying or is just going into egg production will have large heavy bones, and the marrow cavity will be nearly obliterated by the thick bone cortex and the broad trabeculae. As the laying process progresses, the bones become smaller, the walls of the bones become thinner, and the trabeculae are reduced to mere strands spanning the marrow cavity of the bone. When the calcium reserves in the skeleton are nearly depleted, sufficient calcium for eggshell production is no longer available and soft-shelled eggs are laid.

Swine and poultry are usually fed a concentrate ration. Concentrates are deficient in calcium and contain excessive amounts of phosphorus. If adequate supplies of calcium are not added to the ration, the bones are decalcified. To prevent this skeletal depletion, some readily available source of calcium must be fed to balance the ration and maintain the proper calcium-phosphorus ratio. Limestone is usually fed to swine and oyster shell to poultry to supply the needs for calcium. It must be remembered that bone meal does not supply the necessary calcium because more calcium than is contained within bone meal is needed. If just bone meal is fed, the calcium deficiency is not corrected or is aggravated.

## Phosphorus

In the bones and tissues of animals, phosphorus and calcium are closely linked. In the bodies of adult animals there is a rather constant calcium-phosphorus ratio. Expressed in percentage there is approximately 85 per cent $Ca_3(PO_4)_2$, and 15 per cent $CaCO_3$ and $Mg(PO_4)_3$ combined. Roughages and forage plants are usually low in phosphorus content, while concentrate feeds, particularly cottonseed meal and bran, contain an abundance of phosphorus. Since some of our domestic animals are for the most part herbivorous, while others are chiefly granivorous, the location of these elements in the plant has a direct relationship to the conditions resulting from their deficiency. In this connection it may be said that phosphorus deficiency, or aphosphorosis, is probably the most serious disturbance of mineral metabolism in animals.

Reserve supplies of phosphorus are stored in bone. Like calcium, phosphorus fluctuates with the anabolic and catabolic activities of the body. It too is under the influence of the parathyroid gland, and, since it is deposited in bone along with calcium, it is also influenced by the presence of vitamin D. The blood phosphorus ranges between 4 and 6 mg. per cent. Whenever the fluctuations in blood phosphorus vary from this range, symptoms of a phosphorus-deficiency disease appear. As was indicated in the discussion of calcium, a definite ratio exists between calcium, phosphorus, and other elements in the ration. The calcium-phosphorus ratio for most animals is about two parts of calcium to one part of phosphorus (2:1 ratio).

### EXCESS OF PHOSPHORUS

When too much phosphorus is present in the ration, the calcium-phosphorus ratio is altered and may become 2:2, 2:4, 2:6, or even greater. When this occurs, the blood contains abnormal amounts of assimilated phosphorus. To balance the excessive amount of blood phosphorus, calcium reserves are drawn upon in an attempt to maintain an approximate 2:1 ratio within the blood. This mobilization of calcium results in decalcification (osteomalacia) of the skeleton. The bones become soft, lameness develops, multiple fractures of the skeleton occur, and death as the result of bone fracture is frequent. In young animals there is an improper bone development because the proper calcium-phosphorus ratio is not present.

This type of bone disease is observed in animals fed a concentrate ration that contains an excessive amount of phosphorus and does not contain adequate amounts of additional calcium needed to balance the ration. It is extremely common in cattle fed large amounts of cottonseed meal or cake. In the southern states, when a farmer says he is feeding livestock he frequently means he is only feeding cottonseed meal or cake. It is

relatively cheap, readily available, and makes an ideal range ration. Since phosphorus is present in cottonseed meal, it is fed extensively in the South to prevent a phosphorus deficiency, but if excessive amounts are fed, decalcification of the skeleton occurs. If bones become decalcified, they can no longer withstand excessive exertion. When cattle with soft bones begin to frolic or fight, fractures of the skeleton occur as the result of violent muscular contraction. Fracture of the back is especially apt to occur when calves run and gallop across the pasture. The bones of these animals are so soft, as the result of decalcification, they can be cut with a knife or broken by hand.

Bran is a substance that also contains an abundance of phosphorus. Bran has always been used in equine husbandry for its mildly laxative and conditioning effect. Excessive amounts of bran are fed frequently to young colts. This causes improper calcification of cartilage and bone as well as abnormalities in skeletal conformation.

Bone weakness and locomotor disturbances are observed in swine fed a concentrate ration if the excessive phosphorus is not balanced with limestone or some other source of calcium. If there is violent muscular contraction, as occurs when the animals come in contact with an electric fence, multiple fractures of the skeleton occur.

Multiple fractures of the femur and pelvis are observed in sows whose osseous skeletons have been depleted by multiple pregnancies, multiple lactation periods, and a ration deficient in calcium and containing excessive amounts of phosphorus. It is one of the causes of a condition (when a sow is no longer able to stand) known as downer sow.

The high-concentrate ration ordinarily fed to chickens must be balanced with ample amounts of oyster shell if alterations in the calcium-phosphorus ratio are to be prevented. If calcium is not added to the ration, rapid depletion of the reserve calcium within the bones occurs, soft-shelled eggs are laid, and the birds are unable to stand or have difficulty in moving about as the result of osteomalacia.

### DEFICIENCY OF PHOSPHORUS

Aphosphorosis occurs in many sections of the United States and in Canada. It has been reported from several of the North Central States, some of the Gulf States, from the semiarid regions of the West and Southwest, and from Manitoba. The reason for the deficiency is revealed in the low phosphorus content of the hay and grasses in these areas. Rainfall above normal increases the phosphorus in the forage in these regions, and drought decreases it, but even during seasons of normal rainfall the amount is too small for the best conditions of growth, fattening, lactation, and reproduction. During these normal seasons, growing dairy heifers and feed-lot steers do not make the proper gains. The flesh of the latter is not of the best quality. The quantity of milk produced by dairy cows decreases, the period of lactation is shortened, and the calf crop is reduced. In the case of dairy cows the demand for phosphorus is extremely great because the amount required for lactation and reproduction is in excess of that needed for body maintenance. When the supply in the feed falls below the amount required for maintenance plus lactation and reproduction, the signs of aphosphorosis begin to appear. The inorganic phosphate in the blood plasma drops. Evidence of phosphorus deficiency can be detected in the blood of cattle before they show symptoms of its lack. Less than 4 mg. per 100 cc. of blood indicates a deficiency. In calves the bones become soft and flexible due to retarded ossification. In older animals the bones also become soft and flexible or porous due to the withdrawal of phosphorus from them. Since pregnancy and lactation call for greater quantities of this element, these physiologic states accentuate the already serious pathological condition.

There may be a connection between phosphorus deficiency and ruminant digestion. Hay from phosphorus-poor soil is deficient in sugar and phosphate, both of which are essential for the optimum conditions of life for the fauna and flora of the rumen. As a consequence, the numbers and activity of the protozoa, fungi, and bacteria decrease. This affects digestion in the rumen to the extent that it contributes to the general malnutrition characteristic of aphosphorosis.

Although a bone disease involving many animals in a local area had been recognized in the United States (Texas) for many years, the importance of aphosphorosis as the cause of this bone disease became evident following the Spanish-American War when military horses from the United States were taken to the Philippine Islands.

A few months after the cavalry mounts arrived in the Philippines the animals became lame and various bone diseases (splints, spavins, ringbones, etc.) appeared. The native ponies did not show these locomotor disturbances. If the military horses were fed rations brought from the United States no osteopathy occurred. As a result, to maintain healthy horses all of the feed was shipped from the United States to the Philippines. This entailed a tremendous amount of shipping because hay and straw are bulky substances. Later, intensive investigation revealed the bone diseases were due to a deficiency of phosphorus, and the vegetation of the Philippine Islands was deficient in this mineral because there was a phosphorus deficiency in the soil. Although the native animals were small, they did not have bone diseases because over a period of many years they had adjusted themselves to the phosphorus deficiency. The larger animals from the United States had a higher phosphorus requirement and therefore developed bone diseases.

Phosphorus deficiency is one of the most serious animal husbandry problems in the cattle raising areas of the world. It is of special concern in beef animals because they are usually raised on marginal or submarginal land that is unprofitable for more concentrated types of agriculture. In general, waste land is deficient in phosphorus. The problem of phosphorus deficiency is particularly serious in the arid areas of southwestern United States, most of Africa, many areas in the Orient, and subglacial regions. The cattle in these areas show poor growth and development, lamenesses of various types, bone diseases, reproductive disorders, and depraved appetites.

The importance of aphosphorosis as a cause of retarded reproduction and sterility in dairy cattle was well exemplified by the experience in Singapore. Cows were brought to Singapore from the United States to supply milk for the European families living there. A milking herd could not be maintained without numerous replacements from the United States because the cows would not reproduce. Each year it was necessary to bring a new supply of pregnant cows to Singapore. The cows calved in Singapore, were milked until their lactation was no longer profitable, and then were sold for beef. When it was discovered that aphosphorosis was the cause of the reproductive disorders, and when the ration was supplemented with phosphorus, it was no longer necessary to bring new herds of cattle from the United States each year.

The monumental work of Sir Arnold Theiler, done at the Amoedsvlakte Experiment Station in the Union of South Africa, showed the importance of phosphorus in the ration of livestock and the part it played in the diseases of South Africa. The word Amoedsvlakte means poverty land, so named because on these acres it was extremely difficult to raise livestock, and livestock is wealth in range country. Here Theiler showed that the bone disorder observed in cattle was due to a deficiency of phosphorus in the soil. The vegetation found on this soil was also deficient in this element, and since the amount of phosphorus in the plants was inadequate, it was not available to the livestock grazing on these acres.

Because of the mineral deficiency the cattle had depraved appetites and chewed bones, sticks, stones, and other objects in an attempt to obtain phosphorus. A depraved appetite is called *pica*. The term pica is often used erroneously as a synonym for phosphorus deficiency. Pica is a symptom shown by animals when a variety of substances (calcium, phosphorus, iron, salt, protein, etc.) are deficient in the ration and, in an attempt to obtain the deficient ingredient, the animals chew various objects. The pica test is used to measure the degree of depraved appetite. When a phosphorus deficiency is suspected, a method for testing the animals is as follows: Four corrals are constructed next to each other and a trough is placed in each corral. Rotten bones with small amounts of decaying flesh attached are placed in the trough in the first corral. Sweet bones obtained from a freshly killed animal are placed in the second corral. Old dry bones are placed in the third corral. Fresh bone meal of good quality is placed in the fourth corral. The cattle are driven into the first corral containing the rotten bones. If they are extremely phosphorus deficient, they will lick and chew the decaying bones. If they do not show any interest in the rotten bones, they are driven into the next corral and observed. The same procedure is followed with the remaining two corrals. Depending upon which bones the animals chew, they are classified as pica I, II, III, IV, or pica negative if they show no interest in the bones or bone meal, thus indicating no phosphorus deficiency.

In cattle in the area around Amoedsvlakte there was a very high mortality rate that somehow seemed to be associated with the phosphorus deficiency. The disease had a sudden onset, a rapid course, and was characterized by a flaccid paralysis and death. Because of the paralysis the disease became known as lamsiekte or paralysis disease. (A similar disease had been observed in Texas, where it was known as loin disease.) After a tremendous amount of work, Theiler showed the paralysis was caused by the toxin of *Clostridium botulinum.*

When *Cl. botulinum* is grown in meat or other protein, it produces one of the most lethal toxins known. It is so toxic that if a housewife tests home-canned food for spoilage by tasting and detects an undesirable flavor, even though she spits the food from her mouth, there is enough remaining in her oral cavity to cause her death. In establishments where botulinum antitoxin is prepared, the men and women working with the toxin wear protective clothing and dust masks since the inhalation of even a dust particle of the toxin would cause their death.

*Cl. botulinum* was present in the soil and in the digestive tracts of animals in South Africa. When an animal died, the clostridia invaded the cadaver and produced the potent toxin. Since the cattle in the area were deficient in phosphorus, they chewed meat or bones in an attempt to obtain the phosphorus. When the bones contained the toxin of *Cl. botulinum*, the toxin was extracted, absorbed by the digestive tract, and in a few hours the typical paralysis occurred and was usually followed with death.

A little land turtle, measuring about four inches across the shell, was particularly dangerous in causing botulism. The cattle while grazing would step on the turtle accidentally and kill it. The dead turtle was invaded with *Cl. botulinum* and the potent toxin was produced. A few days later, when the cattle regrazed the area, they would find the dead turtle, chew it, and extract the toxin which caused botulism.

A vaccine that will prevent botulism is now available. It is unfortunate this vaccine was developed because farmers in the area are neglecting to feed phosphorus to their cattle and are not adding phosphorus to the soil to correct the phosphorus deficiency and improve plant growth. It is true that vaccination reduces the mortality from botulism but it does not correct the retarded growth and osteopathy caused by the deficiency of phosphorus.

## Magnesium

Magnesium is usually present in adequate amounts in the soil, water, and vegetation. Magnesium is of importance in bone development (especially bone hardness) and is also concerned with the regulation of muscle contractability. A definite magnesium-calcium ratio, one part of magnesium to 3.5 parts of calcium (1:3.5), must be maintained for proper bone growth.

### EXCESS OF MAGNESIUM

Excessive amounts of magnesium in the ration interfere with proper bone formation. The bones are soft because magnesium has an antagonistic action against calcium, and therefore ossification does not occur. It is only in exceptional cases that the magnesium content of the ration is great enough to cause a bone disease. When it does appear, it is usually observed as a leg weakness or as a deformity of the leg bones of chickens. The disease in chickens is associated with the feeding of large amounts of dolomitic limestone because it contains large amounts of magnesium.

### DEFICIENCY OF MAGNESIUM

In the wheat-growing areas of the southern and southwestern states, where it is customary to pasture cattle during the fall and winter months — late September to March — a peculiar nutritional disturbance occurs. It is generally called wheat poisoning in cattle but it is known by other names in different localities, such as grass tetany and railroad sickness. Incoordination and tetany are the characteristic symptoms shown by the affected cattle. Railroad sickness has been applied to it because of the unusual circumstance under which the disease sometimes makes its appearance. It comes on while animals are in transit to feed lots and packing houses after the excitement of loading. Excitement precipitates the condition in animals that have pastured on wheat. There are reports that 20 to 40 per cent of the animals in some shipments have died of the disease.

Wheat poisoning does not make its appearance until after the cattle have been on pasture for 60 to 90 days. It should be stated here that animals pastured on other young grains and grasses (rye, oats, barley, Austrian winter peas, and Bermuda grass) at times have the same disease. Cows in advanced pregnancy and early lactation are usually the first animals to show symptoms of the poisoning. Later, symptoms may appear in steers and unbred heifers, but ordinarily not until they have grazed on the wheat for four months. In the early stages the animals are excited and in some respects act as though they had rabies. Later the symptoms resemble those of milk fever.

The cause of the disease is not exactly known but is associated with magnesium metabolism. Chemically, the young wheat plant is rich in protein, calcium, phosphorus, and potassium, but poor in sodium. The blood of the affected cattle is low in sugar (hypoglycemia), magnesium (hypomagnesemia), and calcium (hypocalcemia). Not only is there a reduction in the magnesium and calcium content of the blood but there is also a very marked change in the relative proportions of the two elements. The normal magnesium-calcium ratio is 1:3.5, but in wheat poisoning it is 1:14. The biochemist looks with suspicion on this disturbed ratio and the reduction in the blood concentration of the two elements as having much to do with the cause of the condition.

Hypomagnesemia occurs in calves fed a ration consisting entirely of milk since milk is deficient in magnesium. As soon as calves begin to consume forage crops or concentrate feeds, adequate amounts of magnesium are obtained to prevent the tetany associated with this deficiency. Calves having a magnesium deficiency exhibit excitement, tetany, and convulsions. Death is often the termination of one of these periods of violent muscular contraction. Whenever calves showing convulsions and fits are observed, magnesium sulfate should be given intravenously in an attempt to correct the possible magnesium deficiency before death occurs. Small amounts of magnesium sulfate should be included in the milk of calves maintained on a total milk ration for a prolonged period of time.

Hypomagnesemia is observed in ewes on pasture. The condition seems to be related to the mineral content of the forage. In England animals on pastures that have been treated with fertilizers rich in nitrogen and potassium most frequently develop the condition.

### Manganese

Ample amounts of manganese are found in most soils. As a result, natural feeds contain an adequate amount of this mineral. Whole oats, oat hulls, and rice bran are very good sources of manganese.

#### EXCESS OF MANGANESE

The amount of manganese obtained from forage crops or grain does not produce any disease in our domestic animals. Manganese poisoning does occur when excessive amounts of the mineral are accidentally or intentionally fed to animals. Potassium permanganate is often used as a drinking water antiseptic for poultry, and if excessive amounts are placed in the water, acute poisoning may occur. At times crystals of potassium permanganate are spilled in the feed or on the floor in preparing these antiseptic solutions. When the chicks consume these crystals an acute toxemia may result.

#### DEFICIENCY OF MANGANESE

An osteopathy of the legs of battery-fed chickens 3 to 7 weeks of age is attributed to a manganese deficiency. It is also observed in young turkeys, pheasants, grouse, and quail. Apparently the disease perosis (*peros*, meaning maimed), or slipped-tendon, in poultry is the result of a deficiency of manganese, choline, and biotin, and the feeding of excessive amounts of calcium, phosphorus, and corn.

Perosis of growing poultry is characterized by a shortening of the long bones, an increasing diameter of the long bones, and a flattening of the articular surface of the distal end of the tibia and the proximal end of the metatarsus. Along with the deformed but calcified bones there is often lack of union between the distal articular cartilage of the tibia and the bone. As a consequence, the cartilaginous disc may slip slightly out of place. The changes in the shape of the bones and in the position of the articular cartilage permit the gastrocnemius tendon to slip out of the shallow, longitudinal groove of the tibial condyles. Because of this displacement of the tendon the condition is often called slipped tendon. At 12 weeks of age the articular cartilage should become thoroughly united to the bone in normal chickens. In chickens with slipped tendon the cartilage and bone remain disunited. Because of the stiff and deformed legs there is loss of locomotion, and the birds die of starvation.

A chondrodystrophy occurring in chicken embryos is characterized by an abnormality in the shape of the beak and has been named parrot beak. In addition to the deformity of the beak, a deficiency of manganese causes a low hatchability of the eggs.

## Iron

The soil usually contains adequate amounts of iron for the needs of animals. There are a few areas in the world (white sandy soils along the sea) where there is an iron deficiency in the soil.

The total amount of iron in the body is not great. The quantitative distribution of this small amount probably varies among the species. In the dog, Hahn gives the location and amounts as follows: 57 per cent in the hemoglobin of the blood, 7 per cent in the myoglobin of muscle, 16 per cent in the tissues in general (parenchymal iron) as cytochromes, catalase, and peroxidase, and 20 per cent in storage in the liver, spleen, and bone marrow as ferritin and hemosiderin.

This widespread distribution of iron in the tissues gives some indication of its importance in the body. Very little of the element is excreted, which means that the amount present in the body is rigidly conserved and re-used time and time again. There are occasions, however, in the husbandry of animals when even the meager required intake may not meet the needs of the body. When this occurs, the most important disturbance which arises concerns the formation of hemoglobin.

### EXCESS OF IRON

A liberal amount of iron in the water and ration of animals does not cause a metabolic disturbance. However, when excessive amounts of iron are present a serious bone disease may result. The reason for this is that iron combines with phosphorus to form an insoluble phosphate. In this form, phosphorus is no longer available to the animal and a mineral deficiency is the result.

A definite amount of iron is needed for the proper metabolism of the erythrocyte. Too little iron results in anemia since it is needed for the production of hemoglobin. Too much iron is extremely toxic to the erythrocyte and the hemopoietic tissues. A severe anemia frequently occurs in baby pigs following the administration of injectable iron.

### DEFICIENCY OF IRON

In the production of hemoglobin not only is iron necessary but also a minute quantity of copper. The copper acts as a catalytic agent. A deficiency of these two elements in the ration gives rise to a disturbance in mineral metabolism characterized by anemia. Since sow's milk does not contain iron or copper, the baby pigs must obtain it from some other source. Baby pigs require 10 to 15 mg. of iron per day. If iron is not available, the reserve supply is depleted and anemia occurs when the pigs are about 21 days of age. The farmer must supply iron (such as crude ferrous sulfate) in some readily available form if anemia is to be prevented. Under natural conditions the baby pigs root in the dirt, eat some of it, and the iron in the soil provides the small amount needed for hemoglobin formation. In the South, where suckling pigs are kept off the soil in order to prevent an ascarid infestation, and in the North, where spring pigs are kept indoors on wood or concrete floors because of the inclement weather, anemia becomes a serious problem unless some form of iron is available. Many pigs die as the result of the anemia. Pneumonia and enteritis are very common in anemic pigs because the body defense mechanism has been impaired by faulty nutrition and oxygenation of the tissues.

The decrease of iron in the blood can be detected before visible clinical manifestations appear. The anemia is the result of a marked fall in hemoglobin (oligochromemia) and a slight decrease in the erythrocytes (oligocythemia). When the hemoglobin value drops to 60 per cent as determined by the Tallqvist and Dare methods, a slight anemia exists. When the reading falls as low as 40 per cent, a serious state of anemia is present.

In some infections plasma iron diminishes in the blood (hypoferremia) because the iron-binding capacity of the globulin has been delayed or impaired. This condition has nothing to do with the dietary supply of iron. It is an endogenous, not an exogenous, deficiency of iron. This is believed to be the underlying factor in the anemia associated with severe infections such as tuberculosis, pneumonia, lung abscesses, gangrene, osteomyelitis, and tularemia.

The seat of origin of this type of anemia may be the adrenal cortex. It is believed that this structure regulates the plasma iron level of the blood. When the function of the adrenal cortex is disturbed, as it may be in acute and chronic infections (stress), the plasma iron level may be depressed. There is some evidence that under these forms of stress the reticuloendothelial system removes the iron from the plasma under the influence of the cortical hormones of the adrenal. Accompanying the hypoferremia there is also a decrease in the number of eosinophils and lymphocytes.

In Florida a nutritional anemia called salt sick, resulting from an iron and copper deficiency, occurs in cattle raised on the white and gray sandy soils and on the residual muck and peat soils that are not subject to overflow from more fertile soil. It is said to be the greatest single cause of loss among cattle in that state. It reduces the calf crop, retards growth, reduces the production of beef, and causes many deaths. Both the hemoglobin and the quantity of blood are reduced. Cattle whose hemoglobin value falls as low as 3.02 grams per 100 cc. of blood (normal = about 11 or 12 grams) usually recover when iron and copper are administered.

## Copper

Copper is found in adequate amounts in most soils, but there are a few areas of the world in which a copper deficiency exists.

Copper functions as a trace mineral in at least four ways: (1) It is a component of the terminal respiratory enzyme, cytochrome oxidase; (2) it enters into the makeup of mitochondria; (3) it influences the rate of phospholipid synthesis; and (4) it plays an important role in hemoglobin formation.

### EXCESS OF COPPER

Acute copper poisoning may occur in exhausted or heavily parasitized sheep that are drenched with copper sulfate for stomach worms. Under these conditions the recommended dose of copper sulfate will cause a severe gastritis, enteritis, and death. Sheep are often transported by truck or train for several hundred miles, perhaps from a ranch in Montana or Texas to a farm in the Midwest. In an effort to control gastrointestinal parasites and, at the same time, to save labor, the farmer drenches the sheep with copper sulfate as he removes them from the train or truck. The sheep are exhausted by the long trip and are extremely susceptible to the effects of copper. Under these conditions a severe toxemia occurs, and death of the entire flock may result.

Smaller amounts of copper administered over a long period of time will cause chronic copper poisoning. Copper is easily assimilated by the animal but is very slowly eliminated. As a result, toxic amounts of copper accumulate within the individual.

A number of years ago certain commercial companies made a copper sulfate-salt mixture designed to control gastrointestinal parasites in sheep. A few months after this mixture appeared on the market, a peculiar sheep disease was observed which was characterized by a severe anemia, icterus, hepatic degeneration and necrosis, and kidneys that had a chocolate-brown color because of the elimination of hemoglobin and bilirubin through them. Before the appearance of symptoms and lesions of copper poisoning, some stress factor was needed. This might be exhausting trips by truck or train, fatiguing drives from one pasture to another, strenuous shearing operations, the complicating factors of parturition, or extenuating weather conditions. The disease appeared as an explosive outbreak with many individuals involved simultaneously.

When salt mixtures containing a number of trace minerals are fed to sheep, various flavoring agents, such an anise, are added to the mixture to increase salt consumption. Some sheep seem to like these flavoring agents and consume tremendous amounts of salt. This causes the sheep to drink water, then return to the bunk and eat more salt, and again return to the tank and drink more water, and so the process continues day after day. Even though the copper content of these mineral mixtures is very low, the retention of copper by the sheep eventually results in high copper levels within the tissues, and copper poisoning occurs. A similar type of poisoning occurs in cattle. Copper poisoning associated with trace mineral mixtures is frequently overlooked because the amount of copper in the mineral mixture is so small that it is not believed the cattle will consume enough of it to cause toxicity.

Certain forage crops, particularly subterranean clover, have the ability of storing copper. If the soil on which these plants are raised has a high copper content, the plants will contain excessive amounts of copper. When sheep consume this forage, the copper is readily assimilated but is slowly eliminated. Toxic amounts of copper are eventually stored within the tissues of the sheep and copper poisoning is the result.

### DEFICIENCY OF COPPER

Although copper is present in adequate amounts in the soil of most areas of the world, there are a few regions in Europe, the United States, Africa, and Australia where copper deficiencies exist. Copper deficiency is particularly prevalent in sheep because they are often grazed on the poorer land where a deficiency of copper is apt to exist.

A small amount of copper is needed as a catalytic agent in the formation of hemoglobin and must be included in the ration along with iron. This can usually be provided if a small amount of crude ferrous sulfate is fed because it contains traces of copper.

There is an interrelationship in the action of copper and molybdenum. Molybdenum accelerates the excretion of copper from the liver. If, in the diet, the quantity of molybdenum is high and the amount of copper is low, the accelerated release of copper from the hepatic tissue may result in a deficiency. Investigation of a copper deficiency in lambs in Colorado revealed that the ration of the lambs was low in copper and high in molybdenum — an unfortunate situation. Manganese counteracts the effect of molybdenum on the copper reserve.

A deficiency of copper occurs in swine when baby pigs are raised on concrete or wooden floors where they cannot come in contact with soil. Sow's milk does not contain copper, and the copper reserves of the baby pigs become depleted in about three weeks. Unless additional copper is given, a severe anemia will result.

A copper deficiency is present in the white sandy soil along the coast of Florida. Cattle grazing on the vegetation growing on this soil suffer from an anemia that is locally referred to as salt sick. The copper deficiency is complicated by an iron deficiency in the same area. The erythrocytes are deficient in hemoglobin because copper is needed for its formation. A similar disease is observed in subglacial areas (Scandinavian countries) where it is known as Skravelsjuka (wasting disease).

Copper is needed for the proper development of the central nervous system in ruminants. The disease is most commonly observed in lambs and is known as swayback because of the incoordination that is present in affected lambs. (See discussion in Chapter 20.)

## Cobalt

Cobalt is a normal constituent of the soil. If adequate amounts of cobalt are present in the soil, the plants grown in the area will contain a sufficient quantity for the needs of the animals grazing on the vegetation. Fortunately cobalt is available in adequate amounts in most parts of the world but tends to be absent in the soil of sea coasts, lake shores, and subglacial areas.

### EXCESS OF COBALT

Cobalt does not occur in excessive amounts in a ration composed of roughages and grains. However, cobalt poisoning may occur if too much cobalt is placed in a mineral mixture used as a ration supplement.

### DEFICIENCY OF COBALT

Cobalt is essential for the maintenance of the normal rumen flora. It is essential in the metabolism of rumen microorganisms. These organisms are necessary for cellulose digestion. If cellulose is not converted into a usable carbohydrate, starvation occurs.

During the stall-feeding period of some years in certain sections of the northern part of the lower peninsula of Michigan, dairy cattle become progressively emaciated and weak, their hair becomes rough, their mucous membranes pallid, they have partial anorexia, and blood examination reveals anemia. Because of the geographical prevalence of the disease in Michigan, cattle owners call it Grand Traverse disease and Lake Shore disease. The deficiency also occurs in cattle in Florida (hill sick), Massachusetts, Wisconsin, Alberta, and Nova Scotia. It has been reported in sheep in Alberta, Wisconsin, and New Hampshire.

Ruminants apparently are the only domestic animals that are subject to cobalt deficiency. It affects cattle of all ages, and those affected most severely usually die unless supplied with a small amount of cobalt orally (not parenterally). The feeding of an amount as minute as 13 milligrams of cobalt chloride each day to an affected cow will bring about a decided improvement in her physical condition in 3 to 10 days. The hay on farms where the disease exists contains one-third to one-half as much cobalt as it does on farms where the disease is not present.

The pathogenesis of cobalt deficiency has not been completely solved. The element is known to be present in the vitamin $B_{12}$ molecule. Since only ruminants seem to need dietary cobalt, it is probably required in the rumen for the synthesis of vitamin $B_{12}$ by the microorganisms normally present there. A deficiency of cobalt in the diet then would lead to a vitamin $B_{12}$ deficiency. Vitamin $B_{12}$ is necessary for hematopoiesis. A deficiency of it results in anemia. The hemoglobin content of the blood declines to 8 to 10 grams per 100 cc. in cows showing mild symptoms of the deficiency, and to 6 to 8 grams in those exhibiting severe symptoms (normal, 12.03 grams per 100 cc.).

## Iodine

Iodine is necessary for the proper functioning of the thyroid gland, which plays an important role in regulating the rate of metabolism, especially in pregnant animals and in the growing young. It also plays a part in the nourishment of the skin and hair, and in the assimilation of minerals and nitrogen.

### EXCESS OF IODINE

Ordinarily there is no nutritional problem as far as excessive amounts of iodine are concerned. If toxic amounts of iodine are present in the ration, the food is so unpalatable the animals will not eat it and

iodine poisoning is prevented. When iodine is used as a therapeutic agent (potassium iodide or organic iodide) and
large amounts are given over a considerable period of time, symptoms of iodine
poisoning will appear. These consist of
hyperkeratosis, excessive desquamation
of dandruff, conjunctivitis, lacrimation,
and a slight rhinitis. Iodine administration should be discontinued when these
symptoms are observed; otherwise the animals lose weight and may eventually die
from iodine poisoning.

DEFICIENCY OF IODINE

A deficiency of this element occurs in
the soil and, therefore, in the water and
plants of the Great Lakes region, the
northwestern states, and the northern
plains region of the United States and
Canada extending from the Great Lakes to
the Rocky Mountains. In Indiana, over 60
per cent of the sheep that are not fed an
iodine supplement have thyroid hyperplasia (simple goiter), and the iodine
content of most of the thyroids is below
normal. In the same state 30 per cent of
the thyroids of swine are hyperplastic, 39
per cent contain only a trace of iodine,
and 45 per cent show only a trace of colloid.

Iodine deficiency is so widespread in the
United States that potassium iodide is
included in the salt of both man and
animals in an attempt to prevent the occurrence of goiter. This has caused a
marked reduction in the incidence of
goiter throughout the country.

Normal thyroids store extremely small
amounts of the iodine taken into the body
in feed and water. A deficiency of iodine in
the feed and water leads to a decrease in
the iodine content of the thyroid which
in turn results in an enlargement of this
gland (simple goiter). Histologically, the
thyroid follicles show three characteristic
changes: (1) There is proliferation of the
epithelial cells; (2) the epithelial cells become tall and columnar; and (3) colloid
is absent or scarce.

The incidence of thyroid cancer is in
direct proportion to the incidence of goiter
and the degree of iodine deficiency in the
area. Goiter, which is a hyperplasia and
hypertrophy of the thyroid gland, is a disturbance of growth. Once this growth disturbance has been initiated, control of the
extent of cellular growth may be lost.
When this cellular growth becomes excessive and is no longer under control, a
thyroid carcinoma appears in the gland.

The most serious effects of this disturbance in iodine metabolism are seen
in young animals that are born in the
early spring. Chemical analyses of the
thyroids of adult animals show that these
glands contain the least iodine from December to March, when the animals are
fed indoors and watered from wells. In
adult animals there may be no clinical evidence of this deficiency, or there may be
only an enlarged thyroid. Affected pregnant animals, however, may give birth to
offspring that show serious nutritional disturbances from this deficiency. In the
newborn of the different species of animals the manifestations of this lack of
iodine vary somewhat, but in general there
is goiter, alopecia, weakness, and high
mortality. The thyroid gland in fetuses
may become so enlarged that the distended
neck of the fetus is larger than the pelvic
canal. At parturition a dystocia results because the enlarged neck of the fetus will
not pass through the pelvic girdle surrounding the vagina.

On some farms where symptoms of an
iodine deficiency appear, chemical analysis indicates there is an abundance of the
element in the feed. This sugests that
some other element may be needed for
its assimilation. There are several goitro-
genic plants (cabbage and cauliflower)
that produce enlargement of the thyroid
independent of the amount of iodine present in the ration.

Iodine deficiency in hens affects the
embryos and the hatchability of the eggs.
The hatching time is prolonged and the
absorption of the yolk sac is retarded. The
thyroid of the affected chicks is enlarged
even though the amount of colloid in

the follicles is small. The increase in size of the gland is due to hyperplasia and hypertrophy of the follicular cells.

## Zinc

Zinc is present in the soil and in the vegetation grown upon it. Excessive calcium and phosphorus interfere with the action of zinc and may cause a zinc deficiency.

### EXCESS OF ZINC

Excessive amounts of zinc in the ration of domestic animals do not occur when the usual roughages and grains are fed. Zinc poisoning may occur if an error is made when additional amounts of zinc are added to the ration in the form of a mineral mixture. When animals are exposed to fumes from welding operations involving zinc metals or galvanized iron, a fatal toxemia may result.

### DEFICIENCY OF ZINC

A deficiency of zinc results in an imperfect keratinization (parakeratosis) of the skin in rats and pigs. The disease occurs in pigs when excessive amounts of calcium and phosphorus are added to the ration in the form of a mineral mixture. (See Chapter 22.)

## Fluorine

Fluorine is found in the soil and is made available to animals when water and vegetation are consumed. Fluorine is concerned with the metabolism of osseous structures and teeth. The amount of fluorine required by the body is rather critical. An excessive amount or a deficiency of fluorine results in bone and teeth defects. According to Groenewald, "Sodium fluoride is more soluble than calcium fluoride and as a result it is also more toxic. It has been established that 100 p.p.m. (0.01 per cent) is the maximum amount of fluorine to be allowed in the dry ration of cattle, sheep, and pigs; 350 p.p.m. may be allowed in the rations for poultry. An intake of 25 to 100 p.p.m. over a period of three to five years can stain teeth. No more than 50 p.p.m. may be allowed in the rations of breeding stock."

### EXCESS OF FLUORINE

Excessive amounts of fluorine may be obtained when the water or vegetation consumed by animals comes from soil that contains an abundance of fluorine. Fluorine poisoning may also occur when rock phosphate, which contains considerable fluorine, is fed to animals in an attempt to correct a phosphorus deficiency. Rock phosphate is used because it is cheap, while bone meal, the usual source of phosphate, is very expensive.

The lesions of chronic fluorine poisoning are found in the teeth and bones. The teeth show various enamel defects as indicated by opaque areas that resemble chalk in appearance but not in consistency, discolorations known as mottling in which areas of yellowish-brown or greenish-black appear in the enamel, and multiple pits indicating areas where enamel was not formed during the developmental stage of the tooth. It must be remembered that once the tooth is completely formed it is not affected by excessive amounts of fluorine. Because of the enamel defects, excessive wear of the teeth occurs and multiple caries may develop.

The bones are shorter and broader than normal. The marrow cavity is smaller than normal because of the enlargement of the cortex and trabeculae of the bone. In addition to the alterations in size, the bones show variations in consistency depending upon the fluorine salt consumed. The bones may be unusually hard with exostoses or they may show osteomalacia and osteoporosis. Because of the alterations in the bone, lameness and stiffness are often observed.

Acute fluorine poisoning may occur when sodium fluoride is administered to swine and poultry in the control of ectoparasites and endoparasites. Sodium monofluoroacetate (a rat poison called "1080") is becoming a serious problem in domestic and game animals because of its extreme toxicity. It produces repeated attacks of excitement, vomiting, convulsions, and violent forced movements. Death occurs after several convulsive seizures.

## DEFICIENCY OF FLUORINE

A trace of fluorine is required in the development of teeth and bones if normal hardness is to be attained. The fluorine is needed during the period when teeth and bone are developing, and it exerts no influence once the teeth and bones have formed.

## VITAMINS

Among the known vitamins, there are at least eight — A, members of the B complex (thiamine, riboflavin, niacin, pantothenic acid), D, E (alpha tocopherol), and K — whose deficiency in the food of livestock and pet animals may occur and give rise to serious pathological disturbances. Each vitamin has a specific biologic action which is absolutely necessary for the well-being of one or more species of animals. As with hormones, only extremely small quantities of each are necessary. Unlike carbohydrates, fats, and proteins, they are not structural materials for cells. Neither do they furnish energy, but they are necessary for the conversion of metabolites into energy and secretory products. At present it seems certain that the lack of any particular vitamin probably results in a suspension of a specific intracellular chemical activity which is important for the tissue involved and indirectly, perhaps, for all of the tissues of the body.

## Vitamin A

Vitamin A is formed in the body from carotene and cryptoxanthin, which are present in plants. All species of domestic animals possess the ability to convert these pigments into vitamin A with the possible exception of the cat. Breeds of cows such as Jerseys and Guernseys which give milk that is somewhat yellow

are less able to form vitamin A from these pigments than the breeds which produce almost pure white milk.

As just stated, the source of the precursors of vitamin A is plants. Carotene occurs in green plants, yellow roots, and yellow corn. Cryptoxanthin is found in yellow corn along with carotene. Field-curing of hay is injurious to carotene and even destroys much of it. Herbivora and omnivora which pasture on green forage or are fed silage or yellow corn obtain an abundant supply of the pigments. Carnivora which are fed liver and other glandular organs, fish-liver oils, or fish-liver oil concentrates secure a sufficient supply of the vitamin itself.

The specific chemical function of vitamin A is not yet fully known. It is certain that it is necessary for adequate growth and for the maintenance of a high state of health. With this high state of health there is an increased resistance to bacterial infection; hence, it is sometimes called the anti-infection vitamin. The reason it aids in preventing the invasion of bacteria is that it assists in maintaining normal epithelial membranes in the body, especially the epithelium lining the respiratory, digestive, and genito-urinary tracts.

## EXCESS OF VITAMIN A

When large amounts of carotene and cryptoxanthin are fed, an excessive orange pigmentation is observed. The mentally deranged human being may consume carrots to such an extent that pigmentation of the skin and other tissues occurs. Likewise the human being who works in canning factories and peels large numbers of carrots may have a yellow or orange pigmentation of the hands and face due to the continuous contact with carotene.

The tissues of domestic animals show variations in color depending upon the amount of carotene present. Nonlaying hens consuming an abundance of carotene have bright yellow beaks and shanks. The body fat of horses and Jersey and Guernsey cattle varies with the amount of ingested pigment.

DEFICIENCY OF VITAMIN A

A-avitaminosis is most apparent in poultry fed for a period of 2 to $3\frac{1}{2}$ months on a ration which is deficient in yellow corn and green feed, in young turkeys kept under dry range conditions, in hogs deprived of pasture and fed on grain alone, and in range cattle pasturing on dry forage in the semi-arid regions of the Southwest. In poultry its most prominent manifestation is an enzootic coryza, usually called **nutritional roup,** in which there is emaciation, weakness, nasal discharge, swelling of the face, conjunctivitis, keratitis, and distention of the glands of the mucous membranes of the mouth, esophagus, crop, and sometimes the proventriculus with plugs of desquamated epithelium. In swine the chief signs of A-avitaminosis are diarrhea, emaciation, muscular incoordination, osteopathy, blindness, and sometimes dermatitis with intense itching. In range cattle during long dry-feed seasons, A-avitaminosis makes itself apparent in the birth of dead or weak calves with or without eye lesions and associated with retained placenta in the dam. Weak, newborn calves have a severe diarrhea, and immature animals in particular show ophthalmia. In feed-lot cattle showing signs of vitamin A deficiency, edema of the brisket and, in some cases, anasarca have been reported.

Histologically, the chief reason for these manifestations of vitamin A deficiency is that the normal cuboidal and columnar epithelium in the ducts of many glands, in the glands themselves, and in many of the mucous membranes atrophies and is replaced by a stratified keratinized epithelium. In the parotid gland the main duct and its interlobular branches are so consistently affected in this manner that the lesion is considered pathognomonic for a vitamin A deficiency. This is especially true in cattle. This metaplasia is often ac-

companied by inflammation. The mucosa of the gastrointestinal tract and the epithelium of the liver and kidneys apparently do not share in these changes. Immediate return of the affected epithelium to its normal type follows the addition of vitamin A to the ration.

While the specific chemical function of vitamin A is not completely understood, there are indications that it stabilizes the proteins of epithelial cells. When there is a deficiency of vitamin A these proteins deteriorate and columnar epithelial cells are replaced by keratinized stratified squamous epithelium. There is experimental evidence that vitamin A plays a major role in directing the differentiation of ectoderm in the embryo. The effects of the deficiency are most marked if they occur at the time organs are being formed, and when this happens anomalies of various kinds are the result.

In chlorinated naphthalenes the toxic substance which causes hyperkeratosis in cattle has an antivitamin A effect. It causes such pronounced decrease in the vitamin A concentration in the plasma of affected cattle that some workers believe many of the alterations in hyperkeratosis may actually be the result of a vitamin A deficiency.

Vitamin A is concerned with the growth and development of bone. When a deficiency of vitamin A is present, mature cartilage is not invaded by the capillaries, and osteoblasts do not appear in the zone where active bone formation normally occurs. If capillary invasion of cartilage does not occur and if osteoblasts do not appear, then no bone is formed and the skeleton does not grow. The amount of skeletal growth depends upon the degree of vitamin A deficiency that is present. Since the development of the nervous system is independent of the growth of bone, the volume of the central nervous system soon becomes too great for the osseous structures that contain it. The pressure causes a distortion of the brain, and the cerebellum and the medulla oblongata are pushed posteriorly into the foramen magnum. The spinal cord becomes too large for the vertebral canal and when removed has a molded appearance. The foramina of the skull and the vertebral column are too small for the nerves that pass through them, and as a result a constriction and pressure atrophy of the cranial and spinal nerves occur at the point where they pass through the foramina. The constriction of the optic nerves as they pass through the sphenoid bone causes hypoplasia of the eyes and blindness (Fig. 4.1).

Vitamin A is concerned with the formation of visual purple in the retina. In the rods of the outer segment of the retina the vitamin is used in the synthesis of rhodopsin. A deficiency of vitamin A results in structural deterioration of the rods which is manifested by night blindness (nyctalopia). Night blindness occurs in all domestic animals but is most commonly observed in horses and cattle.

### Thiamine

Thiamine plays a physiological role in carbohydrate metabolism. When it is ab-

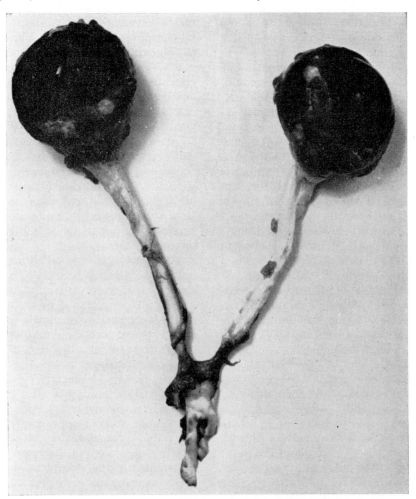

Fig. 4.1 — Constriction of the optic nerves associated with vitamin A deficiency in a calf. Pinching occurs in the optic canal of the sphenoid bone. (Department of Veterinary Pathology, Michigan State University.)

sent or deficient, there is imperfect utilization of lactic acid which is formed in the muscles during carbohydrate metabolism. As a consequence, the lactic acid is not resynthesized into glycogen in the normal manner but accumulates in the body.

Thiamine is present in adequate amounts in normal rations containing whole grain and green feed such as leafy alfalfa. Processed grains, milk, and meat scrap are deficient.

## EXCESS OF THIAMINE

Excessive amounts of thiamine in the ration do not cause any injury to domestic animals.

## DEFICIENCY OF THIAMINE

Except in ruminants, thiamine must be taken into the body preformed. In ruminants this vitamin is synthesized by microorganisms in the rumen. If a deficiency of thiamine should occur naturally in ruminants, it would likely be in very young calves and lambs before the rumen develops. Thiamine deficiency appears in chickens, pigeons, and pigs whose rations lack whole grains, mill-feed by-products, or green feed. Animals subsisting on tankage, meat scraps, dried skim milk, and processed grains which do not include the germ or bran show the effects of the deficiency. Symptoms of the lack of thiamine appear in dogs that are fed prepared foods of poor quality or foods which have been processed too much.

Manifestations of thiamine deficiency in general are: loss of appetite, slow growth in young animals, and loss of weight in adult animals. In addition, in dogs there are convulsions and paralysis marked by rigidity of the muscles and heightened tendon reflexes. In chickens there are nervous symptoms, chief of which are continuous muscular spams of the neck so that the head is drawn back, and also leg weakness. These nervous symptoms are the result of degenerative changes in the neurons of the peripheral nervous system, particularly in the ganglia connected with the dorsal spinal root, and also degeneration of the peripheral nerve fibers within the sciatic nerve.

Some fur-bearing animals (foxes, mink, and ferrets) when fed continuously a ration containing certain frozen fish such as carp, Great Lakes herring, Atlantic herring, Pacific mackerel, mullet, northern pike, smelt, and suckers display the following symptoms: anorexia, weakness, emaciation, diarrhea, and paralysis terminating in death. Because the symptoms of paralysis are so prominent, and because the disease was first recognized on the Chastek Fur Farm in Minnesota the disease is usually referred to as Chastek paralysis. The species of fish named above are not deficient in thiamine but they contain, in some but not all parts of their bodies, an enzyme which destroys the thiamine before the fish are fed. If the fish are ground, the enzyme is distributed throughout all of the meat and the enzymatic action can take place more completely. A similar disease is observed in the domestic cat fed a ration consisting of fresh or canned fish which is not adequately fortified with thiamine supplements. Focal areas of degeneration and hemorrhage are found in the gray matter of the brain.

A thiamine deficiency occurs in horses with bracken or equisetum poisoning. Extracts of equisetum will destroy thiamine.

Thiamine deficiency in swine causes acute cardiac dilatation that results in sudden death. Microscopic areas of necrosis are present in the myocardium. Occasionally they are large enough to be seen macroscopically. Extensive scarring of the myocardium is present when the deficiency has existed for a long period of time. Edema and congestion of the lungs are observed as the result of the cardiac failure. Sows farrow 4 to 16 days prematurely and there is a high baby pig mortality. The offspring show liver and kidney abnormalities, hernias, kinked tails, and enlarged forelegs.

## Riboflavin

Riboflavin is abundant in green grass, hay, and animal by-products, such as meat scrap and skim milk, but is rather low in grains and grain by-products.

### EXCESS OF RIBOFLAVIN

Excessive amounts of riboflavin in the ration of domestic animals apparently cause no abnormalities.

### DEFICIENCY OF RIBOFLAVIN

Chickens and turkeys fed exclusively on grain and grain by-products may show riboflavin deficiency. In poults the chief symptom is a dermatitis. In chicks there is no dermatitis, but growth is slow, there are diarrhea and emaciation, and the development of a "curled toe" paralysis which causes the chicks to walk on their hocks with their toes curled inwardly. In adult fowls egg production is not as seriously affected as the hatchability of the eggs. The principal tissue changes in affected chicks occur in the peripheral nerve trunks. They show degenerative changes in the myelin sheath, proliferation of the cells of the neurilemma, and swelling and fragmentation of the axis cylinder.

A deficiency of riboflavin is a problem in feeder pigs because they are fed a ration consisting primarily of grain and grain by-products. The hair coat of these animals is thin, rough, and dry. Erythematous eruptions, scaling, and ulceration of the skin are found on the snout, behind the ears, along the mid-line of the back, in the inguinal region, and over the abdomen. Ulcers may be present in the region of the coronary bands. The hoof walls show ridging and thickening. Hyperemia of the conjunctiva and edema of the eyelids are observed. Photophobia and lacrimation are seen, and there is a narrowing of the palpebral fissure. Corneal opacities and cortical cataracts may be present. A catarrhal enteritis is observed. There is a slowly progressive normocytic anemia of moderate degree. The pigs have a stiff, mincing, hesitant gait and appear to walk on their toes. The sows farrow 4 to 16 days prematurely and there is a high baby pig mortality. The offspring show liver and kidney abnormalities, hernias, kinked tails, and enlarged forelegs. All of the baby pigs are dead or dying within 48 hours after birth. A hypoglycemia is present and is associated with the collapse manifested by these animals.

## Niacin (Nicotinic Acid)

Niacin is another vitamin B component necessary for health. In some kinds of animals when it is not supplied as such, it can be synthesized from the amino acid, tryptophane, provided it is present in sufficient amount in the protein portion of the ration. This is especially true in the bovine, in which niacin is not necessary in the ration at all since the adult animal can synthesize it in the rumen from tryptophane. Even calves can synthesize it before the rumen is developed, but in them the process occurs in the tissues. In other animals the enzyme systems necessary for this conversion of tryptophane to niacin are supppplied by the bacterial flora of the intestine.

Niacin is found in adequate amounts in alfalfa and animal by-products. It is lacking in corn, oats, and milk and therefore is a problem in fattening livestock unless alfalfa and protein are added to the ration.

### EXCESS OF NIACIN

Excessive amounts of niacin in the ration cause no abnormalities in domestic animals.

### DEFICIENCY OF NIACIN

The two kinds of animals which are most frequently the victims of niacin deficiency are the pig and the dog. Both are subject to it under the influence of the same kind of diet, namely that of corn. Corn contains some niacin but not enough for the needs of the body. Corn is also deficient in tryptophane. Therefore, when corn is the chief ingredient of a diet, there is a niacin deficiency in the body. Since human pellagra has a similar causation, one can readily understand why swine pellagra and canine pellagra are names sometimes applied to this deficiency disease in animals.

In young pigs, those under 60 pounds, the deficiency gives rise to a type of intestinal lesion called nutritional enteritis. It occurs in these pigs, which are mostly in the weanling stage, when they are fed a ration composed entirely of corn, or largely of corn supplemented with only a small amount of protein. After a few weeks on this ration the pigs develop a chronic diarrhea, have diminished appetite, become emaciated and dehydrated, and grow very poorly. A severe anemia is present.

The lesion responsible for the diarrhea and the general state of malnutrition is a severe mucous degeneration of the epithelium of the colon and cecum. At first the areas of degeneration have a localized distribution. Goblet cells are prominent in the epithelium (Fig. 9.4). The gland lumina are distended with plugs of mucus which are being extruded into the intestinal lumen. The collections of mucus on the surface are attached to the plugs in the glands. The surface mucus is stained pale yellow with bile. The mucosa undergoes necrosis, becomes infiltrated with

neutrophils, and may be invaded by *Salmonella choleraesuis*, *Spherophorus necrophorus*, and *Balantidium coli*. The localized necrotic areas enlarge and coalesce with adjacent ones and the result is a diffuse necrotic enteritis (Fig. 4.2).

Dogs fed exclusively on a cereal diet, such as corn bread or johnny cake, develop a niacin deficiency disease called **blacktongue.** Affected dogs display a variety of symptoms, chief of which are: anorexia, salivation, bloody diarrhea, vomition, emaciation and dehydration, convulsions, and finally fever when bacterial infection contributes to the fatal termination.

The lesions underlying this chain of symptoms are those of a very severe intoxication with most of the changes centered in the digestive tract and the peripheral nerves. Petechial and ecchymotic hemorrhages, and inflammation occur throughout the alimentary tract, but the appearance of the tongue attracts particular attention. It is cyanotic with erosions along the edge. The color suggests the name blacktongue for the disease. With the lesions of the digestive tube there may be myelin sheath degeneration of the peripheral nerves, and in 40 to 50 per cent of the cases a scrotal dermatitis.

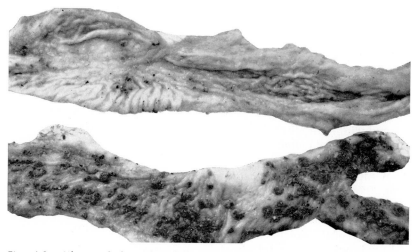

Fig. 4.2 — Ulcers of the colon following focal mucous degeneration of the epithelium in a pig with experimental niacin deficiency — so-called nutritional enteritis. (Department of Veterinary Pathology, Michigan State University.)

## Pantothenic Acid

Pantothenic acid is widely distributed in animal feeds and is found in adequate amounts in alfalfa hay and in most cereals. Storage and processing often destroy or remove the vitamin. It is deficient in corn, and since swine are fattened on corn, a deficiency is often a problem in this species.

### EXCESS OF PANTOTHENIC ACID

Excessive amounts of pantothenic acid cause no abnormalities in domestic animals.

### DEFICIENCY OF PANTOTHENIC ACID

A deficiency of this vitamin in ducks affects the synthesis of hemoglobin. It functions in the synthesis of aminolevulinic acid, which is a precursor of heme. Reduction in the amount of heme results in microcytic anemia.

A deficiency of pantothenic acid in swine produces a hair coat that is thin and rough over the rump and center of the back. Eventually there is a patchy alopecia that is most pronounced on the rump. The skin is redder than normal and somewhat scaly. A catarrhal inflammation of the intestinal tract appears early in the course of the disease. As the disease progresses, it may develop into a necrotic enteritis and occasionally a hemorrhagic enteritis. In the more severe cases ulcers are present in the mucous membrane of the intestinal tract. The lesions are most severe in the colon. Microscopically, there are atrophy and necrosis of the cells of the intestinal mucosa. The surface of the intestine is covered with a diphtheritic membrane. Hyperplasia of the lymphoid tissue in the wall of the intestine may be quite pronounced. A moderate normocytic anemia is present.

The gait of these pigs consists of a jerky goosestep movement. This is caused by a demyelinization of the dorsal columns of the spinal cord and a chromatolysis of the cells of the gray matter. The dorsal root ganglia show chromatolysis followed by necrosis. There are demyelinization and axis cylinder degeneration of the peripheral nerves.

A deficiency of pantothenic acid in pigs produces by far the most severe impairment of growth of any member of the B complex. Deficient pigs have extremely low plasma chlorides. A hypoplasia of the genital organs is found in growing pigs. Gilts become pregnant, but there is early fetal death, and macerating fetuses are found in the uterus.

Pantothenic acid deficiency in chicks causes a retardation in the growth rate. Likewise, feather development is retarded, and the rate of feather growth on various parts of the individual is not normal and uniform, giving the birds a very rough or unkempt appearance. Focal areas of alopecia occur. A necrotic dermatitis involves the eyelids, the corners of the mouth, the area around the vent, and the bottoms of the feet in the vicinity of the articulations. These areas of necrosis appear as raised scabs or crusts. Stomatitis and proventriculitis are also present. The internal organs show degenerative alterations which are most severe in the liver. Myelin degeneration, which results in incoordination and inability to move about in a normal manner, occurs in the spinal cord and peripheral nerves. The deficiency is of little concern in hens, but if pantothenic acid is not present in the ration, there is a marked decreased in the hatchability of the eggs.

Rats, foxes, and dogs show premature graying when pantothenic acid is deficient in the ration. This can be of considerable concern in foxes where grayness in a black pelt is undesirable.

## Pyridoxine

Pyridoxine is abundant in most cereal grains, and therefore a deficiency is not likely to occur with normal rations.

### EXCESS OF PYRIDOXINE

Excessive amounts of pyridoxine in the ration cause no abnormalities in domestic animals.

## DEFICIENCY OF PYRIDOXINE

Chicks with a pyridoxine deficiency have a slow rate of growth and show anorexia. Because of myelin degeneration in the spinal cord and peripheral nerves the birds have a jerky, incoordinated movement of the legs when they attempt to walk. The nervous manifestations become progressively more severe. Finally the birds exhibit spasmodic convulsions, and one of these convulsions terminates in death.

Pigs with a pyridoxine deficiency appear unkempt. The hair is untidy and curled and appears to be longer than normal. Some animals show photophobia and appear to be partially blind. A severe microcytic anemia is present. Hypochromatosis and a marked anisocytosis are observed. Poikilocytosis is rare. There is a reticulocytosis of 10 to 12 per cent. Numerous normoblasts are present. The blood serum contains an abundance of iron. Hemoglobin values as low as 2 to 4 grams per 100 cc. of blood are encountered. There is hemosiderosis of the spleen, liver, and bone marrow. Hyperplasia of the bone marrow is observed. Involvement of the central nervous system is manifested by a stiff, jerky movement together with a twisting of the legs and a swaying of the posterior extremities as the animal attempts to walk. As the disease progresses convulsions are observed. There are demyelinization of the peripheral nerves and degeneration of the axis cylinder. Atrophy and necrosis of the cells of the dorsal root ganglia are present. Degenerative changes are found in the dorsal columns of the spinal cord. Demyelinization of the sensory tracts in the medulla oblongata is present. Degenerative alterations are found in the parenchymatous organs and are most pronounced in the liver where they occur as a fatty degeneration.

## Vitamin C (Ascorbic Acid)

Vitamin C is present in green leafy plants (alfalfa) and is especially abundant in fresh fruits. Citrus fruits contain the greatest amount of vitamin C. Because domestic animals consume an abundance of green feed and since most domestic animals are capable of synthesizing vitamin C, a deficiency is seldom observed. Vitamin A and vitamin C complement each other. If an abundance of vitamin A is present, the amount of vitamin C required by the individual is reduced.

## EXCESS OF VITAMIN C

Excessive amounts of vitamin C in the ration cause no abnormalities in domestic animals. If faddist diets consisting of citrus fruits are consumed by the human being in excessive amounts, digestive disturbances may result, and a stomatitis with focal ulcerations in the oral mucous membrane may be present.

## DEFICIENCY OF VITAMIN C

Vitamin C deficiency has plagued sailors and explorers for centuries. Prior to the advent of refrigeration and transportation, fresh fruits and vegetables were not available during the winter months or could not be carried by sailors at sea or explorers in inaccessible areas such as the arctic regions. When it was shown that vitamin C would prevent the disease known as scurvy, sailors tried to include citrus fruits in their ration. The British Navy was one of the first to employ citrus fruits. It fed its sailors limes and, as a result, the British sailor was nicknamed the "limey." The ability of the British Navy to control scurvy was probably one of the reasons why it came to dominate the high seas.

In man the disease is characterized by capillary fragility. When an injury is received, there is excessive capillary hemorrhage into the tissue. This is especially prominent in the gums and the periarticular tissues — areas of the body that are especially subject to trauma. The gums are swollen, bleed excessively, and ulcers appear in the mucous membrane. Later the teeth become loose, alveolar periostitis occurs, and the teeth fall out. Hemorrhage may occur into the synovial sac of the joints, and a deforming arthritis may result. Faulty bone development occurs in younger individuals.

A similar disease is observed in the guinea pig. Seven days is about the maximum period of time a guinea pig can subsist without vitamin C in the ration. When it is not provided there are progressive loss of weight, hemorrhages in many tissues (especially in the vicinity of joints), and complicating diseases such as pneumonia, enteritis, and salmonellosis.

Angioblasts, fibroblasts, osteoblasts, and odontoblasts seem to be affected most by a deficiency of vitamin C. It is believed the deficiency causes a decrease in the respiratory activity within the cells. This belief is substantiated by the disappearance of cytochrome oxidase in osteoblasts in experimental scurvy and its reappearance when vitamin C is administered. The function of these cells to form intercellular collagen is impaired or prevented. The chief lesions appear in capillaries, bone, teeth, and in areas where wound healing is occurring.

The alterations in bone are very similar to those observed when a deficiency of vitamin A is present. The major difference in vitamin C deficiency is an increased capillary fragility, with excessive hemorrhage in areas where bone growth is taking place. When a complete vitamin C deficiency is present, capillary buds fail to develop and penetrate the mature cartilage, and the endothelial cells forming the capillary buds fail to differentiate into osteoblasts. When a deficiency of vitamin C is not complete, various gradations of capillary fragility, angioblast proliferation, and differentiation into osteoblasts are observed. The osteoblasts fail to produce osteoid tissue, which is the ground substance for the deposition of mineral. Mineralization is not impared and would occur in the normal manner if osteoid tissue were present. Because of the inability of the capillaries to invade cartilage and produce osteoid tissue, bone growth does not occur or is impaired. The formation

of cartilage, which is independent of vitamin C, continues at a normal or near normal rate. Since it is not invaded by capillaries and bone is not formed, great enlargement of the ends of the bones occurs. This distortion of the bone is often erroneously called rickets.

Similar alterations occur in teeth. Odontoblasts undergo degeneration and necrosis, ameloblasts disappear or become keratinized, and cementoblasts fail to function. As a result, dentine, enamel, and cement are not formed or are formed in inadequate amounts. This results in a failure of the teeth to develop, or the normal growth is impaired. If teeth do develop properly, there are defects in their structure. When enamel is defective, caries appear later life.

Wound healing is impaired or does not occur because fibroblasts remain immature and fail to form collagen. Angioblasts do not proliferate and form new capillaries, do not invade degenerating or necrotic tissue, and do not produce the additional capillary bed needed to bring oxygen, nutrient, and cellular constituents to the area of inflammation to effect healing and repair the damaged area. The capillaries are unusually fragile, and excessive hemorrhage in the area of injury occurs. The proliferation of macrophages is impaired, and therefore the cellular defense in the area is inadequate.

### Vitamin D

There are six or eight forms of vitamin D, all having the same chemical structure but differing slightly in certain portions of the molecule. The function of this vitamin is to promote growth and to aid in the proper mineralization of bones and teeth. This function is closely related to the metabolism of calcium and phosphorus. Just how it acts in this function is not fully understood. It is believed that it promotes the absorption of calcium and phosphorus from the intestine. While the manner in which vitamin D exerts this action is not fully known, the effects of this action are well known. Vitamin D does at least three things: (1) It increases the amount of calcium and phosphorus retained in the body on any given diet. (2) It controls the concentration of calcium and phosphorus in the blood. (3) It brings about a deposition of calcium and phosphorus in the bones. Its functions are associated with sunlight or other sources of ultraviolet rays. It seems proven that these rays form the $D_2$ vitamin from ergosterol which is present in very minute amounts in the tissue of plants. Vitamin $D_3$ — that is, activated 7-dihydrocholesterol — is the form present in animal tissues. It is the form of vitamin D fed to poultry, since this species does not use vitamin $D_2$ advantageously. The deficiency problem here, then, is quite complex because it involves four factors: (1) The formation of vitamin D in sun-cured food plants, (2) the formation of it in the skin of animals by the same means, and the necessary intake of (3) calcium and of (4) phosphorus.

This vitamin is deficient in cereal grains but abundant in sun-cured forage; hence, its deficiency is most noticeable in granivorous animals such as swine and poultry. In herbivora it occurs to a limited extent in calves in the northern states during the fall, winter, and spring when these animals are fed liberally on concentrates. It is a deficiency also in carnivora (puppies in particular) that are raised on a cereal diet. In all animals its occurrence is associated with confinement indoors or with the seasons of the year when the ultraviolet waves of the sunlight are so short that they are of little value in generating vitamin D. Vitamin D is abundant in fish and fish oils (cod-liver oil).

Vitamin D and the parathyroid glands apparently cooperate in controlling the calcium balance in the blood. In this connection the parathyroids act as the governor. If the intake or the assimilation of calcium falls, the parathyroids exert their influence so that the mineral is obtained by withdrawing it from the osseous tissue. This is what happens in adult animals when there is a decreased calcium assimiliation due to a deficiency of vitamin D in the body. This withdrawal of calcium from the bone matrix produces a condition called **osteomalacia.**

## EXCESS OF VITAMIN D

Hypervitaminosis produced experimentally in dogs by administering large doses of calciferol (vitamin $D_2$) is characterized by necrosis of the media of the arterioles of the kidneys and inflammation of the glomeruli, tubules, and interstitial tissue of the same organ. These alterations are attributed to the profound changes occurring in the blood. In this hypervitaminosis a hypercalcemia arises. Excessive excretion of calcium through the kidneys apparently damages the renal arterioles, parenchyma, and interstitial tissue. A renal insufficiency results, which is indicated by the symptoms of uremia. In rats given an excess of irradiated ergosterol (vitamin $D_2$), ossification occurs at an increased rate at the epiphyseal-shaft junction in the zone of temporary or provisional calcification. Besides this, there is metastatic calcification in the kidneys, blood vessels, myocardium, pylorus of the stomach, and bronchi. There are atrophy of the thymus and spleen and the formation of urinary bladder calculi.

A mineral disturbance occurs in calves that are fed excessive amounts of fish oil and fish scrap. In northern areas where the fear of a deficiency of vitamin D is always present, and in the vicinity of fisheries where fish oils and fish by-products are cheap, excessive amounts of products containing vitamin D are often fed to domestic animals (especially calves). The oil removes the fat-soluble vitamins from the ration and a deficiency of vitamin E occurs. Coagulative necrosis of skeletal and cardiac muscle occurs when vitamin E is no longer present to control the metabolic activity of muscle. Since necrotic muscle is an ideal matrix in which minerals can be deposited, calcification of the damaged muscle occurs. Mineralization occurs quickly because there is an abundance of vitamin D.

## DEFICIENCY OF VITAMIN D

Very little vitamin D is transferred from the mother to the fetus. Because of this the newly born individual must have a supply of vitamin D which must be provided through the food or by exposure to sunlight. In confined or dark-skinned animals all of the vitamin D must be provided through the feed because irradiation of the skin sterols by ultraviolet light is prevented by the confinement or by the melanin in the skin.

The symptoms of a vitamin D deficiency in young animals consist of a retarded rate of growth, weakness, deformed skeleton, and soft bones. The epiphyseal plate of the long bones is unusually broad and exhibits a lateral protrusion.

The basic lesion consists of the inability of the body to mineralize cartilage and osteoid tissue. Cartilage is produced in a normal manner, and the mature cartilage cells are invaded by the angioblasts which later differentiate into osteoblasts. The osteoblasts produce adequate amounts of osteoid tissue. Since the cartilaginous trabeculae as well as the osteoid trabeculae are not mineralized, they are not strong, sturdy, and resistant to compression. The weight of the individual causes a compression of both the cartilaginous and osteoid trabeculae, and this in turn produces a lateral protrusion of cartilage and osteoid tissue in the vicinity of the epiphyseal line. When vitamin D is supplied, mineralization of the cartilage and osteoid tissue occurs, and although repair is never complete, great improvement in bone structure, growth, and function occurs.

## Vitamin E

Vitamin E is found in adequate amounts in green plants and in the seed germ of grains. The vitamin is not stable in storage and diminishes in amount or disappears after a period of time. Vitamin E is found in inadequate amounts in processed feeds because the germ is removed. Since vitamin E is very soluble in oils, most of it will be removed whenever extraction methods are used to remove oil from feed (extracted cottonseed meal). When excessive amounts of oil (cod-liver oil and mineral oil) are present in the feed, vitamin E is oxidized or removed and is no longer available to the animal.

## EXCESS OF VITAMIN E

Excessive amounts of vitamin E in the ration cause no abnormalities in domestic animals.

## DEFICIENCY OF VITAMIN E

Vitamin E was originally regarded as being important only as an antisterility factor. Experimentally it was demonstrated that succeeding generations of individuals from a vitamin E-deficient parent would develop sterility problems. Later it was shown that vitamin E was much more important as a regulator of metabolic activity and that it prevented diseases of the brain, muscle, and fat of domestic animals.

Vitamin E is essential for the regulation of the rate of metabolic activity in striated and cardiac muscle. The disease is prevalent in nursing animals because milk is a poor source of this vitamin. It is also observed in animals that are starved during periods of drought. The deficiency affects lambs (stiff lamb disease or white muscle disease) that are not more than one or two months of age. Calves a few days old to as much as six months or a year of age are involved. Even adult cattle may have a vitamin E deficiency during periods of severe drought.

The outstanding clinical characteristics of the disease are locomotor disturbances consisting of a reluctance to move, stiffness, inability to stand, and death. Some animals are only moderately stiff but die suddenly as the result of cardiac lesions. The affected skeletal and cardiac muscle contains white, gray, or yellow foci and streaks which run parallel with the fibers. The muscle is dry, firmer than normal, and appears as if it were cooked. The degenerative and necrotic alterations in the muscle are bilaterally symmetrical and are most severe in the muscles of the legs.

No muscles are exempt from injury, and lesions are found in the muscles of the shoulder, rump, intercostal spaces, and neck. All bundles of the same muscle are not equally affected. The deeper muscle bundles show the greatest alteration.

In cardiac muscle the coagulative necrosis is most severe in the ventricular myocardium and especially in the muscle of the wall of the left ventricle. As a result of the cardiac lesions, there is passive hyperemia and edema of the lungs. A complicating pneumonia often develops if the animal survives for a few days.

Histologically, the cardiac and skeletal muscle cells show coagulative necrosis. The architectural design of the muscle persists but the cellular detail is lost. The cytoplasm of the muscle cells is homogeneous and stains pink with eosin. Cohnheim's fields and the muscle columns of Koelliker are no longer visible. Leukocytes (primarily macrophages) invade the necrotic muscle, if the animal survives, and remove the dead tissue. The injured muscle cell may regenerate if the sarcolemma is not destroyed. The space formerly occupied by muscle cells that did not regenerate is filled in with connective tissue and adipose tissue.

In both calves and lambs the degeneration of cardiac and skeletal muscle causes a release of the tissue enzyme glutamic oxalacetic transaminase into the blood stream. Its presence in the serum can be detected by a chemical test and used as an aid in diagnosis. Values of more than one hundred units of the enzyme per milliliter of serum are interpreted as significant.

All muscular dystrophy characterized by coagulative necrosis in calves and lambs is not due to a deficiency of vitamin E. In western United States a selenium deficiency will produce similar lesions.

Coagulative necrosis of the gizzard musculature of turkeys is observed when a deficiency of vitamin E exists in the ration. In ducks a vitamin E deficiency causes coagulative necrosis of the skeletal muscle.

A deficiency of vitamin E causes nutritional encephalomalacia in baby chicks. The disease is usually the result of too much oil (especially cod-liver oil) in the ration. The oil removes vitamin E from the feed and a deficiency is the result. Areas of necrosis containing hemorrhage are found in the cerebrum, midbrain, cerebellum, and medulla oblongata.

Vitamin E is an antioxidant for lipids in various body tissues. When it is absent from the ration of some animals (rat, chick, mink, cat, and pig), symptoms arise which appear to result from the abnormal oxidation of depot and liver fat. Some fats (lard, cod-liver oil, and other highly unsaturated fats) oxidize vitamin E. If the level of these fats in the ration is extremely high even when the amount of vitamin E would generally be considered adequate, symptoms of a deficiency may occur. The symptoms result chiefly from the loss of the antioxidant action of the vitamin. As a consequence, body fat is abnormally oxidized, pigmentation occurs in the adipose tissue, and vitamin A in the liver is destroyed. It is interesting in this connection that selenium is in some way related to vitamin E metabolism. The two (selenium and vitamin E) have mutual sparing effects. In this relationship selenium is an essential trace mineral.

In young minks a condition characterized by a yellowish-brown pigmentation of fat ("yellow fat") is associated with feeding a ration low in tocopherols and high in unsaturated glycerides. Rations containing a high proportion of fresh frozen fish scrap are linked with this condition. A similar disease may occur in cats fed fish-base commercial canned cat food and in pigs fed the waste from a mink ration or refuse from salmon canneries.

In minks, cats, and pigs the subcutaneous and mesenteric fat in particular shows the alterations characteristic of this deficiency. The color of the adipose tissue may vary from bright yellow to yellowish brown. The discoloration may not be uniform. Microscopically, in the interstices of the adipose tissue there is a deposition of foreign fat globules, some of which contain an acid-fast pigment which may be polymerized fatty acids. Fat-laden macrophages are plentiful, and an occasional foreign body giant cell may be present. The adipose tissue cells themselves are not affected. In the subcutaneous fat, foci of inflammation characterized by collections of macrophages, neutrophils, and eosinophils may be prominent between the fat cells. This foreign body reaction in the fat is the basis for applying the name steatitis to this condition.

## Vitamin K

The vitamin K requirements of herbivora and omnivora are easily satisfied because of the abundance of the vitamin in green leaves, especially in alfalfa. These animals and other mammals appear to be assured of an adequate supply of vitamin K due to the fact that the material is synthesized in the intestine by bacterial action. The requirements of chicks, ducklings, and goslings are met in ordinary poultry feeds, but when these birds are reared on a very restricted ration they may show evidences of a deficiency. The feeding of ½ per cent alfalfa leaf meal in the ration prevents the deficiency.

At least four factors are necessary for the coagulation of blood besides thromboplastin and calcium. They are designated: (1) prothrombin, (2) kappa factor, (3) delta factor, and (4) V factor. In vitamin K deficiency the delta factor is absent. The main characteristics of the deficiency are a prolonged blood-clotting time and multiple hemorrhages throughout the tissues of the individual. The hemorrhages cause anemia which may result in the death of the animal.

### EXCESS OF VITAMIN K

Excessive amounts of vitamin K in the ration cause no abnormalities in domestic animals.

### DEFICIENCY OF VITAMIN K

A hemorrhagic syndrome is observed in commercial broiler plants when birds are fed a restricted ration consisting of large amounts of corn and soybean oil meal. The bleeding tendency is greater if solvent extracted meal is fed instead of expeller meal. The bleeding tendency is apparently due to a deficiency of vitamin K.

The addition of chemical compounds, such as sulfaquinoxaline, to the ration in an attempt to control coccidiosis may prevent the synthesis of vitamin K in the intestine by destroying the bacterial flora. The resulting deficiency of vitamin K causes multiple hemorrhages throughout the individual and a general anemia.

A similar bleeding tendency is observed in swine that are fed rations containing sulfonamide drugs or in pigs that are medicated excessively with these drugs. The animals bleed from the nose, and excessive hemorrhage occurs from any wound (castration or wounds produced by fighting) that may be present. Postmortem examination reveals, throughout the cadaver, multiple hemorrhages, that may be confused with those of a septicemic disease such as hog cholera.

Newborn animals tend to have a deficiency of vitamin K. It is not uncommon to encounter litters of pigs that bleed excessively from the umbilical cord or from any injury received at the time of birth or shortly thereafter. Fatalities as the result of this hemorrhage may occur. If bleeder pigs are encountered, it is advisable to institute vitamin K therapy to the mother and the baby pigs as well as to the other sows that are due to farrow on the farm.

In dicoumarol poisoning (sweet clover poisoning) the administration of vitamin K will partially correct the inability of the blood to coagulate. This indicates that the etiology of this disease is more than just a deficiency of vitamin K.

# CHAPTER 5

# Extrinsic Cause of Disease of A Physical, Chemical, and Viable Nature

## PHYSICAL INFLUENCES

Physical influences of a mechanical nature may injure the body in four ways: (1) **Trauma.** A traumatic injury is produced by a sudden, violent, physical force which results in a crushing or separation of the tissues. (2) **Pressure.** A pressure injury is caused by a less violent physical force which exerts its influence over a comparatively long period of time and causes a compression of the tissues. (3) **Obstruction.** An obstructive injury is produced when the lumen of a hollow organ is closed and the normal flow of fluids through the part is prevented. (4) **Malposition.** An injury caused by malposition occurs when organs rotate around their attachment, around their long axes, invaginate into themselves, or protrude into unusual locations in such a manner that a disturbance in circulation is the result. The mechanical injuries will be discussed as injuries due to trauma, pressure, obstruction, and malposition.

## Injuries Due to Trauma

The etiology of the various traumatic injuries is quite varied, but the basic pathologic changes in tissue are quite similar. It matters little whether the injury is produced by a stone ax, knife, bullet, whip, truck, or jet plane; the tissue alterations are approximately the same. Tissues are crushed and torn, many cells die, and blood escapes from the damaged vessels into the surrounding tissue spaces. If large vessels are cut or torn, severe **hemorrhage** takes place which may result fatally. When the injury is located internally, the blood collects in the body cavities or in hollow organs. **Shock** may follow severe injury, especially when much tissue has been crushed, and when the thorax and abdomen are involved. **Bacterial infection** of the site is a frequent complication of traumatic injury.

From the standpoint of meat production, traumatic injuries often are of considerable economic importance. For instance, in a Chicago meat packing house it was once determined that 39 per cent of a lot of over 1,000 hogs which had been shipped by rail and by truck had traumatic injuries that depreciated their value to the extent of about 50 cents per head. About half of these injuries occurred on the farm before the animals were shipped. Among the kinds of trauma were bruises due to whips, canes, clubs, kicks, prods, crowding, and trampling, and punctures due to nails and forks.

A **contusion** is an injury in which the integument is not broken but the underlying tissues are injured, capillaries are broken, and blood escapes into the surrounding tissues. It is caused by the least violent physical forces. The injury is commonly known as a bruise. At first the injured area is red due to the hemorrhage that has occurred. As the blood disintegrates and is phagocytosed, various color combinations of black, blue, green, and yellow appear. The ordinary black eye is a good example of a contusion.

An **abrasion** is an injury that is similar to a contusion but in which the integument is broken. It is produced by a slightly more severe physical force than that which produced a contusion.

An **incision** is a smooth, long, narrow, clean type of wound produced by a sharp object such as a knife. Tissue damage is minimal. The injured cells are confined to a relatively narrow zone along the line of injury. An incision is the type of wound the surgeon strives to produce because tissue damage is minimal and wound healing is rapid.

A **laceration** is a wound characterized by a tearing of the tissues and is produced by a relatively blunt object. Lacerations occur when the legs of horses become entangled in wire and a tearing type of injury is produced. Lacerations are also observed as the result of automobile accidents when tissues are torn asunder, or when horses run into fence or gate posts and masses of tissue are torn away.

A **perforation** is a wound in which the point of entry of the mechanical force is narrow. It is the type of injury produced by a bullet or nail. This wound is especially dangerous because anaerobic bacteria (*Clostridium tetani* and *welchii*) may be carried into the wound and there, in the necrotic tissue, they find a suitable medium for growth.

A **rupture** is an injury in which the tissues are stretched until the fibers part. It is caused by a severe crushing blow or excessive distention. The rupture may involve the wall of a hollow organ (urinary or gall bladder), the capsule of a parenchymatous organ (liver or spleen), or tissues such as muscles, tendons, and ligaments.

A **fracture** is an injury of bone, cartilage, tooth, hoof, horn, or claw in which the continuity of the hard structure is broken. If the injury involves osseous tis-

sue and the skin is not broken, it is called a simple fracture. If the integument is broken, it is termed a compound fracture. The cutaneous defect enables bacteria to enter the area, and the resulting inflammation interferes with bone healing. When the fracture is incomplete and the bone is bent, it is termed a greenstick fracture. This type of fracture is common in young animals. A comminuted fracture occurs when the bone is shattered into numerous fragments. Fractures of this type are frequently observed in the horse because the bones of the horse are more brittle than those of other animals. The second phalanx of the forelimb of the horse is often involved and has been known to shatter into as many as 135 pieces. When the impact of injury drives one portion of bone into another it is designated as an impacted fracture.

**Concussion** is a term used to describe a functional disturbance of the central nervous system which may or may not be associated with loss of consciousness, following a severe jarring injury to the head. The cranial vault may or may not be broken and hemorrhage may or may not occur. The jarring initiates pressure waves that rebound back and forth through the semifluid nervous tissue. These waves injure neurons and nerve tracts, resulting in unconsciousness or incoordinated movements of the animal.

A **sprain** or **strain** is an injury of a joint in which the anatomic relation of the bones is maintained but the supporting ligaments around the joint have been stretched or torn slightly.

A **luxation** or **dislocation** is an injury of a joint in which the anatomic relation of the bony structures is not maintained and ligaments supporting the joint are torn.

### Injuries Due to Pressure

A pressure injury is caused by a less violent physical force acting over a considerable period of time. Usually the damage to tissue from pressure alone is not great; but when the thin-walled capillaries and veins in the area are compressed and blood is prevented from flowing through the area, then severe injury from inadequate nutrition occurs, hypoxia is present, and metabolic waste materials accumulate in the area. As a result, atrophy or death of tissue occurs. If the pressure is exerted slowly over a considerable period of time, the principal tissue alteration is atrophy, but if the pressure is relatively sudden and intense, the cells will die. Lesions of this type are seen near tumors, abscesses, and cysts.

Pressure applied to extremities causes ischemia or local passive hyperemia, depending upon the amount of pressure applied. If great pressure is used, as occurs with the improper use of a tourniquet, the arteries are compressed, ischemia results, and necrosis of the extremity occurs. If less severe pressure is applied, the veins are compressed but the arteries are not, and the result is acute or chronic local passive hyperemia. This occurs when rubber bands, cords, or bandages are placed around tails, ears, or legs. Necrosis of the extremity will result if complete venous stasis is accomplished. If partially restricted circulation is present, edema, connective tissue proliferation, and atrophy of the extremity occur.

When animals are recumbent, the circulation of blood through the skin and subcutaneous tissue pressed against the floor is impaired. This impairment is greatest over the bony body protuberances (stifle, wing of the ilium, zygomatic arch, point of the shoulder, or wherever bone is close to the surface of the body). These bony body protuberances covered by skin support most of the weight of the recumbent animal. When these pressure points are pressed against the floor or the bedding, ischemia occurs and the tissue dies from the accumulation of the waste materials of metabolism and a deficiency of nutrient and oxygen. These focal areas of necrosis are known as decubital ulcers or bed sores. To prevent these cutaneous injuries, animals that are recumbent must be turned frequently and the pressure points must be massaged to aid in restoring circulation to the area. In animals with a failing circulation in which the blood pressure is low, this type of injury is especially apt to occur because of the sluggish circulation.

Mild pressure exerted over a long period of time, particularly if of a rubbing nature, causes hyperplasia and hypertrophy of structures. The result of this type of injury is observed as calluses on the workman's hands or as corns or bunions on the feet of an individual wearing ill-fitting shoes. The effects of pressure are observed on the lateral surface of the stifle and the posterior surface of the elbow of old dogs that remain recumbent for long periods of time. The pressure of the tissue against the floor results in hyperplasia and hypertrophy of the cutaneous structures in the region. The calluses observed at the commissures of the mouths of horses due to the pressure of bits, on the skin of horses where saddles or harnesses rub, and on the knees of dairy cattle that are kept on concrete floors are examples of this stimulated growth.

### Injuries Due to Obstruction

An obstruction is the type of mechanical injury produced when the lumen of a hollow organ is closed and the normal flow of fluids through the part is prevented. The cause of the obstruction may be a foreign body within the lumen of the organ, alterations within the wall of the organ which reduce the diameter of the lumen, or the pressure of objects from without that cause a narrowing of the lumen.

Obstruction to the flow of the contents of hollow organs, regardless as to whether the organ is a salivary duct, the esophagus, a bronchus, the intestine, a ureter, or a lactiferous duct, results in pathological changes which are basically similar. Some of these obstructions arise because of the presence of foreign bodies such as concretions (hair balls in the intestine, calculi in the ureters), parasites (lungworms in the bronchi, and roundworms in the bile ducts of pigs), objects that enter by accident (rubber ball in dog's stomach), objects that are introduced by someone (broken urinary catheter), or ones that are aspirated into the respiratory passages (feed, water, exudate, and medicine).

Within the wall of the organ, alterations that result in a narrowing, or **stenosis,** of the lumen of the organ are caused by contracting scar tissue, inflammation, or neoplasms. The stenosis caused by connective tissue is called a **stricture.** Stenosis may also be caused by external pressure upon the organ exerted by tumors, abscesses, accumulation of ingesta, secretions, excretions, exudate or transudate in adjacent organs or tissues, or the presence of a fetus in the uterus, or because of any other enlargement of an organ. In the intestine, because of the looseness of the attachment and the freedom of movement of the organs, special forms of obstruction take place which differ somewhat from those in other hollow organs. These are discussed under injuries due to malposition.

### Injuries Due to Malposition

Through physical influences the position of organs or parts of the body may become displaced. The change of position referred to here is an acquired one, that is, it takes place after the viscus is formed. It does not refer to a congenital disturbance in the development of an organ. These acquired displacements owe their origin to various physical influences such as increased pressure within a body cavity, unnatural body postures and movements, faulty innervation, the presence of abnormal growths or tumors, and the existence of abnormal openings in a body cavity. Among the malpositions of this nature are the following:

A **volvulus** is a rotation of an organ, such as the small intestine, around its mesenteric attachment.

A **torsion** is a twisting of an organ upon itself or around its long axis as occurs with the large intestine of the horse or the uterus of the cow.

An **intussusception** is a telescoping or an invagination of one portion of the intestine into the immediately posterior portion of the gut.

A **prolapse** is the appearance of an organ or a portion of an organ at a natural or artificial body opening. The term prolapse means "to fall" and implies the effect of gravity on an organ. The term originally was intended to apply to the human. In this sense the term is more correct when the upright position of the human is considered. Then the term has more meaning — the falling or prolapse of the vagina or uterus through the vulva or the protrusion of the rectum through the anus. There are several terms that are associated with specific types of prolapse.

When the rectum turns inside out and protrudes through the anus, or when the vagina turns inside out and protrudes through the vulva, the malposition is called an **eversion.** When a portion of the intestine or other organ protrudes through a rent in the ventral abdominal wall, as might be produced by a horn thrust, the protrusion of the viscera is called an **eventration.** The term **ptosis** is sometimes used to indicate a prolapse of an organ or a portion of an organ, but it usually implies the drooping or falling of the dorsal eyelid as the result of paralysis of the levator palpebrae muscle.

A **hernia** is the protrusion of an organ through a natural or artificial body opening in the wall of the structure that contains it, e.g., cerebral, inguinal, ventral, umbilical, or diaphragmatic hernia. The protruding viscera must be covered by skin, pleura, peritoneum, or meninges. The opening through which the viscera passes is the **hernial ring.** The saccular protrusion formed by the skin or membrane which contains the viscera is the **hernial sac.** The terms hernia and prolapse can often be used to describe the same malposition.

**Strangulation** occurs when the veins of an organ are compressed by the malposition of the viscera and an acute local passive hyperemia is produced. Unless the malposition can be corrected, necrosis of the viscera frequently complicated with gangrene, is the result.

## Injuries Due to Changes in Temperature
### EXCESSIVE HEAT RETENTION

As a result of metabolism, heat is produced, and the body has a very efficient mechanism for getting rid of the excess. The chief heat-regulating center is located in the hypothalamus but is assisted by other nervous mechanisms such as (1) the vasomotor centers, (2) the sweat centers, (3) the respiratory center, and (4) the pilomotor mechanism. The combined mechanisms function so that normally about 75 per cent of the excess heat is eliminated by radiation, conduction, and convection, and a very much smaller amount by vaporization from the skin and respiratory tract. A still smaller amount is lost in the feces and urine.

When the environmental temperature becomes the same as the body temperature, loss by radiation, conduction, and convection ceases, and loss by vaporization is brought into play. This is accomplished by sweating and an increased respiratory rate (polypnea). The latter is carried to the point of panting in some species. As the environmental temperature increases above the body temperature, the greater becomes the necessity for vaporization to occur. This in turn calls for greater consumption of water. The loss of water by sweating is accompanied by the loss of sodium chloride.

Animals react differently to increasing environmental temperatures than does man. In man, body temperature and rate of breathing are little affected, but the pulse rate increases, whereas in animals the immediate effect of exposure to heat is a rise in body temperature and rate of respiration while the pulse is little affected. Man tolerates heat better because his heat-dissipating mechanism is more efficient. Whereas man relies on bringing blood to the skin by a well-adjusted vasomotor apparatus and then cooling the surface by sweating, most animals depend on cooling by evaporation from the respiratory tract. To increase vaporization many of them resort to panting. Ventilation from the tongue increases the rate of evaporation. It is said that the blood flow in the tongue of the dog increases sixfold during hyperthermia. The turbinates of most animals are provided with subepithelial venous, sinus-like structures which facilitate evaporation.

Among animals it is surprising that sheep tolerate heat best, followed in order by the cow, dog, calf, pig, and cat. Among cattle, breeds with short, flat, glossy coats like the Brahma tolerate heat much better than those that have a curly, wooly coat like the British beef breeds. The American Brahma-shorthorn cross, the Santa Gertrudis, possesses the heat tolerance characteristic of the Brahma.

Under certain environmental conditions of temperature, humidity, wind velocity, and movement of air, usually but not always coupled with strenuous muscular exercise, retention of body heat may occur. This is called **heat stroke** or **sun stroke**. Formerly it was customary to distinguish one from the other, but it seems now as though there is no essential difference between them. The overheating occurs during hot, humid weather, either indoors or outdoors, and even in cloudy weather. Under these conditions, if an animal is working in the field, confined in a hot building, or crowded into a stock car, truck, or shipping crate with other animals, the possibility of overheating is even greater.

**Signs of heat stroke.** The stroke usually occurs at the time of overheating but may be postponed a few hours. The early symptoms are dullness and depression, staggering, palpitation of the heart, rapid and weak pulse, difficult respiration, reddened mucous membranes, and a moderate elevation of temperature. Soon the mucous membranes become pale, even blue, and the temperature rises. The animal trembles, later falls, and dies in convulsions.

**Tissue changes.** The post-mortem changes are not particularly characteristic. The skin is red; the blood coagulates slowly; there is dilatation of the right side of the heart; and the lungs, liver, kidneys, and brain show congestion, hemorrhages, and edema. All of these changes indicate circulatory failure and are attributed to shock, which is secondary to the primary effect of the excessive heat. The most important primary injury caused by the hyperthermia is degeneration of the nerve cells in parts of the brain.

## EXCESSIVE HEAT APPLICATION (BURNS)

Heat produces varying degrees of injury to the tissues, depending upon its intensity and duration. A lesion produced by heat is designated a **burn**. For convenience, burns are graded according to the extent of damage produced. A **first-degree burn** is one showing simply reddening of the skin due to an excess of blood in the capillaries (hyperemia or erythema). In it there is mild inflammation of the epidermis which subsides in a day or two and is followed later by a slight peeling of the superficial layers of the skin. A **second-degree burn** is characterized by the formation of a blister or vesicle. The heat causes the epidermis to die and appear coagulated (coagulative necrosis) and also gives rise to an inflammation in which so much lymph is poured out into the tissue that a blister (hydropic degeneration) results. There is much destruction of epidermal cells in the area of the vesicle, but living cells around and beneath it are the source of new cells which fill the gap (regeneration), so that complete recovery soon occurs. In a **third-degree burn** there is complete necrosis and severe inflammation, and the dead tissue sloughs, leaving an ulcer which heals slowly by the formation of connective tissue rich in blood vessels (granulation tissue) which later shrinks, becoming less vascular and very dense (scar tissue). This substitute tissue is covered with poorly nourished epithelium which can be easily abraded. In the **fourth-degree burn** the tissue is blackened and charred; it is carbonized.

**Effects of burns.** If burns are extensive, one-fourth to one-third of the body surface, even if only a first- or second-degree burn, death occurs within 24 hours. In the most severe burns, death occurs within an hour. The animal shows difficult respiration, heart weakness, and a fall in temperature. These symptoms are like those of traumatic shock. In less severe burns, death may be postponed several days. There are frequent convulsions, much lymph in the lungs, and inflammation of the kidneys.

**Reasons for death.** Histamine and histamine-like substances are formed in the burned tissue and, when absorbed, produce the cardiovascular reaction known as shock. In shock the capillaries dilate and become engorged with blood. The walls of the capillaries become more permeable, and plasma flows out of the vessels and into the tissues, resulting in hemoconcentration which in turn reduces the blood volume. In addition, the formation of blisters and the weeping and evaporation of fluid and plasma from the burned areas cause still more hemoconcentration. Because of hemoconcentration and capillary dilatation, an insufficient amount of blood is present in the heart and major blood vessels to maintain blood pressure and normal circulatory time. As a result, the tissues of the body undergo degeneration and necrosis because of inadequate amounts of oxygen and nutrient and accumulation of metabolic wastes.

The injured skin surface is easily invaded by bacteria, and a suppurative dermatitis is the result. Bacterial toxins may be absorbed from the area of inflammation, and bacteria may overcome the body defenses, invade the blood stream, and produce a septicemia which often results in death.

## EXCESSIVE COLD

During exposure to cold the heat-regulating mechanism of animals is very effective. The reasons are, first of all, that animals develop a winter coat of hair or feathers which protects their bodies against excessive radiation of heat. Second, heat production is increased because their appetites become keener, which in turn improves their state of nutrition. Third, when allowed freedom they increase heat production by exercise, and when deprived of exercise they increase heat production by shivering. Even with this effective mechanism, however, there is a limit to the protection it can give the body when the external temperature is lowered excessively or when the animals are subjected to prolonged exposure, especially if there is decreased heat production as a result of insufficient or in-nutritious feed during severe cold weather. Under these circumstances the animals' legs get stiff; therefore, they move with difficulty. This diminution of muscular activity simply aggravates the condition, because with its decline there is also a drop in metabolic processes which results in a still further drop in body temperature. The cold drives the blood from the skin into the interior of the body. As a consequence the heart is burdened with an excess of blood. The cooling of the blood evidently depresses the heart and respiratory centers in the brain. Heart and respiratory actions slow down, and at this point the temperature continues to fall until it reaches 85 to 70° F., when the animal usually dies. Cattle on the range, and horses, cattle, and hogs in transit sometimes die in this manner.

**Local effects of cold.** The local effects of low temperatures vary according to the duration and degree of cold. The tissue changes in some respects resemble those produced by heat. At first there is a contraction of the blood vessels (local anemia), followed later by a paralysis so that they become dilated with blood (hyperemia). If at this point heat loss is prevented, the area returns to normal. If the area is not protected and the temperature of the tissues remains for a short time slightly under the freezing point, the vessel walls suffer injury and inflammation of the tissue (swelling and redness of the skin) develops. If the temperature falls still lower, the blood and lymph stop circulating and the tissue dies. The dead or necrotic areas are sharply demarcated from the healthy tissue. This dead tissue may later become dehydrated (dry necrosis) or may putrefy from bacterial infection (gangrene).

**Parts affected.** Local freezing is usually confined to the extremities. In veterinary literature such freezing is reported for the following parts of the body: the scrotum of steers, the feet of dogs, the teats of short-legged dogs, the combs, wattles, and toes of roosters and hens, the tails of cows, and the fetlocks, pasterns, and coronary bands of horses.

**Mechanism of freezing.** There are four explanations for the effect of freezing: (1) Ice crystals form in the cells and cause mechanical tearing of them. (2) Upon freezing, the water in the cells forms crystals around which salt concentrates. (3) Water is withdrawn from the cells to form ice. (4) With a mild degree of cold the cell colloids approach the gelstate. Frozen tissue becomes firmer, more doughy, and less elastic. This colloidal change is reversible so long as the colloids do not coagulate. That is, recovery occurs when the exposure ceases if the biochemical change has not progressed beyond the gel state. If, however, the temperature drops further, the colloids coagulate. This process is irreversible, and the cells die.

**Histological changes.** The fundamental tissue changes in frostbite involve the blood vessels. Blood clots (thrombi) form in them. These clots obstruct the local circulation so that blood accumulates in the vessels behind the thrombi. This causes the endothelium of the vessels to become more permeable to plasma, leukocytes, and erythrocytes. The poorly nourished tissue dies and becomes a suitable medium for the growth of saprophytes which convert the necrotic tissue into a decomposing mass (gangrene). The necrotic or gangrenous area becomes bordered by a zone of inflammation.

**Chilling.** Chilling by a cold rain, by being confined to cold, damp stables, by lying or standing in strong drafts, by falling into ice water, or by being dipped for external parasites in the winter is a predisposing factor to bacterial infections of the respiratory tract. When the body surface becomes chilled, the temperature of the nasopharynx also falls. This results in a local anemia of the mucous membrane of this organ — a reflex vasomotor constriction of the capillaries. The protective action of the cilia of the respiratory epithelium apparently becomes slower. The leukocytes probably become sluggish and less phagocytic. Saprophytic bacteria with disease-producing potentialities, which are normally present on this mucosa, are afforded an excellent opportunity to invade the tissues and produce disease. Catarrhal inflammation of the respiratory passages of several species of animals may originate in this manner. The reason a sweaty horse which stands in a strong draft may develop colicky pains is not fully explained.

**Hibernation.** It is difficult to understand why hibernating animals can survive when their body temperature goes down almost to freezing. Reports indicate that when their temperature falls only to 44 or 42 degrees F. they do not go sound asleep, but when it falls to about 35 degrees F. they become fast asleep and yet live. Their pulse drops to only 8 to 10 per minute. Respiration becomes extremely slow. The displacement of the lungs by the action of the heart aids in the slight exchange of gases in the lungs.

BENEFICIAL EFFECTS OF COLD

Reasonably cool temperatures have a stimulating and invigorating effect on animals. Cattle and hogs fatten well during the cooler months. They are able to consume large amounts of concentrate, convert it into fat, and do not experience the discomfort of fat animals during warm weather. On the other hand, extremely low temperatures interfere with fattening because the animals will not consume the cold feed and water. In addition much of the consumed feed is required for the maintenance of body temperature and is not converted into fat.

Properly controlled low temperatures have a therapeutic value when used to control the severity of inflammation, relieve pain, and aid in regulating a fever.

Horses afflicted with laminitis obtain considerable relief if they are allowed to stand in cool water. Animals experiencing heat stroke recover much more quickly if proper amounts of cold are applied to the external surfaces of the body. The local application of extremely low temperatures is used for local anesthesia (ethyl chloride and carbon dioxide).

## Injuries Resulting From Alterations in Atmospheric Pressure

EXCESSIVE ATMOSPHERIC PRESSURE

When human beings or animals are placed in caissons, diving bells, or diving suits under increased atmospheric pressure, necessary for withstanding the tremendous external water pressure, the blood and tissues contain an increased amount of the gases found in air. The principal gas present is nitrogen since it is most abundant in the air and is not used by the body in metabolism. The saturation is directly proportional to the degree of atmospheric pressure. If these individuals are suddenly removed from the area of high atmospheric pressure, bubbles of gas appear in the tissue and the blood vessels. The gas in the blood vessels forms emboli which obstruct the flow of blood through the capillaries. The gas in the tissues causes distention and distortion of the cells. Both of these factors interfere with the nutrition and oxygenation of the cells, and pain and severe cramps in the muscles occur. The gas in the stomach and intestine may so distend these organs that they will rupture. The disease is known as the bends or caisson disease. The condition can be prevented by reducing the atmospheric pressure slowly over a considerable period of time (3 to 6 hours), enabling the respiratory system to eliminate the gases contained within the tissues gradually so that they will not produce bubbles and excessive distention of organs.

LOW ATMOSPHERIC PRESSURE

In the Rocky Mountains, particularly in Colorado, Wyoming, and New Mexico, about 1 per cent of the cattle die annually when they are moved from lower altitudes, where they have been raised, to an altitude of 8,000 feet or more. The condition is called brisket disease (Fig. 5.1). It is apparently caused by the lowered atmospheric pressure with its consequent deficiency of oxygen. This produces alterations in the lungs and heart that eventually lead to pronounced general circulatory disturbances. Naturally, when the atmospheric pressure is lowered, respiration must be increased due to hypoxemia. This increases the cardiac function. As a consequence, the myocardium of the right heart increases in thickness (hypertrophy) and later the myocardium and tricuspid valve ring lose tone and stretch (dilatation) (Fig. 14.5). The exhausting exercise coincident with grazing in the mountains still further increases the work of the heart and aggravates the condition. Eventually, the general passive hyperemia makes itself apparent and causes edema in the body cavities and in the subcutaneous connective tissue, particularly of the brisket, the throat region, the neck, and the legs. Death from cardiac exhaustion occurs in two weeks to three months.

## Injuries Due to Light

### EXCESSIVE LIGHT

Overexposure to sunlight an be exceedingly serious. Death from sunburn occurs in the human being but is seldom observed in domestic animals because the skin is usually pigmented or is covered with hair, fur, or feathers which shield the skin from the effects of the sun's rays. The amount of injury is increased at high altitude when the screening effect of the atmosphere is reduced, or in the vicinity of water, snow, or white sand where the exposure to sunlight is increased as the result of the reflected light.

Continuous burning by the sun, probably as the result of the ultraviolet rays contained within the sunlight, causes various skin diseases. Skin carcinoma and abnormal cutaneous pigmentation are extremely common in farmers and sailors who are constantly exposed to the rays of the sun. Carcinomas of the vulva and eyelids of cattle are the result of solar injury. Excessive sunbathing or excessive exposure to ultraviolet lamps should be avoided because of the danger of cutaneous injury.

A severe retinitis occurs when the

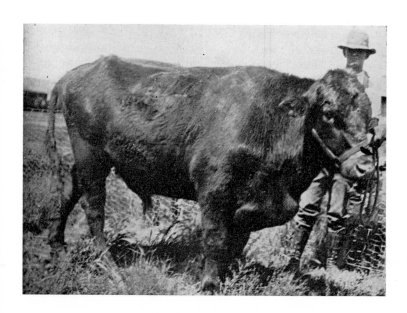

Fig. 5.1 — Brisket disease. Extensive edema of the brisket is present. (Glover and Newsom, Colo. Agr. Exper. Sta., Bul. 229.)

retina is subjected to very intense light. This is commonly observed in man and animals exposed to bright sunshine when snow is on the ground or when they are in areas of white sand where the reflection of the rays of the sun makes the sunlight very intense. Drugs (atropine) or toxic plants (Jimson weed and belladonna) that cause a dilatation of the pupil may cause a severe retinitis when animals are placed in the bright sunshine. Retinal injury may also occur when animals are excessively exposed to ultraviolet lamps, or when pets are exposed to the light rays of arc welding.

There are several substances called fluorescent or photosensitizing agents which, when present in the body, make the tissues more sensitive to light. Those of importance in animal pathology are porphyrins which are derived from the chlorophyll and certain other pigments found in plants (buckwheat, clover, and St. John's-wort). When white-skinned animals eat these plants, if the weather is cloudy or if they are in the shade, no deleterious effects occur, but if the animals are allowed to run in strong sunlight, a condition sometimes called **light sickness** or **photosensitization** occurs. This is characterized by a dermatitis that involves the unprotected or unpigmented portions of the skin. Animals usually recover if placed again in the shade. The photosensitizing agent remains in the body for as long as three to four weeks after the animals cease eating the plant. In extremely bright, hot, and dry summers this condition is often prevalent among sheep in the corn-belt area where it is called big head because of the severe subcutaneous edema of the head. It is believed that the ordinary grasses growing in stubble fields, grasses closely related to Sudan grass, contain the light-sensitizing substance.

Collies and Shetland sheep dogs are reported to be occasional victims of a chronic solar dermatitis. The irritation produced by the sunlight is confined mostly to the nose and eyes and is commonly called collie nose. The affected surface becomes red (erythema), the hair falls out (epilation), scabs form (encrustation), and the skin pigment disappears (depigmentation). The disease may be associated with the metabolism of porphyrins.

## INADEQUATE AMOUNTS OF LIGHT

Light, probably in the form of ultraviolet rays, is necessary for metabolism. Ultraviolet light activates ergosterol in the skin and thereby produces vitamin D which is required for normal bone growth and calcium metabolism. Animals raised in dark surroundings develop skeletal, endocrine, and hemopoietic diseases unless well-balanced rations are fed. However, well-fed mules can be kept for years in mines without any serious metabolic disturbances. Species of fish reared for generations in dark caves have only rudimentary eyes. It has been suggested the eyes have disappeared because of disuse atrophy since the fish have been reared in darkness for many generations.

Sunlight has drying and disinfecting properties. Dark barns, shady barn yards, and wooded areas are damp and wet. Various infectious and parasitic agents survive in these surroundings. Most pathogenic bacteria and parasitic larvae are destroyed in a matter of a few minutes when exposed to direct sun rays.

## Injuries Due to Electricity

Strong electrical currents from artificial sources or from lightning cause burns or result in death (electrocution). An animal produces a short circuit with his body between two conductors whether the electricity is artificially produced or is a discharge of lightning from a cloud to the earth.

Animals occasionally get shocked along street car and interurban lines where the third-rail system is used. Animals may come in contact with high-tension wires which have been torn down as a result of severe wind or sleet storms. Occasionally animals become electrocuted by becoming entangled in high-voltage electric fences. Livestock which have taken shelter under trees during an electrical storm may get struck by lightning.

**Effects of electricity.** The effects of artificially produced electrical current and lightning are the same, except that in the latter there are usually so-called lightning figures which are tree-shaped, branching, reddish or reddish-blue streaks on the skin. Along these streaks the hair is singed, the skin is scorched, and the cutaneous vessels are paralyzed. These arborescent figures may fade out in a few hours, or they may persist for two or three days if the animal survives.

Severe electrical shock usually terminates in death. It is surprising how easily an animal may be electrocuted. When either the positive or negative wire of an ordinary extension cord is applied securely to a moistened area at one end of an animal and the wire carrying the opposite charge at the other end, and a 110- to 120-volt alternating current is turned on, the animal becomes shocked immediately. It falls forcefully and lies outstretched on its side with all its muscles in a state of intense contraction. Usually in less than a minute, if the current is continuously applied, the muscles gradually relax and the animal is dead. By the proper control of such a current, however small, animals can be anesthetized for short periods (electroplectic anesthesia). In abattoirs it is sometimes used to anesthetize pigs before they are bled.

Local effects of an electrical current may be entirely lacking, or they may be seen both at the point of contact where the current entered and at the point of exit, usually near the feet. At these places the skin and subcutaneous tissues show deep burns, even to the bone. The surrounding hair is singed, the bordering tissue scorched, and peripheral radiating lacerations may be observed. These burns are more serious than they appear because, when the animal survives, they are difficult to heal.

General effects may not be prominent, but usually there are pinpoint hemorrhages on the serous membrane of the internal organs. In swine electrocuted in abattoirs, minute pulmonary hemorrhages are usually the only signs of electrical injury. If the animal lives for a period of time after electrical shock, there may be pulmonary edema and terminal dilatation of the right side of the heart. The blood is black and liquefied. Blood vessels are good conductors of electricity and are therefore severely injured. Some are ruptured, while others contain ante-mortem clots (thrombi).

The cause of death is not usually apparent. It is probably due to an arrest of several body functions, most important of which are the cardiac and respiratory. There is cessation of the normal contractions of the cardiac ventricles and a setting up of fibrillary contractions which are ineffective in maintaining circulation. Paralysis of the respiratory center of the medulla also occurs. If cardiac and respiratory arrest continue, vital cells die from oxygen starvation (hypoxia) and somatic death ensues.

### Injuries Due to Ionizing Radiation

The types of nuclear radiation most often utilized for therapeutic and military purposes are: (1) particles designated alpha, beta (electron), proton and neutron, and (2) rays called gamma. X-rays (roentgen rays) do not originate in the nucleus but arise when atoms are bombarded by high-speed electrons. They are otherwise identical with gamma rays. All of these forms of radiation cause ionization in the tissues only if "absorbed." Since the method of absorption varies, the degree of ionization also varies with the different types of radiation. Furthermore, the effects produced by any one of the forms are variable depending upon (1) the rate and degree of exposure, (2) the energy of the ionizing agent, (3) the lapse of time existing since the exposure, (4) the kind of tissue involved, (5) the extent of body exposure (total or partial), and (6) the species of mammal exposed. In the latter regard, swine and man are considered by some authorities to be in about the same range of sensitivity.

Injury due to radiation is not always

immediately apparent either at the site of primary injury or elsewhere in the body. Some latent period must elapse before changes become visible, although tissue alterations must obviously begin at the moment when the radiation is absorbed. It may be days, weeks, months, or years before the peak of the reaction is reached.

The cellular structures most affected by ionizing radiation include the genetic material (genes, chromosomes, plasmagenes) and probably the Golgi apparatus and mitochondria where many of the enzyme systems are concentrated. The chromosomes and genes are much more readily studied and more easily understood than the cytoplasmic inclusions. Therefore more is known about their response to radiation. The cell membrane seems to be less susceptible to damage than the cytoplasm or nucleus.

The radiations cause damage to the cell structures both directly and indirectly. Direct damage is the result of interaction between the radiations and certain essential molecules of the cell — impacts which might cause either (1) fragmentation of the larger protoplasmic molecules or (2) polymerization of somewhat smaller molecules to form more complex polymolecular aggregates. Changes occur in the nucleus and to a lesser extent in the cytoplasm.

Indirectly, radiations injure cells by causing ionization of the water molecules which constitute such a high percentage of the cell protoplasm. These products have been shown to inactivate a number of labile cell enzymes. They also produce a number of other biochemical alterations in the cell. Thus indirect effects are initiated by ionizations which occur at some distance from the ultimately affected molecule. It has been observed that both the direct and the indirect action of ionizing radiations can bring about chromosome and gene aberrations, with subsequent disturbances in mitosis. These effects upon mitosis range from simple chromosome fragmentation with repair, to complete dissociation and subsequent cell death associated with inability of the cell to reproduce normally before degenerating.

If the nuclear changes are not severe enough to cause death immediately, smaller disturbances persisting into future generations of the cell may gradually result in cytoplasmic changes which are not apparent until long after the primary injury has been produced. For instance, if a single chromosome were damaged by radiation, no visible effect might be noticed until after a number of succeeding mitoses had been completed. By that time a cell may have been developed whose form and function have been considerably altered. It is necessary to postulate such events during the long latent period of skin cancer (carcinoma) which appears in careless radiologists after they cease to use the X-ray apparatus.

It is generally believed that sufficient radiation injures the cell membrane, causing its permeability to become altered. Cytoplasmic vacuolization often appears in radiated cells. It is probable that the passage of electrolytes, nutrients, oxygen, and water through the cell membrane is affected. It is known too that the mitochondria and Golgi apparatus frequently appear damaged.

The degree of sensitivity of the different cells and tissues to radiation is not the same. The order of sensitivity from most to least stands approximately as follows: (1) lymphocytes and germinal cells, (2) granulocytes and erythrocytes, (3) epithelial and endothelial cells, (4) smooth muscle, (5) fibroblasts and their derivatives, and (6) neurons.

Vascular changes are prominent in radiation injury because the endothelial cells are especially sensitive. These cells swell when radiated. This is frequently followed by the formation of blood clots within the vessels (thrombi) which partially or completely obstruct the vessels. If the thrombi are in the veins, blood accumulates in the capillaries back of the obstruction, causing capillary dilatation (telangiectasis). The connective tissue around the vessels undergoes a change called hyalinization — a condition in which the collagen fibers fuse, become homogeneous, and in sections take the eosin stain rather deeply. This occurs as a late effect of radiation. All of these vascular effects interfere with circulation to the organs.

Since the skin is most often exposed to radiation, it is not surprising that it frequently shows evidences of damage following excessive therapeutic use of ionizing radiations or following its use in warfare. Rather severe exposures cause redness of the skin (erythema) in 24 to 48 hours. This fades temporarily, but reappears in 10 to 28 days as a result of the vascular changes described above. Finally this redness disappears, leaving the skin pigmented with melanin. If the exposure is more severe, the skin becomes inflamed (dermatitis) and filled with lymph (edema). There is then loss of hair (epilation). If the hair comes back it is usually coarse because it develops from deep follicles which were not killed. If all of the follicles are destroyed, the loss of hair is permanent. The sebaceous and sudoriferous glands are also destroyed, and become homogeneous masses of pink-colored material (hyalin) in sections stained with eosin. The surface layer of the epidermis becomes more heavily keratinized, dry, and scaly. The scars of X-ray burns are sometimes the seat of skin carcinomas.

At Hiroshima in 1945, one-third of the army animals exposed to the atomic bomb blast died of burns caused by the flash, or resulted from fires that followed the explosion. Those that survived the flash developed edema of the skin. Later there was loss of hair, or the hair which remained faded, presumably as a result of the destruction of the cutaneous enzyme which forms melanin (Fig. 5.2). Where parts of the body were protected by harness, collar, or blanket the damage was less. In animals that were more severely radiated, small areas of bleeding (purpura) occurred under the skin. Local tissue death (necrosis) followed in these spots, resulting in ulcers. Saprophytic bacteria grew in the ulcers, converting them into areas of putrefactive flesh (gangrene). In the heart, lungs, kidneys, and brain there were tiny hemorrhages (petechiae). The mucosa of the gastrointestinal tract became inflamed. The lymphoid tissues were swollen and soft at first but later underwent shrinkage (atrophy). Hemorrhage occurred in the bone marrow.

In the Bikini bomb tests in 1947, swine showed the greatest histological changes in the lymphoid organs such as the lymph nodes, spleen, thymus, tonsils, and Peyer's patches. Lymphocytes in the peripheral

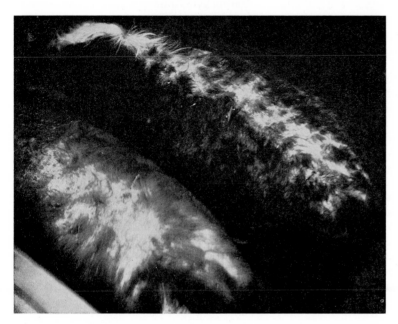

Fig. 5.2 — Beta radiation burns on backs of cattle caused by deposition of fission products f r o m cloud produced by Alamogordo atomic bomb test. (Wright H. Langham, Univ. of Calif., Los Alamos Scientific Lab.; Proc. U.S.L.S. Sanit. Assn.)

blood were likewise structures showing the greatest injury.

Thirty per cent of the Bikini animals died within a month. Death in the majority of them was due to ionizing radiation. Ten per cent were killed by the air blast. Flashburn was not important because the hair coat afforded protection.

The ionizing effects were exerted chiefly upon the blood elements — the erythrocytes, the leukocytes, and the platelets. As a result there was loss of blood from the vessels (hemorrhage). Lack of platelets in the blood (thrombocytopenia) resulted in failure of the blood to coagulate. Loss of blood with its red cells gave rise to anemia. The destrution of leukocytes (leukopenia) robbed the animals of antibodies and phagocytes so that they became victims of infection, particularly in the lungs (pneumonia).

## CHEMICAL INFLUENCES

Life depends upon chemical reactions, but in these reactions the chemical substances must be beneficial to the cells. If injurious chemical substances combine with the protoplasm of cells so as to produce structural and functional changes in them, the condition is called poisoning, intoxication, or toxicosis. Poisons which enter the body from the exterior are called **exogenous**; those arising within are **endogenous**.

### Exogenous Poisons

Exogenous poisons belong in the realm of either inorganic or organic chemistry. Many of them are familiar inorganic acids, bases, and salts such as sulfuric acid, potassium hydroxide, and mercuric chloride. Organic poisons are derived from flowering plants, molds, fungi, and bacteria, and from certain parasitic and venomous animals. The poisonous properties of plants are mostly alkaloids, glucosides, resinoids, phytotoxins, and organic acids. Bacteria possess exotoxins and endotoxins. Parasitic animals such as ascarids, tapeworms, and bots produce toxic substances. Some snakes form venom, a most potent zootoxin.

The effects of these toxic agents upon tissues are almost as varied as the substances themselves, but in general it can be said that according to their action they may be classified under four headings. (1) They exert a corrosive or caustic action, or (2) they produce degenerative changes in the so-called parenchymatous organs such as the liver, kidneys, and heart, or (3) they excite, depress, or paralyze the nervous system and heart, or (4) they alter the blood.

**Corrosives** include the caustic alkalies, e.g., sodium hydroxide (caustic soda), potassium hydroxide (caustic potash), calcium oxide (quick lime), and barium chloride; the corrosive salts of heavy metals, e.g., mercuric chloride and zinc sulfate; and corrosive acids, e.g., nitric, sulfuric, hydrochloric, oxalic, acetic, and carbolic. These substances act locally by producing burns which vary in their intensity from simple hyperemia to severe inflammation, even to necrosis and ulceration, depending upon the quantity, the concentration, and the place of contact of the particular agent. The necrosis is the type in which the affected tissues are coagulated or liquefied. The dead tissue sloughs, leaving behind ulcers which may heal with the formation of scar tissue.

**Parenchymatous poisons** cause regressive disturbances of cell metabolism, principally in the liver, kidneys, and heart. Phosphorus, arsenic, lead, mercuric chloride, and silver nitrate are examples.

**Nerve poisons** either overstimulate, depress, or paralyze nerve cells. Some of these act as nerve stimulants at first but later as paralyzers. Among these poisons are the narcotics, strychnine, atropine, pilocarpine, physostigmine, the toxins of *Clostridium tetani* and *Clostridium botulinum*, and snake venoms.

**Poisons affecting the blood** prevent the red cells from carrying oxygen, either by forming stable compounds with the hemoglobin or by destroying the erythrocytes and liberating the hemoglobin (hemolysis), or by inhibiting the coagulation of the blood, or by causing agglutination of the erythrocytes (hemagglutination).

Carbon monoxide is an example of a poison combining with hemoglobin. It forms a relatively stable compound which renders the hemoglobin incapable of combining with oxygen. The affinity of hemoglobin for carbon monoxide is from 200 to 300 times greater than for oxygen.

OCCURRENCE OF EXOGENOUS POISONING

In human pathology the detection of tissue changes produced by some chemical substances has a medicolegal aspect because these agents are commonly used in homicides and suicides. The medicolegal importance of determining the results of malicious poisoning of animals is not very great. Accidental poisoning, however, is of greater importance. It is not difficult to understand its rather common occurrence when one considers the multitude of opportunities animals have of ingesting toxic substances. A partial list of poisons together with the occasion for their ingestion could include the following:

**Livestock in general:** various toxic chemicals that are used in the mass treatment of animals for parasites; toxic freshwater algae from drinking the water of certain lakes; alkaloids, glucosides, and saponins from eating poisonous plants; hydrocyanic acid from eating the sorghums and Sudan grass during certain seasons; lead or arsenic from drinking various dips and insect sprays and from eating grasshopper bait; selenium in the north central Great Plains from ingesting selenium-bearing vegetation growing on arid and semiarid grazing lands; the nitrate or chlorate of sodium or calcium from eating fertilizer or weed killers.

**Cattle and sheep:** lead from licking freshly painted surfaces and from eating the contents of discarded paint pails; the presence of dicoumarin in damaged sweet clover; sodium mono-fluoroacetate (compound 1080) and thallium sulfate in prairie dog bait (Fig. 5.3); chlordane used as an insecticide dip.

**Sheep:** copper from the mass treatment for stomach worms with copper sulfate in grain, or from long-continued use of salt mixtures containing copper sulfate.

**Cattle:** fluorine from raw rock phosphate used as a mineral supplement.

**Swine:** lye improperly used in the treatment of infectious necrotic enteritis; various toxic agents in table refuse used on garbage-feeding farms; various mineral salts from the injudicious use of mineral mixtures; ethyl mercuric phosphate (ceresan) in treated seed oats left over from planting.

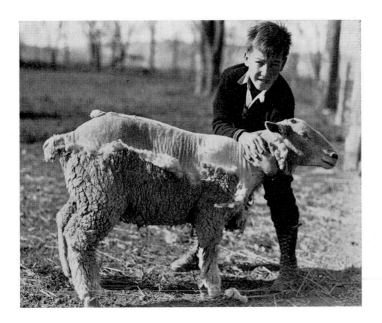

Fig. 5.3 — Thallium sulfate poisoning. The loss of wool from the head and back resulted from eating oats mixed with thallium sulfate (prairie dog poison). (Newsom and Loftus, J o u r . A.V.M.A.)

**Dogs:** phosphorus, arsenic, alpha-naphthyl thiourea (antu) and thallium used in rodent baits.

**Poultry:** toxic weed seeds and ergot from feeding grain screenings; a toxin, possibly a neurotoxin, from eating rose chafers; formaldehyde from eating seed grains treated for smut.

**Wild waterfowl:** lead from eating birdshot from the bottoms of lakes.

POISONOUS PLANTS

The toxic principles in poisonous plants include alkaloids, glycosides (glucosides), organic acids, minerals (nitrates, selenium, molybdenum), resins or resinoids, phytotoxins, and substances causing photosensitization. These toxic principles act in various ways to cause disease.

**1. Alkaloids.** For the most part they affect the nervous system, but the manner in which they do this is not completely understood.

**2. Glycosides.** Some glycosides yield hydrocyanic acid when hydrolized in the rumen by the enzymes of the microflora. The hydrocyanic acid inhibits the activity of the cell enzyme, cytochrome oxidase. Since the function of this enzyme is to aid in cell respiration, the inhibition of it results in cell death. Common plants containing this glycoside are wild cherries, Johnson grass, Sudan grass, arrow grass, and sorghum.

Other plant materials contain saponins which are glycosides that hemolize erythrocytes. Sweet clover (Fig. 5.4) contains coumarin in combination with a glycoside. In spoiled sweet clover the coumarin is released from the glycoside and becomes dicoumarin, an anticoagulant, which lowers the prothrombin level of the blood and causes prolonged bleeding following surgery.

Oleander contains a cardiac glycoside which causes livestock losses in the southern states.

**3. Organic acids.** In the West oxalic acid in halogetin is present in the soluble form (sodium and potassium). In this form it is easily absorbed and combines, in the blood, with the calcium and is precipitated. This lowers the calcium ion content of the blood (acute hypocalcemia). Furthermore, when the calcium oxalate is excreted in the kidneys, oxalate crystals occlude the uriniferous tubules.

**4. Mineral poisons.** Crop plants and weeds during certain seasons or when fertilized with liberal amounts of nitrate fertilizer may contain excessive amounts (more than 1.5 per cent dry weight) of nitrate. The use of the herbicide 2,4-D causes some weeds, such as pigweeds, rag-

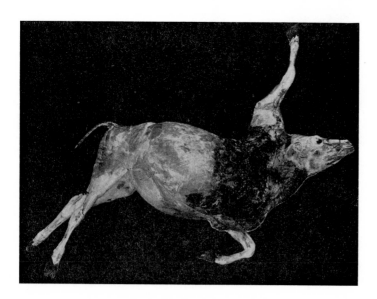

Fig. 5.4 — Sweet clover poisoning in a calf. The toxic agent in the damaged hay caused fatal hemorrhage. (Roderick, Jour. A.V.M.A.)

weeds, and Jimson weed, which are generally unpalatable, to become palatable. It also causes them to accumulate nitrate to a toxic level. When they are ingested, especially by ruminants, much of the nitrate is converted to nitrite, which is about 10 times more toxic than nitrate. Nitrite interferes with the transport of oxygen in the blood. The nitrite oxidizes ferrous hemoglobin to ferric hemoglobin (methemoglobin), which cannot carry oxygen. The blood, consequently, becomes chocolate-brown in color. Death is due to hypoxia, and occurs when about three-fourths of the ferrous hemoglobin has been converted to methemoglobin.

In the north central Great Plains there are areas where the soil is rich in selenium and where the plants grown on the soil absorb enough of the element to poison livestock. Farmers call the acute type of poisoning blind staggers and the chronic form, alkali disease. Technically it can be designated selenosis. Chicks which hatch from eggs laid by hens that have been fed selenium-containing grain are sometimes malformed.

In the San Joaquin Valley of California and in Manitoba, during certain years, grazing cattle develop diarrhea, rough coats, and lose weight. The hair may change color in spots and in severe cases may fall out, leaving dry, red areas of skin which have a tendency to crack. Calves, mostly, are affected, but sometimes dairy cows also show evidences of the condition by failing to conceive, or if they do conceive, they abort. This poisoning is due to an excess of molybdenum, which is absorbed more by the leguminous plants than by the nonlegumes. Alkalinity of the soil seems to favor absorption of the chemical by the plants.

5. **Resins or resinoids** directly affect nervous and muscle tissue by causing irritation. Water hemlock is a widely distributed plant in the United States and it contains a resin causing such injury.

6. **Phytotoxins** (toxalbumins), such as ricin in the castor bean, cause hemolysis.

7. **Porphyrins,** contained in some plants, sensitize animals to sunlight.

## POISONS IN PROCESSED FEEDS

For many years in the United States agene (nitrogen trichloride) was used as a bleaching agent in the milling of flour. During that period some dogs were subject to a peculiar nervous disorder called running fits, canine hysteria, or fright disease. Agene in the flour was not toxic for man, but when bread or biscuits containing it were fed to dogs continuously, even when they received other food, the nervous disturbance sometimes appeared. It was believed that the toxicosis resulted from an interaction of agene and the essential amino acid methionine. Agene is no longer used as a bleaching agent for flour, but many veterinarians still have vivid recollections of its effects on dogs.

In the extraction of oil from soybeans one chemical employed has been trichloroethylene. The meal, which is a by-product of the manufacture of the oil by this process, causes lesions and symptoms of intoxication when fed to cattle. When the amount fed daily and continuously does not exceed one pound, the poisoning does not occur. The lesions displayed by the animals resemble those of bracken poisoning — principally hemorrhages widely distributed throughout the body and associated with a rapidly progressive and fatal aplastic anemia.

In the two examples of poisoning by processed feeds just described, traces of the toxic agent used in the processing were left in the finished product. In the next example, that of cottonseed meal poisoning, the toxic principle, gossypol, is present in the raw material (cottonseeds) and is not removed by the hexane method of extracting the oil. Gossypol is a normal constituent of the pigment glands of the seeds. It is a polyphenol which is difficult to extract with oil solvents. In some instances it remains in the meal. It depresses the appetite and therefore inhibits the growth of animals which consume it. It is especially toxic for chickens and swine.

Poisoning by processed feeds contaminated with machine lubricants containing highly chlorinated naphthalenes occurs mostly in young cattle 6 to 12 months old.

The skin of the neck, back, and rump becomes thick and crusty. Later this dermal thickening extends down the sides. Wartlike growths on the oral mucosa make mastication difficult. Lacrimation is often prominent. Other symptoms are loss of weight, diarrhea, and polyuria. Hyperkeratosis is the name used because this is the most prominent lesion.

### POISONS FROM INDUSTRIAL PLANTS

The origin of another kind of poisoning of livestock is more varied than any of those just mentioned. This is poisoning with fluorine compounds (fluorosis). It occurs from the drinking of water high in fluorine content, grazing on forage contaminated by smoke and dust from certain kinds of industrial plants, and from the long continued feeding of rock phosphate. It occurs mostly in cattle and sheep.

The intake of a small amount of fluorine is beneficial and reduces the incidence of dental caries. Water which contains 1.5 to 2 parts per million will cause mottling of the teeth. Most water in the United States contains less than 1 part per million. In parts of the United States, particularly in the Southwest, water may contain 6 or more parts per million, and forage crops irrigated by that water may contain as much as 15 to 25 parts per million. Cattle can tolerate 1 mg. of fluorine per kilogram of body weight per day for 5 years with no apparent effect on the body outside of discolored teeth. When the amount ingested per day reaches or exceeds 2 mg/kg of body weight per day over long periods, symptoms of fluorine poisoning begin to appear.

Fluorosis occasionally occurs in the vicinity of manufacturing plants which discharge fluorine compounds into the air from smoke stacks. Industrial plants which have been known to contaminate nearby pastures have been aluminum reduction plants, steel and enamel work, brick factories, and electric power stations. The source of the fluorine is the bauxite, cryolite, feldspar, fluospar, or sodium fluoride used as a flux, or the coal used for generating power.

The long continued feeding of rock phosphate containing as much as $3\frac{1}{2}$ per cent fluorine causes damaging fluorosis.

Usually, poisoning with fluorine has occurred from carelessness in handling superphosphate for fertilizing land. This fertilizer contains 18 per cent fluorine as against 1 to 3 per cent in rock phosphate. Cattle that have had access to places where it is unevenly distributed have been known to develop fluorosis.

The first evidences of fluorosis are mottling, and increased and uneven wear of the incisors. Next the animals show stiffness and become unthrifty, even to the point of showing mild emaciation. This may be accompanied by diarrhea. Examination of the blood reveals a state of anemia, and a urine analysis shows the presence of more than 10 parts per million of fluorine. Eventually exostoses appear on the long bones, the mandible, and ribs. The hoofs become long and ridged. The fluorine content of the bones is increased 5 or 6 times beyond the normal limit.

Fluorine is not the only toxic substance which is known to contaminate pastures by way of the air in the vicinity of industrial plants. Molybdenum from plants which use this mineral in manufacturing aluminum and steel alloys has caused chronic toxicosis in cattle and sheep. The high intake of molybdenum on such pastures reduces the copper storage ability of the liver and results in copper deficiency. The symptoms displayed by the animals are those of **hypocuprosis,** but the intoxication is called **molybdenosis.** The cattle and sheep scour and become unthrifty. The cattle resemble those having Johne's disease.

**Body defenses against poisons.** To a certain extent the body can defend itself against poisonous substances. Vomiting, increased peristalsis resulting in diarrhea, the production of large amounts of mucus by irritated mucous membranes, and excretion by way of the kidneys and lungs are examples of this defensive function of parts of the body. The body has a special means of defense, which belongs in the field of immunology, against some poisons such as snake venom, bacterial toxins, and some phytotoxins, as ricin and abrin.

### Endogenous Poisons

The nature of endogenous poisons is not so well known as that of the exogenous ones. It is known, however, that toxic substances originate within the body wherever there is disintegrating necrotic tissue such as occurs in severe burns, in areas of gangrene, and in regions of the body affected by extensive intravital blood-clot formation in the vessels. Endogenous intoxication also results from suppressed function of organs as occurs in the condition called uremia. This arises in connection with severe renal damage or with obstruction of the urinary tract. Endogenous intoxication is sometimes associated with perverted metabolism of the cells which exists in disturbances of some of the glands of internal secretion. An example is the formation of the toxic beta-oxybutyric acid in diabetes mellitus.

## VIABLE INFLUENCES

### Bacterial and Viral Forms of Plant Life

An infection, from the standpoint of pathology, is understood to be an invasion of the body by pathogenic organisms. They grow in the fluids and tissues of the body to such an extent that the fluids and tissues undergo alterations either by the mechanical action of the bacteria themselves or by the chemical action of their toxins. An infection produced quite consistently by a particular organism is called a specific infectious disease. While one particular microorganism is the cause of a specific infectious disease, there are instances where secondary invaders may change the appearance of the disease so that field cases may look quite different from laboratory-induced cases. Examples of such diseases are swine influenza, canine distemper, and hog cholera.

**Nomenclature.** There has been no uniform or prescribed method of naming the specific infectious diseases. In many cases the name is descriptive of one of the most prominent lesions of the disease; e.g., in horses: suppurative arthritis, vesicular stomatitis, encephalomyelitis, epizootic periodic ophthalmia; in cattle: granular vaginitis, blackleg, icterohemoglobinuria; in sheep: caseous lymphadenitis; in swine: necrotic enteritis; in dogs: blacktongue; in the domestic fowl: laryngotracheitis. Several diseases have received their names by combining the name of the causative organism with the termination -osis, denoting disease or pathologic process, e.g., tuberculosis, paratuberculosis, brucellosis, pasteurellosis, salmonellosis, actinomycosis, actinobacillosis, psittacosis, and staphylococcosis. The names of two diseases, tetanus and rabies, are derived from their principal symptoms. Two others, colibacillosis and necrobacillosis, get theirs by combining the species name of the organism with the word bacillosis, meaning a state of bacillary infection. In necrobacillosis, *necro* is a contraction of necrophorus. In one case (tularemia) the root of the species name is combined with -emia, signifying the presence of the causative organism in the blood of the infected animal. The meanings of a few names are not very significant and sometimes not so apparent, for example, glanders and strangles of horses, influenza of horses and swine, distemper of horses and dogs, cholera of swine and chickens. The famous bacteriologists and pathologists, Bang, Johne, and Aujeszky, are memorialized in the names of the diseases for which they discovered the cause by simply using their names with the word "disease" — Bang's disease, Johne's disease, Aujeszky's disease. In a different way, which has already been noted, the names of Bruce, Pasteur, and Salmon are associated with diseases for which they discovered the cause. An error in etymology occurred when the fowl disease caused by *Salmonella pullorum* was named pullorum disease. The use of pullorum in this manner is incongruous since the word pullorum is the Latin genitive of *pullus* and means "of young fowl."

**Etiology.** The causes of the diseases described in this book, as far as they are known, have already been studied in detail in courses in bacteriology which have preceded this course in pathology. It will not be necessary therefore, here or later, to do much more than name the causative organism or organisms in connection with each disease. The student, however, will find it advantageous to refer to a textbook of bacteriology frequently because certain peculiar characteristics of some microorganisms have a direct bearing on their ability to invade the body, on their distribution after entering the body, on the nature of the lesions they produce, and consequently, on the termination of the disease. A list of these special characteristics which aid microorganisms in producing disease would include size, motility, capsules, spores, hemolysins, aggressins, and endo- and exotoxins.

The specific infectious diseases are transmitted by mediate (indirect) or immediate (direct) contact of affected animals with susceptible animals. Whether the contact be direct or indirect, the infective discharges must reach and enter the body of the susceptible animal. Several factors operate to establish different degrees of contagiousness. Among these factors are: (1) the number of organisms which escape from the body of a sick animal, (2) the number of organisms which enter the body of the susceptible animal, (3) the effectiveness of the defense mechanism of the susceptible animal, and (4) the virulence of the organism.

Naturally the number of microorganisms which leave the body of an infected animal is dependent upon the distribution of those organisms in the body. If they are localized, their chance of leaving the body is much less than if they are distributed widely as they are in the septicemias. The septicemic diseases as a rule are much more contagious than the localized infections. Examples of such septicemias are equine influenza, hog cholera, canine distemper, and fowl typhoid. Examples of localized infections are staphylococcosis of horses, streptococcic mastitis of cows, actinomycosis of the mammary gland of

sows, and pullorum disease of hens. An exception to the above rule occurs with relation to localized specific infectious diseases of the digestive and respiratory tracts. Because the infective discharges from the nose, mouth, and anus can so readily contaminate the feed and water of susceptible animals, diseases of the respiratory and digestive organs may be highly contagious. Examples of such diseases are strangles of horses, foot-and-mouth disease of cattle, contagious ecthyma of sheep, swine influenza, and laryngotracheitis of chickens.

The number of organisms which enter the body of the susceptible animals in a herd or flock is influenced by the methods of husbandry and sanitation. Superior methods of husbandry and sanitation in one group of animals may limit the spread of the infection as compared with inferior methods in another. The incidence of infection may be so low in the herd under good management that one is tempted to say the disease is less contagious than in the herd under poor management.

The effectiveness of the defense mechanism of an animal may be so perfect that for this particular animal the disease in question is not at all contagious. Other animals in the same herd or flock may be in an excellent state of health, and as a consequence their defense mechanism may function so well that only a few contract the infection. A still smaller number may be undernourished or parasitized. Their defenses against infection may be so weak that pathogens can invade their bodies and produce disease. In this herd, then, contagiousness of the infection is a relative matter. The fault with the above illustration is that sometimes the best animals in a herd for some unknown reason die of the infection first. This is especially true of animals that are affected with viral diseases.

The virulence of the organism is an important factor in the production of an infection as has already been pointed out in the course in bacteriology. It would be natural to suppose that low and highly virulent strains of the same organism would give rise to mildly contagious and highly contagious infections. This is borne out experimentally and is even made use of to some extent in some forms of immunity production.

A few diseases which apparently are rather highly contagious experimentally do not seem to be so in nature. Some of these, such as tularemia of wild animals, equine encephalomyelitis, equine infectious anemia, and hog cholera, may depend upon insect vectors for their transmission. The contagiousness of these diseases often varies considerably. This may be partly explained by the fact that the vectors may or may not be plentiful. In this case, then, it is not a matter of degree of contagiousness but a question of incidence or occurrence of the disease which is dependent upon the prevalence of the vector.

**Channels of infection.** In the spread of a specific infectious disease the etiologic microorganisms must leave the body of the diseased animal and enter the body of the susceptible. The escape may be from any of the natural body openings, or from wounds, abscesses, and ulcers on the surface. The organisms may be present in the normal body excretions or in inflammatory exudates which are being discharged from the body. To complete the cycle of infection these organisms must enter the body through one of the natural body openings, through breaks in the continuity of the body covering, through the conjunctiva, or by way of the umbilicus in fetuses and newborn animals.

The feeding and drinking habits of animals, which of course are imposed upon them by nature or by man, make it easy for infection to enter the body by way of the digestive tract. Much of their feed and drink must be taken directly from the ground or from utensils placed close to the ground where the danger of contamination with body discharges is constantly present. Fetal calves furnish an interesting example of alimentary introduction of infection when they drink amniotic fluid contaminated with *Escherichia coli* and develop a prenatal enteritis.

Infectious agents may adhere to dust particles or be present in droplets of exudate floating in the air. Organisms clinging to dust particles may come from any of the infectious discharges. Those in the air-borne droplets are forcefully expelled from the respiratory organs by sneezing or coughing. Air in poorly ventilated, insanitary buildings housing diseased animals with susceptible ones may be the means of transmitting an infection by the respiratory system. The organisms of glanders in horses, tuberculosis in cattle, influenza in swine, distemper in dogs, and laryngotracheitis in chickens are believed to enter the body often by this avenue of infection.

The urinary system, as a portal of entry for microorganisms, is not nearly as important as the digestive and the respiratory. There are two reasons for this. First, it is entirely an excretory system. Secondly, infection from without must ascend the tract against the flow of the excretion. Such ascension occurs more frequently in the female because the urethra is comparatively short and its lumen is large. Furthermore, it terminates in the vagina which is quite often the seat of infection. Organisms occasionally are introduced directly into this system by means of surgical instruments. *Corynebacterium renale* in cows and sows is one of the very few specific infections which has the urinary system as its portal of entry.

The genital system is the avenue of entrance for a small group of infectious agents. The most prominent organisms in the group are *Brucella abortus*, *Brucella suis*, *Vibrio fetus*, *Trichomonas foetus*, *Trypanosoma equiperdum*, and *Streptococcus genitalium*. These are all abortion-producing organisms.

The intact skin for the most part is an effective barrier against the entrance of microorganisms. *Brucella abortus*, however, has been shown experimentally to be able to invade the uninjured skin. It and other organisms may enter through the conjunctiva. Some of the clostridia such as the ones of tetanus, malignant edema, and blackleg enter through wounds in the surface of the body. Often, however, no apparent surface injury can be found in connection with *Clostridium chauvoei* infection. When these anaerobes are introduced into wounds they are usually accompanied by aerobes which use up the oxygen and thus aid in making conditions suitable for the growth of the clostridia. Three organisms which produce necrosis and in most cases chronic suppuration with the formation of tumor-like masses of granulation tissue, depend upon wounds, mostly by penetrating objects, for their introduction into the skin. They are *Actinomyces bovis, Actinobacillus lignieresi,* and *Staphylococcus aureus. Mycobacterium tuberculosis* sometimes enters through wounds on the legs and teats of cattle. Puncture wounds inflicted by the teeth of rabid animals are the avenue of entrance peculiar to rabies virus. Insect vectors, however, introduce several organisms through punctures of the skin as in anthrax, tularemia, equine encephalomyelitis, fowl pox, equine infectious anemia, and possibly hog cholera.

In mammals either during intra-uterine life or right after birth the umbilical vessels or the navel may admit the entrance of infectious agents. This may occur in any of the domestic mammals but is more prevalent in colts and calves. In colts *Shigella equirulis, Streptococcus genitalium, Streptococcus pyogenes, Salmonella abortivoequina,* and *Corynebacterium equi* may enter here either singly or in combination. In calves *Escherichia coli, Streptococcus pyogenes, Corynebacterium pyogenes,* and *Brucella abortus* enter in a similar manner. In bird embryos *Salmonella pullorum* and related organisms, which are present in the vitelline substance of the egg yolk, are already present in the young at the time of hatching. This is a mode of entrance of infection comparable but not exactly like intra-uterine infection in mammals.

**Defenses against infection.** Just as microorganisms have qualities which favor their invasion into the body, so does the body have means of hindering their entrance. In the stomach the hydrochloric acid, and in the intestine the high carbon dioxide content resulting from fermentation of ingesta inhibit the development of some microorganisms like *Bacillus anthracis.* Some organisms irritate the stomach mucosa and are removed to a large extent by emesis. Others irritate the intestinal mucosa and are pushed along the tract by accelerated peristalsis and washed out with increased secretions. In the respiratory organs the entrance of bacteria is opposed by the action of the cilia, the sticky adhesive mucus, phagocytes on the epithelium, and the reflexes of sneezing and coughing. The flow of urine down the urinary tract is usually quite effective in washing out infection. In the vagina the mucus and the reaction of the secretion prevent the entrance of many kinds of bacteria. During pregnancy the constriction of the cervical canal and the presence in it of an albuminous and mucous plug further prevent the invasion of bacteria. If the organisms evade these primary defenses of the body, they must then encounter the secondary defenses — the antibodies and the phagocytes. The action of these infection-fighting agencies is supplemented by the inflammatory reaction and fever.

**Period of incubation.** The time elapsing from the entrance of pathogenic microorganisms into the body until the appearance of the first symptoms is the period of incubation. In general each specific infectious disease has a more or less constant period of incubation. Most periods are measured in days. Some, however, run for weeks and months. Regardless of whether the periods are measured in days, weeks, or months, they are variable in length. When stating the duration of the periods, minimal and maximal lengths, or average lengths, are given. Minimal lengths for several diseases with short periods are: anthrax, fowl cholera, enteritis of sucklings, swine influenza — 1 day; vesicular stomatitis of horses and cattle — 2 days; foot-and-mouth disease, blackleg, swine erysipelas, equine encephalomyelitis — 3 days; canine distemper and strangles

— 4 days. Extremely long periods of incubation are present in leukosis of the domestic fowl — usually about 3 months; tuberculosis, glanders, actinomycosis, actinobacillosis, staphylococcosis, and bovine brucellosis — several weeks or months; and Johne's disease — perhaps 2 to 3 years. The length of the period of incubation is dependent upon the virulence of the organism, the amount of infection entering the susceptible animal, the mode of infection, and the resistance of the animal.

**Pathogenesis.** If pathogens evade the body defenses and establish themselves in the tissues and fluids, they increase in numbers and begin to injure the tissues. The step-by-step development of the whole series of changes which occur in the body is designated pathogenesis. The pathogenesis of a given specific infectious disease is rather constant, but that for the whole group of diseases is quite variable. Even different species of bacteria within a genus may produce diseases the pathogenesis of which are very dissimilar.

In general the mode of development of a specific infectious disease depends upon whether the organism remains localized after it gains admission to the body or whether it invades the blood stream. If the infection enters the blood vascular system, the character of the disease is governed principally by the number and virulence of the organisms present. If the number remains small, widespread injury to the body does not result. This condition is termed **bacteremia**. On the other hand, if the organisms increase rapidly in the blood stream and produce tissue damage over wide areas of the body, the resultant condition is called a **septicemia.**

In the bacteremias the disease processes which arise are conditioned by the type of bacteria which enters the blood stream. For instance, *Brucella abortus* causes a bacteremia in cows which soon terminates in localization of the organism in the pregnant uterus and udder. Because of the nature of the organism, only a mild suppurative inflammation ensues. In navel ill of foals, on the other hand, a bacteremia may occur in which pyogenic bacteria are carried to various parts of the body where they localize and form abscesses. Even in septicemias the tissue changes can be quite dissimilar. For instance, some septicemias are characterized by vascular disturbances — hyperemia, edema, hemorrhages — e.g., hog cholera, swine erysipelas, icterohemoglobinuria, and anthrax. Others have mild inflammation of the various mucous membranes as their prominent lesion, e.g., equine influenza and canine distemper. Some diseases begin as a septicemia but cease to be after the causative organism localizes, e.g., foot-and-mouth disease, canine distemper, and equine encephalomyelitis.

The viruses likewise cause specific infectious diseases with localization of the virus in parts of the body and also with its distribution throughout the blood. Among the viruses which localize are those of cow, swine, and fowl pox, both foot-and-mouth disease of cloven-footed animals and equine infectious encephalomyelitis after a short initial septicemic stage, vesicular stomatitis of horses and cattle, equine contagious pneumonia, avian infectious laryngotracheitis, and swine influenza.

Viruses which produce septicemias are those of equine infectious anemia and influenza, hog cholera, canine distemper, and fowl pest. A study of the pathogenesis of the viral diseases indicates that the viruses have affinity for certain tissues and organs. As a consequence, they have been classified according to the principal tissue or tissues they attack, hence the designations epitheliotropic, neurotropic, viscerotropic, and pantropic viruses.

The pathogenesis of the dermotropic, epitheliotropic, and neurotropic ultraviral diseases needs special consideration. With regard to the first two, namely the dermotropic and epitheliotropic diseases, there seem to be three stages of development. These three stages may overlap so much that it may not be possible to determine where one ceases and another begins, but in general they can be said to exist. Furthermore, these stages do not always appear with the same intensity. Their variability creates the distinguishing characters of the diseases in which they occur. The three stages are marked by the following changes:

1. Stimulation and proliferation of the epithelium.
2. Degeneration and necrosis of the epithelium.
3. Inflammation of the subepithelial tissues.

Stimulation and proliferation of the epithelium are especially prominent in the poxes of cattle, swine, and birds, in infectious myxomatosis of rabbits and infectious papillomas of cattle, dogs, and rabbits. Degeneration and necrosis are particularly marked in foot-and-mouth disease, vesicular stomatitis, and avian laryngotracheitis. They appear to occur so rapidly that proliferation of the epithelium may not take place at all. In the poxes, degeneration and necrosis occur slowly enough so that the epithelial proliferation is apparent. In infectious papillomas, degeneration and necrosis are absent. Inflammation, when it occurs, is probably secondary to the degeneration and necrosis. The inflammatory reaction is greatest in those diseases in which epithelial damage is most severe, and vice versa.

The development of the histological changes in the neurotropic viral diseases is apparently controlled by the avenue of entrance of the virus, by its affinity for a specific tissue, and also by its virulence. The portal of entry may be by the axis cylinder of a peripheral nerve to the nerve root ganglion cells, then to the cord, and eventually to the brain as in rabies. It may, however, be by the lymph channels along the olfactory nerve to the cerebrospinal fluid and thence to the brain substance as in some cases of equine encephalomyelitis. Then again it may be by the general circulation to the brain.

The changes in the central nervous system are inflammatory and degenerative. One may not always be able to ascertain which occurs first. The inflammatory reaction is characterized by two cellular changes, infiltration and proliferation. The infiltration is a vascular and perivascular accumulation of neutrophils, lymphocytes, plasma cells, and macrophages. The proliferation is of the astrocytes and microglia. They may have a diffuse or focal distribution. Focal collections of glia around degenerating and dead nerve cells are indicative of neuronophagy. The degenerative changes are in the neurons. They may occur before or after the infiltrative and proliferative changes.

In the pathogenesis of some viral diseases, cell inclusion bodies appear. They are variable in size up to that of a neucleolus or larger. Some are located within the cytoplasm and others within the nucleus. The location and also the number is rather characteristic for each disease in which they occur. They appear in epithelial cells more often than in others. Their staining qualities are not uniform. Whether these bodies are the etiological agent itself or material produced by it, or whether they are products of cytoplasmic and nuclear degeneration due to the virus has not been determined. No one explanation of their origin is satisfactory for all of them.

**Lesions.** The changes which take place in the tissues and body fluids in the specific infectious diseases are nothing more than various combinations of lesions which have already been studied in general and systemic pathology. When these changes are grouped together in rather definite combinations, they constitute the lesions of the specific infectious diseases.

**Course.** The variableness of the duration of a specific infectious disease can be indicated by the application of the following words: peracute, acute, subacute, subchronic, and chronic. In the order given, these words signify gradations in the duration of a disease ranging from the exceedingly short course with relatively severe manifestations to the long course with perhaps less alarming characteristics. It is not always possible to make such fine distinctions in the course of a disease. One can rather easily distinguish between an acute and a chronic infectious disease.

**Termination.** A specific infectious disease may terminate in one of three ways: (1) death after a short duration, (2) death after a period of invalidism, or (3) recovery after repair of the damage done in the body has been accomplished.

The septicemic diseases and the neurotropic viral diseases often terminate in death. Death in these diseases may result from the effects of the organisms and their toxins upon the central nervous system. Vascular and cellular infiltrative changes in the brain parenchyma and degenerative changes in the nerve cells and fibers of the cardiac and respiratory centers disturb the functions of these centers so that hypoxia occurs. Hyperthermia may be a contributory factor to death when the heat-regulating center is seriously upset. In infectious anemia of horses and infectious icterohemoglobinuria of cattle, there is such a destruction of erythrocytes that hypoxia occurs. In the infectious diseases in which pneumonia is a lesion or a complication, such as equine contagious pneumonia, equine influenza, canine distemper, swine influenza, and fowl cholera, death from hypoxia is due to a hindrance to respiration.

In diseases with localization of the infection the termination is variable. When the upper respiratory organs and trachea are the seat of the infection, such as is the case in strangles of horses, "diphtheria" of calves, avian laryngotracheitis, and fowl pox, death results from hypoxia due to respiratory interference. Inanition usually occurs in actinomycosis and actinobacillosis in and around the oral cavity, foot-and-mouth disease, vesicular stomatitis, avian diphtheria, and oral papillomas in puppies because of difficulty in mastication. The same thing may be said about tetanus and equine encephalomyelitis, but the reason for the wasting of the body is the inability of the animal to swallow as well as to chew. Starvation may occur in chickens afflicted with a neurolymphosarcoma, not because the affected birds do not want to eat but because they cannot move about to get food, and sometimes cannot see. Death in infectious enteritis of cats, infectious necrotic enteritis of swine, and paratuberculous enteritis (Johne's disease) of cattle is preceded by a period of emaciation and general tissue dehydration because of failure to absorb nutrient material and water from the intestine.

In the specific infectious diseases, such as strangles and navel ill, which are characterized by localized suppurative processes, the infection may metastasize so that the animal may eventually die of a generalized infection.

Specific infections of the generative organs usually do not terminate in death, but the affected animals often become unserviceable as breeders either temporarily or permanently. Infectious granular vaginitis, Bang's disease, and vaginal trichomoniasis of cattle, brucellosis of swine, and infectious abortion and dourine of horses should be mentioned here.

### Protozoan and Metozoan Forms of Animal Life

Lower forms of animal life which infest higher animals live either on the surface or in the interior of the body. Zoologically, the external parasites are either insects or arachnids belonging in the phylum Arthropoda. Most of the internal parasites belong in the phyla: (1) **Protozoa** (trichomonads, coccidia, leukocytozoa, trypanosomes, and piroplasmata), (2) **Platyhelminthes** (trematodes and cestodes), and (3) **Nemathelminthes** (nematodes). These animal parasites cause lesions in much the same manner as do the lower forms of plant life, i.e., by mechanical injury and by their toxins. The injuries produced can be grouped like those resulting from bacterial and viral infections.

**Anemia.** General anemia is due to (1) loss of blood, either by blood-sucking parasites or through wounds made by the parasites (stomach worms of sheep, hookworms of dogs, strongyles of horses, ticks of various animals), and to (2) the destruction of erythrocytes (babesia and anaplasma infections). Local anemia is caused by pressure exerted by encysted parasites (tapeworm larvae).

**Hemorrhage.** The manner in which animal parasites cause hemorrhage has just been noted. Often the loss of blood is out of proportion to the size of the wounds because the parasites causing the wounds produce anticoagulants. Experimentally it has been shown that a dog given 2,000 infective hookworm larvae loses one liter of blood (his total blood volume at any one time) in 16 to 27 days.

**Swelling of the spleen.** Engorgement of the spleen with broken-down erythrocytes is produced by some protozoa (babesia).

**Degeneration and death of cells.** This occurs when parasites (1) invade cells (erythrocytes, leukocytes, and epithelial cells invaded by protozoa), (2) when they feed on tissues of the host (liver flukes in cattle and sheep, strongyles in the horse, maggots in the wounds of various animals), and (3) when the presence of a large parasite exerts considerable pressure on the surrounding tissues (kidney worm in the dog), or (4) when large parasite cysts act in the same manner (tapeworm larvae).

**Tissue proliferation.** Increase in cells as a result of parasitic invasion occurs in various parts of the body such as in the lymphatic tissue (trypanosomes in horses), in and around bile ducts (coccidia in rabbits), in the gastric mucosa (*Habronema megastoma* in horses), in the intestinal wall (nodule worms in sheep, thorny-headed worms in swine), and around the portal canals in the liver (ascarid larvae in pigs).

**Mechanical obstruction of hollow organs.** This is due to the presence of (1) large numbers of relatively small parasites (lungworms in bronchi and bronchioles of several species of animals, heartworms in the right cardiac chambers in dogs, flukes in the bile ducts of cattle and sheep) and to the presence of (2) a few large worms (adult ascarids in the bile ducts of swine, and tapeworms in the same ducts of sheep). In the horse a small number of strongyle larvae often obstruct the branches of the anterior mesenteric artery by producing a thrombus and an arteritis.

The defense reactions of the body against the lower forms of animal life are quite similar to those exerted against low forms of plant life but differ in degree.

## STRESS

In this chapter the various physical influences, chemical agents, microbiologic and lower animal forms which cause disease have been described. It has been noted that these specific causes produce rather specific tissue alterations.

One cannot predict what organ may be the site of these changes or what kind of change will be produced, but many of the vital organs are known to be the seat of these changes, and many of the tissue alterations studied in general pathology occur. These reactions are called **stress** responses. The causes of them are referred to as **stressors**. The process occurring within the body is an adaptive one by which the animal is attempting to preserve body structure and function in an environment which is constantly changing. Stress becomes apparent when the environmental changes become extremely severe and the responses of the body exceed those which are considered physiologic.

There are differences of thought relative to the way in which these responses are brought about. If the responses proceed in the usual manner, they are the result of stimuli to the central nervous system. The pathway then seems to be to the hypothalamus, to the pituitary, and from it to the various endocrines and organs. Among the reactions the release of an adrenocorticotrophic hormone (ACTH) causes the excretion of steroids by the adrenal cortex. The release of these steroids may or may not be the all-important aspect of the reaction. Regardless of whatever the mechanism of the stress response may be, the most important thing seems to be that stress causes a derangement of the adaptive mechanism of the body and that the various nonspecific structural and functional disorders result in the important systems of the body. Furthermore, stress is a predisposing factor to some of the infectious bacterial, viral, protozoan, and metazoan diseases.

# Part III

# Basic Vascular
# and Cellular Alterations

| # Disturbances of Development

The study of the disturbances of development occurring during embryonic or fetal life constitutes the science of **teratology**. The curiosities and oddities of medicine were of great interest to ancient civilizations, and many of their myths were based upon these malformations. The myth concerning Cyclops was based upon an individual who had only one eye. The god Janus was the result of a malformed individual who had two heads fused along their posterior surfaces with their faces pointing in opposite directions.

The early compilers were more concerned with the curiosities and oddities of medicine than they were with the sound basic facts that constitute an organized study of pathology. William Harvey was the first individual to recognize that abnormalities of growth were due to defects in development of the embryo and fetus. Prior to his time, these teratological abnormalities were thought to be the result of Divine displeasure. Another theory was that some pregnant individuals were frightened by strange creatures or objects during gestation and that the impression was so great as to be transposed to the fetuses.

## ANOMALIES

**Definition.** An anomaly is a disturbance of development that involves an organ or a portion of an organ.

The causes of anomalies are not always known. Embryologists state that most of them have their origins within the first few weeks after fertilization. Some, however, may develop later in pregnancy. Studies by geneticists indicate that many even have their inception in the germ plasm — that is, they are hereditary.

### Heritable Malformations

Heritable defects are the result of definite elements in the germinal makeup. They are transmitted in accordance with the Mendelian laws of inheritance, and in many instances their mode of inheritance has been definitely determined. As in the case of other hereditary characters, certain defects are inherited in a simple fashion, while others are due to larger gene complexes. Most hereditary defects appear to be recessive, but there are a few which behave as dominant characteristics.

Hereditary defects also differ widely in their effect on the individual. Some, for example, destroy the life of the individual in early development, whereas others are hardly of sufficient importance to affect materially the economic value of an animal. If the character of the genes results in the death of the fetus or newborn, such genes are known as lethal (Fig. 6.1). Many such factors have been encountered in the various domestic animals, but since they manifest themselves prior to birth

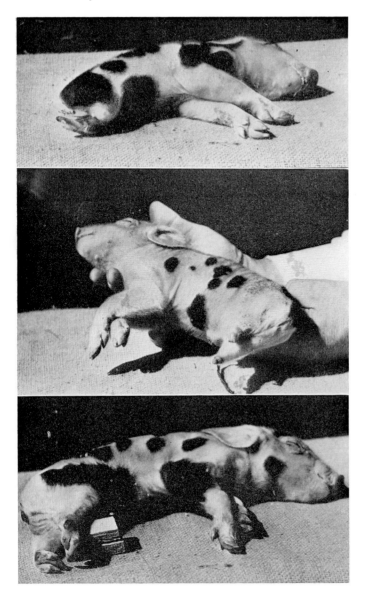

Fig. 6.1a — Malformed male pig with undersized testes, no anus, crooked tail, and only partially developed hind legs.

Fig. 6.1b — Male pig with same malformations as in 6.1a.

Fig. 6.1c — Female pig with normal external genitals and anus, crooked tail, and legs more nearly developed than the two males. These three pigs were litter mates. (Hughes, Jour. A.V.M.A.)

and result in death of the fetus or newborn, they usually attract little attention.

A specific example of such a lethal factor is provided by Dexter cattle, an English breed with short legs, closely related to the Kerry breed. Dexter cattle when mated *inter se* never breed true, but they follow the Mendelian law and give birth to offspring according to the following ratio: 1 bulldog, 2 Dexter, 1 Kerry (normal). Bulldog calves are always stillborn and show features characteristic of a condi-

tion known as achondroplasia. The explanation of this phenomenon is that in the Dexters shortleggedness is due to a dominant lethal gene which, if inherited both from the sire and the dam, causes their offspring to be stillborn. A similar defect has been observed in the Telemark breed in Norway. This type of achondroplasia, however, is recessive, since normal individuals may have defective offspring.

In some of the beef breeds of cattle, especially in Herefords in the United

States, a latent lethal defect which is a form of dwarfism occurs. Genetically it is conditioned by a simple, autosomal, recessive gene. These dwarfs seldom reach reproductive age.

A dwarf gene-carrier bull when introduced into a dwarf gene-free herd will not get dwarfs in the first generation of calves, but 50 per cent of the calves will be dwarf gene-carriers. In the second generation, dwarf gene-carrier females which are mated with dwarf gene-carrier males produce dwarfs according to the characteristic Mendelian ratio.

Abnormalities in size and shape of certain bones give these dwarfs a characteristic appearance. The head appears too large for the body. Due to a shortening of the premaxillae and maxillae, the face is slightly dished below the eyes. The lower jaw is somewhat undershot. The front cannon bones are shortened, which makes the front quarters lower than normal. The bodies of the last 4 or 5 thoracic vertebrae and all of the lumbar vertebrae are compressed anteroposteriorly. This makes the back short where the longissimus dorsi and psoas major muscles are located. The ventral surface of the bodies of normal vertebrae in this area arches dorsally. In the compressed vertebrae the bodies are shorter anteroposteriorly than normal and deeper dorsoventrally. The ventral line of the body becomes straighter and ridged. In some cases the lateral aspects of the transverse processes of the lumbar vertebrae curve forward in the fashion of a hook. Also, in some animals there is an overgrowth of the dorsal articulations of the lumbar vertebrae and a pinched condition of the occipital condyles.

Some of the animals have a peculiarity in breathing which has led to designating these dwarfs as "snorters." They usually stand with the head and neck lowered and extended. This position seems to facilitate breathing. So-called snorters are diabetic, which means that they do not utilize glucose as do normal cattle. Some of these animals have a ball-shaped heart. The condition basically is a congenital

abnormality in bone formation resulting from a defect in interstitial cartilage growth in some bones. Because there is a depression of interstitial growth of articular and epiphyseal cartilage but not of the normal growth by apposition, certain bones, especially those of metacarpal and metatarsal regions, become shorter than normal but have the usual width. There is also premature fusion of the sphenooccipital synchondrosis.

Lethal characters have also been found in other domestic animals. In the horse, for example, a lethal character is known which causes complete closure of the ascending colon in the region of the pelvic flexure. This condition, known as atresia coli, was observed among the descendants of a Percheron stallion imported into Japan from Ohio in the latter part of the last century. The lethal characters just referred to are only a few examples of several which have been encountered among domestic animals.

There are a few heritable defects which are not lethal in character yet are of considerable economic importance. Two of these occur in swine — cryptorchidism and scrotal hernia. (1) In the cryptorchid pigs the undescended testicles make the animals worthless as breeders. Furthermore, pork derived from their carcasses is likely to have an undesirable sex odor. (2) The pigs with scrotal hernia have large inguinal canals. A special technic must be used when they are castrated and the operation always involves a certain risk.

Another nonlethal characteristic is of importance to the breeders of collies. It is the deafness which is occasionally found in white collies. It, however, is not confined to white collies but appears sometimes in other white breeds of dogs, white cats, and other white animals.

## Heritable Blood Defects

While emphasis is usually placed upon the defects which occur in the connective tissue, epithelium, smooth muscle, and nervous tissue, it must be pointed out that the elements of the blood are not immune to the laws of heredity. For instance, the clotting mechanism is governed by heredity. A good example of a pathologic condition of the blood of man which is heritable is hemophilia. It is a defect in coagulation which is transmitted through female carriers and is therefore designated a sex-linked recessive character. When females which carry this gene and the character it induces are mated with normal males, half of the male offspring should be bleeders (hemophilic); that is, they should have a prolonged clotting time. It is not certain just what the basic factor behind the defect is, but it seems most probable that it is a deficiency of readily available thromboplastin, which in turn may be due to the platelets being less fragile than normal. Resistant platelets do not disintegrate quickly enough during hemorrhage to release the thromboplastin necessary for rapid clotting.

In New York a transmissible hemophilia has been reported in a kennel of purebred dogs. As in man, the male individuals that are the offspring of female carriers are the victims of the disturbance. During play, or as a result of being handled, or even at rest, hemorrhages occur to such an extent that massive blood cysts (hematocysts) form and fatal bleeding ensues.

In Missouri, in a herd of swine severe bleeding occurred whenever certain animals were injured (ear notching, ringing, castrating, tusk nipping, and bruising) or when the vagina was traumatized in coitus or at the time of parturition. It again is a heritable defect in coagulation which is transmissible, but is not sex-linked — it is transmissible to both sexes.

A heritable defect in the formation of hemoglobin occurs occasionally in cattle and swine. It is called "congenital porphyria." The defect seems to lie in the enzyme system of the bone marrow cells which form porphyrin. The place the porphyrins occupy in the synthesis of hemoglobin is shown in the following summary of the steps occurring in the process: pyrrole $\times$ 2 = pyrromethene $\times$ 2 (types I and III) = porphyrin (types I and III,

protoporphyrin) + ferrous iron = heme + denatured globin = hemochromogen of hemoglobin.

In this metabolic process it is believed that the enzyme system responsible for the conversion of porphyrin to heme is defective. As a result not all of the porphyrin is converted to heme, and the young erythrocytes are given a mixture of porphyrin and hemoglobin. Many of these porphyrin-laden cells apparently become hemolyzed before they can leave the bone marrow. This releases the pigment, porphyrin, into the plasma, and as it circulates in the blood it becomes deposited in the dentine of teeth and in bone. Both tissues become discolored with shades of reddish brown. The tooth discoloration has given rise to the name "pink tooth."

The pigment is also excreted in the urine and feces, imparting a reddish brown discoloration to the urine (porphyrinuria). The presence of the porphyrins in erythrocytes, plasma, bone marrow, bone, dentine, feces, and urine can be detected by viewing these tissues under ultraviolet light. This light causes the porphyrins to display a reddish fluorescence.

In congenital porphyria there is a great diminution in the number of erythrocytes. Many of those which reach the peripheral circulation are immature, and many are oversized but contain the normal amount of hemoglobin. The total amount of hemoglobin in the blood, however, is decreased. This constitutes a state of anemia which is designated macrocytic normochromic. It contributes to retarded growth of affected animals.

**Nonheritable Malformations**

The origin of malformations which are not heritable can sometimes be traced to abnormal influences present during intrauterine life such as the separation of the embryo from its attachments and abnormal pressure upon the fetus. When the embryo becomes separated from its attachment, its nutrition is disturbed and premature expulsion is usually the result. If the separation is only partial, the disturbance in the nutrition of the fetus may give rise to abnormalities in its development. Such separation may be due to concussion of the abdomen, the effect of toxic inorganic and organic agents on the blood vessels of the maternal and fetal placentae, nutritional and vitamin deficiencies, tumors, and bacteria and their toxins. Increased pressure may be the cause when there is a deficiency in the amount of amniotic fluid. In this case the fetus is not protected against the pressure exerted by the uterus and the fetal membranes. The result may be deformity of the extremities, neck, and spinal column. Pressure produced by an excess of amniotic fluid is also held to be a factor in the development of hemicephalus, hydrocephalus, and in most fissure formations. Adhesions between the amnion and the surface of the embryo are responsible for some anomalies. In addition, it is recognized that disturbances in the endocrine system may directly affect growth and development. In this connection the relationship of congenital thyroid deficiency to dwarfism and pituitary hyperplasia to giantism is emphasized.

Malformations have been produced in some of the lower vertebrates by radically changing the environment at critical times in the development of the embryo. By temporarily lowering the surrounding temperature or by directly cutting off the supply of oxygen, deformities have been caused in embryos. While the growth of an embryo is continuous, it is not at a uniform rate in all its parts. At one time the cells which are predestined to become a particular organ are rapidly proliferating and differentiating while others are more or less quiescent. If the embryo is subjected to an adverse influence at this particular time, the rapidly developing part ceases to grow and develop or develops abnormally. It is believed that this offers a rather valid reason for the appearance of many malformations.

Experimentally, congenital malformations can be produced in mammals by making the diet of the pregnant dam deficient in such nutritive substances as vitamins A, B, D, and E. With vitamin $B_{12}$ deficiency must be included riboflavin, folacin, and pantothenic acid deficiencies. It appears now that the malformations caused by maternal vitamin deficiencies are due to a lack of specific chemical substances whose functions in intra-uterine development are not yet understood. Some of these substances are more necessary at one stage of gestation than at another. For instance, riboflavin and folacin seem to be required in greater amounts for tissue differentiation and organ development than for growth of the embryo and fetus.

The end results of the maternal nutritional deficiencies and abnormal genes are quite similar. That is, the malformations resulting from either are similar in morphology and in their mechanism of development. Both factors may operate in the same way. They may depress or inhibit certain enzymatic processes which are necessary for tissue differentiation and organ development. In a sense they act as blocking agents.

A nonheritable deforming condition of calves which is due to malnutrition is of special interest to veterinarians practicing in the foothill areas of the Sierra Nevada Mountains of California. It occurs in dry years in animals which have been on poor pasture for a long time. The deformed offspring of the deficient cows are designated "acorn calves" by cattlemen. This designation is given because the condition is associated with the feeding of acorns when pasture is short.

Unlike the heritable defect of bulldog (Dexter) calves in England, this nonheritable California condition is not lethal. The calves are carried full-term, are born alive, will live if helped, and will mature and reproduce, giving birth to normal calves if fed adequately.

Deformed calves have short legs, arched backs, may or may not have malformed heads, and sometimes are subject to chronic bloat. The malnutrition giving rise to this nonheritable defect is believed to be due to a lack of vitamins and protein in the diet of the dam.

Some geneticists think that this defect may be due to the combined effects of a genetic factor and a nutritional deficiency. They suggest that genes act by determining the presence of enzymes in the embryo. It may be that in these calves there is a mutation of enzymes that affect the metabolism in embryonic development, and that the lack of the normal enzyme does not make its appearance until the animals are on a deficient diet. In fact, three types of malformations occurring naturally in domestic animals belong in this category. Appropriate examples are: malformations in chicken embryos resulting from necrosis caused by selenium transmitted in the egg; disturbed development of pig fetuses farrowed by vitamin A-deficient sows; and anomalies in pigs carried by sows during hog cholera virus infection.

### Classification of Anomalies

DISTURBANCES IN DEVELOPMENT

**A. Arrest of development**

    1. *Agenesia* — incomplete and imperfect development of an organ or

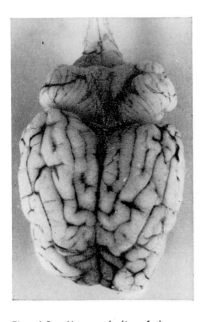

Fig. 6.2 — Hypocephalia of the vermis of the cerebellum in a lamb. (Department of Veterinary Pathology, Michigan State University.)

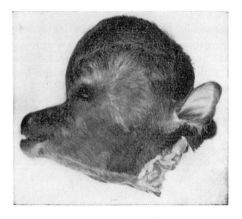

Fig. 6.3 — Hydrencephalocele, defective skull with brain protruding. Ventricles distended with fluid. (Department of Veterinary Pathology, Michigan State University.)

part; and *aplasia* — absence or imperfect development of an organ or part.

**Acrania,** absence of most or all of the bones of the cranium.

**Anencephalia,** absence of the brain.

**Hypocephalia,** incomplete development of the brain (Fig. 6.2).

**Hemicrania,** absence of half of the head.

**Exencephalia,** defective skull with brain exposed or extruded. If the protruding brain contains a ventricle which is filled with excessive amount of fluid, the malformation is a hydrencephalocele (Fig. 6.3).

**Arhinencephalia,** absence or rudimentary development of the olfactory lobe with corresponding lack of development of the external olfactory organs.

**Agnathia,** absence of the lower jaw (first visceral arch).

**Anophthalmia,** absence of one or both eyes.

**Abrachia,** absence of the forelimbs.

**Abrachiocephalia,** absence of forelimbs and head.

**Adactylia,** absence of digits.

**Atresia,** absence of normal opening, e.g., atresia ani (Fig. 6.4).

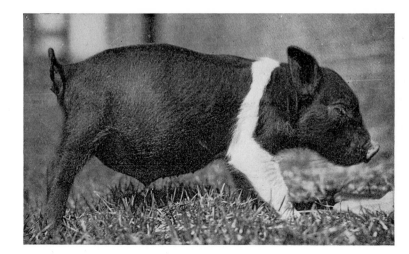

Fig. 6.4 — Anal atresia in a 3-week-old male pig. Note distention of abdomen and protrusion in anal region. (Department of Veterinary Pathology, Iowa State University.)

**Microphthalmia,** incomplete development of the eye resulting in an abnormally small organ of vision (Fig. 6.5).

2. *Fissures* on the median line of the head, thorax, and abdomen.

**Cranioschisis** (skull).

**Cheiloschisis** (lip), often referred to as harelip.

**Palatoschisis** (oral cavity), often called cleft palate (Fig. 6.6). Harelip and cleft palate result from faulty development of the maxillary process derived from the first visceral arch.

**Rachischisis** (spinal column).

**Schistorrachis or spina bifida** (spinal column).

**Schistothorax** (thorax or sternum).

**Schistosomus** (abdomen).

**Schistocormus** (thorax, neck, or abdominal wall). Results from arrested development of the amnion.

3. *Fusion* of paired organs.

**Cyclopia** (eyes).

**Ren arcuatus** (kidneys), often referred to as horseshoe kidney.

Fig. 6.5 — Microphthalmia, incomplete development of the eyes. (F. W. Schofield.)

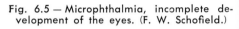

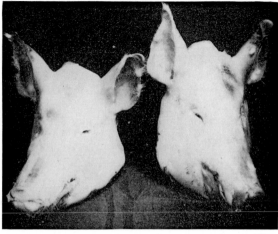

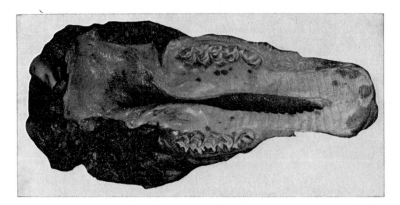

Fig. 6.6 — Palatoschisis in a 6-week-old Holstein heifer calf. (Department of Veterinary Pathology, Iowa State University.)

B. Excess of development.
1. *Congenital hypertrophy* (Fig. 8.1).
Hemihypertrophy (partial).
2. *Increase* in the number of a part.
Polyotia (ears).
Polyodontia (teeth).
Polymelia (limbs).
Polydactylia (digits) (Fig. 6.7).
Polymastia (mammary gland).
Polythelia (teats).

## DISPLACEMENTS DURING DEVELOPMENT

A. Displacements of organs.
Dextrocardia, transposition of the heart to the right side.
Ectopia cordis cervicalis, displacement of the heart into the neck.
B. Displacements of tissues.
Teratoma, inclusion of an abortive fetus within a normal individual.
Dermoid, inclusion within a normal individual of a tumorous, cystic mass containing skin, hair, feathers, or teeth, depending upon the species.
Dentigerous cyst, a displaced dental follicle containing fluid and teeth.

## PERSISTENCE OF FETAL STRUCTURES

This includes the foramen ovale, ductus arteriosus, urachus, Wolffian ducts (mesonephric ducts), the vitelline duct (Meckel's diverticulum), and branchial clefts.

## FUSION OF SEXUAL CHARACTERS

Hermaphrodite, an individual having both testicular and ovarian tissue.
Pseudohermaphrodite, an animal having unisexual development of the sex glands (either testicular or ovarian tissue), but having also either a unisexual or bisexual development of the other parts of the genitalia. If the development of the external genitals is unisexual, the glands do not correspond in sex with the remainder of the genitalia (Fig. 6.8). *Freemartin*, a female calf having arrested development of the sex organs and being the twin of a perfect male. A freemartin is sometimes incorrectly called a hermaphrodite, but this type of malformation is not a fusion of sex organs; it is characterized simply by a lack of development of these organs. There is a rudimentary vagina and uterus; the vulva is small or absent; the urethra often opens in the perineal region; there may be an enlarged clitoris; the gonads are so undeveloped that they

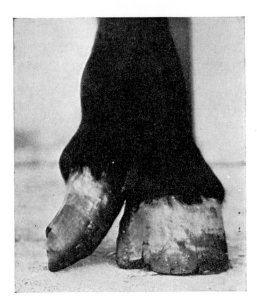

Fig. 6.7 — Polydactylia in a 7-month-old colt. (Iowa State University Veterinarian.)

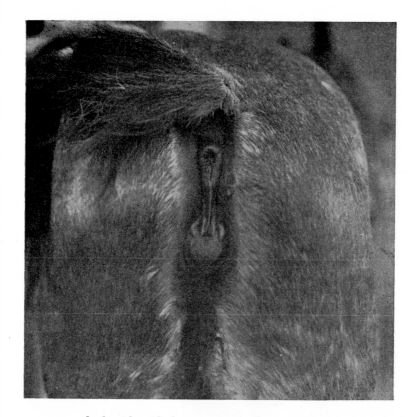

Fig. 6.8 — Female - like external genitals of a pseudohermaphro d i t e horse which had male gonads. Testicles were poorly developed, and one was undescended. (Department of Veterinary Pathology, Iowa State University.)

can scarcely be identified as ovaries; the udder is small; and the parenchyma is not clearly differentiated from the surrounding adipose tissue. A similar arrest of development of the sex organs also occurs in other species but not with such regularity as in the bovine. The most plausible explanation for the origin of a freemartin is based upon the following facts: (1) In the bovine in twin pregnancy there is usually fusion of the chorions and anastomosis of the circulation of the fetuses. (2) Sex hormones appear earlier in the male fetus than in the female. (3) When one fetus is a male and the other a female, the male hormone circulating in the blood of the female twin stimulates the recessive male characters in the female before the dominant female characters are stimulated by her own hormones. The result is a sterile female with internal genitals predominantly male in character, and external genitals mostly female in type. So frequent is freemartinism that it is said that a normal female may be expected only about once in 12 cases of twinning in which both sexes are represented.

## MONSTERS

**Definition.** A monster or monstrosity is a disturbance of development that involves several organs and causes great distortion of the individual. For the most part monsters possess a duplication of all or most of the organs and other parts of the body. They develop from a single ovum. They are therefore the product of incomplete twinning. The conjoined pair have a single chorion and are of the same sex. In a kind of sea minnow called Fundulus, complete and incomplete twinning can be caused by subjecting the embryos to adverse conditions during the late cleavage stages. In birds, double chicken embryos have been produced by a similar procedure at about the time of gastrulation. It is believed that these experiments throw some light on the etiology of monsters, although what the cause of any particular monstrous individual may be can rarely be stated with surety.

## Classification of Monsters

### TWINS ENTIRELY SEPARATE

Although separate, these twins are in a single chorion. One twin as a rule is well developed; the other is malformed (acardiacus). In the malformed fetus there is more or less arrested development of the heart, lungs, and trunk. Such monsters may lack a head (acephalus), limbs, and other recognizable features (amorphus), or the trunk (acormus).

### TWINS UNITED

These twins are more or less completely united and are of symmetrical development.

**A. Anterior twinning.**

The anterior part of the individual is double, the posterior single.

1. *Pygopagus* — united in the pelvic region with the bodies side by side.

2. *Ischiopagus* — united in the pelvic region with the bodies at an obtuse angle.

3. *Dicephalus* — two separate heads; doubling may also affect the neck, thorax, and trunk. According to the number of posterior and anterior extremities present, dicephalus is given the added designations tetrapus, tripus, dipus, tetrabrachius, tribrachius, and dibrachius.

4. *Diprosopus* — doubling in the cephalic region without complete separation of heads; only the face doubled. Added designation depends upon the number of (a) eyes (tetrophthalmus, triophthalmus, diophthalmus), (b) ears (tetrotus, triotus, diotus), (c) mouths (distomus, monostomus), and (d) forelimbs (tribrachius, dibrachius).

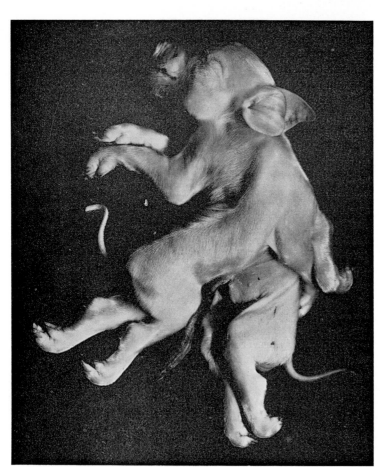

Fig. 6.9 — A pig monstrosity of the type designated dipygus tetrabrachius. (Department of Veterinary Pathology, Iowa State University.)

**B. Posterior twinning.**

The posterior part is double, the anterior single. The position of human monsters relative to each other may be dorsal (back to back), lateral (side to side) or ventral (abdomen to abdomen). The position of monsters of domestic mammals is practically always ventral.

1. *Craniopagus* — brains usually separated; bodies as a rule at an acute angle. Depending upon the place of attachment, the following forms are recognized: parietalis, frontalis, and occipitalis.

2. *Cephalothoracopagus* — union of head and thorax.

3. *Dipygus* — doubling of posterior extremities and posterior part of body. Dipygus may have the form dibrachius or tetrabrachius (Fig. 6.9).

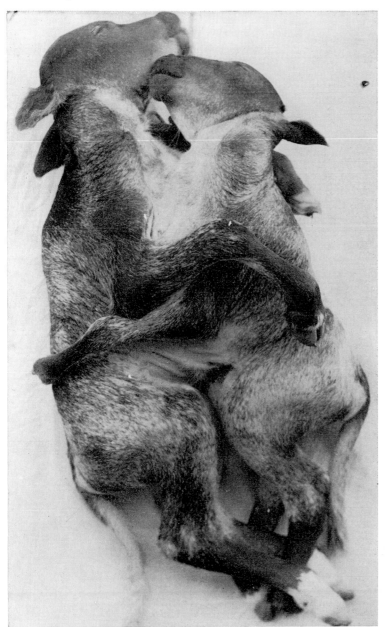

Fig. 6.10 — Incomplete twinning with union at the thorax (thoracopagus). (Department of Veterinary Pathology, Michigan State University.)

**C. Twinning almost complete.**

Duplication of the whole trunk or the anterior or posterior extremities with parallel, ventral arrangement of the fetuses. The pair is joined in the region of the thorax, often also in the abdominal region.

1. *Thoracopagus* — united only by the thorax. Again the number of fore and hind extremities determines the complete designation of the monster (Fig. 6.10).
2. *Prosopothoracopagus* — besides the union of the thorax and abdomen, the head and neck are united.
3. *Rachipagus* — thoracic and lumbar portion of the spinal column united.

All of the double monsters thus far mentioned have symmetrical development. They may also have asymmetrical growth; that is, one of the pair may be smaller and less well developed than the other. This one is called the parasite and the more normally developed one the autosite. Often the parasite is partially embedded in the autosite.

## REFERENCES

Eaton, O. N.: 1937. A summary of lethal characters in animals and man. Jour. Hered., 28:320.

Emerson, M. A., and Hazel, L. N.: 1956. Radiographic demonstration of dwarf gene-carrier beef animals Jour. A.V.M.A. 128:381.

Field, R. A., Rickard, C. G., and Hutt, F. B.: 1946. Hemophilia in a family of dogs. Cornell Vet., 36:285.

Fourie, P. J. J.: 1936. The occurrence of congenital porphyrinuria (pink tooth) in cattle in South Africa (Swazeland). Onderstepoort Jour. Vet. Sci., 7:535.

Gruenwald, P.: 1947. Mechanisms of abnormal development. I. Causes of abnormal development in the embryo. II. Embryonic development of malformations. III. Postnatal developmental abnormalities. Arch. Path., 44: 398, 495, and 648.

Hutt, F. B.: 1946. Some hereditary abnormalities of domestic animals. Cornell Vet., 36:180.

Muhrer, M. E., Hogan, A. G., and Bogart, R.: 1942. A defect in the coagulation mechanism of swine blood. Amer. Jour. Physiol., 136:355.

Tyler, W. S., Julian, L. M., and Gregory, P. W.: 1957. The nature of the process responsible for the short-headed Hereford dwarf as revealed by gross examination of the appendicular skeleton. Amer. Jour. Anat., 101:477.

| # Disturbances in Circulation

The description of the circulation of the blood by William Harvey was the most important single contribution to anatomic pathology. Without an understanding of the circulatory system and how the blood progresses through it, the major alterations in pathology could not be explained. Terms such as hyperemia, hemorrhage, thrombosis, embolism and metastasis would have no meaning. The distribution of oxygen and nutrient through the body as well as the removal of waste material could not be explained. Since hyperemia is the most basic of these alterations, it will be discussed first.

## HYPEREMIA

**Definition.** Hyperemia is an increased amount of blood in any portion of the circulatory system.

The circulation of blood through the tissues is governed principally by (1) the action of the heart, (2) changes in the diameter of the lumen of the vessels, and (3) the amount of blood. With regard to local disturbances in circulation, the alterations in the diameter of the vessel lumen are of most importance. The smaller arteries and arterioles are supplied with vasomotor fibers, and some of these apparently supply the capillaries also. The amount of blood passing through the vessels depends upon the action of

these nerves. Under normal or physiologic conditions there are marked variations in the amount of blood passing through the tissues. Most organs are made up of units. In organs at rest, the flow through the units which are functioning is very abundant, and very little flows through the inactive ones. In active organs, however, the increased blood supply has a more diffuse distribution. This constitutes physiologic hyperemia. It occurs in the stomach and intestines which contain ingesta, in the spleen at more or less periodic intervals, in the lactating mammary gland, in the so-called sexual skin of female monkeys during the menstrual cycle, in the testicles of sexually mature cockerels, in active muscles, and in the skin during periods of increased heat production. Hyperemia becomes pathologic when the changes are excessive and lasting.

### Active Hyperemia

**Definition.** Active hyperemia is an increased amount of blood in the arterial side of the vascular system. Usually it is due to inflammation in the tissue or organ.

It is caused by the direct action upon the vessel walls of various physical and chemical irritants and by many bacteria and their toxic products. Heat and trauma are examples of physical causal agents. Various acids, bases, and their salts exert a similar action. Active hyperemia is always one of the several changes which are present in an acute inflammation.

Grossly, the affected area is red and swollen. If it is on the surface of the body it is warmer than normal. Microscopically, hyperemia is recognized by the presence of capillaries distended with blood. In normal tissues blood is not conspicuous in these tiny vessels. The erythrocytes, which are the most prominent element in the blood, usually flow through the capillaries in single file. In hyperemia, however, several erythrocytes, 10 to 20 or even more, may be counted across the diameter of a capillary.

### Passive Hyperemia

**Definition.** Passive hyperemia is an increased amount of blood in the venous side of the vascular system due to some form of hindrance to the flow of blood from an organ or region. The word congestion is sometimes used to indicate passive hyperemia; however, the term hyperemia is preferable.

The condition is general if the impediment is central, i.e., in the heart or lungs, and local if in the vein of an organ or part of the body. It can be acute or chronic, but the latter is of greater frequency.

#### ACUTE LOCAL PASSIVE HYPEREMIA

**Definition.** Acute local passive hyperemia is a temporary increase in the amount of blood in the veins of a portion (foot, tail, kidney, spleen, etc.) of an individual as the result of an obstruction to the flow of blood from an organ or region.

In the acute form the venous obstruction which gives rise to the condition is either (1) an intravenous clot (thrombus), or (2) it is caused by sudden pressure exerted upon the vessel as occurs in intestinal displacements (strangulation, torsion, volvulus, and invagination). The first-mentioned condition, thrombosis, usually affects large vessels. In special pathology it will be noted that certain veins in particular species of animals are more subject to this obstruction than others. In the second condition, that of sudden obstruction due to pressure, the hyperemia is extreme for two reasons. First, the veins, being thin-walled, are compressed more than the thicker-walled arteries. This allows blood to continue to enter the area, but its exit is seriously interfered with. Secondly, the sudden onset of the condition allows no time for collateral circulation to develop. When the obstruction arises slowly, anastomosing veins can become large enough to take care of the extra volume of blood, and hyperemia is scarcely noticed.

Microscopically, the venules and capillaries are stuffed with blood. In severe cases some may be ruptured. The tissue spaces are filled with lymph. Macroscopically, the affected part or organ is dark red in color, rather cold, edematous, and enlarged.

#### CHRONIC LOCAL PASSIVE HYPEREMIA

**Definition.** Chronic local passive hyperemia is an increase in the amount of blood that persists for a long time in the veins of a portion of the body and causes permanent tissue alterations in the area.

Chronic local passive hyperemia is due to venous obstruction produced by pressure exerted by tumors, enlarged lymph nodes, aneurysms, parasitic cysts, and extensive perivascular fibrosis, e.g., hepatic cirrhosis. The results are not so severe as in the acute forms, because opportunity is given for collateral circulation to develop. In the more severe forms, because of the decreased supply of oxygen and food, and also because of the pressure exerted by the accumulated blood, the parenchyma of the part is damaged. Lack of nutrition and the accumulation of waste products disturbs its function. Pressure produced by the excessive amount of blood may cause atrophy and even death of the parenchyma. Later these cells may be replaced with connective tissue if they cannot regenerate.

#### ACUTE GENERAL PASSIVE HYPEREMIA

**Definition.** Acute general passive hyperemia is an increase in the amount of blood in the venous side of the circulatory system due to a sudden obstruction to the flow of blood in the heart or lungs. The hyperemia involves the entire venous side of the circulatory system.

Acute general passive hyperemia results from interference with the functioning of one or more of the so-called blood pumps, namely, (1) the heart, (2) the movements of respiration including the diaphragm, and (3) the movements of muscles. Regardless of which one of the pumps is incapacitated, the end result is that venous blood stagnates because its onward flow is impeded.

1. Disturbances of the heart which result in general passive hyperemia are those in which there is myocardial weakness, or constriction or leakage of the valves on the right side. Myocardial weakness is often due to severe acute general bacterial or viral infections such as anthrax and canine distemper. It may also be caused by chemical poisons such as lead and arsenic. Since the myocardial degeneration usually occurs late in these intoxications, general passive hyperemia frequently does not occur until near the time of death and is often the final pathological change necessary to bring about death.

2. The respiratory (diaphragmatic) pump may inadequately aid circulation whenever the lungs cease to function normally, as in hydrothorax, or when painful diseases of the thoracic wall cause breathing to be shallow, as in fracture of the ribs or acute inflammation of the pleura.

3. The help which muscular movements give to circulation is diminished in animals which are in a state of coma, as in milk fever and ketosis of cows.

CHRONIC GENERAL PASSIVE HYPEREMIA

**Definition.** Chronic general passive hyperemia is an increase in the amount of blood in the venous side of the circulatory system that persists for a long period of time and results in permanent alterations (atrophy and fibrosis) in various tissues and organs throughout the body.

The cardiac lesions which give rise to this form of hyperemia are (1) either changes in the amount of valvular clearance due to narrowing of the openings (stenosis) or to inability of the valves to close the opening completely (insufficiency or incompetence), or (2) diminished heart power due to myocardial weakness or failure. In the case of the valvular lesions there is a constant obstruction to the flow of blood. In the majority of cases this obstruction is at the left atrioventricular (mitral) valve. Obviously, this results first in an accumulation of blood in the left atrium, then in the lungs, later in the right chambers of the heart, and eventually in the venous system.

In the case of diminished heart power due to myocardial weakness or failure, the congestion is brought about in a different manner. The weakened myocardium fails to force enough blood into the aorta. Consequently the arterial blood pressure falls. To overcome this, the arterioles contract. The end result is that the volume of blood in the venous system is increased.

In the lungs the chief causes of the obstruction are (1) chronic emphysema (heaves in horses), and (2) fibrosis resulting from chronic pulmonary infections. In the case of emphysema, the alveoli become ballooned and may rupture. As a consequence the capillaries in their walls are stretched and compressed, and many are destroyed. The whole process acts as a hindrance to the flow of blood through the lungs from the right side of the heart. Its accumulation here leads to its accumulation in the venous system. In the case of pulmonary fibrosis, connective tissue replaces the lung parenchyma and its very extensive capillary bed. This acts as an impediment to the flow of blood into the lungs. Its accumulation in the right side of the heart is eventually felt in the venous system.

**Effects of chronic general passive hyperemia.** Since the lungs are usually involved in this condition, a description of the effects should begin with them. With the accumulation of blood in the venules and capillaries the circulation slows down. Naturally, this means that the margin of safety of oxygen is lowered, and the concentration of carbon dioxide in the blood increases. The increased carbon dioxide stimulates the respiratory center and causes labored breathing (dyspnea). The decrease in oxygen results in an increase in reduced hemoglobin which in turn makes the blood more venous in appearance. The visible mucous membranes have a purplish or bluish tinge (cyanosis) because their capillaries are distended with this venous blood.

The accumulation of blood deficient in oxygen and excessively rich in carbon dioxide probably has an injurious effect on the walls of the veins which permits plasma to escape from them into the surrounding tissues (edema). This is especially true in dependent parts of the body, i.e., those farthest removed from the heart, such as the legs. Another, and probably even more important factor, contributes to the edema in these regions. It is the increased intercapillary blood pressure (hydrostatic pressure) due to the circulatory obstruction. Fluid escapes not only into the tissues but also into the serous cavities (hydropericardium, hydrothorax, and hydroperitoneum).

**Macroscopic and microscopic appearance.** In the early stages of passive hyperemia the part affected is somewhat increased in size and dark red to purplish red in color because the capillaries and venules are distended with venous blood. If the part is an organ which normally has sharp borders, the borders become rounded. When cut, dark red blood flows freely from the surface.

As the process continues, the presence of the large amount of venous blood causes nutritional and pressure atrophy of the parenchymatous cells, and at the same time favors the proliferation of connective tissue which nearly always thrives under conditions unfavorable to the more highly specialized, but less resistant, parenchyma cells. The behavior of fibroblasts and parenchyma cells under these conditions reminds one of the relationship of quack grass to grain under bad weather conditions or on infertile soil.

The connective tissue gradually increases, and as it matures it shrinks. This causes the blood volume in the part to decrease, the consistency to become more firm and tough, and the size to diminish. It also changes the color from dark or purplish red to a grayish red or grayish blue.

### Hypostatic Congestion

**Definition.** Hypostatic congestion, or hypostasis, is a special form of hyperemia that occurs in the dependent parts of the body of recumbent, weak, sick animals and in animals a short time before death, probably due to a loss of vascular tone or cardiac weakness. It also occurs after death in the lowermost parts of the body due to the settling of the blood by gravity.

### ISCHEMIA

**Definition.** Ischemia (local anemia) is a deficiency of arterial blood in a portion of an organ or region.

The chief causes of ischemia are: (1) external pressure upon an artery, (2) narrowing of the lumen of an artery, and (3) diversion of blood from one part of the body to another (collateral anemia).

With reference to the first cause, that of external pressure upon an artery, it should be mentioned that when such pressure is exerted upon an artery the effect upon the accompanying vein is even more pronounced than upon the artery, and as a consequence a passive hyperemia or hemorrhagic infarction is the result rather than anemia. But if the pressure is great enough, as when a tourniquet is tightly applied, the result is local anemia. Similarly, a rapidly growing neoplasm, the accumulation of large amounts of exudate or transudate in a serous cavity, or the distention of a hollow organ causes anemia in adjacent structures. The pressure resulting from the contact of external bony prominences of recumbent, debilitated, emaciated animals with a hard floor or the ground results in ischemia which eventually leads to local tissue death (decubital ulcer).

The second cause, that of a narrowing of the lumen of an artery, has not the same significance in animal pathology that it has in human pathology. The reason is that animals are seldom affected with arteriosclerosis which is the principal cause of the narrowing of arterial lumina in man. The classic example of a narrowing of an arterial lumen in animals is furnished by the horse in which verminous thrombosis and embolism of branches of the anterior mesenteric artery occur. Here, however, because of the extensive anastomosis, closure does not result in total anemia but in the formation of a hemorrhagic infarct which may be just as serious in its end results.

The third cause, namely the sudden diversion of blood from one part of the body to another, affects the brain chiefly. Brain anemia occurs following the rapid removal of large quantities of pleural or peritoneal exudate or transudate, or the sudden relief of ruminal tympanites in cattle by trocharization.

**Effects of local anemia.** The effects of local anemia are varied. They depend upon the size of the occluded vessel, the degree of occlusion, the rate of closure, the amount of anastomosis, and the kind of tissue affected. In the study of systemic pathology this subject will be considered in detail. Here it need only be said that if the closure is rapid and anastomosis is absent or poor, necrosis occurs. If the closure is slow and anastomosis absent or deficient, atrophy and perhaps some necrosis of the parenchyma occur. The tissue which dies is replaced with connective tissue (fibrosis). If the closure is gradual and anastomosis good, no effects may be apparent. Grossly, the anemic part or organ is paler than normal, often tinged slightly with yellow, the temperature is lowered, and the volume diminished.

## HEMORRHAGE

**Definition.** Hemorrhage is the escape of all of the constituents of the blood from any portion of the blood vascular system.

Obviously, escape of the blood constituents can take place when there is a break in the continuity of the wall of a vessel or the heart. This is designated hemorrhage by **rhexis**. The escape may occur, however, when there is no apparent microscopic anatomic alteration in the vessel wall, particularly in capillaries and venules. This is called hemorrhage by **diapedesis**.

**Etiology of hemorrhage.** Breaks in the continuity of the walls of the cardiovascular system which result in hemorrhage by rhexis are: (1) trauma such as cuts, bruises, lacerations, and punctures, including those made by certain bloodsucking parasites; (2) erosions such as occur in intestinal ulcers, rapidly infiltrating tumors, and rapidly developing nodules of tuberculosis and glanders; (3) diseases of the vessel walls which weaken their structure as, for example, calcification and aneurysm; (4) increased blood pressure from excitement or in acute passive hyperemia; and (5) deficiency of oxygen in the blood (hypoxia) such as occurs in asphyxia.

Hemorrhage that occurs through the apparently unruptured walls of capillaries and venules is caused by mechanical and toxic influences. All the elements of the blood escape as in hemorrhage by rhexis, but the designation hemorrhage by diapedesis is supposed to indicate the manner in which the erythrocytes leave the vessels. The designation, however, is incorrect because only certain of the leukocytes possess ameboid movement which permits them to escape in this way. Just how the erythrocytes escape has not yet been completely explained. Some believe they find their way out between the endothelial cells of the vessel walls, but reasons for this permeability have not been fully determined. Some physical chemists attempting to explain this on the basis of the properties of colloidal particles suggest that the erythrocytes pass directly through the endothelial cells like droplets of a dense colloidal material through one of less density (a drop of mercury through a mass of gelatin). Regardless of whether the red cells pass out between the endothelial cells or through them, it seems likely that certain injurious influences damage the walls of the capillaries and venules to such an extent that they become more permeable. Thus hemorrhage occurs in chronic passive hyperemia, a mechanical condition, but the actual reason for the escape of blood may be a nervous influence, a vasomotor paralysis. This type of hemorrhage also occurs in poisoning with some inorganic chemical substances (phosphorus), and in many bacterial and viral infections, especially in those of a septicemic nature (pasteurellosis, anthrax, blackleg, hog cholera, canine leptospirosis).

Hemorrhages are characteristic lesions of an intestinal toxicosis (enterotoxemia) of feeder lambs and nursing lambs, kids, calves, and pigs (Fig. 7.1). The intoxication is caused by the toxins of certain types of *Clostridium perfringens*.

The toxin apparently is produced by the microorganism in the small intestine, principally in the jejunum and ileum. Conditions are most favorable for the

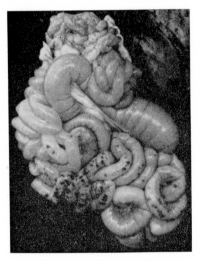

Fig. 7.1 — Hemorrhages of various sizes in the small intestine of a lamb with enterotoxemia. (Department of Veterinary Pathology, Michigan State University.)

toxin production when the intestine contains much milk or other highly nutritious feed. The results of injury of the blood vessels caused by the toxin are seen most often in the peritoneum, epicardium, endocardium, thymus, and diaphragm, where petechiae, ecchymoses, and even suffusions may occur.

Hemorrhage is a prominent characteristic of the disease purpura hemorrhagica which occurs chiefly in horses. Hemorrhages and edema appear in many parts of the body but are most constant in the subcutaneous and submucous connective tissue. The cause of the condition has not been determined for certain. Circumstantial evidence points toward it being the result of a septic bacterial intoxication following an active microbic infection in which there is much suppuration and necrosis. Most often it is a postinfection intoxication associated with strangles, pneumonia, and various pyogenic infections but especially with those produced by streptococci. It seems likely that the bacterial toxin still present in the blood after the infection has disappeared can damage the venules and capillaries so that hemorrhages and edema result.

Hemorrhage is also a prominent characteristic of sweet-clover disease of cattle which results from the continuous feeding of toxic sweet clover. At times sweet clover produces this disease because it contains a toxic coumarin compound. The hay containing dicoumarol must be fed continuously for about a month to cause the intoxication. Although there is a massive escape of blood from the vessels into the tissues and body cavities, no alterations have been discovered in the vessel walls. In this disease the blood which escapes from the vessels does not coagulate, hence the bleeding is a rather continuous process and usually results in the death of the animal. Failure of the blood to coagulate is due to its low prothrombin content. Whether the decrease in prothrombin is the result of the destruction or inactivation of prothrombin, or of interference with the mechanism which is responsible for its formation has not been determined. Inadequate calcium concentration of the blood may be a contributing factor. In sweet-clover poisoning, hemorrhages may occur in almost any part of the body but they most frequently occur in the subcutaneous and intermuscular fascia, and in the serous membranes. In the latter they are especially prominent in the epicardium, diaphragm, and rumen (Figs. 5.4 and 7.2). Horses seem to resist the effects of the anticoagulant. Link suggests that their digestive tracts may not be sufficiently alkaline for absorption of the coumarin compound or that rapid and efficient detoxification takes place.

**Classification of hemorrhages.** Hemorrhages are classified according to the source of the blood in them, the size of the collection of extravasated blood and the location of the bleeding in the body. The adjectives arterial, venous, and capillary when applied to hemorrhages naturally indicate the source of blood. Size and shape of hemorrhages are most accurately

expressed in exact measurements and by description, but adjectives such as petechial and ecchymotic give some indication of both of these factors. Petechial hemorrhages, or petechiae (singular, petechia), are tiny and punctate, having a diameter not larger than one millimeter (Fig. 7.3). Ecchymotic hemorrhages (Fig. 7.4), or ecchymoses (singular, ecchymosis), are circumscribed hemorrhages only a few millimeters in diameter. For convenience of classification one can limit their size to 10 millimeters.

Small hemorrhages the size of petechiae or small ecchymoses, arising just prior to death and in association with the death struggle, are called agonal hemorrhages. They are a sign of asphyxiation (hypoxemia). Hemorrhages which appear as lines, most often on the crests of folds in the mucous membrane of the gastrointestinal tract and on the serous surfaces of some organs, are called linear hemorrhages (Fig. 17.25). Diffuse, flat, often irregular-shaped areas of bleeding are

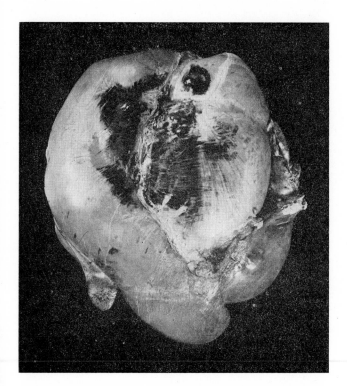

Fig. 7.2 — Diffuse hemorrhage in the serosa of the rumen of a cow with sweet-clover poisoning. (Roderick, Jour. A.V.M.A.)

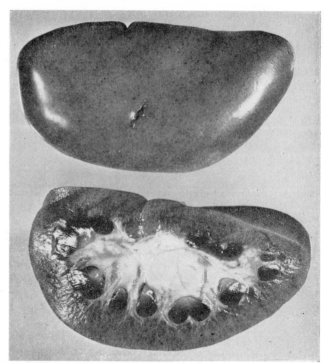

Fig. 7.3 — Petechial hemorrhages in the kidney of a pig with hog cholera. (Department of Veterinary Pathology, Michigan State University.)

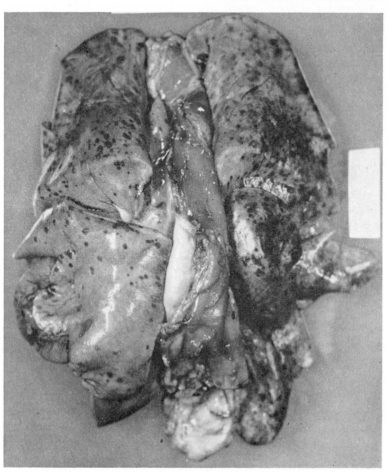

Fig. 7.4 — Ecchymotic hemorrhages in the lung of a dog with severe staphylococcic infection. (Department of Veterinary Pathology, Michigan State University.)

termed suffusions (Fig. 7.2). If the extravasated blood collects in a spherical-shaped mass in the tissues, it is designated a hematocyst or hematoma (Fig. 7.5). The latter term is a misnomer, and its use is often misleading to the student. The suffix -*oma* is used in connection with the names of tumors. Its use with reference to a collection of blood may give the impression that the mass is a blood tumor, which is incorrect. Large collections of blood of this nature often occur in sweet-clover disease of cattle where their volumes at times may be as much as twelve quarts. When such hematocysts appear they are usually located in and between muscles, under the scapula, or around the esophagus.

According to location, hemorrhages can be around structures, under membranes, within the parenchyma of organs, underneath their capsules, or in body cavities. With this in mind, the significance of the following designations for hemorrhages is quite obvious: perivascular, perirenal, subserous, submucous, parenchymatous, subcapsular, hemothorax, and hemometra.

Bleeding from various body openings is given special designations such as epistaxis (nosebleed), hemoptysis (spitting blood), hematemesis (vomiting blood), entorrhagia (intestinal hemorrhage), metrorrhagia (uterine bleeding), and hematuria (discharging bloody urine).

**Changes in extravasated blood.** In small hemorrhages the erythrocytes are removed by macrophages and the serum is absorbed into the lymphatics and veins. In large hemorrhages there is hemolysis. The hemoglobin is split by ferments into a soluble protein (globin) and an insoluble iron-containing pigment (hematin). The latter disintegrates into hematoidin and hemosiderin. Hematoidin is iron-free and is deposited in the tissues as granules or rhombic crystals or is converted into soluble bilirubin which is carried away in the lymph. Hemosiderin contains iron, appears as amorphous granules, is phagocytized by macrophages, and is carried to the lymph nodes.

**Arrest of hemorrhage.** There are two steps in the arrest of hemorrhage. (1) A

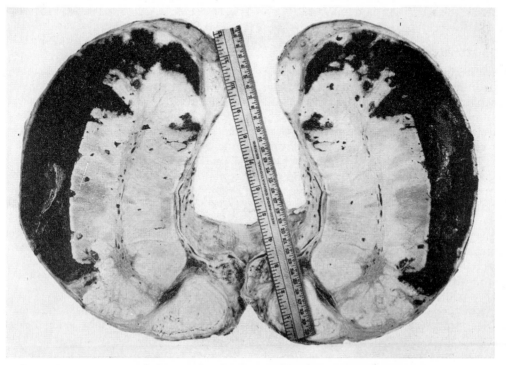

Fig. 7.5 — Hematocyst of the testicle of a boar infected with **Brucella suis.** The cyst contained almost a liter of coagulated blood. (McNutt, Jour. A.V.M.A.)

temporary clot forms, which is nature's way of supplying a first-aid plug to a ruptured vessel. At first the clot is red (erythrocytes and fibrin). Later it becomes white, sticky, soft, and jelly-like (mostly platelets). (2) Following the initial clot formation, the margins of the opening in the vessel wall exhibit an inflammatory process which is accompanied by an outgrowth of newly formed connective tissue and capillaries into the temporary clot. This permanently arrests the hemorrhage and repairs the damage insofar as it can be repaired. This is called organization of a hemorrhage.

Massive hemorrhage into the body cavities undergoes a similar sequence of changes. After the formation of the clot, fibroblasts and angioblasts originating in the serous membranes (parietal and visceral) push out into the clot and organize it. In time the newly formed connective tissue shrinks, leaving the adjacent serous surfaces firmly adherent (adhesions) or covered with fibrous tags. Hematocysts in the subcutis or in muscles terminate in a similar manner, but the final marker to indicate their location is a mass of tough scar tissue.

## SLUDGED BLOOD

**Definition.** The sludging of blood is the conglutination of erythrocytes within the vascular system of the living individual.

In normal circulating blood the erythrocytes repel each other slightly. They are not coated with any apparent protein precipitate which would tend to cause them to agglutinate. Neither do these cells adhere to the endothelium of normal vessels because the endothelium is smooth and clean. In normal flowing blood the cells form a central core in the lumen surrounded by a peripheral layer of plasma. The cells in the center of the core move more swiftly than those at the periphery.

In healthy animals the size of the lumina of the small vessels (arterioles, capillaries, sinusoids, and venules) is in a constant state of fluctuation to accommodate the physiologic needs of the tissues relative to nutrients, the removal of metabolites, and heat. These small, normal vessels in most tissues and organs do not permit much loss of blood fluid so the blood is in a constant liquid state — that is, there is no hemoconcentration. Neither is there an accumulation of lymph outside the vessels (edema) because the normal endothelium allows only enough leakage to nourish the tissues.

In man and animals, in a great variety of disease conditions, it has been observed that important changes occur in the circulating blood — changes which become apparent in the physical relationship of the blood cells. The cells cease to repel one another. Instead, they agglutinate so that a circulating sludge is formed. The cells adhere to each other because they become coated with a thin film of plasma protein.

Conglutination of erythrocytes (sludged blood) has been observed in the vessels of the exposed conjunctiva of living, unanesthetized, unoperated animals and humans, using binocular dissecting microscopes with special light. They are not changes which can be demonstrated in microscopic sections such as are studied in the laboratory.

This state of the blood has been studied in various inflammatory and noninflammatory processes resulting from almost all classes of etiological agents (physical, chemical, and biological). It is known that such a hematologic change also occurs in the circulating blood of domestic animals under similar conditions. It has been found in acidentally ill, unanesthetized, comatose rabbits and cats, and has been studied in the blood of pigs experimentally infected with hog cholera virus.

The effects of the agglutination of the blood cells are very grave. First, clumping of the erythrocytes in the pulmonary capillaries interferes with oxygen intake by the blood. Furthermore, sludged blood flows more slowly. The combined effects of these two changes result in hypoxia of the tissues of the body and may lead to degenerative changes. Secondly, the agglutinated erythrocytes act as emboli and plug small arterioles and capillaries. The emboli may give rise to areas of focal necrosis or to the formation of intravascular clots (thrombi) which in turn lead to large areas of necrosis (infarcts). Third, since sludged blood flows more slowly, the oxygen supply of the capillary endothelium becomes inadequate. The poorly nourished and degenerating endothelium becomes more permeable, and edema results. This loss of fluid leaves the blood in the vessels in a state of greater concentration. Fourth, if the sludging is very extensive, death occurs within a few hours.

In nonfatal cases where sludged blood occurs, the agglutinated erythrocytes are phagocytized by the reticuloendothelial cells of the liver, spleen, and bone marrow.

## THROMBOSIS

**Definition.** Thrombosis is the formation of a clot from the elements of the circulating blood within the vascular system. This clot is designated as a thrombus (plural, thrombi).

Some pathologists like to call a thrombus "an intravital, intravascular clot." All the elements of the blood take part in the clotting but in varying proportions. Platelets and fibrin enter into the process to a greater extent than do the erythrocytes and leukocytes.

**Pathogenesis of thrombosis.** Three factors are involved in the formation of a thrombus: (1) injury of the intima, (2) a slowing of the blood stream, and (3) alterations in the blood which favor coagulation.

The first factor, injury to the intima, is produced by (a) mechanical force, (b) infection, and (c) parasites. (a) Mechanical forces which cause severe contusion or crushing of tissues together with traumatic injury of the vessels of the region, and slow penetration of vessels by foreign bodies such as sometimes happens in the posterior vena cava and in the portal vein in cattle are examples. (b) Infection reaching the affected spot by way of the blood stream (thrombosis of the heart valves in chronic swine erysipelas), or by extension into a vessel from an adjacent inflammatory area (thrombosis of the uterine veins in septic metritis), or by direct entrance from without (veni-puncture of the jugular) are examples. (c) Irritation of the intima with resulting thrombosis of the anterior mesenteric artery and its branches or of the external iliac artery of horses caused by the larvae of *Strongylus vulgaris* is an example.

The second factor, slowing of the blood stream, permits the platelets to collect along the lining membrane of the cardiovascular system (endocardium and intima). Thrombosis, however, does not occur unless at the same time there is injury to the lining membrane which permits the platelets to cling and conglutinate. Places where the blood flows slowest, and consequently places where thrombi are most commonly encountered, are in the veins during passive hyperemia, in the arteries in aneurysmal dilatation, and in the heart in the auricular appendages and intratrabecular spaces.

The third factor, alterations in the blood which favor coagulation, exists whenever foreign substances appear in the blood stream. Occasionally heartworms (*Dirofilaria immitis*) in the pulmonary artery of dogs make conditions favorable for intravascular intravital clot formation. Fragments of heart valve thrombi and clumps of bacteria originating in an area of infection may act in a similar manner.

**Formation of a thrombus.** When the above-mentioned requisites for thrombus formation are present, the process begins at the point where the intima is injured. Platelets collect and conglutinate at this roughened spot. Masses of them form ridges on the vessel wall transversely to the blood stream. They fuse so tightly that their outlines cannot be seen in sections. They appear simply as pink-staining granular masses. When they conglutinate they liberate thromboplastic substances. As a result of this, fibrin is formed so that at this stage the clot consists only of platelets and fibrin. It is therefore white in color. With the formation of fibrin, numerous erythrocytes and leukocytes are trapped in its meshes. At this stage the falling out of erythrocytes is facilitated because the clot slows the flow of blood. The accumulation of erythrocytes then makes the clot appear red. Eventually the lumen of the vessel may be completely closed with the thrombus, and the red portion may extend up the vessel in the direction from which the blood flows. In time all the elements fuse into a more or less hyaline mass.

Physical chemists explain thrombus formation on the basis of colloidal flocculation. Their evidence seems to indicate that the flocculation of colloidal particles and the formation of fibrin are quite similar. Both apparently belong to the group of surface phenomena. The formation of fibrin (flocculation) depends upon influences which cause cytolysis of platelets and also upon changes in the surface composition of the blood as, for example, the presence in it of foreign colloidal substances which possess active internal surfaces. According to this theory, there is in the process of thrombus formation a conversion of fibrinogen (sol state of fibrin) into fibrin (gel state). This is brought about by the introduction and action of substances with great surface activity, around which fibrinogen (fibrin sol) will concentrate, adhere, and flocculate (change from the sol to gel state). Such surfaces are provided (1) whenever the inner lining of the heart (endocardium) or of the vessels (intima) is injured, (2) whenever foreign substances such as bacteria, products of bacterial or cell disintegration, and certain animal parasites appear in the blood, and (3) whenever the rate of blood flow is decreased.

Since thrombi vary in color, location, and composition, they may be classified in the following ways:

**Classification According to Location Within the Blood Vascular System**

(1) **Cardiac thrombi** are located in the heart. The thrombi may be attached to the valves (valvular thrombi) or walls (mural thrombi). Cardiac thrombi must not be confused with post-mortem clots, especially when the sedimentation rate of the blood is rapid and the blood has arranged itself, prior to clotting, into cellular and plasmatic components. Valvular thrombi are most commonly observed in the pig when the valve is invaded with *Streptococcus pyogenes* or *Erysipelothrix rhusiopathiae*. *Corynebacterium pyogenes* in cattle and *Streptococus equi* in horses are causes of valvular thrombi. Mural thrombi are most frequently observed in *Clostridium chauvoei* infections in the bovine and are particularly common on the wall of the left atrium. An acute fibrinous endocarditis with mural thrombosis is considered to be pathognomonic of blackleg.

(2) **Arterial thrombi** are located within arteries and are more frequently observed in domestic animals than are cardiac or venous thrombi. The thrombi that form in the anterior mesenteric artery of the horse as the result of injury produced by migrating *Strongylus vulgaris* larvae are excellent examples of this vascular alteration.

(3) **Venous thrombi** are found in veins. They are not as important in animals as they are in man because diseases of the veins which produce thrombosis are relatively uncommon in animals as compared to man. In addition, all animals, even when ill, move about, thus preventing sluggish circulation in injured veins. In contrast, when the human being is ill, he goes to bed, the circulation is sluggish, and this slowing of the blood stream favors thrombosis. A contributing factor to the high incidence of venous thrombosis in man is his erect position, particularly when a general passive hyperemia is present. This causes an unusual distention of veins afflicted with phlebitis. The sluggish circulation through these damaged veins favors the formation of thrombi. Venous thrombi in man are particularly common in the femoral vein of elderly bedridden individuals. Venous thrombi

in domestic animals are most frequently observed in the nasal vascular sinuses of the cow and horse, the veins of the broad ligament of the uterus of the cow, and in the scrotal plexus of the horse.

(4) **Capillary thrombi** are located within the capillaries. They are most frequently associated with inflammation because the etiologic agent injures the vascular endothelium. Structureless masses, commonly known as hyaline thrombi, are frequently observed in capillaries. These are not true thrombi because they are not composed of platelets and fibrin. They consist of a mass of agglutinated erythrocytes resulting from the intravenous administration of incompatible blood. They are also observed when conglutination of the erythrocytes associated with the sludging of blood is present. As a matter of differentiation, it must be remembered that post-mortem clotting of blood does not occur in the capillaries.

## Classification According to Location Within the Heart or Blood Vessel

(1) **Mural thrombi** are attached to the wall of the heart or blood vessel.

(2) **Valvular thrombi** are attached to the heart valves.

(3) **Lateral thrombi** are attached to one side of a vessel wall.

(4) **Occluding thrombi** are attached to the entire endothelial circumference of the vessel.

(5) **Saddle thrombi** straddle the bifurcation of blood vessels just as a saddle straddles the back of a horse.

(6) **Canalized thrombi** result when intravascular clots have been partially repaired and new blood channels have been formed through the clot, thus allowing a partial restoration of the circulation of blood through the vessel.

## Classification According to the Infectious Agent

(1) **Septic thrombi** are those intravascular clots that contain bacterial organisms.

(2) **Parasitic thrombi** are those intravascular clots that contain parasites (*Strongylus vulgaris* larvae in the horse and *Dirofilaria immitis* adults in the dog).

(3) **Aseptic thrombi** are those intravascular clots that do not contain bacteria or parasites.

## Classification According to Color

(1) A pale or **white thrombus** is buff or white in color and is composed almost entirely of platelets. It is observed in the heart and blood vessels (aorta, carotid, and femoral arteries). A white thrombus forms because platelets are sticky, and when they are swept along in the swiftly moving blood stream and come in contact with damaged endothelium, they are able to adhere to the site of injury. Fibrin is not deposited in a vessel that contains a swiftly moving stream of blood because an interval of time is required for the formation of fibrin. When the thrombokinase liberated by the damaged endothelium and disintegrating platelets comes in contact with the plasma of the blood, a chemical reaction occurs between thrombokinase, calcium ions, and fibrinogen. This chemical reaction is not instantaneous but requires as much as four minutes or even longer to take place. During this interval of time, the chemical constituents that were to form fibrin have been swept away by the blood stream, and the resulting fibrin, if it does form, is not able to attach to the site of injury. If fibrin were able to attach to the site of injury, erythrocytes would become entangled in the fibrin net and this would impart a red color to the thrombus. Since erythrocytes are not held in the area by platelets, the color of the thrombus remains white.

(2) A **red thrombus** is red in color and is composed of platelets, fibrin, erythrocytes, and leukocytes. The red color is due to the presence of erythrocytes entrapped in the meshwork of fibrin. A red thrombus is most frequently observed in

veins or in partially obstructed arteries where the flow of blood is sluggish or is near a state of stasis. In an area where the circulation is sluggish, the interval of time required for the formation of fibrin from thrombokinase, calcium ions, and fibrinogen is sufficient, and, as a result, fibrin becomes attached to the site of injury. A red thrombus may be confused with a post-mortem clot unless careful consideration is given to the characteristics of each.

(3) A **mixed thrombus** is composed of both white and red intravascular clots and is the most common type. The white portions are formed when the flow of blood through the area is rapid, and the red portions are formed when the circulation is sluggish.

(4) A **laminated thrombus** (Fig. 7.6) is a type of mixed thrombus composed of alternating layers of white and red constituents. This lamination is the result of variations in the rapidity of the flow of blood through the vessel. The factor determining whether the flow of blood is rapid or slow is the need for blood in the area vascularized by that vessel. When there is an increased metabolic activity in a limb as the re-

sult of exercise, the rapidity of blood flow through the leg is increased, and a white thrombus is formed. When the animal is at rest, the rate of flow is slow because less oxygen and nutrient is required in the area, and a red thrombus is formed.

**Fate of Thrombi**

There are various possibilities in the fate of a thrombus. The most favorable fate is lysis with repair of the endothelium. If, however, the thrombus is septic it may soften, disintegrate, and even become an abscess. Portions of it (infected emboli) may be transported by the blood to other parts of the body where new foci of infection develop (pyemia). Sometimes the infected thrombus furnishes the source of a general bacterial infection of the blood (bacteremia). The changes occurring in an aseptic thrombus are quite different. After it forms, it contracts due to the fibrin. Next there is a disintegration and a hyalinization of the mass. The disintegration is a digestive process carried on by the proteolytic enzymes of the leukocytes. The liquefied portion of course is easily disposed of without harm, but disinte-

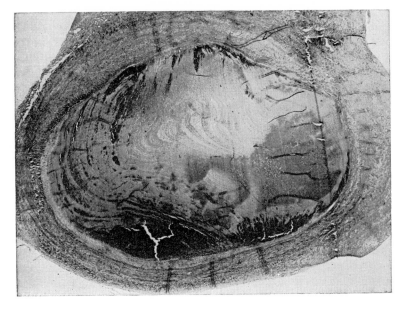

Fig. 7.6 — A mixed laminated thrombus of the splenic vein of a horse. The thrombus had its origin on the intima in the upper right quadrant of the vein as shown in the illustration. Organization had already begun at the point of origin. Some blood was still able to pass through the vessel ventrally to the thrombus. ×8. (Department of Veterinary Pathology, Iowa State University.)

grating fragments (emboli) may be carried away in the blood stream and become the origin of secondary thrombi.

Large thrombi cannot be removed in this manner. They become organized (Fig. 14.3). The organization takes place somewhat as follows: Fibroblasts and angioblasts originating from the connective tissue and capillaries at the place where the thrombus is attached to the vessel wall proliferate and push their way into the slowly disintegrating mass. The fibroblasts construct a loose reticulum in which the angioblasts form new capillaries. These two thus organize the thrombus. It is more easily understood if one assumes that the young, vascular connective tissue replaces the thrombus. Later the newly formed, very vascular connective tissue becomes less vascular, more collagenous, and shrinks (scar tissue). If it shrinks enough, circulation is re-established and the vessel remains only partly occluded. If the thrombus completely fills the vessel and if there is injury of the intima entirely around it, the termination is slightly different. Newly formed vascular connective tissue penetrates the thrombus at many points at its periphery. As the newly formed capillaries of this granulation tissue anastomose, blood is forced through them from upstream until they enlarge greatly and their walls become thicker. Circulation is thus partly re-established, and the thrombus is said to be **canalized.** Occasionally a venous thrombus becomes calcified. If it does, and if the calcified portion becomes free, it constitutes a venous concretion (phlebolith).

**Difference between a thrombus and a post-mortem clot.** In post-mortem examinations the beginner often has difficulty in distinguishing between a thrombus and a post-mortem clot. This is particularly true when he examines the large clots which appear in the heart and the large vessels. A thrombus is inelastic, soft, friable, granular, adheres to the endocardium or intima, and when removed leaves a roughened spot at the place of attachment. Post-mortem clots in the heart may be red, soft, elastic, and moist (currant-jelly clot), or yellow, firm, elastic, and moist (chicken-fat clot). The red clots form rapidly, the yellow ones slowly.

**Results of thrombosis.** Thrombosis is evidently one of the manifestations of the defense mechanism of the body. It appears to be one of nature's methods of localizing and preventing the spread of infection from heart lesions, of preventing ruptures at weak places in the blood vessels, and of diverting blood from areas where disturbances might easily result in fatal hemorrhage. Along with these advantages, however, come certain disadvantages, viz., embolism, secondary thrombosis, infarction, edema, gangrene, aneurysm, bacteremia, and pyemia.

## EMBOLISM

**Definition.** The process of a foreign body moving through the circulatory system and becoming lodged in a vessel causing obstruction is known as embolism. An embolus (plural, emboli) is any foreign body in the blood stream that is transported from one part of the circulatory system to another.

### Location of Emboli

The embolus will always lodge in an artery or a capillary since the diameter of these vessels decreases in width as the terminal branches of the vessel are reached. An embolus does not ordinarily lodge in a vein because the flow of blood in a vein is always into a vessel of increasing diameter, and therefore there is nothing within the lumen of the vein to prevent the passage of the foreign body. Embolism may also occur in the lymph vascular system. The emboli originate in the lymphatics and becomes lodged in the sinuses of the lymph nodes.

**Kinds and importance of emboli.** The most common emboli are detached portions of thrombi. They usually constitute the largest of the emboli and cause obstruction at their site of lodgement. Bacteria in clumps are dangerous emboli in such infectious diseases as anthrax (Fig. 7.7), swine erysipelas, and bovine and ovine vibrionic abortion because they are responsible for some of the most important lesions which characterize these diseases. When malignant tumors erode vessels, detached tumor cells become emboli and are transported to other parts of the body, where they lodge and furnish the beginning of other new growths similar to the parent one (Fig. 7.8). Protozoan and worm parasites constitute an important group of emboli in domestic and wild animals. Especially important among these parasites are the amoeba of enterohepatitis of turkeys, larval forms of microfilaria and hookworms in dogs, ascarids in swine, and strongyles in horses.

Fat-droplet emboli originating from traumatized fat cells of fractured bones which contain fatty marrow probably do not have the same significance in veterinary pathology as they do in human pathology. Only in pet animals in which such fractures are frequently reduced is there a possibility of excessive manipulation of the broken bones that is necessary for the

liberation of fat emboli. Fat emboli may cause serious pulmonary disturbances. Air-bubble emboli injected intravenously are usually of no importance, contrary to former belief. The introduction of large quantities of air is necessary before there is interference with circulation. A large volume of air will accumulate in the right heart and displace the blood in the ventricle, which prevents filling of this chamber.

**Source and route of emboli.** Emboli may originate in any part of the circulatory system, except perhaps in the capillaries. Arterial emboli arise on the arterial side of the circulation, often in the left side of the heart, and are carried to the parenchymatous organs (brain, kidneys, liver, and spleen) where they lodge. Heart-valve thrombi in chronic vegetative endocarditis are fairly common in animals in chronic navel infection, chronic swine erysipelas, and in chronic infections with streptococci, *Corynebacterium pyogenes*, and occasionally with members of the Pasteurella group. These thrombi are friable, fragment readily, and therefore result in

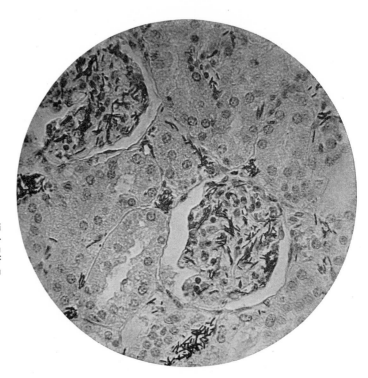

Fig. 7.7 — Bacterial emboli (**Bacillus anthracis**) in capillaries of the kidney of a guinea pig. ×400. (Department of Veterinary Pathology, Iowa State University.)

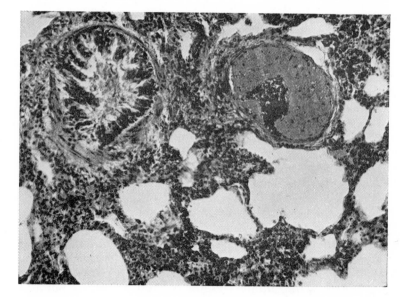

Fig. 7.8 — Tumor-cell embolus in a small blood vessel in the lung. The primary tumor was a melanosarcoma located in the inguinal region of a gray gelding. ×165. (Department of Veterinary Pathology, Iowa State University.)

embolism. The best example of arterial embolism is furnished by the larvae of *Strongylus vulgaris* in the horse, as has been previously stated. These occur principally in the anterior mesenteric and external iliac arteries and their branches. Arterial emboli are usually arrested at the bifurcations of the vessels.

**Effects of embolism.** The effects of embolism depend upon (1) the character of the emboli and (2) the vascular arrangement of the part involved. With reference to the character of emboli, they are either infected or noninfected. Infected ones contain pyogenic or nonpyogenic organisms. Large emboli containing pyogenic bacteria (septic emboli) result in the formation of infarcts which are accompanied by an inflammatory process and may terminate in abscess formation. If the emboli are so small that they are not arrested in the arteries or arterioles, they pass into the capillaries and produce tiny abscesses without the formation of infarcts. These are called metastatic embolic abscesses. Probably the best example of infected emboli containing pathogenic, but not pyogenic, bacteria is seen in swine erysipelas. Infarction is the result of the lodging of these emboli, particularly in the kidneys. Noninfected (bland) emboli lead to infarction which will be discussed later.

The second factor which determines the effect of embolism is the arrangement of the vessels in the part affected. This will be described more fully under infarction. For the present it need only be said that when noninfected emboli are arrested in arteries, they immediately become surrounded by a thrombus. The thrombus plugs the vessel, which in turn gives rise to a cone-shaped area of ischemia in the tissues supplied by it. If anastomosis in the affected area is abundant, the circulation is re-established, and little or no harm is done. If the anastomosis is deficient, the ischemia persists, or the area may become stuffed with venous blood. This may terminate in necrosis and eventually in replacement of the dead parenchyma with newly formed connective tissue. In the liver and lung this seldom happens because both organs are supplied with a double source of blood.

## INFARCTION

**Definition.** An infarct is a local area of necrosis resulting from ischemia due to an obstruction in the arterial tree.

The word infarction is derived from the Latin *infarcire,* meaning "to stuff." In most infarcts there is at some time an actual stuffing with blood.

**Location of infarcts.** In domestic

animals infarction is more or less dependent upon the localization of certain bacterial and animal parasites in parts of the circulatory system. Since the place of localization varies with the different parasitic forms and also with the species of animals invaded, it is obvious that there is considerable variation in the place of location of infarcts. In general pathology, it is sufficient to say they are fairly common in the spleen (Fig. 7.9), kidneys (Fig. 7.10), intestine, and mammary gland, and less common in the liver (Fig. 17.35), lungs, and brain. They are rare in the heart, which is a condition quite unlike that in the human where coronary thrombosis so frequently leads to infarction.

In the kidneys, spleen, intestine, and mammary gland, infarcts are of greatest significance. In the kidneys they are characteristic of chronic swine erysipelas in which they often accompany chronic valvular endocarditis. In the spleen in acute hog cholera, infarcts originate because of endothelial proliferation of the follicular branches of the splenic artery. The hog cholera virus is believed to be responsible for the endothelial proliferation of the vessel intima. The masses of proliferating cells more or less completely block the lumen of the follicular branches of the splenic artery and lead to the formation of infarcts in the areas supplied by the occluded vessels. The effect of blocking these small arteries is similar to that caused by thrombi. In the large intestine of horses, infarction is a sequel to verminous embolism or thrombosis of the anterior mesenteric artery and its branches. In the mammary gland of dairy cattle, infarction results from thrombosis of branches of the mammary artery or vein in severe mastitis as a result of extension of the inflammatory process from the parenchyma into the vessel walls.

**Pathogenesis of infarcts.** The sequence of changes which occurs in an infarct is, in general, as follows: An embolus or thrombus suddenly occludes an artery. As a consequence the area supplied by this vessel is deprived of blood from its usual source but gets some from neighboring arteries through anastomosing capillaries. The amount that is supplied by these sources depends upon the extensiveness of their anastomoses. In any event the blood pressure is not great enough to force all of this blood out of the area after it enters, so it accumulates and greatly distends the arterioles, capillaries, and venules.

At this stage the area constitutes a red infarct (Fig. 7.9). The stagnated blood in the infarct soon becomes deficient in oxygen and heavily charged with carbon dioxide and other waste products of cell metabolism. This lack of nutrition and ac-

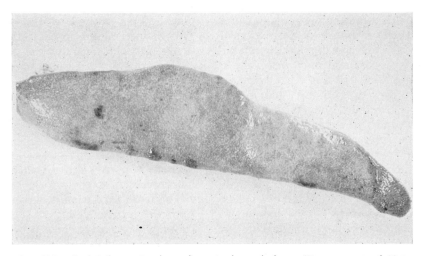

Fig. 7.9 — Red infarcts in the spleen in hog cholera. (Department of Veterinary Pathology, Michigan State University.)

cumulation of waste products are injurious both to the capillary endothelium and the parenchyma of the part affected. The damage to the capillary wall permits edema and hemorrhage by diapedesis to occur. The injury to the parenchyma leads to cell death (necrosis). In this type of necrosis the cells and the tissues formed by them retain their form and relative positions. Their cytoplasm, however, appears coagulated. This coagulative necrosis begins in the center of the area within 24 hours after the onset and extends towards the periphery so that within 48 to 72 hours the whole area is necrotic. The erythrocytes become hemolyzed and the hemoglobin is removed.

What was earlier a red infarct is now a pale one (Fig. 7.10). The dead tissue gives rise to toxic substances which in turn induce an inflammatory reaction in the sur-

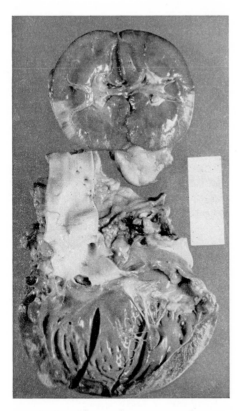

Fig. 7.10 — White infarcts in renal cortex and myocardium of a dog. (Department of Veterinary Pathology, Michigan State University.)

rounding tissue. This is indicated by the narrow zone of inflammation which surrounds the necrotic area. This zone is characterized by dilated capillaries and a collection of leukocytes. A moderate number of the latter infiltrate the infarct. The necrotic cells in the infarct gradually undergo autolysis and disappear. Newly formed connective tissue replaces them. Later it contracts and only a scar remains. Thus the termination of an infarct is similar to that of a thrombus — it becomes organized, and as the vascular connective tissue ages, it becomes a cicatrix.

**Macroscopic appearance of infarcts.** Most infarcts, particularly those in the spleen, kidneys, lungs, and brain, are cone shaped, with the apex of the cone at the point of embolism or thrombosis and with the base at the surface of the organ. Sections cut from the apex to the base then will be wedge or fan shaped. In the early stages the area is swollen and dark red due to the distention of the capillaries with blood. Usually, after 48 to 72 hours it becomes pale with a red margin (Fig. 7.11). This is the result of the necrosis and inflammatory border. Infarcts in the lung and liver usually remain red because the affected areas have two sources of blood. The double blood supply also accounts for the rarity of infarcts in these two organs. In the lungs they can hardly occur unless, in addition to the usual etiological factors necessary for their formation, there is also a passive congestion in the organ due to lesions in the left heart which hinder circulation. Under these circumstances there is weak arterial pressure and strong venous pressure. It requires a combination of these two factors to provide favorable conditions for pulmonary infarct formation. In the intestines the infarcted area is dark red (never pale), swollen, and the peritoneal surface rough and dull. In later stages the necrotic tissue becomes soft and putrid.

**Results of infarction.** The function of an infarcted area is lost. The dead tissue becomes a menace to the animal because it is subject to infection. If pyogenic microorganisms invade the dead tissue,

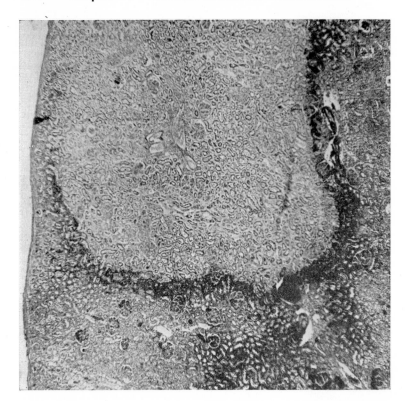

Fig. 7.11 — An infarct of the kidney of a goat. The infarcted area has undergone coagulative necrosis. A zone of hyperemia and leukocytic infiltration borders the infarct. ×27. (Department of Veterinary Pathology, Iowa State University.)

suppuration ensues. If saprophytes enter the area, putrefaction (gangrene) occurs. Sometimes when infarcts occur in such organs as the kidneys, liver, spleen, lungs, and heart, the termination is favorable enough so that the animal survives. In these cases the favorable termination is organization of the infarct. The dead tissue undergoes autolysis and is absorbed. Newly formed connective tissue and newly formed capillaries rapidly grow into the area and fill the gap left by the disintegrated tissue. The dissolving and absorbing processes and the filling-in process go on simultaneously. Finally, the young vascular connective tissue matures, becomes less vascular, and shrinks, forming a dense, tough, grayish-white scar.

Infarction of the intestine is practically always fatal. The animal dies (1) from shock due to absorption of toxic substances formed in the dead tissue, or (2) from acute anemia as a result of extensive loss of blood by transudation from the infarct into the abdominal cavity, or (3)

from peritonitis resulting from the invasion of the infarct with pyogenic bacteria, or (4) from intestinal rupture made possible by the gangrene.

### EDEMA

**Definition.** Edema is a condition in which there is an excessive amount of fluid in the intercellular spaces or body cavities.

When an animal consumes water, it is absorbed from the intestine into the blood. From the blood, part of it passes out of the capillaries into the interstitial tissue and from the interstitial tissue into the cells. Therefore, water in the body may be said to have a tripartite distribution: (1) intravascular, (2) interstitial, and (3) intracellular. Water in the natural body cavities is considered to have an interstitial distribution. In the present discussion it is not important to know what portion of the total amount of body water is located in each of the three places, but it should be borne in mind that the percentage distribution in each of the places remains more or less constant in normal animals.

The vascular and interstitial fluids are practically one and the same fluid, the essential difference between them being that the vascular fluid contains considerable protein (plasma protein) whereas the interstitial fluid has very little. There is a constant flow of the two fluids to and fro between the capillaries and the interstitial tissue. This occurs between the two ends of the capillaries — the arterial end and the venous end. At the arterial ends of the capillaries the blood filtration pressure (hydrostatic pressure) is constantly forcing some fluid into the interstitial tissue. At the venous ends of the capillaries where the hydrostatic pressure is reduced, there is a return of fluid to the vessel. In this short detour the fluid carries nutrients to the interstitial and parenchymatous cells, and metabolites from these cells to the capillaries.

What has just been said is not the whole explanation for the to-and-fro movement of water from the capillaries into the interstitial tissue and back to the capillaries. In the vessels the plasma proteins have a certain water-binding power. They act like a sponge, and are said to be hydrophilic. At the arterial end of the capillaries this water-binding power is a little less than the capillary filtration pressure (hydrostatic), and as a consequence some water can leave the vessel, as stated previously. At the venous end where the capillary filtration pressure has become reduced, the colloid osmotic pressure can assert itself and suck the fluid back into the capillaries. The plasma proteins have assistance at this point too because the blood is more concentrated, having lost some of its water at the arterial ends of the capillaries. This hemoconcentration favors the hydrophilic action of the plasma proteins.

If more fluid enters the interstitial tissue from the arterial ends of the capillaries than can be carried away at the venous ends, the fluid has an alternate route of escape through the lymph capillaries (lymphatics). This is the route which is traversed by the fluid containing a larger amount of protein than can readily enter the venous end of the capillary.

While the amount of interstitial water remains more or less constant in health, there are pathologic states in which it may be increased or decreased. If it is increased, the condition is called edema; if decreased, dehydration. The present discussion is concerned only with edema, a circulatory disturbance. Dehydration is a disturbance due to a water deficiency and has been discussed in Chapter 4.

The amount of interstitial water depends upon (1) the amount ingested, (2) the condition of the tissues, (3) the condition of the capillary walls, (4) the condition of the kidneys, and (5) the activity of the mechanism which regulates the water balance in the body. Whenever any one of these factors is disturbed so that an abnormal amount of fluid accumulates in the tissue spaces, lymph vessels, and serous cavities, accompanied by varying degrees of increased fluid content of the cells, the condition is called edema (Fig. 7.12). The distribution and quantity of this fluid accumulation can vary much. It may be simply a localized collection as in a blister or a bee sting, or it may be more or less generalized as it is in chronic heart and kidney diseases.

In edema the fluid in general resembles lymph. Edema fluid, however, is not uniform in composition. Its characteristics and content depend upon its cause. If it originates because of a condition not characterized by inflammation (a transudate), it differs somewhat from that occurring in inflammatory processes (an exudate). The distinguishing characteristics between the two are shown in Table 7.1 (page 135).

Names are applied to the various collections of edematous fluid. The terms hydrocephalus, hydrothorax, hydropericardium, and hydroperitoneum are self-explanatory. Ascites is a synonym for hydroperitoneum. *Hydrops*, the Latin for edema, is used in conjunction with the names for edematous collections in several parts of

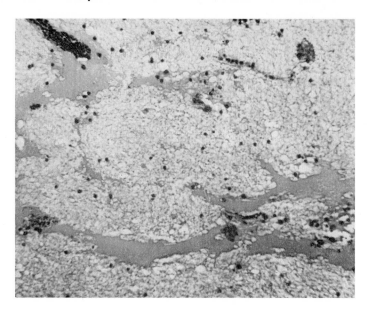

Fig. 7.12 — Edema of the brain from moldy corn poisoning. ×200. (Schwarte, Biester, and Murray; Jour. A.V.M.A.)

the body, such as hydrops abdominis, amnii, and tubae. Hydrocele refers to a local accumulation of serous fluid in the tunica vaginalis of the testicle. Anasarca is a generalized subcutaneous edema.

### Causes of Edema

The causes are explained by a combination of the theories of the physical chemists. At least five principal factors are involved: (1) increased permeability of the capillary walls, (2) increase of the capillary blood pressure, (3) decrease of the colloid osmotic pressure of the plasma proteins, (4) disturbed tissue nutrition, and (5) lymphatic obstruction.

**Increased permeability of the capillary walls.** The normal capillary wall is a membrane with varying degrees of permeability through which water and salts pass readily in either direction. Alterations in this membrane have no marked effect on the passage of these materials. Their passage is governed chiefly by forces either within or without the vessel. This is not the case with the blood proteins which are colloidal. Their diffusion depends upon the condition of the membrane. Normally, in all parts of the body except the liver and the intestines, plasma proteins, partly because of the size of their molecules, are

held back almost completely by this membrane. But when the wall is injured by any toxic agent or by insufficient oxygen (hypoxemia) as occurs in venous obstruction, its permeability becomes increased.

There are numerous agents which may injure the capillary endothelium so that loss of fluid from the vessels may occur. Experimentally, bacterial filtrates and extracts of bacteria have been proven to cause edema. It is not surprising then that bacteria in some septicemic diseases cause generalized edema. *Clostridium hemolyticum, Bacillus anthracis,* and *Pasteurella multocida* produce this type of widespread edema. The clostridia of blackleg and malignant edema cause a more circumscribed infiltration of fluid. Edema may be a postinfection phenomenon also as it is in horses in purpura hemorrhagica. It has already been stated that this condition seems to be an intoxication following a severe streptococcic infection. Besides bacterial toxins, other substances of importance in producing injury and increased permeability of blood capillaries in animals are foreign sera, snake venom, and ether. In an area of local inflammation the nitrogenous compound leukotaxine, which results from necrosis or injury of tissue, is believed to be the impor-

TABLE 7.1
DISTINGUISHING CHARACTERISTICS OF A TRANSUDATE AND AN EXUDATE

|  | Transudate | Exudate |
|---|---|---|
| Specific gravity....... | 1.006–1.015 (average about 1.013). | Over 1.018 (average about 1.022). |
| Coagulation......... | Usually absent or slight.  None occurs in serous cavities. | Usually occurs because of presence of fibrinogen.  May occur in serous cavities.  More marked when withdrawn. |
| Albumen........... | Under 3% | Over 3% |
| Reaction........... | Alkaline | Acid |
| Cytology........... | Mesothelial cells with large nuclei and some lymphocytes. | Polymorphonuclears in acute inflammations; lymphocytes in chronic. Flocculi of fibrin. |
| Bacteriology........ | Usually sterile. | Bacteria usually present. |

tant factor in increasing the permeability of capillary and venule endothelium so that edema results.

Special mention should be made of the toxin produced by a hemolytic strain of *Escherichia coli* of a particular serotype. In the intestines of pigs it produces a toxin which, when absorbed, apparently alters the permeability of the capillary endothelium in various parts of the body (eyelids, face, ears, stomach, mesocolon, body cavities, some lymph nodes) so that edema occurs. Some organic chemical compounds also cause edema. Of particular interest is the drug alpha-naphthyl thiourea (ANTU) which is used as a rodent poison. Dogs which consume rat bait containing this chemical may develop severe pulmonary edema.

Venous obstruction sufficient to cause edema may be due to venous thrombosis, torsion of the intestine, thrombosis of the tricuspid valve in chronic valvular endocarditis, chronic inflammation of the liver with connective tissue increase in the organ, and heaves in horses in which there is great destruction of the capillary bed and pressure upon the branches of the pulmonary vein by the ballooned air sacs.

Capillary endothelium normally permits only water, crystalloids, and a minute amount of plasma proteins to pass out of the vessels.

As previously stated, the injury to the capillary endothelium makes the membrane more permeable to proteins. The escape of the proteins is further favored by the dilatation of the capillaries in the area of obstruction. The proteins diffuse into the tissue spaces, and if the injury also involves the capillaries of the renal corpuscles, protein will appear in the urine (albuminuria). The diffusion of the proteins into the tissue spaces raises the extravascular colloid osmotic pressure, and their disappearance from the blood decreases the intravascular colloid osmotic pressure. This shift in colloid osmotic pressure permits an increase in the transfer of fluid from the plasma to the tissues. Briefly, then, the whole process is a cycle which may be summarized as follows: Increased permeability of the capillary walls permits the diffusion of blood proteins into the tissues. This in turn reduces the colloid osmotic pressure in the capillaries, which allows water to escape into the tissues.

**Increased capillary blood pressure.** Capillary blood pressure (filtration or hydrostatic pressure) has been determined by physiologists to be approximately equal to the colloid osmotic pressure of the blood proteins, i.e., somewhere between 20–30 mm. Hg. This means, then, that when the capillary wall is impermeable to the plasma proteins, the colloid osmotic pressure counterbalances the capillary filtration pressure, and there is little or no lymph produced by filtration. On the other hand, there normally may be some absorption of lymph by the capillaries at their venous ends because at this point the capillary blood pressure may be below the colloid osmotic pressure. Whenever, therefore, the capillary blood pressure is increased to the point where it is greater than the colloid osmotic pressure, fluid passes from the capillaries into the tissues. The capillary filtration pressure is increased in any part of the body whenever there is an obstruction to the venous flow. The consequent increase in venous pressure is felt also in the capillaries. This is one of the reasons why edema accompanies passive hyperemia as it does in cardiac weakness, valvular lesions, and venous thrombosis.

**Decreased colloid osmotic pressure of the plasma proteins.** This third factor in the cause of edema has already been mentioned. Before discussing it further, we should be reminded that physiological chemistry teaches that the blood proteins, by means of their colloid osmotic pressure, are important agents in governing the retention of water in the vessels. In some forms of kidney disease there is such a loss of plasma proteins through the urine that the colloid osmotic pressure of the blood is greatly reduced. The loss of albumin is greater than the loss of globulin and fibrinogen because the molecules of albumin are smaller and can escape more easily through the "pores" of the glomerular filter. Since the osmotic activity of albumin is much greater than that of the other two plasma proteins, its loss allows fluid to leave the blood and pass into the tissues. Hence, edema may accompany any renal disease in which there is albuminuria. Blood protein deficiency is also the reason for the edema that characterizes many cases of long-continued anemia.

This is probably the reason why sheep that are heavily infested with stomach worms show marked edema of various parts of the body.

**Disturbed tissue nutrition.** An important added factor in the cause of edema is disturbed tissue nutrition in an organ or part. In venous obstruction, for instance, the tissues that are in contact with the stagnated blood suffer in two ways: (1) they are poorly nourished, and (2) they are injured by irritating metabolites which accumulate in the area. As a consequence the cells undergo degenerative changes, and carbonic and other organic acids accumulate in them. The acids, both in the cells and in the intercellular spaces, cause the colloids of the tissue to become water-imbibing (hydrophilic). Thus, passive hyperemia contributes to the formation of edema in three ways: (1) by increasing the permeability of the capillary walls as a result of hypoxia, (2) by increasing capillary pressure, and (3) by making the tissues hydrophilic.

**Lymphatic obstruction.** Since lymph leaves an area by way of the lymphatics, it is obvious that any obstruction to these vessels results in edema. In this case the accumulation of lymph has a local distribution. Anything which can exert pressure upon a lymph vessel or obstruct it from within may cause the condition. Such obstructions may be caused by enlarged lymph nodes, tumors, distended hollow organs, and inflammatory processes in the lumen of or around the lymphatics.

### Varieties of Edema

Edema is either local or general in distribution in the body. Furthermore, it is either inflammatory or noninflammatory in origin.

**Inflammatory edema** is always local in distribution although several areas in the body may be affected simultaneously with the same condition. Edema accounts for much of the swelling in an inflamed area. Leukotaxine originating from the injured tissues causes the capillary endothelium to become more permeable to plasma. The fluid is so rich in fibrin that it is held in the inflamed area and does not gravitate.

**Noninflammatory edema** is either local or general in its distribution. Locally, it is observed most often in the subcutaneous fascia of the limbs. In these places it is either caused by obstruction to the flow of lymph in the lymphatics or of blood in the veins. It is said to be obstructive in origin. It should be stated here that often in animals an edema of the fascia of the throat region, brisket, and ventral thoraco-abdominal wall occurs which has the appearance of a true local edema but in reality is a partial manifestation of a more general edema. An example is the throat and brisket edema in sheep heavily parasitized with stomach worms. This is not an obstructive edema but is one related to hypoproteinemia.

Local noninflammatory edema appears when there is interference with the passage of lymph through lymph nodes or lymphatics by tumors, abscesses, or fibrosis resulting from chronic inflammation, or when the nodes are surgically removed. Local obstructive edema can also have a venous origin. It is likely to arise whenever local increased venous pressure occurs. The most frequent causes of increased local venous pressure are thrombi in large veins or pressure on such veins by tumors or abscesses.

Obstructive edema of either lymphatic or venous origin imparts coolness and doughiness to the tissues. The condition is seen most often in the limbs. The fluid is loose in the tissues because of the absence of fibrin, and consequently is easily influenced by gravity.

There is a form of local edema which is neither inflammatory nor obstructive in origin. It occurs in the limbs of animals. In the limbs conditions are such that one could expect local edema to occur quite readily. The principal factor which could be responsible for such edema is high venous pressure in the extremities. The hydrostatic pressure necessary to support a column of blood in a vein coursing from a foot to either vena cava is much greater than the colloidal osmotic pressure of the plasma in the vein. This pronounced difference in the two pressures should interfere with the takeup of interstitial fluid at the venous ends of the capillaries in the limb and result in edema. Normally this condition is prevented by (1) valves in the veins, (2) the pumping action of the movements of the limb muscles, (3) the increased flow of lymph, and (4) increased tissue pressure due to the structure of the limbs (small diameter, high volume of firm tissues such as bone, tendons, and ligaments, low volume of soft tissue such as skeletal muscle, and a dense covering of thick, tight skin). Even with these factors for the prevention of fluid accumulation in the tissues of the limbs, a state of physiologic edema occurs in the larger animals during periods of inactivity. If the animal is customarily a very active one, such as a work, saddle, or race horse, even the idleness of one day may result in a very conspicuous state of physiologic edema. The legs are said to be stocked. The condition disappears with exercise.

**General edema** in animals is usually cardiac, renal, or parasitic in origin.

**Cardiac edema.** Underlying the cardiac form is some long-continued impediment to the passage of blood through the heart (valvular lesions or progressive heart weakness) which leads to general chronic passive hyperemia (Fig. 16.7). Here again the increased venous and capillary pressure and the capillary dilatation provide the setting for edema. Both the tissues and the serous cavities become filled with fluid. On the surface of the body the edema is most noticeable in the limbs (stocking). Apparently the fluid collects here readily because the capillaries are subjected to the full filtration pressure of the column of blood due to the effect of gravity. There is reason to believe, though, that it may be formed in other parts of the body as well and then gravitate down the limbs. If the seat of the trouble is in the left heart, there is also pulmonary edema.

Renal edema. Renal edema is a characteristic of kidney disease in which the outstanding pathological changes are (1) degenerative changes in the renal filter, or (2) inflammatory swelling of the glomeruli which reduces the blood flow through the kidneys. It is associated with albuminuria. The loss of plasma albumin in the first-mentioned condition reduces the colloid osmotic pressure of the blood so that water passes from the capillaries into the tissues. This water transfer is facilitated somewhat by the retention of sodium chloride in the tissues. The reason for the latter is not fully understood. The second-named condition raises the capillary filtration pressure in other parts of the body and at the same time results in retention of injurious waste products in the blood which may increase the capillary permeability. The characteristics of the resultant edema are similar to those of the cardiac form.

Parasitic edema. It has already been said that edema is associated with decreased colloid osmotic pressure as a result of loss of plasma proteins. This is also a general edema. Such an edema appears in some parasitic diseases in which there is a constant loss of plasma proteins through numerous small puncture wounds produced by the parasites. This is particularly true in heavy stomach worm infestation of sheep. With the continuous loss of plasma proteins through tiny wounds in the stomach, generalized edema appears. This is especially pronounced in the region of the throat and neck and along the brisket. The pleural and peritoneal cavities and the pericardial sac practically always contain a variable amount of clear, serous fluid. Severe pulmonary edema may be the direct cause of death. The edematous lung may have the appearance of that of a drowned animal.

Appearance of edematous tissue. The appearance of edematous tissue is dependent upon whether the type of edema is inflammatory or noninflammatory and whether it is acute or chronic. A part of the body displaying acute inflammatory edema is hot and firm — firm because the fluid is contained within the meshes of a fibrin network and cannot be moved. A chronically inflamed area will be moderately warm and will be characterized by the presence of very little edema because vascular changes are not prominent in chronic inflammation.

An area of noninflammatory edema has a different appearance. It is cold to the touch and "pits on pressure." Subcutaneous edematous tissue gives up considerable fluid when cut. Excised portions are rather solid, heavy, and moist. When squeezed in the hand, water flows as from a sponge. Excised pieces left untouched for an hour or less shrink rapidly due to loss of fluid. A chronically edematous area, however, contains less fluid and more connective tissue. A fibrosis has occurred. Therefore the tissue becomes more firm and less doughy.

Microscopically, in sections stained with hematoxylin and eosin, the tissue elements are separated by a pale, pink-staining, finely granular material. The intensity of the pink staining depends upon the amount of protein in the fluid. In inflammatory edema a fine fibrin network is quite likely to be present. The cells are swollen, and their cytoplasm stains less pink than that of normal cells.

## SHOCK

Definition. Shock is a circulatory disturbance characterized by decreased total blood volume, decreased volume flow, and by hemoconcentration.

In animals shock usually occurs soon after severe injury in which there has been either hemorrhage or crushing of tissues. Consequently we speak of **hemorrhagic** and **traumatic** shock. In shock there is a deficiency of blood in the heart and large vessels and an excess of it in the capillaries and venules. It has been said that the animal literally bleeds into its own capillaries.

Causes of shock. The cause of shock is not fully understood. In dogs it can be produced by crushing large masses of muscles of the rear limbs. When this is done, shock is more liable to occur if the dog is anesthetized with ether or a barbiturate. Shock can also be induced in dogs by bleeding but the total volume of circulating blood which can be removed before shock occurs varies widely in dogs. As in traumatic shock, unanesthetized dogs tolerate bleeding better than anesthetized ones. It is conjectured that the anesthetics further diminish the blood volume in the heart and large vessels. This is attributed to spasm of the hepatic and pulmonary veins caused by the anesthetic. The venous spasm results in the accumulation of blood in the liver and lungs and further depletes the already diminished quantity of blood in the heart and large vessels. Sick dogs are more subject to hemorrhagic shock than well ones, due apparently to the reduced blood volume accompanying dehydration.

A special study has been made of fatal surgical shock such as follows repeated hemorrhage after an operation. If the hemorrhages occur more often than every two hours, the lost blood cannot be replaced adequately. Fluid in the tissues surrounding the vessels passes into the venous ends of the capillaries to compensate for the fluid loss. To be effective this fluid must contain protein to maintain the colloid osmotic pressure of the blood. Albumin is more effective than globulin for this purpose, but in surgical shock resulting from repeated hemorrhage, albumin is not replaced as rapidly as globulin. This acute hypoalbuminemia is in turn responsible for the failure to compensate for the loss of blood.

Shock can also be caused by the prolonged manipulation of the small intestine. Because of this it is reasoned that this type of shock is induced by overstimulation of the autonomic nervous system.

It is also believed that shock is due to substances that are derived from extensive destruction of tissue as occurs in trauma from crushing and in severe burns. Experiments do not confirm this belief. Blood from the crushed limb of one dog perfused through the vessels of the limb of a second dog does not cause a fall in blood pressure or vasodilation, both of which are indications of shock.

It has been contended also that histamine or a histamine-like substance originating in crushed muscles causes shock. While shock can be induced by histamine, it requires an amount greater than that present in the entire musculature of the body.

**Lesions in shock.** In shock there is a dilatation of capillaries and venules (vasodilation). As a consequence these vessels hold an increased amount of blood, which means that blood is diverted from the heart and larger vessels. In dogs in experimental traumatic shock, the blood pressure falls to 70 mm. of mercury or less (normal = 150–190), and the concentration of hemoglobin averages 137.7 per cent in contrast to the normal 100 per cent. The dilated vessels become more permeable to fluid, and edema results. Edema is especially pronounced in the traumatized area in traumatic shock. The dilatation of the small vessels also increases the volume capacity of the vascular system. Furthermore, the loss of the fluid reduces the total volume of blood. The combined result of the dilatation of the small vessels and the loss of fluid is that the volume flow of blood is reduced and the concentration of the blood is increased. Death comes because of failure of the cardiovascular system.

A peculiar phenomenon has been observed in the blood in traumatic shock. Normally, erythrocytes in the circulating blood repel each other and do not agglutinate, but in areas of crushed muscle a precipitate forms between and around erythrocytes and coats them. This precipitate binds them together into semirigid wads. This changes the circulating blood into a thick, mucklike sludge. The initiator of this sludging of blood may be related to substances capable of initiating the clotting of blood. An injury capable of releasing the initiator needs only to be severe enough to cause a local transudation of plasma containing a few erythrocytes. The conglutinated erythrocytes are ingested by phagocytes of the spleen, liver, and bone marrow. So much of the blood may be- come sludged that anemia results. In extensive tissue injury enough of the initiating substance may be released to cause sludging of all of the circulating blood.

## REFERENCES

Knisely, M. M., Bloch, E. H., Eliot, T. S., and Warner, L.: 1947. Sludged blood. Science, 106:431.

Moon, V. H.: 1948. The pathology of secondary shock. Amer. Jour. Path., 24:235.

———: 1937. Shock: Its mechanism and pathology. Arch. Path., 24:642 and 794.

Welch, W. H.: 1920. Embolism. Papers and addresses by William Henry Welch. Johns Hopkins Press, 1:193.

———: 1920. Hemorrhagic infarction. Papers and addresses by William Henry Welch. Johns Hopkins Press, 1:66.

———: 1920. The structure of white thrombi. Papers and addresses by William Henry Welch. Johns Hopkins Press, 1:47.

———: 1920. Thrombosis. Papers and addresses by William Henry Welch. Johns Hopkins Press, 1:110.

# CHAPTER 8

# Disturbances in the Nutrition and Growth of Cells

Normal adult cells of a given tissue have a rather definite size which does not vary appreciably in the different species of animals. The cells of the same tissues in a cat are approximately the same size as those in a horse. The difference in size of the two animals is dependent upon the total number of cells in their bodies. Alterations in nutrition, however, can cause some change in the size of the cells. With diminished nutrition they shrink, and with good nutrition, accompanied usually by some other factors, they may enlarge somewhat. These deviations are designated as aplasia, hypoplasia, atrophy, hypertrophy, hyperplasia, and metaplasia.

## APLASIA

**Definition.** Aplasia is the complete failure of an organ or tissue to develop. This disturbance of growth occurs in the embryo and fetus during intra-uterine development.

**Etiology.** The cause of this disturbance of growth is apparently due to three factors: (1) **Hereditary defects** in the germ plasm that may or may not be sex-linked. This subject is studied in genetics. (2) **Accidental death** of a cell at some critical point in the development of the individual. The earlier this occurs in fetal life, the more likely there will be a serious defect in the mature individual. The death of a single cell in the near-mature fetus is not apt to be serious, but in the embryo this failure of development may be very serious because subsequent generations of cells which should have been derived from the lost cell cannot appear. As an example, if the cell that forms the arm or leg bud should die, then that limb will not develop. (3) **Diseases,** particularly viral, of the dam during gestation may invade the fetus and cause cellular damage. If cells are injured in particularly critical periods of embryonal or fetal life, tissues or organs may not develop.

**Macroscopic appearance.** There is a total absence of a tissue or organ. At times, in the area where the structure should have been, there is a mass of fat or connective tissue, and the blood vessels and nerves that were to supply the organ may be readily discernible in the area. Whether aplasia will be lethal or not depends upon which organ is involved. If the heart or brain fail to develop, the animal will not live. The failure of major blood vessels or major endocrine glands (pituitary) to appear will result in the death of the individual. Aplasia of a kidney, an adrenal, or a testicle (paired organs) is not as serious because the remaining organ is capable of undergoing hypertrophy and hyperplasia and assuming the function of the organ that fails to develop.

Microscopic appearance. None of the missing tissues or organs are present.

## HYPOPLASIA

Definition. Hypoplasia is a failure of cells, tissues, or organs to attain their mature size. It differs from atrophy in that atrophic cells have attained their adult size prior to their regression to a diminutive form.

Etiology. The etiology of hypoplasia is as follows:

1. **Congenital anomalies.** There are many examples of hypoplasia associated with congenital anomalies, and these may be observed in all organs. Hypoplasia of the kidney can occur in all animals and is the failure of one or both kidneys to develop to their adult size (Fig. 8.1). Hypoplasia of one or both eyes is very common, especially in pups, baby pigs, and Jersey calves. Hypoplasia of the cerebellum is frequently observed in kittens, lambs, and calves.

2. **Inadequate blood supply.** If there is an obstruction to the flow of blood through an artery that supplies blood to an organ of a growing individual, the part vascularized by this vessel cannot develop normally and, as a result, hypoplasia of the part occurs.

3. **Inadequate innervation.** One of the best examples of this defect is the faulty innervation of a limb or organ following infantile paralysis in man. When this occurs in a young individual, that part does not develop properly and the individual has a short or distorted leg.

4. **Malnutrition.** The young growing animal, if lacking adequate nutrition, does not have the essential nutrients required for growth, and as a result is stunted in size. Malnutrition may involve a few critical cells, an organ, or the entire individual.

Macroscopic appearance. As the definition indicates, hypoplasia is a less severe disturbance in development than is aplasia. Some of the tissue or organ is present

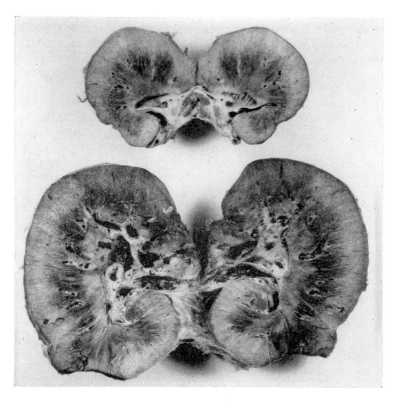

Fig. 8.1 — Atrophy and compensatory hypertrophy of the kidneys of a horse. The atrophic kidney was one-half normal size; the hypertrophied one was more than twice normal size. (Department of Veterinary Pathology, Michigan State University.)

but it never attains its normal adult size. This variation in size can be determined by weight, volume, or measurement when compared with normal tissues or organs. Hypoplasia may involve one or many organs of the body and does not necessarily result in death of the individual if sufficient vital parenchyma or special structures such as nerves and blood vessels are present. The color of hypoplastic tissue may be normal as compared with normal control organs or it may lack color intensity and have a fish-flesh appearance. Hypoplasia is recognized by a disproportion in the size and conformation of organs and tissues. Because of their diminutive size, they lack normal strength and function. If it involves the skeletal musculature, such as the muscles of a limb, the individual may have difficulty in moving about or may move at a slower pace than is normal. If hypoplasia involves a secretory organ (pancreas, salivary gland, or pituitary gland), there is a diminished amount of secretion, and malnutrition or improper development of the individual is evident.

**Microscopic appearance.** In hypoplastic tissue the cells are not as large as normal, may be fewer in number, or there may be a disproportion of the cells in that particular organ or tissue (too few parenchymatous cells for the amount of connective tissue present). Quite frequently there is an excessive amount of connective tissue and fat in the hypoplastic area that fills in the space normally occupied by that tissue or organ.

**Result.** The damage is permanent since the disturbance of growth cannot be corrected.

## ATROPHY

**Definition.** Atrophy is the diminution in the size of cells that have reached their full or mature development. This is not to be confused with hypoplasia, which is a failure of cells to attain their adult size.

There are complex synthetic and decomposition processes going on constantly in the cells. When the optimum conditions prevail for the maintenance of these processes, the cells are in their normal state, but if they receive insufficient nutrition or their metabolic processes are upset, they diminish in size and, sometimes, also in numbers but may not show conspicuous degenerative changes. This change, called atrophy, may be a physiologic process, as it is in the thymus of an animal approaching maturity, in the uterus following parturition, or in the mammary gland at the end of the lactation period. All of the minor and major involutionary processes that occur in the body, beginning in the prenatal period and extending through old age to death, are examples of physiologic atrophy. In addition to this old-age or senile atrophy, in pathology we are interested in the forms caused by malnutrition, disuse, disturbed innervation, and toxins.

### Senile Atrophy

Senile atrophy, like malnutrition atrophy, is a generalized condition. Its characteristics, which give it the name of **emaciation,** are of a more serious nature than those of malnutrition atrophy. There is flabby skin with wrinkles, much desquamation, and loss of elasticity. The subcutaneous adipose tissue disappears and the skeletal muscles shrink. Sunken eyes, outlines of conspicuous bony prominences and ribs, sway-back, and pronounced weakness complete the external picture. The bones become rarefied so that they break more easily when the animal falls or is restrained for an operation. In some species the teeth loosen and fall out. The liver diminishes in size and is of firmer consistence. Because of the atrophy of its parenchymal cells, its connective tissue elements become more prominent. This may give the organ the appearance of an increase in connective tissue. In hogs the normal fat deposits are replaced by a loose yellowish or reddish, moist, and often jelly-like tissue. This is called serous atrophy of fat. The fat is absorbed and the space it occupied is filled with serous fluid. The condition is essentially an interstitial edema although the cytoplasm of the fat cells also participates in the storage of water. In old dogs, and sometimes in old swine, there is atrophy of the spleen accompanied by areas of compensatory hyperplasia. A similar condition is observed in the prostates of aged male dogs. In the myocardium, masseter muscles, and muscles of the cervical region of old cattle, especially if they have chronic wasting diseases, the muscle cells are greatly reduced in thickness and have accumulations of granular, brown pigment (lipochrome) at the poles of the nuclei. This condition is designated brown atrophy.

### Starvation Atrophy

Starvation atrophy is a characteristic often displayed by farm animals in drought-stricken areas. It consists of a generalized atrophy of the skeletal muscles and subcutaneous tissues. It is a generalized atrophic condition of otherwise healthy animals. The fatal termination of this type of atrophy can be postponed by supplying water. Tissue dehydration resulting from lack of water is even more serious than lack of nutrient. In starvation atrophy, the stored substances of the body waste first, i.e., fat and glycogen. Next come the tissues themselves, beginning with those that are least active. The central nervous system, heart, and bones withstand the lack of nutrient longest. Sick and aged animals may show a wasted condition of the body called emaciation. It is probably due to malnutrition and is characterized by an atrophy of adipose as well as muscle tissue. When it becomes extreme, as it may in severe carcinoma and in some chronic infectious diseases such as paratuberculosis, tuberculosis, and anaplasmosis, it is designated **cachexia**. Formerly it was believed to be due to toxic substances present in these diseases and was called toxic atrophy, but it is now considered to be a form of malnutrition atrophy.

### Disuse Atrophy

Disuse atrophy is a local condition, whereas the two previous atrophies discussed were general. Inactivity, as occurs when the fractured leg of a dog is immobilized by a rigid splint or the hind limb of a horse is prevented from flexing at the hock as the result of a spavin, leads to atrophy of the muscles of the affected members. Similar atrophy accompanies the inactivity that is attendant upon disturbed innervation of a part. Examples in the horse are atrophy of the supraspinatus and infraspinatus muscles following injury of the suprascapular nerve, and of the left laryngeal muscles in injury of the recurrent laryngeal nerve (Fig. 16.4). A neurotrophic factor probably operates in conjunction with disuse in these cases. With inactivity the individual muscle cells shrink until they are reduced to mere remnants. Many completely disappear and are replaced by connective and adipose tissue. Atrophied laryngeal muscles have the appearance of, but are tougher than, fish flesh. Some muscle cells among the shrunken ones show degenerative changes and autolysis. The replacement connective tissue often undergoes mucoid degeneration.

### Pressure Atrophy

Pressure atrophy results when force is applied continuously to tissues in such a manner that the blood supply to them is diminished to the point where they shrink from lack of nutrition. The best example of this is probably the zone of atrophied cells which surrounds a tumor, an accumulation of fluid (Fig. 7.5), or a parasitic nodule (Fig. 8.2). Another example is furnished by glands whose secretory ducts are obstructed by concretions, inflammatory swellings (Fig. 8.3), or tumors. The accumulated secretions exert the pressure which results in the atrophy of the gland parenchyma.

### HYPERTROPHY

**Definition.** Hypertrophy is an increase in the size of a tissue or organ without an increase in the number of cells.

This disturbance of growth often owes its origin to increased functioning of an organ and to the heightened metabolic processes occasioned by this work. This is evidenced by the well-developed muscles of draft horses, the enlarged heart of racing dogs and horses, and the hypertrophy of the musculature of the pregnant uterus. These are examples of physiologic hypertrophy.

Hypertrophy, however, may arise from certain pathological processes. Cardiac hypertrophy, for example, may occur whenever there is some long-continued obstruction to circulation. The increased work placed upon the heart in forcing blood past the obstruction causes the myocardial fibers to increase in size. A healthy kidney becomes hypertrophied when the corresponding one either ceases to function or has its function diminished. Since the healthy kidney undergoes increased size to compensate for the loss of function of its opposite, this is termed compensatory hypertrophy.

## HYPERPLASIA

**Definition.** Hyperplasia is an increase in the size of a tissue or organ as the result of an abnormal increase in the number of cells. Hyperplasia and hypertrophy are frequently found together in the same structure (prostate) and are difficult to distinguish from each other.

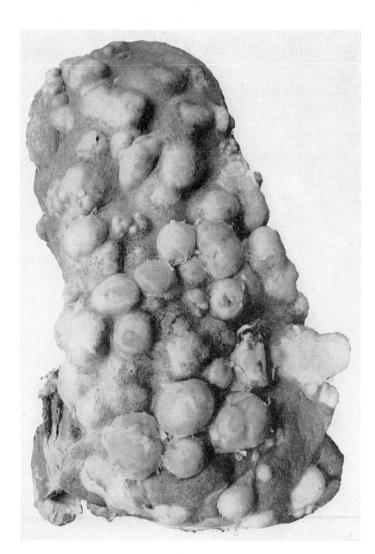

Fig. 8.2 — A lobe of the liver of a hog. Extreme pressure atrophy due to Echinococcus cysts. (Morris, Jour. A.V.M.A.)

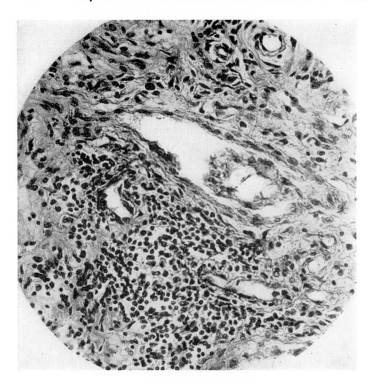

Fig. 8.3 — Atrophy of a convoluted seminiferous tubule of a testicle of a bull. This resulted from fibrosis caused by chronic **Brucella suis** infection. (Mathews and Roberts, Jour. A.V.M.A.)

The numerical increase in cells is, first of all, one of the most important characteristics of tumors. Every kind of cell in the body has the potential ability to undergo hyperplasia to form tumors. The inciting factor for the hyperplasia is not always known, but in the case of some epithelial tumors (infectious warts of cattle and dogs) it is a virus. In rabbits an interesting hyperplasia of the gall bladder and bile duct epithelium is caused by a protozoan parasite — a coccidium. Hyperplasia of cells of the reticuloendothelial system occurs in the presence of certain bacteria, fungi, and protozoa such as *Mycobacterium tuberculosis*, *Blastomyces dermatitidis*, and *Toxoplasma canis*. Surrounding the bone ends after a fracture has been reduced, a hyperplasia of osteoblasts forms a callus. On the skin at places where constant pressure or friction occur, due to bits, bridles, halters, harness, saddles, stanchions, or even the bare floor, a hyperplasia of the epithelium results which is also called a callus.

Often when a solid tissue undergoes atrophy its place becomes filled with adipose tissue. This occurs physiologically in the marrow of the long bones of young animals. In the development of the blood-cell-forming tissue in the marrow, the active cell-forming areas become atrophied in the diaphysis and become concentrated in the epiphyses. The atrophied hematopoietic tissue in the diaphysis becomes replaced with adipose tissue. This is an illustration of atrophy of one tissue followed by hyperplasia of another. This same combinaton of atrophy of blood-cell-forming tissue and hyperplasia of adipose tissue occurs in the hematopoietic areas of the marrow in some forms of anemia.

## METAPLASIA

**Definition.** Metaplasia is the transformation of one type of tissue into another, such as white fibrous connective tissue changing into bone or columnar epithelium changing into stratified squamous epithelium (Fig. 8.4). The transformation

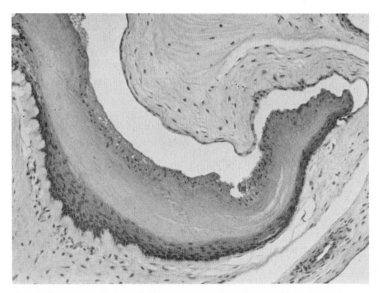

Fig. 8.4 — Metaplasia of the amnion of a lamb. Note the change from simple squamous epithelium to stratfied squamous epithelium.

occurs only to cell types of the same germ layer and is an alteration from a less specialized cell type to a more specialized cell type (cuboidal epithelium to columnar epithelium, columnar epithelium to stratified squamous epithelium, white fibrous connective tissue to bone, cartilage to bone).

Metaplasia should not be confused with anaplasia. **Anaplasia** is the reversion of a more highly specialized cell type to a less highly differentiated cell type. Anaplasia represents the reversion of normal tissue to a more embryonal cell type and is the type of cell alteration observed in tumors. The subject of anaplasia will be discussed in the chapter on neoplasms. It must be remembered that in both metaplasia and anaplasia the cell itself does not undergo transformation, but, rather, the new cells in the area appear as a replacement of a different cell type.

The cause of metaplasia is not known. The stimulus which is responsible for it may vary in different pathologic states.

Three excellent examples of metaplasia are supplied by (1) aged animals in which cartilage is replaced by bone, (2) a tumor of the bone in which the cells may form fibrous connective tissue, mucoid connective tissue, cartilage, and bone, and (3) a mammary gland tumor of bitches in which similar forms of connective tissue appear in the stroma. These examples emphasize the rule for the occurrence of metaplasia, which is that when the change occurs it is confined to cells which are closely related, i.e., have their derivation in the same type of parent cell.

Epithelium undergoes a transformation which is usually classed as metaplasia. It occurs where surface epithelium is exposed constantly to a rather mild irritation. Mild bacterial infection in the trachea, bronchi, or lactiferous ducts (Fig. 8.5), over long periods, or the presence of concretions in a hollow organ such as the gall bladder or urinary bladder constitute such forms of irritation. The change occurring in the epithelium is actually a proliferation with metaplasia, because an epithelium which is normally simple, cuboidal, columnar or a pseudostratified columnar, or transitional becomes a stratified squamous epithelium, sometimes even with a cornified layer.

In Vitamin A deficiency, metaplasia of the stratified epithelium is a common

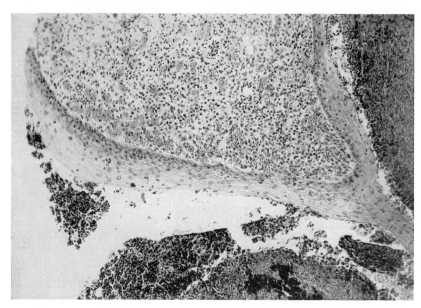

Fig. 8.5 — Metaplasia of epithelial lining of lactiferous duct in chronic mastitis in a cow. (Department of Veterinary Pathology, Michigan State University.)

lesion. The particular cells which become affected are those that not only cover a surface but also have a secreting function and do not have the power to divide. The affected surface cells undergo atrophy first. This is followed by proliferation of the underlying basal cells. These proliferating basal cells grow and differentiate into a new, highly keratinized epithelium. Such metaplasia may occur in parts of the digestive, respiratory, urinary, and reproductive systems.

# CHAPTER 9

# Disturbances of Cell Metabolism

Our understanding of the disturbances of cell metabolism which are called **degenerations** and **infiltrations** has been extended considerably by the use of the electron microscope. For many years, with the light microscope and proper staining techniques, it has been possible to recognize the nuclear membrane, nucleus, nucleolus, chromosomes, centrosome, centrioles, mitochondria, and Golgi complex. With the more recently developed physical and chemical techniques, not only has the ultrastructure of these intracellular components been made more apparent but a new "'cell organ" has been discovered — the endoplasmic reticulum. The expanded knowledge of cell structure has made it possible for the biochemist to better correlate intracellular structure and function. For instance, the mitochondria now appear to be the "power plants" of the cells. They are the centers of carbohydrate and fat metabolism. They are believed to contain many enzymatic systems and are the source of energy. The more recently discovered endoplasmic reticulum appears to be vitally concerned with synthesizing protein for secretion. It seems reasonable to believe that whenever cells are injured, these delicate intracellular mechanisms may be deranged and, as a consequence, disturbances of cell metabolism may arise.

The exact type of degeneration or infiltration resulting probably depends upon the nature of the injury and the specific function of the cells.

Injury to cells which upsets their metabolism may be due to any one of the various etiological factors already discussed in previous chapters. When the specific effect of any of these factors upon the cells is considered, it becomes apparent that the injury is actually the result of (1) a change in the environment of the cells, (2) contact of the cells with chemical agents or physical influences which alter their structure and therefore their function, or (3) withholding from the cells nutrients which are necessary for their normal existence.

The lesions caused by these injuries may vary in intensity from the mere accumulation of certain substances in the cells to complete destruction of the cells. The terms **degeneration** and **necrosis** are used to designate these two extremes. In degeneration the injury is usually only severe enough to cause the cells to "sicken." Similarly, as the metabolic processes as a whole are disturbed when animals are sick, the processes of anabolism and catabolism are disordered when the cells are ill. The result is that the food of the cells or their metabolites accumulate in them.

In necrosis the injury is so great that the structure of the cells is destroyed. The cells are dead.

Degeneration and necrosis are not the only manifestations of disturbances in cell metabolism. In some disease conditions, disturbances in cell metabolism are characterized by a deposition, either within or between the cells, of a substance natural to the cells or the part of the body but in excess of the normal amount. Examples of such substances are fat, glycogen, calcium, melanin, bilirubin, and hemosiderin. In other instances, the substance deposited, in this case extracellularly, is foreign to the part of the body. Examples are amyloid and urates. This deposition of substances is designated **infiltration.**

This chapter will deal with the following disturbances of cell metabolism: (1) protein, (2) carbohydrate, (3) fat, (4) mineral, and (5) pigment.

## DISTURBANCES OF PROTEIN METABOLISM

### Gout

**Definition.** Gout is the condition associated with the deposition of sodium and calcium urate in connective tissue and serous membranes. It is a disturbance of protein metabolism which is of greater importance in fowls than in mammals.

The etiology and pathogenesis of gout are not completely understood. With reference to chickens and turkeys we have the following knowledge.

There are two known forms of the disease, **articular** and **visceral.** The articular form has been experimentally produced by feeding a meat diet exclusively, and the visceral form by interfering in various ways with the functioning of the kidneys so that uric acid normally excreted in the urine is retained in the blood (hyperuricemia). This acid is derived from the catabolism of nucleoproteins of food (exogenous purines) and body tissues (endogenous purines). Normally, uric acid is present in the blood in small amounts (more in birds, however, than in man), and is excreted in the urine either in its pure state or in the form of its salts (urates). When the amount of uric acid retained in the blood becomes excessive, as it is in gout, it is deposited in the tissues. Indications of its retention and deposition are present in the joints and on the serous surfaces of the abdominal and thoracic cavities.

Birds affected with gout lose their appetite (anorexia) and become emaciated and weak. The leg and wing joints occasionally swell. In and around these joints there are deposits of white chalklike material (tophus, plural tophi). The articular form of gout in fowls is less common. In the visceral form, which is the more common, the serous membranes are covered with white, flaky deposits that look like fine frost. The ureters are filled with chalky-white, soft plugs of urates. Microscopically, the deposits and infiltrations consist of needle-shaped crystals and radiating bundles of monosodium urate or calcium urate. These are made visible by special staining methods.

In the primates (man, apes, and monkeys), in the catabolism of nucleoprotein, uric acid is oxidized to urea and excreted in the urine. In human gout this latter change does not take place completely and the uric acid is converted into sodium urate which accumulates in cartilage and connective tissue, especially in and around joints.

In the usual domestic mammals of veterinary practice the fate of uric acid is different. The tissues of these animals contain an enzyme, uricase, which converts uric acid to allantoin. The latter is excreted in the urine. This conversion of uric acid to allantoin occurs mostly in the liver. The mechanism for this conversion is so efficient that these animals rarely have gout. The Dalmatian dog occupies a peculiar position among these animals however. In this dog the method of catabolism of nucleoprotein is a combination of that of primates and that of the lower mammals. In the Dalmatian only about one-third of the uric acid is converted to allantoin. As a result this dog is subject to the formation of uric-acid urinary calculi, but contrary to expectation apparently does not have gout more often than other breeds.

## Hyaline Degeneration

**Definition.** Hyaline degeneration is the term used to describe a heterogeneous group of tissue changes that have in common that they are translucent, homogeneous, and stain sharply with eosin. Microscopically, they appear smooth, not granular, and with the usual hematoxylin and eosin stain they may vary in color from pale blue to deep pink or red. These staining reactions suggest the idea, which actually is a fact, that the hyaline materials are not a uniform chemical substance. The name, then, simply indicates the physical appearance of the material. Chemically, hyalin is a protein substance, but its composition varies so much that we recognize it in the form of such unrelated entities as mucin, mucoid, colloid, amyloid, and simple hyalin.

In hyaline degeneration we are concerned with simple hyalin. That it is not a uniform chemical substance is evidenced by its staining reaction, which is pink to red with eosin. Ordinarily it is recognized only with the aid of the microscope. Affected cells and tissues lose their structural characteristics and fuse. Evidently there is a coagulation of the cytoplasm at first and then a subsequent coalescing of the cells. The condition remains localized; that is, the hyalin is not transported and deposied as is amyloid.

**Varieties of hyalin.** Hyaline degeneration may occur in epithelial, muscle, and connective tissue. In epithelial cells it appears as droplets or globules, pink with eosin in renal epithelium and as casts in uriniferous tubules in chronic nephritis (Fig. 9.1), and occasionally in acute nephritis. Some pathologists think these droplets are related to the granules of cloudy swelling because they are often found simultaneously. Other examples of epithelial hyalin are the corpora amylacea in the alveoli of the lungs in the region of old infarcts, in the acini of the normal prostate of some species of animals, and in the acini of the mammary glands of cows. These bodies are concentrically laminated accumulations of epithelial hyalin or secretions of a hyaline substance which have been deposited around nuclei of dead cells. Some laminae in them stain blue, others pink. The bodies are stained by iodine and are therefore starchlike but are not related to amyloid. Keratinization of the superficial layers of stratified squamous epithelium is a form of physiologic epithelial hyalinization.

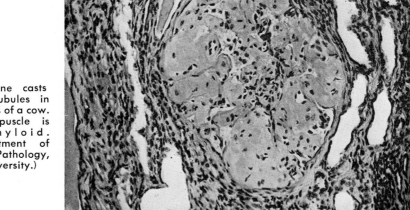

Fig. 9.1 — Hyaline casts in uniferous tubules in chronic nephritis of a cow. The renal corpuscle is filled with a m y l o i d. ×150. (Department of Veterinary Pathology, Iowa State University.)

Skeletal and cardiac muscle fibers may undergo hyaline changes. It is a characteristic change occurring in some of the laryngeal muscles in paralysis of the recurrent laryngeal nerve (hemiplegia laryngis) of horses. In the gluteal muscles of horses it is a prominent lesion in azoturia. (Fig. 9.2) In calves and lambs it is the most important tissue change of so-called white muscle disease (Fig. 9.3). In these animals it appears in the gluteal and intercostal muscles in particular and may also be present in the myocardium. It seems to be related to alpha-tocopherol (vitamin E) deficiency. In the breast muscles of young laying hens it is one of the lesions of avian monocytosis (bluecomb, pullet disease), which is caused by a virus.

Macroscopically, the affected muscle has the appearance of fish flesh and the disease is sometimes referred to as fishflesh necrosis. More often, however, it is called Zenker's necrosis in recognition of the scientist who first described the condition.

Microscopically, the muscle fibers lose their striations, the myofibrillae disappear, the sarcoplasm is fused into a homogeneous mass usually not staining uniformly pink with eosin, and the nuclei undergo degeneration. Often there may be an attempt at muscle fiber regeneration accompanying the necrosis, or collections of macropahges may group around portions of the necrotic material in the process of removing it.

The most common hyaline degeneration is probably that of connective tissue. The fibers become indistinct, fuse, and stain pink with eosin. Nuclei are not numerous and are scattered about in the homogeneous material. The condition is encountered in old tuberculous lesions, in the stroma of some tumors, in the reticulum of lymph nodes draining an area of chronic inflammation, in encapsulated necrotic tissue, in scar tissue, and in organized thrombi. Calcification may accompany hyalinization in these conditions. An unusual and interesting form of hyaline degeneration is that of the connective tissue in the walls of the follicular arterioles of the spleen in hog cholera.

Elements of the blood are sometimes converted into hyalin. Examples are hyaline emboli in capillaries. These are masses of conglutinated erythrocytes. Fibrin may fuse to form hyaline masses. In blood clots, hyaline formation is probably a combination of the two conditions just mentioned.

While hyaline degeneration is the most common reaction of connective tissue to injury there is another reaction which is attracting increasing attention. It is fibrinoid degeneration. In this condition the connective tissue takes on a homogeneous appearance with mixed staining characteristics; that is, it is metachromatic. It

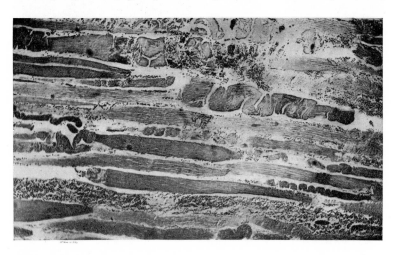

Fig. 9.2 — Skeletal muscle degeneration and hemorrhage in azoturia. Muscle pigment (myoglobin, is released and excreted in the urine, giving the latter a reddish-brown color. (F. W. Schofield, Ontario Veterinary College.)

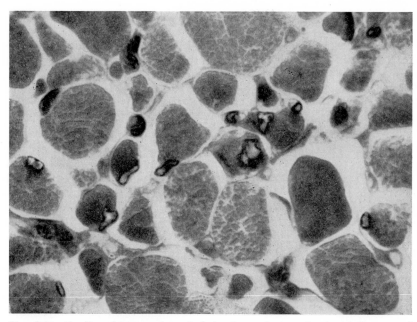

Fig. 9.3 — Hyaline degeneration of skeletal muscle in a lamb. In the normal fibers the Cohnheim areas are especially distinct. The degenerated fibers are more compact, homogeneous, and shrunken. (Department of Veterinary Pathology, Michigan State University.)

may stain eosinophilic like collagen or bluish like fibrin. Furthermore it lacks nuclei. Whether fibrinoid is derived from fibrin, collagen, or smooth muscle is a debated question.

The ground substance of normal connective tissue has a gel-like structure consisting to a large extent of acid mucopolysaccharides, such as hyaluronic acid, and chrondroitin and mucoitin sulfuric acids. When the acid mucopolysaccharide of the ground substance is precipitated, fibrinoid is formed. In many of the conditions in which it occurs the tissues become basic, probably as a result of the liberation of an alkaline substance. In man fibrinoid has been reported in a great variety of pathologic processes involving connective tissue. In veterinary literature little mention of it has been made.

### Amyloid Infiltration

**Definition.** Amyloid infiltration is the deposition, between the capillary endothelium and the adjacent cells, of a homogeneous translucent substance that re-

sembles starch in some of its chemical reactions.

Amyloidosis is the disease characterized by the deposition of amyloid in tissue. Amyloid means starchlike, referring to the brown, blue, or black color reaction when iodine is applied. Amyloid is a translucent, glistening polysaccharide, containing protein, that is more glassy than the other hyalins. It is not normally present in the body. Amyloid is precipitated between cells, not ordinarily within them. Its location, then, is extracellular. This does not mean, however, that fixed and wandering cells of the reticuloendothelial system (phagocytes) cannot engulf the material. Amyloidosis is really an infiltration even though it is sometimes called a degeneration.

The mechanism responsible for the formation of amyloid is not known. Circumstantial evidence seems to indicate that it is a precipitate resulting from an antigen-antibody reaction. When an antigen (in this case bacteria or bacterial products) is injected into an animal, an immune reaction occurs. The antigen stimulates the immune mechanism of the animal to form antibodies. The antibodies are substances which have the capacity to react with antigens so as to neutralize them or prepare them for engulfment by phagocytes. These antibodies are intimately associated with the gamma globulin fraction of the blood serum. It seems quite probable that this fraction of the globulin is increased in the antigen-antibody reaction. It is known that experimental amyloidosis is accompanied by an increase in the total serum globulin content (hyperglobulinemia). Persistent and repeated stimulation of antibody formation is a fundamental factor in the experimental production of amyloidosis. In manufacturing plants where antibacterial serums and antitoxins are produced, the occurrence of amyloidosis in horses supports this theory relative to the cause of the condition.

Amyloidosis is encountered most often in horses used in the production of antiserums and antitoxins for certain infectious diseases of man and animals. More than half of the horses used for the production of scarlet fever serum, and diphtheria and tetanus antitoxin have been reported to show the presence of amyloid. In 100 horses which had been used for serum and antitoxin production for periods of 2½ to 54 months, Doerken discovered that 60 developed some degree of amyloid infiltration in the spleen, liver, adrenals, kidneys, and intestine.

The theory that amyloid infiltration is dependent upon an antigen-antibody reaction for its genesis is supported also by spontaneous cases of the condition. In most animals which show it, there is or has been a chronic infection. Examples of such infections are tuberculosis in chickens and infectious anemia in horses. In dogs renal amyloidosis occasionally occurs in chronic inflammation of the kidneys.

In most instances in veterinary medicine amyloidosis is not diagnosed until the affected animal is examined after death, and not even then unless routine tests for amyloid are applied to the viscera or unless the condition is so far advanced that gross lesions are prominent. More often the condition is discovered when sections made from the organs are studied following the necropsy. By this, one may correctly infer that amyloid infiltration is uncommon.

The type of amyloidosis thus far described is designated secondary. Since 1929 many human cases of primary amyloidosis have been reported. In these cases the deposition of amyloid has been chiefly in the cardiovascular system and in the tissues of mesodermal origin. While it is the rule for secondary amyloidosis to be found in association with chronic infections, this is not the case with the primary form. With it no other disease may be present. In the majority of the cases there has been no involvement of the organs most often affected in secondary amyloidosis (liver, spleen, kidneys, adrenals). The cause of primary amyloidosis is not known yet. Reports of a similar condition in domestic animals are uncommon.

**Location and effects of amyloid.** The organs most subject to amyloid infiltration are the spleen, liver, adrenals, kidneys, and intestine. In the 100 serum and antitoxin horses examined by Doerken the incidence of lesion distribution in the organs was: spleen 100 per cent, liver 44, adrenals 34, kidneys 21, and intestine 12. In eight animals the infiltration led to fatal hepatic rupture.

Regardless of the organ involved, amyloid infiltration always occurs first just outside the endothelium of the blood vessels, i.e., in the tissues immediately surrounding capillaries and in the media of arterioles and venules. It is seldom seen in the larger vessels. Even before its appearance around capillaries and in the walls of small arteries and veins, it is known to be present in fixed and wandering reticuloendothelial cells. The infiltration gradually extends from these original sites into the surrounding tissues so that what was at first a localized deposit may become a diffuse condition.

Two important changes occur in the tissues as a result of the infiltration: (1) The lumen of the affected vessels becomes constricted so that some degree of anemia occurs in the area supplied by them. In the kidney where amyloid between the capillary loops of the glomerulus and the visceral layer of Bowman's capsule squeezes the capillary loops, blood cannot pass through the renal filter. As a consequence toxic waste products are retained in the blood (uremia). Death from this intoxication is the usual termination. (2) Amyloid accumulating between the cells causes degenerative changes and atrophy as a result of pressure. Amyloidosis may not be a permanent condition because in rabbits in which it was experimentally induced in the liver, spleen, and kidneys, the amyloid was later reabsorbed from the liver and spleen but not from the kidneys.

**Appearance of amyloid.** Amyloidosis is rarely diffuse enough to be seen macroscopically, but when it is, the affected organ is enlarged, firm, and pale (anemic), having a tense capsule and rounded edges. On its cut surface the amyloid deposits are more or less waxy, transparent or translucent, and homogeneous. The deposits can be differentiated from other hyaline substances by first smearing the cut surface with acetic acid; then applying Lugol's solution, which imparts a yellowish color to the tissues and other hyalins but stains amyloid a dark or mahogany brown; and finally, touching the surface with a 1 per cent sulfuric acid solution, which changes the color of the amyloid to a brownish blue or bluish black. This is the reaction similar to that for starch but, as stated above, the material is a protein.

In the spleen, amyloid is easy to see. It occurs in a focal and a diffuse form. In the former it collects in the Malpighian corpuscles and causes them to appear as clear, rounded globules which are in marked contrast to the background of red pulp. In the diffuse form the amyloid is distributed throughout the pulp and gives it a lardlike, glistening appearance.

In the liver, if the amount of amyloid is slight, it may be inconspicuous, but if abundant, it is easy to detect. In the horse the liver becomes firm, is easily torn with the fingers, and has a tendency to rupture and permit hemorrhage into the parenchyma or into the abdominal cavity. According to Joest, the reason for this increased friability of the liver is that the amyloid is deposited at the periphery of the lobules so that the parenchyma becomes easily separated from the interlobular connective tissue. Microscopically, in the liver the amyloid appears between the endothelium of the blood sinusoids and the hepatic cells. It compresses the latter.

In the kidney, amyloid is difficult to detect with the naked eye. In sections the deposits appear in the glomerulus between the capillary tufts and the visceral layer of Bowman's capsule (Fig. 9.1), in the walls of the arterioles and venules, and between the collecting tubules. It may result in uremia.

## Mucous and Mucoid Degeneration

**Definition.** Mucous and mucoid degeneration is the excessive accumulation of mucin in cells or tissues and is accompanied by retrogressive alterations within the cell.

Mucin is normally produced by specialized epithelial cells of the mucous membranes, especially by goblet cells. Mucin is a glassy, viscid, stringy glycoprotein similar in appearance to egg white. It is precipitated by dilute acetic acid and stains very faintly with basic dyes (hematoxylin). The excess production of mucin accompanied by degenerative changes in the nucleus constitutes **mucous** (mucinous) degeneration. In some tumors that originate from mucous membranes (carcinoma of the stomach, colon, and mammary gland), a similar mucous degeneration sometimes occurs. In cystic tumors of the ovary (cystadenoma), the cysts may become filled with another glycoprotein, pseudomucin, which is only slightly different from mucin.

Mucous degeneration may occur in the

epithelial cells of a mucous membrane as a result of a rather mild irritation. A good example of the condition can sometimes be found in the respiratory, intestinal, and Fallopian tube epithelium when there is an acute catarrhal inflammation. Another example of it is seen in the colon of pigs which exhibit symptoms of niacin deficiency (Fig. 9.4). Why it occurs is not known.

In mucous degeneration the mucin re-places the cytoplasm of the epithelial cells, pushes the nuclei to the base of the cells, and compresses them so that they atrophy. Normal cylindrical cells become goblet cells. Cell outlines disappear.

Mucoid is another glycoprotein. It is also quite similar to mucin but is formed by mesodermal tissues (chiefly connective tissue) when there is a disturbance of protein metabolism. This histopathological condition is called **mucoid** (myxomatous)

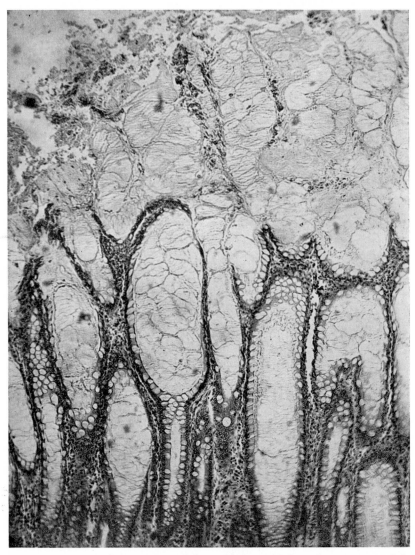

Fig. 9.4 — Mucous degeneration of the epithelium of the colon in niacin deficiency in a pig. (Department of Veterinary Pathology, Michigan State University.)

degeneration. Physiologically, mucoid is present in the connective tissue of the umbilical cord (Wharton's jelly), in joint cavities, bursae, and tendon sheaths. Pathologically, it occurs between the cells in connective tissue tumors (myxomas), in the bone marrow, adipose tissue, and cartilage of malnourished animals, and in the connective tissue of some of the laryngeal muscles of horses that have paralysis of the recurrent laryngeal nerve (roarers). It stains faintly blue with hematoxylin. Soft connective tissue tumors (nasal polyps) often have a mucoid appearance, but the condition is usually a gelatinous, edematous infiltration of the connective tissue and not mucoid degeneration.

## Cloudy Swelling

**Definition.** Cloudy swelling (sometimes called parenchymatous degeneration or albuminous degeneration) is a disturbance in protein metabolism in which the cells swell and the cytoplasm of the cells becomes more granular than normal.

The name cloudy swelling describes the microscopic appearance of the cells of an organ so affected. The organs which show this condition to any recognizable extent are the liver, kidney, and heart. The causes of this disturbance of protein metabolism of cells are toxic substances which may originate outside or inside the body. The condition then is the expression of an intoxication. The most common exogenous toxic agents are those derived from certain pathogenic microorganisms; hence, cloudy swelling is observed to some degree in the liver, kidney, and heart in practically all severe septicemic infections. Chemical poisons such as the salts of some of the heavy metals (lead arsenate, lead carbonate, copper acetoarsenite, selenium compounds) and alkaloids contained in such plants as the senecios (ragworts) in relatively small amounts are examples of other exogenous poisons. Jaundice is a pathologic condition in which a toxic agent that can cause cloudy swelling is produced within the body, particularly in the kidney. Bile salts retained in the blood are believed to be the irritant.

While exogenous and endogenous poisonous substances are considered to be the most common causes of cloudy swelling, they are not the sole causes. Another cause is hypoxia (diminished supply of oxygen). It is proper therefore to say that cloudy swelling is either **toxic** or **hypoxic** in origin.

To explain how hypoxia is a cause of cloudy swelling it is necessary to elaborate a bit on cell oxygenation and the factors which interfere with oxygenation. A prime requirement for cell health is an adequate supply of oxygen. This implies that the respiratory system must receive a sufficient supply of oxygen which it must be capable of transferring to the blood. The blood in turn must contain sufficient hemoglobin to carry the oxygen. Furthermore, the heart must possess strength enough to force the blood through healthy arteries to the cells which are to receive the oxygen and use it.

Cells suffer from hypoxia when:

1. Atmospheric oxygen is insufficient, as in high locations such as the Rocky Mountains.

2. Air cannot reach the pulmonary capillaries as a result of respiratory disease.

3. Hemoglobin is deficient as in the anemias and in hemorrhage, or when hemoglobin is combined with carbon monoxide which prevents the union of hemoglobin with oxygen.

4. Cardiac diseases result in heart weakness.

5. Local disturbances affect circulation.

When any of these five conditions interfere with the oxygen supply of cells, the cell metabolism is upset. It is quite probable that the cell enzyme system fails, and the consequence is that the cells cannot then utilize the usual nutrients brought to them, so the nutrients accumulate in the cytoplasm.

By histochemical means it has been shown that certain enzymes, particularly respiratory enzymes, are concentrated in rather definite zones in liver lobules. Some, for instance, are located chiefly in the peripheral portion of the lobules, others principally around the portal canals, and still others in the center of the lobules around the central vein. It seems quite reasonable to suppose that when injurious influences affect any particular enzyme, disturbances of metabolism should arise in the specific zone where the enzyme is located. This probably accounts for variations in the location of certain disturbances of cell metabolism within hepatic lobules.

Cloudy swelling has been observed to occur in parts of the body in association with several of these hypoxic conditions. These same hypoxic conditions give rise to other disturbances of cell metabolism such as fatty metamorphosis (degeneration) and cell death (necrosis).

**Appearance of cloudy swelling.** Grossly, organs showing this disturbance are usually swollen. The cut surface ordinarily bulges and appears grayish, dull, granular, and rather dry. Various adjectives are used to describe this appearance, viz., cooked, parboiled, boiled, ground glass, and scalded. The tissues are in a state of partial anemia because the swollen cells compress the smaller blood vessels. The microscopic appearance of fresh, unfixed tissue that is examined immediately after death explains its gross characteristics. The cells are swollen. Their cytoplasm appears granular and their nuclei indistinct (Fig. 9.5). In stained preparations this granularity of the cytoplasm is not so apparent, but when pronounced, it is best observed with diminished light. The extreme swelling of the cells accounts for the partial anemia observed in the gross specimens. It has been determined that even though the involved tissues ordinarily contain less blood, their cells actually contain an excess of fluid. .

Autolysis of cells resembles cloudy swelling so closely that one cannot be differentiated from the other. Therefore, it is not safe to speak of cloudy swelling with reference to an organ unless the condition is observed immediately after death. It has been determined in human pathology that six hours after death, even

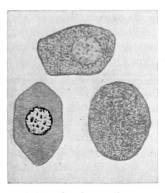

Fig. 9.5 — Cloudy swelling in unfixed hepatic epithelial cells. Upper cell is normal, the cell at right shows moderate degeneration, and the lower cell illustrates marked degeneration. N o t e swelling of affected cells, granularity of plasma, and indistinctness and obscurity of nuclei.

when the body has been held in a refrigerator, autolytic changes occur which obscure and simulate cloudy swellings.

**Nature of cloudy swelling.** While cloudy swelling is the most common of the degenerative changes, there is much concerning its nature that is not yet known. The facts that are known are: (1) It occurs during intoxications. (2) The granules in the cytoplasm satisfy the chemical tests for protein. (3) The alterations in the cells are temporary; that is, the cells recover if the irritant is removed before the damage becomes more than cloudy swelling. The important question which has not yet been answered with certainty is, "Why do the protein granules form?" Virchow thought that their presence and the consequent swelling of the cells was the result of a stimulation of nutrition and an increased absorption of food caused by the irritant. More recently some chemical pathologists have reasoned that the irritant causes the larger protein molecules in the cells to split into smaller ones. These latter increase the colloid osmotic pressure of the cells. In addition to this explanation other chemists suggest that with the disturbance of metabolism there is an accumulation of acid waste products of cell activity. These are hydrophilic and result in swelling of the cell colloids. The third theory used to explain the swelling of the cells is that the causative factor injures the cell enzyme system so that protein metabolism does not proceed normally. As a result, nutritive protein brought to the cells accumulates in the cytoplasm. Regardless of whether there is increased colloid osmotic pressure of the cells or water-imbibing power on the part of the colloids, or injury of the cell enzyme system, it is known that the cells do contain an increased amount of fluid.

**Functional disturbances.** Cells in a state of cloudy swelling do not function normally. In the myocardium they give rise to heart weakness, in the kidney they cannot form and excrete urine in the normal manner, and in skeletal muscles they contribute to the general loss of tone which is observed in severe intoxications.

## Hydropic Degeneration

**Definition.** Hydropic degeneration is a disturbance in protein metabolism in which the cells take on clear fluid to such an extent that they swell and may burst. Hydropic degeneration is primarily a condition involving epithelial cells. It is a cellular change quite closely related to cloudy swelling.

As stated before, in cloudy swelling there is an imbibition of water. In hydropic degeneration the imbibition may become so great that the cells burst. However, cells often display hydropic degeneration in a much less severe form than this. In the mild form the cytoplasm contains numerous minute water-containing vacuoles. In this state hydropic degeneration is closely associated with cloudy swelling, and in fact may be identical to it.

Just what occurs in injured cells to result in hydropic degeneration is not known. The cells imbibe water and swell. The process is probably reversible until the nucleus is injured. After that the imbibition continues; the cells balloon and may burst.

Various kinds of cells are subject to hydropic degeneration but it is best observed in epithelial cells of the skin and glands, nerve cells after nerve section, muscle fibers, and irradiated cancer cells. In veterinary pathology the best examples of it are furnished by the blisters which result from the application of such vesicants as croton oil and cantharides, by the vesicles of the oral mucosa in foot-and-mouth disease and infectious vesicular stomatitis, and by the skin lesions in the various poxes of animals (Fig. 9.6).

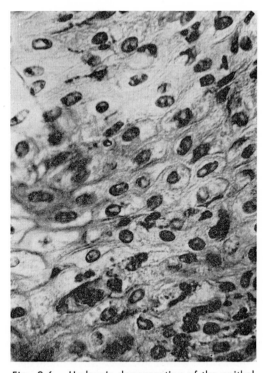

Fig. 9.6 — Hydropic degeneration of the epithelial cells in a swine pox lesion. Lack of staining of the cytoplasm around the nucleus is due to presence of vacuoles filled with fluid. ×620. (McNutt, Murray, and Purwin; Jour. A.V.M.A.)

## DISTURBANCES OF CARBOHYDRATE METABOLISM

### Glycogen Infiltration

**Definition.** Glycogen infiltration is the abnormal accumulation of glycogen in tissues.

Glycogen is the only carbohydrate that can be made visible for microscopic study in the tissues. Even it cannot be demonstrated except by examining the tissues immediately after death and by special technics. The reason the examination must be made right after death is that the glycogen is quickly converted into glucose which is not stainable. Special technics must be used to preserve and stain it. When the usual methods of making sections are employed, the glycogen is dissolved by water, and vacuoles appear in its place. One may not be able to tell whether glycogen or fat has been present. Therefore, to demonstrate glycogen the tissues must be obtained immediately after death, and the fixation must be in absolute alcohol. Following this, the glycogen can be made visible by special staining. Iodine stains it reddish brown, and carmine bright red.

In liver sections of well-nourished animals, fixed and stained by the usual methods, the presence of glycogen causes the cells to be large and the cytoplasm to appear to be quite clear, whereas in sections from poorly nourished animals, such as those which have been sick prior to death, the cells appear smaller and the cytoplasm more condensed due to the lack of glycogen. A similar appearance occurs in the hepatic cells of well-nourished animals if the tissue is not fixed immediately after death. Glycogen disappears most rapidly during the first hour after death. The rate of loss is increased if the tissue is kept warm. The glycogenolysis is caused by enzymes which are normally concerned with carbohydrate metabolism. A researcher becomes quite aware of the presence and absence of glycogen in his animals when he compares the liver sections of healthy control animals with those

which die on an experiment. When skeletal and cardiac muscle, cartilage, and most epithelial cells of well-nourished animals are stained specially, they too usually contain less numerous but nevertheless prominent glycogen droplets.

Pathologically, glycogen infiltration occurs in some rapidly growing tumors, in cells in areas of inflammation, and around areas of dead tissue. In suppurative inflammation the polymorphonuclear leukocytes in the general circulation and in the pus contain many tiny droplets of glycogen.

In man, in diabetes mellitus, the glycogen in the liver and skeletal muscles is so rapidly converted into glucose that its supply in these places is markedly depleted. On the other hand, there is an infiltration of it in the cardiac muscle and in the loops of Henle in the kidneys. The increased presence of glycogen in the cardiac muscle is unexplained, but its infiltration in the loops of Henle is believed to be due to glycogen absorption from the urine, which is heavily charged with it in diabetes. In these epithelial cells it appears in large globules. In animals, so far as we know, diabetes mellitus is not as common as in man. It is seen occasionally in dogs and cats.

In animals that have undergone starvation, have been subjected to violent exercise, or have been poisoned with strychnine, there may be some depletion of glycogen in the tissues which ordinarily contain it.

## DISTURBANCES OF FAT METABOLISM

From the standpoint of pathology it is essential to emphasize that fat has two different types of distribution in the body: (1) in the fat depots and (2) in the cell protoplasm. In the depots it occurs in the form of neutral fat in adipose tissue. Neutral fat is composed of the triglycerides of palmitic, stearic, and oleic acid. In the protoplasm of cells fat occurs in the form of sterols, phospholipids, and glycolipids. There are three disturbances of fat metabolism which concern us: (1) excessive storage (obesity), (2) fatty infiltration, and (3) fatty metamorphosis (fatty degeneration).

### Depot Fat

Depot or neutral fat (adipose tissue fat) is most prominent in the following storage places: (1) the subcutis, (2) the subserosa of the epicardium, omentum, and parietal peritoneum, (3) perirenal region, (4) bone marrow, (5) orbital fossa, (6) the brisket of cattle, and (7) the jowl of swine. In these and other places it serves principally as a reserve food supply, as insulation, and as shock absorbing and protective padding for delicate structures.

As need for protoplasmic fat arises, the depot fat is removed and converted into the form occurring in the colloid of the cell protoplasm. The first step in the preparation of this fat for cell use is transportation to the liver for desaturation and union with choline. After this chemical transformation of the fat has been performed, much of it is released to the cells of the body, but the liver stores a considerable quantity of it.

### OBESITY

**Definition.** Obesity is the excessive storage of fat in adipose tissue.

In the parlance of animal husbandry an obese animal is simply said to be very fat, or perhaps overly or excessively fat. Whereas in man such a condition is undesirable, in food-producing animals it is usually a highly desirable body state. Only when it interferes with body function or appearance for which the animal is kept does obesity constitute a pathologic condition.

In obese animals an excessive amount of fat usually accumulates in the connective tissue which separates the parenchymatous cells, groups of parenchymatous cells, or groups of structures which form lobules. This constitutes **fatty infiltration.** The fat is located in fat cells between the parenchymatous cells. Places in the body where it frequently occurs are the heart and skeletal muscles. In skeletal muscles the presence of the fat cells between the muscle fibers and bundles is referred to as "marbling."

There are a few organs in which fatty infiltration of the parenchymatous cells occurs physiologically. They are the liver and adrenal glands of all species, the kidneys of dogs and cats, and the heart of cats. In the hepatic cells it occurs in pregnant females and in animals that become excessively fat (Fig. 9.7). In the adrenals it is present in the cells of all three zones

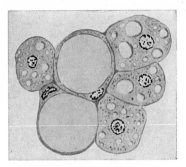

Fig. 9.7 — Fatty infiltration of hepatic epithelial cells. Note accumulation of fat droplets, their coalescence, the displacement and compression of the nuclei which still maintain their more or less normal characterstiics.

of the cortex but is especially abundant in the zona fasciculata. In the kidneys of mature dogs and cats it is present in the epithelial cells of the convoluted tubules and in the arms of Henle's loop. Visible, stainable fat in the cardiac muscle fibers in the cat fluctuates with dietary intake of fatty substances. It is very important to remember that in these organs in these particular species it is often difficult, if not impossible, to distinguish between physiologic and pathologic fatty infiltration.

### Causes of Obesity

1. Excessive intake of fat and carbohydrates, as in animals in the feed lot or in preparation for exhibition.

2. Diminished utilization of fat, as in house dogs, idle horses, stabled male breeding animals, and setting hens.

3. Diminished metabolic rate, as in dysfunction or loss of function of some of the

endocrine glands such as thyroid and pituitary deficiency, or from removal or atrophy of the gonads.

### Effects of Obesity

1. Infiltration of excessive amounts of fat into organs where it interferes with function, such as in the interstitial tissue of the myocardium, or under the epicardium.

2. Increased body weight interfering with body movement, as in old house dogs and in show animals.

3. Diminution of the capacity of the abdominal cavity due to the accumulation of omental and perirenal fat with the consequent interference with the action of the diaphragm and lungs.

4. Overfilling of normal subcutaneous depots resulting in patchiness of distribution of fat in beef cattle.

5. Flabbiness of skeletal muscles.

6. Predisposes to prolapse of the vagina in beef cattle.

The interference with the action of the heart and lungs, together with the added weight carried by the animal and the flabby state of the skeletal muscles, results in increased respiration (polypnea), rapid pulse, and ease of fatigue, and even rupture of an internal organ such as rupture of the liver in fat hens.

### Protoplasmic Fat

The sterols, phospholipids, and glycolipids which comprise the protoplasmic fats are in a colloid state in combination with proteins, carbohydrates, inorganic salts, and water. In such a state they are not recognizable microscopically in ordinarily stained sections nor can they be made visible by the use of stains having an affinity for fat. Neutral fat in adipose tissue, on the other hand, can be seen readily within the cells and can be stained with certain chemical agents.

The important sterols which occur in protoplasmic fat are cholesterol, 7-dehydrocholesterol, and ergosterol. The three phospholipids are the lecithins, cephalins, and the sphingomyelins. The three glycolipids are kerasin, phrenosin, and nervone of nervous tissue.

### FATTY DEGENERATION (FATTY METAMORPHOSIS)

**Definition.** Fatty degeneration is a retrogressive cell change in which fat droplets appear in the cell cytoplasm.

Since the days of Virchow it has been known that when the parenchymal cells of organs such as the liver, kidney, heart, adrenals, and skeletal muscles become "sick" they often contain droplets of fat which are visible with the microscope and which can be stained with special dyes. The presence of visible fat in parenchymatous cells has always been considered pathologic except in the liver of all animals, in the renal epithelial cells of some carnivores, in the adrenal cortex, in the sebaceous glands, and in the epithelial cells of bile ducts in the hepatic trinities of dogs.

The presence of fat in parenchymatous cells has been the subject of research and speculation for years. The causes of the condition are fairly well known. They seem to be (1) various toxic substances and (2) a deficiency of oxygen (hypoxemia). The origin of the fat, however, is puzzling. It can be reasoned that cells subjected to toxic or hypoxic influences may be affected in the following ways with respect to fat metabolism:

1. The colloid of the cell protoplasm becomes disorganized and splits up into its component parts such as fat, protein, and carbohydrate. In this state the invisible fat becomes visible microscopically. This is called fat phanerosis.

2. The cell proteins split up into amino acids which are de-aminized to fatty acids and finally take on the form of visible fat.

3. Neutral fat in transit from the fat depots to the liver is absorbed by cells too sick to discriminate between neutral fat and the fat released by the liver for the use of cells. The injured cells then contain the normal amount of protoplasmic fat plus the added neutral fat. The most

recent researches seem to support this theory. Fatty degeneration in the liver, the myocardium, and the kidney have been shown to be of this nature. Either the lipase of the injured cells is not capable of handling this form of fat or the enzyme has been destroyed. The pathologic change is actually an infiltration of fat.

The question now facing us is what to call the process. While the English researcher who has done much research on this fatty change prefers to call it an infiltration, he sees no objection to calling it fatty degeneration or fatty metamorphosis since the condition is a degenerative change in which the morphology of the cell is changed as a result of disturbed metabolism.

## Causes of Fatty Degeneration

The causes of fatty degeneration are twofold: (1) a diminished supply of oxygen (hypoxia), and (2) certain toxic agents (organic and inorganic chemical compounds).

**Hypoxic causes.** In diseases of the blood such as anemia there is a loss of erythrocytes and hemoglobin, and consequently an interference with the oxygen-carrying capacity of the blood. In diseases of the lungs and cardiovascular system the cells of parts of the body or of the entire body often receive a diminished supply of oxygen. This partly accounts for the fatty changes which occur in areas of passive congestion.

**Toxic causes.** Agents which may be responsible for this disturbance of cell metabolism are various inorganic or organic chemical compounds. Common inorganic toxic substances are certain compounds of phosphorus, lead, arsenic, and antimony. Among the organic toxic agents are chloroform, chloral hydrate, carbontetrachloride, tetrachloroethylene, and phenol. The most common and, therefore, most important of the organic poisons, however, are the bacterial toxins. In this connection it must be said that the action of these chemical agents is quite variable because they are also the cause

of cloudy swelling and necrosis, depending upon their concentration. In fact, cloudy swelling, fatty degeneration, and necrosis may occur simultaneously in the same organ due to the action of the same chemical compound. This suggests that there is a close relationship between cloudy swelling and fatty degeneration. It is believed by some that they are simply manifestations of different degrees of cell injury. Apparently, it requires only a rather mild irritant to disturb protein metabolism but a more drastic one to upset fat metabolism. Frequently, there are evidences that the process begins as cloudy swelling and progresses to fatty degeneration when the irritant continues to operate or when the intensity of its action is increased. Cells thus affected may eventually die.

While the usual causes of fatty degeneration are hypoxic and toxic in nature there is another cause which is demanding increased attention. This cause is a deficiency of choline which can occur in very poorly nourished animals. To understand how this causative factor operates it is necessary to outline some of the important steps in fat metabolism.

Briefly, the metabolism of fat proceeds as follows: Neutral fat is ingested by the animal. It is digested in the small intestine and absorbed by the intestinal mucosa in the form of a water-soluble complex containing bile salts. In the chemical changes which occur in the mucosa much of the fatty acid and glycerol are resynthesized to neutral fat and a lesser amount is converted to phospholipid. In the mucosa almost three-fourths of the fat is transferred to the lacteals of the villi and eventually reaches the blood stream by way of the thoracic duct which terminates in the anterior vena cava. More than one-fourth of the fat is probably transferred to the capillaries of the villi and is transported to the liver by the portal vein. Regardless of which route the fat is carried, much of it is picked up by the liver for temporary storage. Here most, if not all, of the neutral fat is transformed to phospholipid for distribution to the organs and tissues. If this transformation from neutral fat to phospholipid is interfered with, neutral fat accumulates in the hepatic cells. The accumulation can become so great that the condition can be classed as fatty degeneration.

For this transformation of neutral fat to phospholipid, choline is needed. Because this nitrogenous base is necessary for this chemical change, it is called a "lipotropic" agent, meaning that it has an affinity for fats. If choline, or the constituents from which it is made, is lacking in the diet, the conversion of neutral fat to phospholipid does not proceed normally, and neutral fat accumulates in the liver cells. This presence of choline is therefore necessary to prevent fatty livers. It is not surprising, then, that fasting and starved animals have fatty livers. Fatty livers in newborn pigs and calves that have been deprived of colostrum may be attributed to choline deficiency also. The choline requirements of these young animals is very high, and colostrum is an excellent dietary source of this lipotropic factor.

**Appearance of fatty degeneration.** Fatty degeneration can be observed in the parenchyma of many organs of the body, but its presence in the three vital ones, the heart, the kidneys, and the liver, concern us most.

In the **heart,** in gross specimens, the myocardium is soft and flabby. There is a pale yellow, mottled, or streaked appearance of the endocardium, seen best in the walls of the ventricles. Sometimes the streaking resembles the color pattern of a tiger's hide and is referred to as tigroid appearance. Microscopically, the muscle fibers contain very minute fat droplets.

In the **kidney** the gross appearance of the cortex, in particular, is pale yellowish brown in color. This does not mean that the medulla is not also affected, but the normal color of the medulla masks the color of the fat. The organ is not necessarily enlarged unless the fatty degeneration is accompanied by cloudy swelling. This, however, usually occurs. Microscopically, the cells of the convoluted tubules and the thick segments of Henle's loops contain many small fat droplets. At first they are seen only between the nucleus and the base of the cell but later in the luminal end as well. The nuclei may or may not be degenerated. In the collecting tubules these changes are slight or absent. Histochemically, it has been shown that alkaline phosphatase and 5-nucleotidase are markedly decreased before fatty degeneration of the renal epithelium occurs. This decreased enzymatic activity apparently disturbs phospholipid metabolism.

In carnivores one can expect normally to find some fat droplets in cells of the convoluted tubules. The nuclei of these cells are always normal and the fat is present mostly at the luminal end of the cells. In dogs under one year of age no fat at all, or very little, is present anywhere in the tubules, but as dogs age, the amount of normal stainable fat gradually increases in the proximal convoluted tubules and in the ascending and descending arms of Henle's loop. It is not present, however, in these cells in the chronic nephritis of old dogs.

In the **liver,** disturbances in fat metabolism are more complicated and are more difficult to differentiate. The difficulty arises from the fact that normal liver cells frequently contain some fat droplets. This is especially true in very fat animals and in late pregnancy in well-fed females (Fig. 9.7). When the physiological deposition of fat in the liver has added to it a large amount of fat during a pathological condition, the state of hepatic fatty metamorphosis can become extreme. An excellent example of this occurs in pregnant ewes affected with ketosis (pregnancy disease). The fat content may be so greatly increased that the liver is perfectly yellow and excised portions float on water. The cut surface is also yellow and quite greasy. The texture is soft. Microscopically, the hepatic cells contain well-defined globules. Usually there is only one globule; at most, only a few. As they increase in size they displace the nuclei and cytoplasm laterally until they are compressed into crescent-shaped figures at the periphery of the cells. In hematoxylin and eosin-stained sections the fat has been removed by xylene so that only an empty, open, round space indicates its former presence. In sections prepared from tissue fixed with osmic acid, the droplets are black. In those treated with Sudan III, the fat stains red—yellowish red to scarlet. If the nuclei are only slightly compressed, they have almost normal appearance. If squeezed excessively, they become flattened and appear to stain more deeply with hematoxylin. The cytoplasm also appears condensed or may not be recognizable at all. In car-

size of the liver. Its color is dull yellowish brown, and its texture is soft (Fig. 9.8). Microscopically, the nuclei often remain at or near the center of the cells, but show evidences of degeneration. These evidences are usually shrinkage and distortion of the nuclei with a condensation of the chromatin (pyknosis) or a fragmentation of the nuclei (karyorhexis). Occasionally there is dissolution of the chromatin with the nuclear membrane remaining intact (karyolysis). Around the nuclei are numerous small fat droplets, often so nu-

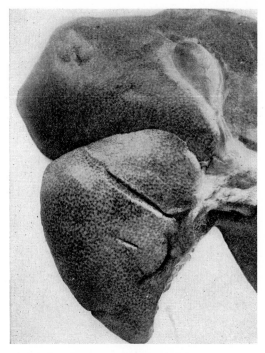

Fig. 9.8 — Fatty degeneration of the liver of a pig with nutritional anemia. The presence of irregularly shaped, grayish-yellow, degenerated areas gives the organ a mottled appearance. (Craig, Jour. A.V.M.A.)

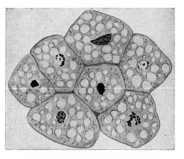

Fig. 9.9 — Fatty degeneration of hepatic epithelial cells. Note distribution of fat droplets, central position of nuclei, and evidences of nuclear degeneration (pyknosis, karyorrhexis, and karyorrhexis, and karylysis). (McCrory and Ward, J o u r . A.V.M.A.)

merous that they give the cytoplasm a foamlike appearance (Figs. 9.9 and 9.10). When the fat is dissolved as it is in hematoxylin and eosin-stained sections, only a cytoplasmic network remains.

**Functional effects.** Naturally, "sick" cells whose colloidal systems are disorganized, and in which there is an infiltration of fat, cannot function normally. With a knowledge of physiology and with a little imagination one can list a series of disturbed functions which would result when the liver, the heart, or the kidneys are affected with fatty degeneration. When one understands that the same irritant may produce the same change in all three of these organs simultaneously, he can realize the seriousness of this disorder of cell metabolism.

bon tetrachloride injury of liver cells the mitochondria are affected before the nuclei. The mitochondria swell.

What has just been described is the fatty metamorphosis characteristic of ketosis in ewes. The more usual appearance — that occurring in hypoxia and in various inorganic and organic intoxications (including bacterial and viral) — is different. There is no appreciable increase in

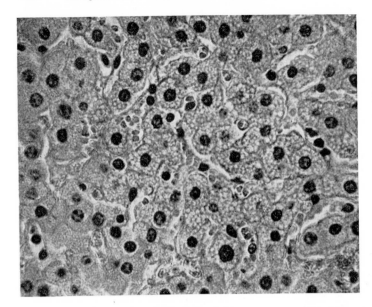

Fig. 9.10 — Fatty degeneration caused by thallium sulfate. Liver of a cow. (High power.) (McCrory and Ward, Jour. A.V.M.A.)

Furthermore, when this disturbance of cell metabolism becomes so extensive that the nuclei degenerate, the cells die. Then one of two things must happen if the animal survives. Either the degenerated parenchymatous cells must be replaced by others of their own kind (repair by regeneration), or if this is impossible, the place left vacant by the parenchymal cells must be filled by newly formed connective tissue cells (repair by substitution). In the latter case the function of the affected organ may never return to its normal level.

### DISTURBANCES OF CALCIUM METABOLISM

In the blood and other body fluids, calcium occurs in combinations not yet fully understood. It is known that the amount present is larger than can ordinarily be kept in solution; that is, the blood is supersaturated with it. One of the explanations of this phenomenon is that the calcium in solution is concentrated around each colloidal particle, and that this state is maintained by the high carbon dioxide content of the blood and tissue fluids. There are, then, three important factors involved in maintaining this supersaturation of calcium: (1) the nature and amount of the colloids, (2) the amount of carbon dioxide, and (3) the amount of

calcium in the blood and fluids. Disorders involving these three factors lead to disturbances in calcium metabolism, the most important of which, from the standpoint of veterinary pathology, are the pathological deposition of calcium called calcification and calcium deficiency. (See Chapter 4.)

### Calcification

**Definition.** Calcification is the deposition of calcium salts in tissues other than osteoid tissue and bone. It should not be confused with ossification, which is the deposition of calcium salts in osteoid tissue and bone. Calcification is of two types, general and local.

#### GENERAL CALCIFICATION

General calcification may follow increased calcium in the blood. When there is hyperactivity of the parathyroid glands, whose function it is to maintain a rather constant calcium level in the blood, this occurs. Maintaining the higher level in the blood is accomplished by withdrawing calcium from the tissues, especially the bones. As a result the bones lose calcium and become soft. The resulting condition is called *osteitis fibrosa* or *osteodystrophia fibrosa*. As a further consequence of the condition there is a deposition of calcium in numerous foci in parenchymatous organs, especially in those which secrete acid, such as the stomach (hydrochloric acid), and those which eliminate acid, such as the kidneys (hippuric and uric acid) and the lungs (carbon dioxide). This statement, that calcification may occur in the lungs where carbon dioxide is eliminated, does not sound compatible with the statement made previously, to the effect that the high calcium concentration of the blood is maintained by its high carbon dioxide content. Neither does it sound reasonable that calcification should occur where acid is secreted or eliminated. The explanation given for its occurrence in these places is that on account of the ready loss of acid, the tissues are supposed to be left in a relatively alkaline state. This explanation is not altogether satisfactory. Getting back to the subject of excess calcium in the blood and fluids, it should be stated that it may occur also as a result of excess vitamin D in the food.

LOCAL CALCIFICATION

Local calcification has no relationship to the calcium content of the blood or to the reaction of the body fluids. It is governed entirely by local conditions in the tissues. The essentials necessary for such a calcium deposition are a ground substance, which can absorb calcium, and deficient circulation. The ground substance, or matrix, consists of degenerating or necrotic tissue such as is found in tuberculous foci (Fig. 9.11), encapsulated abscesses, encysted parasites, scar tissue, poorly nourished tumors, inflammatory exudate of long standing, verminous aneurysms in the arteries of horses, old blood clots, and in foci in the walls of the large vessels of aged animals, especially those with chronic infectious or suppurative processes. In dead and dying tissue the carbon dioxide tension is low because the metabolism of the cells is at a standstill. Under these conditions the soluble calcium salt is precipitated. This process can be duplicated in the laboratory. By placing a

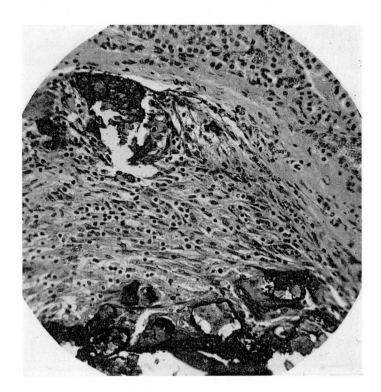

Fig. 9.11 — Calcification in a tuberculous lesion in the testicle of a boar. In the illustration the masses of calcium appear black. (Mathews, Jour. A.V.M.A.)

colloid with smooth surfaces, such as gelatine discs, in an alkaline solution and then reducing the carbon dioxide content, the soluble alkaline salt is precipitated around the discs.

In pathological calcification the ratio of calcium phosphate to calcium carbonate is practically identical with that in physiological calcification (bone formation). In gross appearance the calcium deposits remind one of grains of sand or particles of mortar. In hematoxylin and eosin-stained sections the calcium stains dark blue. It varies from fine particles having the size but not the uniform shape of bacteria up to large, dense, irregular-shaped masses.

## DISTURBANCES OF PIGMENT METABOLISM

Pigmentation of certain cells in the body is a physiological condition. Externally, in the skin, hair, and feathers, it imparts color to animals and serves as a protection against the strong actinic rays of the sun. Internally, the pigment hemoglobin functions in connection with the carrying of oxygen to the tissues and is also concerned in the formation of bile pigments. All of these pigments are endogenous; that is, they are produced within the body by the tissue cells. In pathology we are concerned with two kinds of endogenous pigments: (1) melanins and (2) hemoglobin derivatives. Disturbances in the metabolism of pigments embrace irregularities in their formation and distribution. There may be an overproduction, an underproduction, or an abnormal location of them.

### Melanins

The melanins are a group of black or brown pigments. They occur naturally in the basal layer of the epidermis; in hair; in the choroid coat of the eye; in the aorta, endometrium, and meninges of many sheep; in the oral mucosa and often in the esophageal mucosa of some breeds of dogs, especially in chows; occasionally in the testes of roosters and gobblers; often in the horns, hoofs, and claws of many animals; and in the feathers of birds. The variations in the colors of the species and breeds, and even of individuals within breeds, depend upon variations in the melanins.

The melanin that concerns us in pathology is dark brown or black. Melanin for the most part is produced by specialized cells called melanoblasts which are located mostly in the basal layers of the epidermis. The question as to whether these cells are derived from the epidermis or from the mesenchyme has not yet been settled. The origin and formation of this pigment by these cells is not fully understood either. Biochemists believe that the melanoblasts, by means of an oxidase, convert certain colorless protein derivatives in the blood into melanin. This often contains small quantities of iron and sulfur. In sections the pigment appears as dark brown or black granules. It imparts a black color to the tissue.

Some of the melanin produced by the melanoblasts is passed over to highly differentiated connective tissue cells or connective tissue phagocytes of the dermis. These act as carriers of it and are therefore called chromatophores. When dark or iron-gray horses fade to light gray or white, the melanin is transported from the melanoblasts in the skin to the lymph nodes by the chromatophores.

The most striking example of overproduction of melanin, as well as abnormal location of the pigment, is provided by melanotic tumors. These tumors are formed principally of melanoblasts which originate in the skin (Fig. 9.12). This type of tumor is common in gray and in white horses (Fig. 9.13). It has been stated that 80 per cent of gray horses develop melanomas if they reach old age. It is safe to say that one such tumor contains several hundred times as much melanin as is present in the skin of a coal-black horse. In fact, there may be such an overproduction of pigment that it spills over, so to speak, into the blood (melanemia) and may then appear in the urine (melanuria).

Another striking example of both excessive production and abnormal location of melanin occurs in calves and lambs,

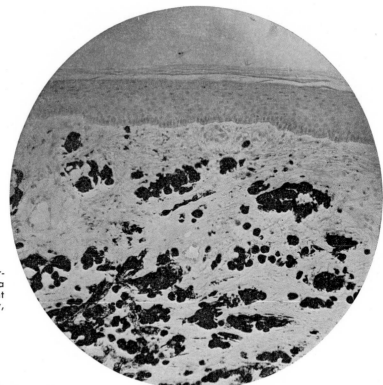

Fig. 9.12 — Melanosarcoma from the skin of a horse. ×140. (Department of Veterinary Pathology, Iowa State University).

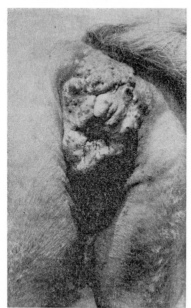

Fig. 9.13 — Melanosarcomas involving the anus and vulva of an aged gray mare. Numerous similar, small, cutaneous tumors appeared elsewhere in the same animal. (Shigley, Jour. A.V.M.A.)

sometimes in other young animals, in the form of **congenital melanosis.** The condition apparently has no relationship to the color of the animal. The pigment appears as jet-black spots upon and in the lungs, upon the epicardium and endocardium, in the liver and kidney (Fig. 9.14), under various mucous membranes, and in the coverings of the central nervous system. The pigmentation has no effect upon the health of the animal. At times it occurs more diffusely distributed and usually disappears with age.

Still another example of misplaced melanin is encountered in the mammary glands and surrounding fat of black or red gilts and sows (Fig. 9.15). This misplacement begins in the fetus. The localized area of epidermis, which proliferates and then invaginates into the corium to form the ducts of the mammary gland, may carry with it some melanoblasts which produce a considerable quantity of melanin in the belly fat. In meat-packing establishments

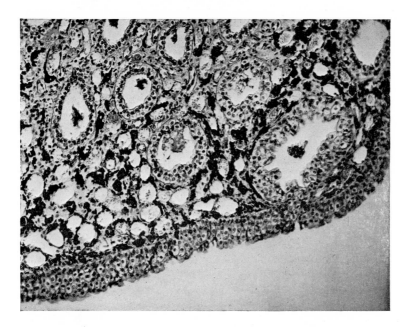

Fig. 9.14 — Melanosis of the kidney of a lamb. The pigment appears between the collecting ducts and capillaries near the pelvis. Casts of melanin lie in the ducts also. ×150. (Department of Veterinary Pathology, Iowa State University.)

bacon bellies which contain fat discolored by melanin originating in this manner are called "seedy bellies, seedy bacon, or seedy cut."

Other unusual sites for melanosis are the testicles of roosters and gobblers, and the uterus and oviducts of ewes. In any part of the body, melanosis, unaccompanied by tumor formation, is of no significance unless the part is to be used for human consumption. Even then it does not affect the wholesomeness of the part for food but is objectionable because of its appearance.

Melanosis of the cornea is reported to be a cause of blindness in some breeds of dogs. It occurs mostly in breeds that have large prominent eyes such as Boston terriers, boxers, and pekingese, but other breeds may have this ocular form of pigmentation. It is usually bilateral and symmetrical. The pigment is believed to originate in the germinal epithelium of the cornea and to become dispersed into the superficial stroma of the cornea.

A deficiency of melanin in domestic and wild animals is of rather common occurrence. Some breeds are characterized by a partial or complete white coat associated with skin that is deplete or at least almost deplete of melanin. Members of other breeds, like the Percheron horse, begin life with pigmented hair but may reach old age with a gray or white coat. One of the most interesting examples of periodic alternate pigmentation and depigmentation is shown by some of the fur-bearing animals which change colors with the seasons. Depigmented patches of skin with white hair are seen often in horses where saddle sores, collar galls, and other injuries to the epidermis have occurred and in the skin of animals exposed to the effects of ionizing radiation. These are localized areas of leukoderma. This is a pathologic state, a lack of pigment in places where it is normally present. It appears that the injured epidermal cells are deficient in the enzyme which is active in producing melanin.

A congenital absence of pigmentation with melanin is called **albinism.** A characteristic sign of albinism is absence of melanin in the iris, retina, and choroid. The eyes appear red because the vascularity of the choroid is not masked by the usual pigment. In albinos the hair is destitute of pigment wherever it is absent in the skin. The condition is common among rats, mice, and rabbits. It is occasionally seen in horses, collie dogs, English bull-dogs, and cats. In the three latter animals it is often associated with deafness.

### Hemoglobin Derivatives

An understanding of the disturbances of pigment metabolism, when the hemoglobin derivatives are involved, calls for a brief review of the fate of erythrocytes and their chemical constituents after the erythrocytes die (Fig. 9.16). When erythrocytes have served their purpose, they are destroyed principally in the spleen, the graveyard for erythrocytes. The reticuloendothelial cells of the spleen (also in the liver and bone marrow) are the actual destroyers of the erythrocytes, and when they perform their function they split the hemoglobin into two pigments, the iron-containing hemosiderin, and the iron-free bilirubin-globin complex, which is also called bilirubin proteinate. It is a large-molecule protein compound which is released into the portal circulation chiefly by the splenic reticuloendothelial cells and is carried to the liver. To differentiate this protein compound of bilirubin from the simpler form of bilirubin execreted by the liver, it seems appropriate to call it **hemobilirubin.** In this discussion we can forget the iron-containing hemosiderin.

The hepatic cells receive the hemobilirubin and split it into **cholebilirubin** and the protein fraction. (Chemically the dif-ference between hemobilirubin and chole-bilirubin is that in the latter form bilirubin is conjugated with glycouronic acid.) We can forget the protein fraction in this discussion. After cholebilirubin is excreted by the hepatic cells, it is conveyed to the duodenum by the system of bile and hepatic ducts. In the intestine, bacteria convert it into urobilinogen, a pigment which has no function in the body but is useful to the clinical pathologist. Part of the urobilinogen remains in the intestine and stains the feces. The remainder is absorbed by the intestine, transported to the liver by the portal system, and re-excreted by the liver.

Even with the normal destruction of an estimated six trillion erythrocytes daily in a horse and a corresponding number in other species, there is no pigmentation resulting from hemoglobin derivatives. It is only when the destruction is far greater than normal or when the pigments cannot be disposed of in an animal in the usual way that pigmentation occurs. Thus, only when there is a general increase of pigments in the blood in diseases characterized by the destruction of erythrocytes, and in conditions in which there is a marked disturbance of liver function or an interference with the excretion of bile, does actual **generalized** pigmentation result. It should be mentioned here, however, that there is a **local** increase of blood

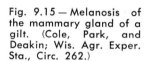
Fig. 9.15 — Melanosis of the mammary gland of a gilt. (Cole, Park, and Deakin; Wis. Agr. Exper. Sta., Circ. 262.)

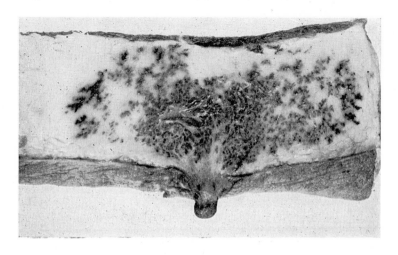

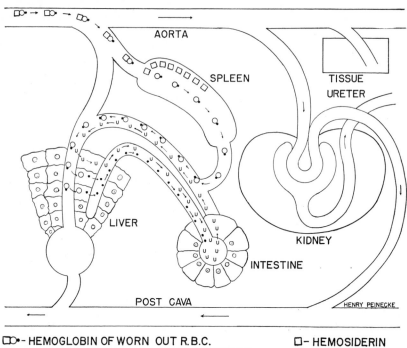

CD•- HEMOGLOBIN OF WORN OUT R.B.C.          □- HEMOSIDERIN
O• - BILIRUBIN PROTEINATE (HEMOBILIRUBIN)   • - CHOLEBILIRUBIN
O - PROTEIN PORTION OF BILIRUBIN PROTEINATE  ᵁ - UROBILINOGEN

Fig. 9.16 — Fate of blood pigments under normal conditions.

pigments in an area of hemorrhage, infarction, or chronic passive hyperemia due to the accumulation of blood pigments.

### ICTERUS (JAUNDICE)

Icterus (jaundice) is a pathologic condition in which there is an excessive amount of either hemobilirubin, or cholebilirubin, or both in the circulating blood (hyperbilirubinemia). When these pigments are present in excess in the blood, they stain the tissues grossly a yellowish hue. Since both forms of bilirubin are soluble in the body fluids they are not usually visible in histological preparations. Only when they are present in massive amounts can they be seen. They then have the form of reddish-brown rhombic plates or needle-like crystals. They are located chiefly between cells, but some may be engulfed by phagocytes.

There are three forms of icterus. To understand them and the uses which can be made of the clinical laboratory tests which are employed for the diagnosis of icterus, one must keep in mind the sequence of events just outlined regarding the fate of erythrocytes. In the first place it becomes apparent that an excessive amount of either hemobilirubin or cholebilirubin, or both, in the blood (hyperbilirubinemia) may result from something that happens (1) before the hemobilirubin reaches the liver, (2) at the time it is in the liver, or (3) after cholebilirubin leaves the liver. Anatomically then, the origin of icterus may be said to be: (1) prehepatic, (2) intrahepatic, or (3) posthepatic.

**Prehepatic icterus.** In prehepatic icterus (Fig. 9.17), quite obviously, the reason for the appearance of an excessive amount of hemobilirubin in the blood must be attributed to something which happens in the first stages of the pigment formation. What happens is that there is an increased destruction of erythrocytes. In domestic mammals the usual causes of the destruction of the erythrocytes are exogenous hemolytic agents such as the virus of equine infectious anemia, certain strains of streptococci, the protozoan blood parasites such as piroplasmata and eperythrozoa, snake venom, and lead salts. Because the hyperbilirubinemia is the result of hemolysis, this condition is also called **hemolytic icterus.**

A most unusual prehepatic icterus has been reported in foals in Kentucky. Occasionally, foals that are normal at birth develop icterus in 24 to 48 hours and die before they are four days old. After they develop icterus they have only 2,000,000 to 3,000,000 erythrocytes per cmm. The serum of the mares which give birth to these colts will agglutinate the erythrocytes of the stallion that sired the foals. The factors which are responsible for the destruction of the erythrocytes are present in the colostrum of the dam. They are antibodies of two types—one that agglutinates

erythrocytes (hemagglutinin) and the other which destroys erythrocytes (hemolysin).

Experimentally, a similar condition can be produced in swine; that is, a sow can be sensitized to the erythrocytes of the boar to whom she was bred. The sow develops hemagglutinins and hemolysins for the boar's erythrocytes. Pigs that inherit erythrocytes similar to the sire's will develop hemolytic icterus and die. This type of iso-immunization of sows also occurs naturally. Pigs farrowed by such sows are born healthy but develop the hemolytic disease within a few hours. In this naturally occurring condition iso-agglutinins, but not isohemolysins, have been found in the sow's serum and colostrum. In spite of isohemolysins not being detectable in the sows, the pigs have a severe hemolytic anemia. The peculiar feature of the anemia is that it may or may not be characterized by icterus.

This condition in domestic mammals

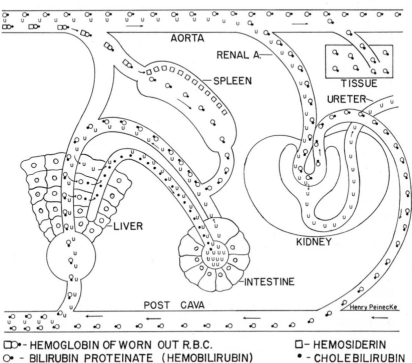

□▶- HEMOGLOBIN OF WORN OUT R.B.C.          □- HEMOSIDERIN
O▶ - BILIRUBIN PROTEINATE (HEMOBILIRUBIN)   • - CHOLEBILIRUBIN
O - PROTEIN PORTION OF BILIRUBIN PROTEINATE  ᵁ - UROBILINOGEN

Fig. 9.17 — Fate of blood pigments in prehepatic (hemolytic) jaundice.

reminds one of the hemolytic anemia and icterus of newborn babies (erythroblastosis fetalis) which occurs when a mother is Rh negative and develops antibodies against the fetus which is Rh positive. In women the antibodies can reach the infant in two ways: (1) directly from the maternal to the fetal circulation, and (2) after birth, in the colostrum. The direct passage from the maternal to the fetal circulation is possible because only three tissue layers separate the two circulations. In the bitch, in which four tissue layers separate the two circulations, it is known that antibodies can pass from the dam to the fetus. In the other species, however, this is apparently not possible because five to seven tissue layers form a natural barrier. In these species the fetus gets the antibodies only in the colostrum.

With the greater destruction of erythrocytes in prehepatic icterus the reticuloendothelial cells of the spleen, liver, and bone marrow discharge increased quantities of hemobilirubin. Furthermore the liver, even though normal, is unable to handle the increased amount of hemobilirubin and leaves part of it in the blood where it circulates and stains the tissues very moderately. The hemobilirubin circulating in the blood cannot pass through the renal filter (glomerulus) because the large protein molecule with which the pigment is combined is too large. The hemobilirubin can be detected in the blood serum by the Van den Bergh test.

In prehepatic icterus the liver attempts to relieve the blood of the excess load of hemobilirubin and, in doing this, it excretes an increased amount of cholebilirubin which in turn is converted into urobilinogen in the intestine. This colors the feces deeply. The intestine absorbs more of the urobilinogen than normally, and when this is transported to the liver by the portal vein, the already overtaxed liver, unable to handle it, leaves it in the blood to be disposed of by the kidneys. Its presence in the urine can be detected by Ehrlich's aldehyde test. Liver function tests show that the liver parenchyma has not been damaged in this form of icterus.

To summarize, the clinical laboratory tests therefore indicate that there is an increased destruction of erythrocytes, and that the liver is functioning normally but its function is overtaxed.

**Intrahepatic icterus.** In intrahepatic icterus (Fig. 9.18) the pathologic changes responsible for hyperbilirubinemia are located in the hepatic cells and bile capillaries. Degeneration and necrosis of the hepatic cells (Fig. 17.34) are the histologic changes responsible for the presence of excessive amounts of bilirubin in the blood. These cellular alterations permit seepage of the pigment from the bile capillaries into the blood sinusoids. The liver damage is caused by various toxic agents, examples of which are the endotoxin of the spirochete *Leptospira canicola*, the virus of infectious canine hepatitis, the salt of a heavy metal like lead arsenate, an alkaloid like that present in the senecios (ragworts), and a mineral such as selenium occurring in plants in the western plains states. Because the condition is usually caused by toxic substances it is also called **toxic icterus.**

In intrahepatic icterus only a fraction of the total number of liver cells are damaged, otherwise the animal would die before the onset of the condition. The hepatic cells which can function convert as much as possible of the hemobilirubin into cholebilirubin. That which is unconverted remains in the blood and can be detected by testing the serum with the Van den Bergh test. Functioning cells convert some of the hemobilirubin to cholebilirubin, but due to disruption of the bile capillaries it is diverted into the blood sinusoids and thence into the general circulation so that its presence can be demonstrated by the appropriate reaction to the Van den Bergh test. Other tests reveal a condition of liver dysfunction.

Some cholebilirubin is excreted by the functioning liver cells. It goes the usual route and some of it returns to the liver in the form of urobilinogen, but the liver is incapable of acting upon it, so it is excreted by the kidneys. The Van den Bergh test will indicate the presence of

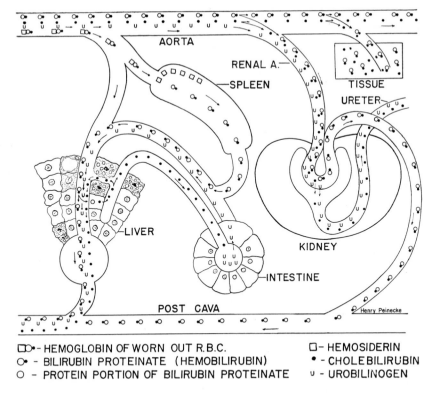

AORTA
RENAL A.
SPLEEN
TISSUE
URETER
LIVER
KIDNEY
INTESTINE
POST CAVA
Henry Peinecke

☐▷• – HEMOGLOBIN OF WORN OUT R.B.C.          ☐ – HEMOSIDERIN
○• – BILIRUBIN PROTEINATE (HEMOBILIRUBIN)    • – CHOLEBILIRUBIN
○ – PROTEIN PORTION OF BILIRUBIN PROTEINATE  ᴜ – UROBILINOGEN

Fig. 9.18 — Fate of blood pigments in intrahepatic (toxic) jaundice.

cholebilirubin in the serum, and Ehrlich's aldehyde test the presence of urobilinogen in the urine.

Circulation of the two forms of bilirubin throughout the body stains the tissues. The tissues stained most conspicuously are the visible mucous membranes and the skin of white animals. The urine is stained distinctly yellow by the cholebilirubin because its small molecule can pass through the renal filter.

To summarize, the clinical laboratory tests in intrahepatic icterus reveal hyperbilirubinemia with both hemobilirubin and cholebilirubin present, and liver dysfunction, and the presence of an increased amount of urobilinogen in the urine.

**Posthepatic icterus.** In posthepatic icterus (Fig. 9.19) the underlying factor responsible for the hyperbilirubinemia is bile passage obstruction (**obstructive icterus**) which may be due to any one of several things. Among them are mature ascarids in swine (Fig. 15.20), fringed

tapeworms in sheep, liver flukes in cattle and sheep (Fig. 15.28), gall stones, tumors of the ducts or of structures adjacent to the ducts, enlarged portal lymph nodes, and inflammatory swelling of the duct wall. Cholebilirubin in the bile and hepatic ducts which cannot leave the passages because of the obstruction is reabsorbed by the blood capillaries along the passages and accumulates in the blood. There is a possibility also that back pressure of bile in the bile capillaries of the hepatic cords may cause leaks or diffusion of the pigment into the blood sinusoids. The circulating cholebilirubin stains the tissues intensely and colors the urine highly. Since in posthepatic icterus bile does not reach the intestine when the obstruction is complete, the feces are clay-colored due to the absence of urobilinogen, and greasy because of incomplete fat digestion.

Since the biliary obstruction may be either partial or complete, the reactions to the usual clinical laboratory tests will be

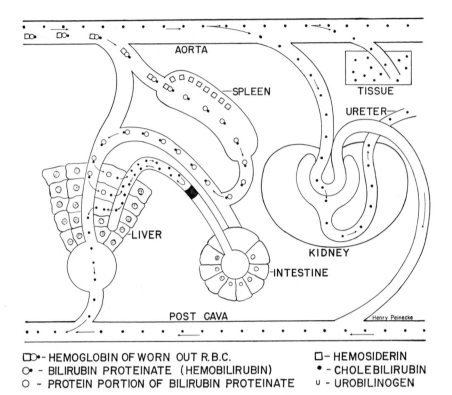

CD•- HEMOGLOBIN OF WORN OUT R.B.C.          □ – HEMOSIDERIN
O• - BILIRUBIN PROTEINATE (HEMOBILIRUBIN)          • - CHOLEBILIRUBIN
O - PROTEIN PORTION OF BILIRUBIN PROTEINATE          ᵁ - UROBILINOGEN

Fig. 9.19 — Fate of blood pigments in posthepatic (obstructive) jaundice.

somewhat variable. In either case the Van den Bergh test will show only the presence of cholebilirubin, and the function tests will indicate no dysfunction. Some urobilinogen will be present in the urine if the obstruction is partial but none at all if it is complete.

In connection with the diagnosis of each kind of jaundice, reference has been made to the use of the Van den Bergh test for the detection of bilirubin in the blood serum. It is appropriate here to summarize this information and elaborate a little regarding the test without describing the technic for conducting it. When the reagent is added to the serum containing cholebilirubin alone (obstructive icterus), an immediate reaction occurs. This is called the direct or immediate Van den Bergh reaction. When the reagent is added to serum containing hemobilirubin (hemolytic icterus), no reaction occurs until cholebilirubin has been freed from the complex globin molecule (hemobilirubin) as a result of the addition of alcohol. This reaction occurs slowly and is therefore called the indirect or delayed Van den Bergh reaction. When the reagent is added to serum containing both hemobilirubin and cholebilirubin (toxic icterus) an immediate and a delayed reaction occur. This is called the biphasic or mixed Van den Bergh reaction.

### HEMOSIDEROSIS

Hemosiderin occurs as fine, amorphous, yellowish-brown granules or crystals under the same conditions that give rise to the presence of bilirubin. The pigment, however, is more frequently seen histologically because it is less soluble in body fluids than bilirubin. It gives the Prussian blue reaction for ferric iron when gross specimens or sections are treated with potassium ferrocyanide and hydrochloric acid. The reticuloendothelial cells of the bone marrow, spleen, liver, and other parts of the body are concerned in its formation. These same cells, along with the epithelial cells of the liver and kidneys, phagocytize the pigment so that it always appears intracellularly. Its presence in an organ or tissue is spoken of as hemosiderosis. In addition to its appearance in old hemorrhages and infarcts, it is seen in the lungs and spleen in chronic passive hyperemia.

Under normal conditions the spleen contains varying amounts of hemosiderin. It is greatest in the horse and least in the dog. In old animals it is greater than in the young. In hemolytic diseases, except in chronic equine infectious anemia, it increases in amount. In chronic equine infectious anemia there is a remarkable disappearance of hemosiderin from the spleen and a just as remarkable increase of it in the liver. It has been theorized that in this disease the spleen relinquishes its function as a destroyer of erythrocytes and concentrates on antibody production. The destruction of erythrocytes is then apparently assumed by the liver because it shows extreme hemosiderosis.

The deposition of iron pigment in the kidneys may occur in animals suffering with diseases associated with intravascular hemolysis. A good example is equine infectious anemia. The hemosiderin accumulates in the epithelial cells of the tubules and interferes with their excretory functions. The deposition of iron pigment in the walls of some of the blood vessels of the brain of healthy horses has been reported by Saunders. In the cerebrums of 15 out of 25 healthy horses over 6 years of age he observed the pigment in the walls and in some cases around the vessels in the places where the wall was pigmented. He concluded that the presence of iron pigment in these places makes the presence of it in the brains of horses which have symptoms of brain diseases of little or no significance.

A brown, sometimes almost black, pigmentation of the bones, called **osteohemochromatosis,** is seen occasionally in cattle and hogs in packing houses and on farms where home butchering is practiced. All of the bones of the skeleton may participate in the discoloration. Spongy bones display a uniform pigmentation, but compact bones show it mostly under the periosteum. In teeth the dentine and cement are discolored but the enamel remains white. Cartilage, ligaments, and tendons are not involved. Sometimes, however, the bone marrow, lymph nodes, kidneys, liver, and spleen show the same pigmentation (hemochromatosis). The pigment reacts to the test for iron like hemosiderin but has the spectroscopic characteristics of hematoporphyrin. Even though the pigment has the characteristics of a porphyrin, the affected animals do not show the symptoms of a porphyria such as sensitiveness of the skin to sunlight. The cause of the pigmentation is unknown. In some animals at least it is apparently congenital.

Fourie, who has made an extensive study of this condition in cattle in South Africa, presents evidence which indicates that osteohemochromatosis may be a misnomer for this disease. While the bones may be discolored by an iron-containing blood pigment, he believes that basically the disease is a disturbance of porphyrin metabolism. The underlying condition he designates **congenital porphyria,** which may be characterized by porphyrinuria and porphyrinemia. In the cases he studied, the teeth had a brownish-pink discoloration which suggests the popular name "pink tooth" for the disease. The bones were mahogany brown. The animals he observed displayed some degree of photosensitization, and several of them were the progeny of one bull.

### Exogenous Pigmentation

Exogenous pigmentation is not a disturbance of metabolism, but for the sake of convenience it will be considered here. Foreign substances entering the body by way of the respiratory and digestive tracts and the skin and subsequently deposited in the tissues constitute this type of pigmentation. In veterinary pathology only exogenous pigmentation of the lungs is of any significance, and even that is not usually serious from the standpoint of the health of animals.

The lung and its lymph nodes are the reservoir for various dust particles which are inhaled in the air. They may be found free in the bronchioles and alveoli, in macrophages in the alveoli, in the alveolar epithelial cells, in the endothelial cells of the peribronchial and interlobular lymph vessels, in the peribronchial lymph follicles, and eventually in the bronchial lymph nodes. In the latter the pigment is located in the lymph cords of the medulla. The dust particles act as mild irritants, and the tissue response to them is a slight increase in connective tissue. The pigment with this accompanying fibrosis is called **pneumoconiosis.** If the pigmentation is the result of coal dust, as it so frequently is in city-reared dogs, and in horses and mules used around and in coal mines, the condition is called **anthracosis.** A similar condition occurring in the lungs of animals living or working in stone quarries and cement plants is designated **silicosis** or **chalicosis** (calcicosis).

Hulse, in England, believes that when inhaled dust particles reach the alveoli they are engulfed by alveolar phagocytes which subsequently become overgrown by other dust-laden phagocytes. This heaping up of phagocytes engorged with dust gives the appearance of the presence of dust in the interstitial tissue when in reality it is in the accumulation of phagocytes.

In man there is a form of exogenous pigmentation with hemosiderin severe enough to be classed as **exogenous hemochromatosis.** It occurs as a result of repeated blood transfusions (approximately 200 or more). At first only the liver, spleen, and pancreas are pigmented, but eventually hemosiderin appears in the dermis and in Brunner's glands of the duodenum. It is not likely that transfusions will be made over a period sufficiently long to cause such an exogenous hemochromatosis in animals.

## LIPOCHROMES

Of much less importance than the melanins are the lipochromes or fatlike substances which contain yellow pigments and occur in natural fats. The pigments in lipochromes may be carotene and xanthophyls present in plants eaten by animals. Some of the lipochromes stain red with Sudan IV. Normally they are present as yellowish granules in the heart muscles, nerve cells, seminal vesicles, adrenal cortex, corpus luteum, and the interstitial cells of the testes. They are sometimes called "wear and tear" pigments because they seem to be produced from the cytoplasm of atrophic cells.

When organs or parts containing the lipochrome granules atrophy, the discoloration due to the granules becomes very prominent. The color may be yellowish, brownish yellow, or almost black. This discoloration constitutes the condition of **lipochromatosis** or **xanthosis.** Meat inspectors observe it most frequently in the lingual, masseter, and cardiac muscles. Sometimes they see it in the diaphragm, neck, and leg muscles and much less frequently in the trunk muscles. In California it is reported to occur about once in 700 head of dairy cattle and about once in 2,000 head of beef cattle. This pigmentation also occurs in the testes of aged dogs. Generally the pigmentation is associated with atrophy of the affected organ or part, and is then designated **brown atrophy.**

Microscopically, brown, iron-free pigment granules are present at the poles of the nuclei of affected muscle cells and in the interstitial cells of the testes.

A peculiar yellow or brownish pigmentation of adipose tissue occurs in mink kits and occasionally in pigs that are fed on fresh fish or fresh ocean fish scrap which has not been supplemented with tocopherol (vitamin E). The pigment, which is acid-fast, accumulates in the fat cells and is also phagocytized by macrophages. Sometimes an inflammation of the adipose tissue (steatitis) accompanies the pigmentation. It is believed that the feeding of excessive quantities of highly unsaturated glycerides along with inadequate amounts of tocopherols is in some way responsible for the condition.

An extremely rare condition of pigmentation in the wattles and skin of white leghorn pullets has been reported. The pigment, which is orange-yellow to yellow in color, occurs intracellularly in the epidermis, dermis, and subcutis of the wattles and in areas on the breast, abdomen, and thighs. The skin of involved areas is thickened and tumor-like in appearance. Microscopically, the swellings consist of foam cells, fibroblasts, lipoid droplets, and lenticular spaces. Histochemically, the lesions yield an abundance of cholesterol, which apparently fills the lenticular spaces. The condition is designated **xanthomatosis.** The cause is not known.

## REFERENCES

Bollman, J. L., and Schlotthauer, C. F.: 1936. Uremia in turkeys. Jour. A.V.M.A., 42:313.

Bruner, D. W., Brown, R. G., Hull, F. E., and Kinkaid, A. S.: 1949. Blood factors and baby pig anemia. Jour. A.V.M.A., 105:94.

————, Hull, F. E., Edwards, P. R., and Doll, E. R.: 1948. Icteric foals. Jour. A.V.M.A., 112:440.

Cronin, M. T. J.: 1955. Haemolytic disease in newborn foals. Vet. Rec., 67:479.

Doll, E. R., and Brown, R. G.: 1954. Isohemolytic disease of newborn pigs. Cornell Vet., 44:86.

Gorham, J. R., Boe, N., and Baker, G. A.: 1951. Experimental "yellow fat" disease in pigs. Cornell Vet., 41:332.

Grayzel, H. G., Jacobi, M., Marshall, H. B., Bogen, M., and Bolker, H.: 1934. Amyloidosis: experimental studies. Arch. Path., 17:50.

# CHAPTER 10

# Death

## NECROSIS

**Definition.** Necrosis is the local death of tissue cells within the living individual.

Disturbances in cell metabolism can be of such a nature that the cell eventually dies after it has gradually passed through such retrogressive changes as cloudy swelling and fatty degeneration. Cells which die and remain in the living body for various periods after their death obviously do not look the same as they did at the time of their death. In view of this we can expect to find a variety of changes in necrotic cells, depending upon the length of time they have been carried in the living body after their death.

### Causes of Necrosis

When cells are denied oxygen or food or have the physical and chemical constitution of their protoplasm altered to such an extent that they cannot adapt themselves to their changed environment, they die. Such death may be brought about by:

1. **Bacterial endotoxins** such as those resulting from infection by *Spherophorus necrophorus, Mycobacterium tuberculosis, Brucella suis, Pseudomonas aeruginosa, Corynebacterium renale,* and *Corynebacterium pyogenes.*

2. **Physical influences** such as heat, cold, electricity, and mechanical forces.

3. **Chemical substances** (inorganic and organic) such as mineral acids, caustic alkalies, and phenol.

### Cellular Changes in Necrosis

Soon after cells die it is believed they liberate thrombokinase which causes coagulation of the fibrinogen in the blood plasma and cells. As a result, the cytoplasm appears granular. Skeletal and heart muscle cells lose their striations and the sarcoplasm often becomes homogeneous. The alterations are not confined to the cytoplasm alone, because any one of three distinct changes occurs in the nuclei: 1. The nuclei may lose their affinity for basic stains and gradually fade until only rings indicating their outlines remain. Finally these too disappear. This, the most common indication of nuclear death, is called **karyolysis.** 2. The nuclei may fragment as they do at the border of an infarct or base of an ulcer (Fig. 10.1). **Karyorrhexis** is the name given to this change. 3. The nuclei frequently shrink and stain deeply with hematoxylin because there is a condensation of the chromatin. This is **pyknosis.**

In sections which have been prepared from animals that have been dead several hours, many of the cells will have undergone self-digestion — autolysis. This is es-

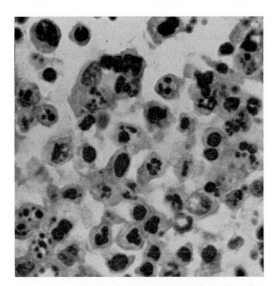

Fig. 10.1 — Karyorrhexis in a lymph node of a dog with infectious canine hepatitis. (Department of Veterinary Pathology, Michigan State University.)

pecially true of glandular epithelium. Postmortem autolytic changes are easily confused with the changes which characterize necrosis. In autolysis, pyknosis of the nuclei occurs similarly as in necrosis. There is at first an abnormal increase of chromatin granules, next a coalescence of the granules followed by shrinkage of the nuclei. The final result is pyknotic nuclei which may contain tiny vacuoles but are otherwise homogeneous. Within a few hours after somatic death the cytoplasm of unfixed glandular epithelial cells becomes granular, similarly as it does in cloudy swelling, but as soon as autolysis occurs the cell membranes rupture or become irregular in outline and the granules undergo dissolution. If tissues are fixed in a preservative such as 10 per cent formalin within one to two hours after death, the autolytic changes do not ordinarily occur. Sections prepared from these tissues are more suitable for study. The student must remember, however, that often material for sections may be obtained only at the time of necropsy, which may be several hours after death.

## Coagulative Necrosis

**Definition.** Coagulative necrosis is local death, within the living individual, of tissue in which the architectural detail of the area persists but the cellular detail is lost.

Up to this point the changes which occur in necrosis are fairly common to all types of cells. Beyond this point other cellular changes can occur, but most necrosis progresses no further than this stage. It characterizes infarcts of the kidney (Fig. 7.11), liver (Fig. 17.35), and spleen, the necrotic areas caused by such caustic chemical agents as phenol and mercuric chloride, by other poisons such as thallium sulfate (Fig. 10.2), and by some bacteria such as *Spherophorus necrophorus* (Figs. 10.3 and 10.4). Grossly, the area of necrotic tissue is yellowish gray or pale yellow in color. It does not shrink at first and may even be increased in volume. While the tissue may appear dry, there is actually no loss of fluid. In fact, this type of necrosis occurs where the tissue is kept moist by the diffusion of lymph. Microscopically, the architectural outlines of the

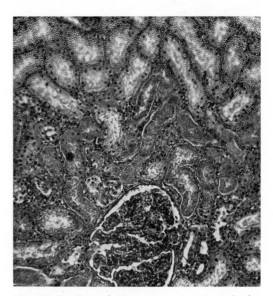

Fig. 10.2 — Coagulative necrosis caused by thallium suflate. Kidney of a cow.
(Low power.) (McCrory and Ward, Jour. A.V.M.A.)

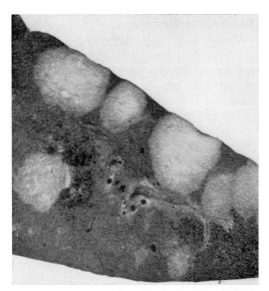

Fig. 10.3 — Areas of coagulative necrosis caused by **Spherophorus necrophorus** in a cow's liver. (Barnes and Brueckner, Jour. A.V.M.A.)

organ are preserved. The cell detail, however, is lost. The granular appearance of the cytoplasm reminds one of cloudy swelling. Pyknosis and karyolysis are prominent in the center of the area and karyorrhexis usually at the border.

## Caseous Necrosis

**Definition.** Caseous necrosis is the local death, within the living individual, of tissue characterized by the absence of both architectural and cellular detail and which is fused into a homogeneous granular mass resembling cottage cheese.

Only fragments of nuclei remain mixed in with the pink-staining, granular cell debris. This type of necrosis is characteristic of the lesions of tuberculosis (Fig. 10.5) and glanders. Probably because of the high hydrogen-ion concentration of these lesions, there is no infiltration of them with polymorphonuclear leukocytes, and, hence, there is an absence of their proteolytic enzymes which have marked ability to produce liquefaction. As a consequence, these areas of dry, cheesy, granular necrotic tissue remain as such for long periods of time.

## Liquefactive Necrosis

**Definition.** Liquefactive necrosis is the local death, within the living individual, of tissue characterized by the disintegration of the necrotic material into a liquid mass in which cellular and architectural detail is lost.

In tissue poor in coagulable albuminous material but rich in lipoids, such as the brain and cord, the necrotic tissue undergoes rapid digestion. This is called liquefactive necrosis but it is actually coagulative or caseous necrosis followed by digestion of the dead tissue. The digestion is carried on by enzymes which are present in the tissue, elaborated by bacteria, or secreted by the larvae of primary blowflies. As stated above, it is the common form of necrosis of nervous tissue (Fig. 10.6). It may follow coagulative necrosis in other tissues, however, especially in those that have undergone fatty degeneration or that have become macerated with serous fluid. In these tissues the digestion is an autolytic process. In liquefactive necrosis the dead tissue has a creamy or

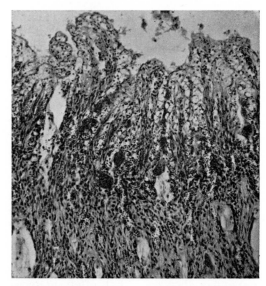

Fig. 10.4 — Coagulative necrosis caused by bacteria in the mucosa of the jejunum of a cat. Note colonies of bacteria at base of a zone of necrosis in which much of the normal architecture persists. ×140. (Department of Veterinary Pathology, Iowa State University.)

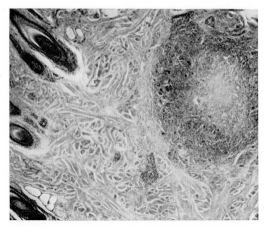

Fig. 10.5 — Caseous necrosis in the center of a cutaneous lesion caused by **Mycobacterium tuberculosis** in a cow. ×25. (Runnells, Jour. A.V.M.A.)

pasty consistency. At its margin there is a zone of hyperemia and inflammation. Bleeding into the area of necrosis naturally changes the color of the liquefied tissue. The focus of liquefaction may be absorbed and a cystlike cavity may remain.

### Fat Necrosis

**Definition.** Fat necrosis is the death of adipose tissue. There are two types: abdominal (internal) and subcutaneous (external).

The abdominal form of fat necrosis has been produced by various experimental procedures such as ligation of the pancreatic duct, temporary obstruction of the pancreatic circulation, sectioning the pancreas, placing fresh pancreas in the abdominal cavity, and the injection intraperitoneally of pancreatic juice, pancreatic emulsion, commercial pancreatin, and lipase. As a result of this experimental production of abdominal fat necrosis it is believed that when pancreatic juice escapes from the pancreas either as the result of injury or inflammation of that organ, the proteolytic and lipolytic enzymes attack the adipose tissue of the abdominal cavity. It seems quite probable that the protease attacks the adipose tissue cells first and kills them, and that the lipase then digests the fat.

Subcutaneous fat necrosis is also called traumatic fat necrosis because it is believed to be due to a mechanical injury of the adipose tissue. The origin of the lipase which is responsible for subcutaneous fat necrosis has been the subject of speculation for a long time. It never has seemed reasonable that it comes from the pancreas. In China it was suggested that its source might be vegetable lipase in the ration of affected animals, but in Missouri the condition could not be produced by feeding soybeans and peanuts which contain lipase. Recently it has been shown that while adipose tissue does not contain lipase, connective tissue does, so it seems probable that when the subcutis is traumatized, tissue lipase (and also protease)

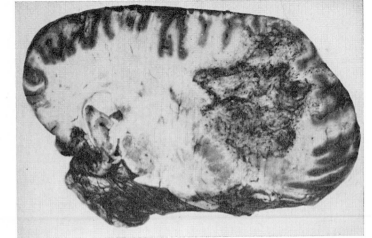

Fig. 10.6 — Liquefactive necrosis such as is found in moldy corn poisoning in the cerebrum of the horse. (Doyle, Jour. A.V.M.A.)

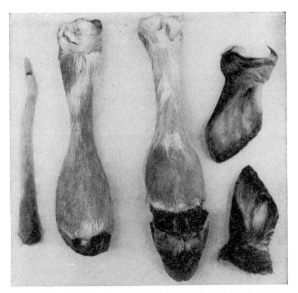

Fig. 10.7 — Dry gangrene of ears, feet, and tail of a month-old calf. This is the type of necrosis occurring in ergotism and fescue-foot. (Department of Veterinary Pathology, Michigan State University.)

is released. To substantiate this theory the skin of young pigs has been pinched with forceps, and fat necrosis has resulted.

The affected fat is split into fatty acids and glycerine. The glycerine is soluble and is removed from the area by the lymph stream. The fatty acids remain in the cells in the form of acicular crystals that are laid down in a very irregular manner (Fig. 10.8). Some of the fatty acid combines with calcium to form calcium soap. Cells containing it are filled with a finely granular or homogeneous bluish-pink material in sections stained in the usual manner. In some of the cells, calcium may be precipitated from the soap. It takes a deep blue stain. At the periphery of the necrotic area is the usual narrow inflammatory zone which surrounds necrotic tissue. Since the necrotic area constitutes a foreign body, it is to be expected that macrophages and foreign body giant cells will appear in this peripheral inflammatory zone.

Grossly, in the normal adipose tissue of the mesentery and sometimes of the omentum and perirenal region, there are pinhead to rather large, sharply circumscribed, yellowish-white to chalky-white, opaque areas. Upon palpation they feel firm and nodular. Their cut surface is dry, hard, cheesy, and opaque. When calcium is precipitated in them, they feel gritty.

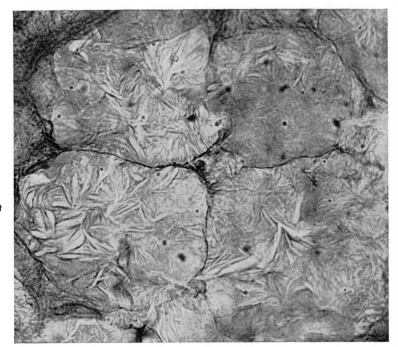

Fig. 10.8 — Fat necrosis of the peripancreatic fat of a pig. Note acicular crystals of fatty acid in the fat cells. ×400. (Department of Veterinary Pathology, Iowa State University.)

Fat necrosis has been reported in most of the domestic mammals. It is seldom diagnosed in life except in cows. In them it is found occasionally when a veterinarian is palpating the reproductive organs for indications of pregnancy or for the causes of sterility. He may even mistake a nodule of fat necrosis for an ovary. In such cows the fat necrosis may have arisen from injury during parturition.

Fat necrosis is detected mostly during post-mortem examinations and is therefore encountered principally by meat inspectors. They observe the condition quite often in cattle. The occurrence of it in the thoracic cavity is occasionally reported by them. They see the condition in swine also, especially in the South, where kidney worms (*Stephanurus dentatus*) cause injury in the perirenal fat, in the pancreas, and in the pancreatic duct. Usually, though, the inspector can not determine the source of the lipase causing the necrosis because the pancreas often appears normal macroscopically and no other source of the enzyme can be detected. The subcutaneous form, which occasionally is seen when animals are skinned, is undoubtedly due to trauma inflicted some time in the past.

## Gangrene

**Definition.** Gangrene is the invasion and putrefaction of necrotic tissue by saprophytic bacteria.

**Etiology.** Gangrene can involve any tissue of the body but is most frequently observed in the lungs, intestine, mammary gland, heavy muscles of the thigh and shoulder, and the extremities. Gangrene of the lung often results from drenching the animal with medicament from a bottle. Whenever an animal is drenched, the head must be held horizontal with the ground, and, in addition, the medicament must be given slowly so the animal can swallow it. If the head is held too high or the medicament is administered too rapidly, the animal is unable to swallow it and, instead of the material going into the esophagus, it flows into the trachea and into the lungs. The medicament is often quite irritating and injures the lung tissue. In addition, it carries bacteria with it into the lungs. As the result of the lung injury and the invasion of the necrotic tissue by saprophytic organisms, gangrene occurs.

Pulmonary gangrene can be caused by improper insertion of a stomach tube. Instead of being inserted into the esophagus and stomach, the tube sometimes is passed into the trachea by mistake, and the medicament is pumped into the lungs rather than the stomach.

Gangrene of the lung is associated with paralysis, anomalies, and infectious diseases of the throat in which the direction of the food passing through the pharynx cannot be controlled, and the food, instead of going into the esophagus, enters the larynx and trachea. As a result, it gravitates into the lungs and gangrene occurs.

Gangrene of the intestinal tract in the horse is usually associated with infarction resulting from a verminous thrombus in the anterior mesenteric artery or is the result of acute local passive hyperemia associated with a malposition of the viscera (torsion, volvulus, or intussusception). The vascular disturbance causes necrosis of the intestinal wall, and the necrotic tissue is then invaded with saprophytic bacteria found in the intestinal content.

Gangrene of the extremities (leg, ear, tail, wattle, or comb) is most frequently associated with freezing. The freezing temperatures cause coagulative necrosis of the tissue that is later invaded with saprophytic bacteria. Certain drugs or plants (ergot and fescue grass) contain active principles which cause arterial spasms to restrict the flow of blood to the extremity, and ischemia is the result. Because of the ischemia, necrosis of the extremity occurs, and later the tissue is invaded with bacteria.

Gangrene of the mammary gland results when the tissue becomes necrotic following a staphylococcic mastitis and is invaded by saprophytic bacteria.

**Macroscopic appearance.** Gangrene may

be divided into two main types, dry gangrene and moist gangrene. Whether a tissue exhibits dry gangrene or moist gangrene depends upon the amount of moisture present as well as the temperature of the tissue.

**Dry gangrene.** Dry gangrene is usually observed in the extremities. When necrosis has occurred, fluid is no longer brought to the area because the circulation to the part is no longer maintained. Then dehydration by evaporation occurs and the necrotic tissue becomes dry. Since bacteria require moisture for optimum growth, the invasion and spread of bacteria in the area are slow. The second factor that determines whether dry gangrene is present or not is the temperature of the extremity. When the tissue is dead and the circulation is no longer maintained, the part becomes cool. The growth rate of bacteria is suppressed when the surroundings are cool, and, therefore, invasion and spread of bacteria through the necrotic tissue are slow.

The area of gangrene is dry and shrivelled and appears to be mummified. This dry shrivelled appearance is the result of dehydration by evaporation. The color of the extremity is reddish brown, green, gray, or black. The color depends upon the pigments liberated by the disintegrating erythrocytes as well as the presence of hydrogen sulfide, resulting from bacterial putrefaction of the dead tissue. When hydrogen sulfide comes in contact with the iron contained within blood pigment, a black pigment (iron sulfide) is produced. The area has a very disagreeable putrid odor as the result of the presence of hydrogen sulfide and other volatile gases produced in the area of decomposition. Although gas from putrefaction is present, it usually exists in such small amounts that it is not observed macroscopically.

Dry gangrene extends along the extremity in the direction of the body until a point is reached where the circulation is adequate to maintain life in the area. At this point, a sharp line of demarkation develops between the living and dead tissue. It is along this line that a severe inflammatory reaction develops when the body defenses attempt to prevent the bacteria from invading the living tissue. In addition, the defense line tries to prevent the entrance of toxins formed in the dead tissue from being absorbed by the living tissue and carried to all parts of the body. Along this line of defense there is an accumulation of neutrophils, macrophages, and other leukocytes as well as lytic enzymes. The leukocytes and lytic enzymes cause liquefaction of the dead tissue along the sharp line of defense. If successful, amputation of the extremity occurs along the defense line. In this manner the body rids itself of the putrefying tissue.

**Moist gangrene.** Moist gangrene usually occurs in the internal organs where there is an abundance of moisture and where the necrotic tissue is kept warm by the surrounding living organs. When optimum conditions of moisture and warmth are present, the growth and spread of saprophytic bacteria are very rapid. Once the bacteria begin to grow and multiply and liberate their toxins, they can no longer be confined within the necrotic tissue and spread to adjacent organs. This is particularly true when the moist gangrene involves the intestinal tract, because numerous bacteria capable of invading the intestinal wall are contained within the content of the intestine. In addition, when the wall of the intestine becomes necrotic, rupture occurs and the fecal content is discharged into the peritoneal cavity, facilitating the spread of microorganisms throughout the viscera. The course of the disease is extremely rapid, and death occurs from septicemia, toxemia, and shock.

Gangrenous tissue is moist and disintegrates readily when handled. The color consists of shades of red, green, gray, or black produced by blood pigments and hydrogen sulfide. The odor is extremely offensive because of the abundance of hydrogen sulfide and other decomposition products associated with putrefaction. The fermentation process, which takes place within the tissue as the result of bacterial invasion, produces gas, and numerous gas bubbles can be observed within the tissues. The intestine is distended with large quantities of gas. There is no sharp line of demarkation between the living and dead tissue. The body defenses are overwhelmed and are not able to establish a defense line.

Specific types of moist gangrene frequently observed in man and animals are known as **gas gangrene, malignant edema,** and **blackleg.** These types of gangrene are due to the invasion of the tissue by various clostridial organisms (*Clostridium welchii, chauvoei, septicum,* and *novyi*). These organisms are inhabitants of the soil and the digestive tract. They are frequently introduced into wounds of various types (shearing, castrating, docking, and ear notching), war wounds, or are injected into tissue by means of the hypodermic syringe. The injury to the tissue results in necrosis, and in this necrotic tissue these organisms grow and multiply. They produce powerful exotoxins that kill the surrounding tissue. When the surrounding tissue is necrotic, the clostridial organisms invade the tissue and in this manner spread throughout the body and bring about the death of the individual. Many of these clostridia are present in tissues of individuals showing no evidence of a clostridial infection (since no tissue of the normal individual is bacteriologically sterile). If some traumatic injury results in the presence of necrotic tissue in the vicinity of these organisms, the bacteria will grow and multiply, and moist gangrene is the result.

A simple laboratory experiment that is often used to demonstrate the presence of these anaerobic bacteria consists of the injection of oleum ricini intravenously into a rabbit. The oleum ricini causes necrosis of skeletal and cardiac muscle, and the anaerobes present in this necrotic muscle begin to grow and multiply. As a result, multiple focal areas of gangrene appear throughout the individual. The same series of events occurs in blackleg and malignant edema in cattle and sheep. If the animals are raised in an area where *Clostridium chauvoei, novyi,* and *septicum* are common in the soil, the muscles of the animals will soon contain many of these organisms. Moist gangrene does not develop in these muscles until necrotic tissue is present. Cattle and sheep frequently receive severe traumatic injuries while moving about on rough terrain. They are also injured by other animals by means of kicks, horn thrusts, or bunts. These injuries cause necrotic tissue to be present in the muscle. The clostridia present in the necrotic tissue grow, multiply, and spread rapidly through the tissue, resulting in the death of the individual. The reason blackleg and malignant edema are most frequently observed in the heavy muscles of the thigh and shoulder is that these are the areas of the body most subject to trauma. Herd outbreaks of blackleg and malignant edema are often observed in which the characteristic swelling of the shoulder or thigh is not present. Instead, multiple small focal areas of moist gangrene are found throughout the entire individual. This suggests that the disease commenced as the result of a general necrosis of the musculature throughout the entire individual just as occurred in the rabbit when oleum ricini was administered. These animals that show multiple-focal areas of gas gangrene frequently have a diffuse coagulative necrosis of the skeletal and cardiac muscles as the result of a deficiency of vitamin E or selenium. This provides the necrotic tissue suitable for the growth requirements of the clostridia.

**Microscopic appearance.** Both dry and moist gangrene have the same basic characteristics. The tissue is necrotic and may or may not have architectural detail, depending upon the amount of putrefaction that has taken place. Since it is necrotic tissue, no cellular detail is visible. Numerous bacteria can be seen throughout the necrotic tissue. Multiple bubbles of gas are present. These are very numerous in moist gangrene but are smaller and fewer in dry gangrene. In moist gangrene, particularly when the gangrene is the result of passive hyperemia, the area is edematous. In dry gangrene, because of evaporation, the area contains little intercellular fluid, and the tissue cells and fibers that are still visible are closer together than normal. An acute inflammatory reaction is observed at the junction of the living and dead tissue.

### Results of Necrosis

Necrosis may terminate in several ways, depending upon the location of the necrotic area and the type of necrosis that is present, as indicated below:

**1. Death of the individual** is the usual result if moist gangrene is present. Since moist gangrene occurs in the viscera and in the heavy muscles of the body where environmental circumstances are ideal for bacterial growth, the body defenses are overwhelmed, and the bacteria spread throughout the individual and cause death. Death of the individual may or may not occur if dry gangrene is present. Whether death occurs or not depends upon the ability of the body defenses to contain or wall off the infection and prevent the extension of bacteria into the living tissue. If the body defenses can amputate the extremity along the sharp line of demarkation between the dead and living tissue, or if the necrotic tissue is removed by surgical methods, the chances of survival are greatly increased. Death or survival with the other types of necrosis (coagulative, liquefactive, caseous, and fat) depend upon the organ involved, the location of the lesion within the organ, and the extent of the damage. If necrosis involves a vital organ (lung, heart, or brain) the chances of survival are greatly reduced.

**2. Sloughing and desquamation** of the necrotic tissue may occur if the external surfaces of the individual are involved. This may also take place in organs, such as the digestive tract, in which the necrotic material is cast off into the lumen of the organ and eliminated from the body. This type of elimination occurs when burns have involved the skin and the necrotic cutaneous tissue is sloughed.

**3. Liquefaction and removal** by the leukocytes, lymph, and blood occur when the area of necrosis is small. When the area of necrosis is large, its entire removal cannot be accomplished in this manner, and methods 4, 5, 6, and 7 are used.

**4. Liquefaction, abscessation, and discharge** of the necrotic material occur when pyogenic bacteria invade the necrotic tissue. The bacteria attract leukocytes (primarily the neutrophil), the enzymes of the leukocytes liquefy the necrotic tissue, and the liquefied material is discharged to the exterior of the individual. This is the type of elimination associated with a boil or an abscess, and the surgeon can aid the body in discharging the liquefied material by incising the area, thereby providing a path for drainage to the exterior.

**5. Liquefaction of the tissue and formation of a cyst** occur when the necrotic tissue has been placed in a fluid state by tissue and cellular enzymes, but the mass is so large it cannot be removed by the leukocytes, lymph, and blood, or cannot be discharged to the exterior. Since this liquid mass of necrotic tissue is irritating, the body forms a protective wall of leukocytes and connective tissue around it, thus enclosing and containing the undesirable material.

**6. Encapsulation without liquefaction** occurs when tissue and cellular enzymes capable of liquefying the necrotic area are not present (coagulative and caseous necrosis). Necrotic tissue is foreign to the body and always acts as an irritant. In response to this irritation, a containing wall of leukocytes and connective tissue is formed around the mass and the area becomes ecapsulated.

**7. Organization** of the necrotic tissue occurs when it is invaded with capillaries, connective tissue, and leukocytes. The leukocytes dissolve and digest the necrotic tissue, the area formerly occupied by the necrotic tissue becomes infiltrated with connective tissue, leaving a scar.

**8. Calcification** of the necrotic material may occur because the two antecedents of calcification — necrotic tissue and impaired circulation — are present.

**9. Metaplasia** may occur in the vicinity of the necrotic tissue. Metaplasia of connective tissue with the appearance of bone is most commonly observed in fat necrosis, especially in the abdominal fat of swine.

## SOMATIC DEATH

**Definition.** Somatic death is the disappearance of life from the entire individual. It should not be confused with necrosis, which is the local death of tissue within the living individual.

Life depends upon the cooperation of all the tissues and organs of the body. A few or even many cells may die here and there throughout the body without causing death of the entire organism. Some organs can even be completely eliminated and yet death may not occur, but when the functions of the heart, the respiratory system, or the brain completely fail, somatic death follows at once. The immediate cause of death can usually be said to be asphyxia, but back of asphyxia may be paralysis of the cardiac and respiratory centers of the brain and still further back may be some influence operating upon the brain. Death, then, may be a chain of influences which eventually completely upset the vital regulating mechanism of the organism but result in a permanent state of anoxia.

### Asphyxia

As stated above, asphyxia can usually be said to be the immediate cause of death. In asphyxia there is a deficiency of oxygen and an excess of carbon dioxide in the blood. The condition makes its appearance with signs of respiratory difficulty. Respiration is forced. There are spasmodic movements of the respiratory muscles. The heart action is accelerated. The whole musculature of the body displays spasmodic quivering. There is loss of consciousness, irregularity of respiratory movements, and cessation of heart action.

If the oxygen deficiency takes place more slowly, these symptoms appear less pronounced. The tissues undergo degenerative changes as a result of the oxygen hunger, the respiratory center loses its irritability, and life ceases, with gradually increasing loss of consciousness and paralysis of the heart. In this dying state, which may be of several hours or even several days duration, the animal is said to be in a moribund condition.

According to the cause and rapidity of death by asphyxia, the post-mortem lesions vary considerably. One of the common changes is the color of the blood to dark red or almost black. This color is due to an excess of carbon dioxide. The blood may be partially coagulated and resemble tar, or may remain fluid. Small hemorrhages are usually present in the lungs and pleura. There are areas of pulmonary emphysema which arise from forced inspiration during the death struggle. White or pale pink froth collects in the trachea and bronchi as a result of pulmonary edema. The right side of the heart is distended with blood (terminal dilatation).

### Post-mortem Changes

As soon as an animal dies, post-mortem changes begin to develop. If the surrounding temperature is high or if the animal has a heavy body-coat, as does a sheep, the changes may develop so rapidly that they overshadow ante-mortem changes even when the post-mortem examination is performed within a few hours after death. To avoid confusion in differentiating ante-mortem from post-mortem changes, it is necessary to know what may happen in a carcass after death. Chief among these changes are rigor mortis, post-mortem blood clotting, decomposition, putrefaction, and rupture and displacement of the gastrointestinal tract.

In **rigor mortis** there is stiffness of the joints due to muscular contraction. The condition affects first the muscles that have been most active and best nourished just prior to death, namely those of the eyelids, heart, diaphragm, thorax, jaws, neck, and finally the extremities. The jaws become set so firmly that they can scarcely be pried apart. The rigor passes off in the same order in which it occurred.

The onset of rigor mortis is hastened by heat and retarded by cold. Usually it comes on within 1 to 8 hours after death and leaves within 20 to 30 hours, sometimes not until more than 50 hours. If the animal dies during violent exercise or as the result of tetanus or strychnine poisoning, the onset is immediate. It develops earlier, is more feeble, and of shorter duration in emaciated, weak, and debilitated animals than in healthy, well-nourished animals.

The condition is looked upon as a colloid swelling phenomenon. In a well-nourished animal, at the time of death there is much lactic acid in the tissues which cannot be removed after circulation ceases. The degree of rigor corresponds with the concentration of this lactic acid which in turn is related to the depletion of the glycogen in the muscle cells. The muscle colloid, myosin, of the individual cells swells, thus causing the entire muscle to become tense. After autolysis and putrefaction begin, myosin loses its colloidal nature and the rigor disappears. Rigor mortis does not return once it has disappeared.

The other post-mortem changes are those which involve the (1) blood, (2) parenchymatous organs, including the skeletal muscles, and (3) organs of the alimentary tract which contain ingesta. **Post-mortem clotting** of blood is most conspicuous in the heart chambers and in the larger vessels. Such a clot has no attachment to the endocardium or intima. It usually separates into an upper chicken-fat clot and a lower currant-jelly clot. A predominance of the first indicates slow death. If there is rapid decomposition of the blood after death or if the animal dies of a septicemia due to hemolytic bacteria, the erythrocytes hemolyze and stain the endocardium, intima, and tissue surrounding the smaller vessels. This is called **imbibition of blood.** If this occurs along the alimentary tract where sulfuretted hydrogen from putrefying ingesta can combine with the iron of the hemoglobin, iron sulfide is formed and stains the tissues grayish blue, green, or black. This condition is frequently referred to as **pseudomelanosis.** It is often seen on the parietal and visceral peritoneum. Immediately after death some of the blood may gravitate into the veins in the lowermost parts of the body; this condition is designated **hypostasis** or **hypostatic congestion.**

In the parenchymatous organs and skeletal muscles a **granular coagulation** of the cytoplasm which resembles cloudy swelling occurs soon after death. Next, the cells undergo **autolysis** and also **digestion** by ferments elaborated by saprophytic putrefactive bacteria. The rapidity with which these changes take place depends upon the location of the tissues in the body and the degree of warmth that prevails. The mucous membranes of the digestive tract naturally show this change first. The mucosa swells, becomes soft, transparent, glassy, and strips with ease from the underlying muscular coats. This is especially noticeable in the forestomachs of ruminants. Saprophytic bacteria entering the blood stream from the intestine near the time of death cause **putrefactive decomposition** of the parenchymatous organs and skeletal muscles which is similar to that in moist gangrene. In the putrefactive process, gas is frequently formed and appears as bubbles in the tissue (**post-mortem emphysema**).

In the stomach and intestine, ingesta continue to ferment after death and cause bloat (**post-mortem tympanites**). It is differentiated from ante-mortem bloat by the absence of passive hyperemia in the other abdominal viscera and in the thoracic organs. The gas may continue to form until **rupture** occurs. Absence of a swollen, hemorrhagic border distinguishes this from an ante-mortem tear. After death, peristalsis may continue for a time and terminate in **intestinal displacements.** These are not accompanied by the vascular and inflammatory changes which characterize ante-mortem displacements. The yellowish or greenish discoloration of the liver and intestines where they come in contact with the gall bladder is due to **imbibition of diffused bile.**

# CHAPTER 11

# The Defenses of The Body Against Injury

## INFLAMMATION

**Definition.** Inflammation is the complicated vascular and cellular reaction of an individual to an irritant.

It is often said that he who understands inflammation understands pathology. This is certainly true because the various circulatory disturbances, degenerative alterations, necrotic changes, and the other lesions studied thus far are all blended together into a heterogeneous mixture of cellular, vascular, and hydraulic phenomena. It is therefore extremely important for the student of pathology to master the basic pathological alterations in tissue before he studies the subject of inflammation. Otherwise he is confused by the structural alterations observed.

Most diseases at some time in their courses are examples of inflammation. All infectious diseases (rhinitis, fowl pox, salmonellosis, streptococcosis, mastitis, brucellosis, etc.) exhibit the alterations associated with inflammation. It is in the study of inflammation that the importance of cellular pathology becomes apparent to the student, and it is then that he appreciates the highly organized cell state of the body in which each integral portion has a very important place in the defense mechanism. It is in the study of inflammation that the student begins to appreciate the monumental contributions made by Virchow, Cohnheim, Metchnikoff, and Celsus.

**Objects of inflammation.** The vascular and cellular response of the body to the application of an irritant has two objects. First, it attempts to destroy and remove the irritant, thus preventing additional injury to the tissue and spread of the irritant to other regions of the body; and second, it endeavors to repair the damage created by the irritant and restore the body to normal.

**Occurrence of inflammation.** There are no living cells or tissues within the body that cannot be involved in an inflammatory process. Certain tissues are more likely to be affected than others because they are located in more vulnerable positions and are more readily exposed to injurious agents. Since the skin is in a very exposed position it is constantly experiencing inflammatory alterations. The gastrointestinal tract, because it may contain injurious food, protozoa, metazoa, bacteria, or toxic compounds, is likewise commonly involved in an inflammatory process.

**Principal phenomena of inflammation.** The reactions of the body to an irritant can be grouped into three major categories which follow each other in a very precise and well-organized manner. (1) **Early circulatory changes.** The first alteration to occur in tissue after the application of an irritant is hyperemia. There must be an increased amount of blood in the area if the cellular and humoral defenses are to be concentrated in that region. This can be compared to an army in the stage of mobilization when the collective forces of the country are being brought to the area where the invader has commenced his attack. (2) **Exudation of protective cells and fluids.** Exudation is the process of cells and fluids pouring into the injured area. The cells are the leukocytes and erythrocytes, and the fluid is the plasma of the blood which contains the humoral defenses. This can also be compared to an army which has been mobilized and now is pouring men and equipment into the conflict, meeting the attacking forces, and driving them out of the country. Survival of the animal or the country depends on whether the invader can be overcome and destroyed. (3) **Repair.** In this stage the dead and injured tissue is removed, and regeneration of cells takes place in an attempt to restore the part to normal. This again can be compared to an army. The conflict is over; the dead must be buried; the houses, the bridges, and the land must be restored if that country is to prosper again.

### Etiology

The cause of inflammation is extremely varied, and a vast number of nutritional, physical, chemical, and viable agents cause a vascular and cellular reaction in the body. It is well to remember that the severity of an injurious agent determines the type of alteration that occurs. When the injurious agent is extremely mild the tissues are stimulated, hypertrophy and hyperplasia are the result, and little if any inflammation is present. This is exemplified by the calluses on one's hands as the result of mild irritation from a pick or shovel handle. If the injurious agent is of moderate to severe intensity, irritation of the tissues is the result and an inflammatory reaction is produced. If the irritant is extremely severe, necrosis of

the tissue occurs, and often the inflammation is directed more towards the necrotic tissue than the irritant which produced the death of cells.

The degree of irritation and the tissue sensitivity determine the course and termination of a disease. In general, bacterial and viral infections produce a moderate to severe tissue irritation, which results in an acute inflammation. The body defenses respond with an intense vascular and cellular reaction. The infectious agent is either overcome by the body or the agent destroys the animal, and recovery or death of the animal occurs in a comparatively short period of time. This is the type of reaction that is observed in pasteurellosis, blackleg, anthrax, and equine viral encephalomyelitis. When an animal is infected with fungi and the higher forms of bacteria, the irritation produced by these organisms is relatively mild. The body defenses are not stimulated enough to cause them to mobilize in sufficient magnitude to bring about the destruction and removal of the irritant. As a result, the vascular and cellular reaction appears slowly and is seldom intense. The body tolerates the presence of the irritant and, as a result, the termination of the disease in recovery or death is delayed and often no termination is achieved. Diseases of this type are actinomycosis, tuberculosis, and blastomycosis. Protozoan and metazoan parasites in general are more perfect types of parasitism. The tissue irritation produced by them is slight, the body defenses are not stimulated to bring about the extrusion of the invader, and as a result there is often no termination of the disease as far as elimination of the infectious agent by the body is concerned. Neither is there much evidence of infection as evidenced by vascular and cellular reactions, merely because the tissues are not stimulated by the invaders. Examples of these types of diseases are malaria, balantidiasis, cestodiasis, and nematodiasis.

Chemical agents cause a somewhat different type of injury in that they often damage the tissues at the site of application as well as at the point of elimination. Mercuric chloride, uranium nitrate, or mushroom poisoning cause a gastrointestinal inflammation when they are ingested. The absorbed toxins are eliminated through the kidney, and as the urine is concentrated by the selective absorption of the tubular epithelium, the toxic substances become extremely injurious to the renal tubular epithelium, and degeneration, necrosis, and nephritis result.

### Cardinal Signs of Inflammation

Five clinical signs must be observed before a diagnosis of inflammation can be made. At times all of the signs are not very apparent and a careful examination must be made before their presence is detected. The cardinal signs of inflammation were first described by Celsus during the first century A.D. He described four, and since then we have added a fifth. The cardinal signs of inflammation are as follows.

**1. Redness.** The redness of the tissue is due to the increased number of erythrocytes in the area as the result of hyperemia.

**2. Swelling.** The enlargement of the area of inflammation is first of all due to hyperemia. There is more blood in the tissues, blood has volume, and therefore the part must become larger than normal. Secondly, humoral and cellular substances in the form of an exudate have accumulated in the area. These substances likewise have volume and the tissue must enlarge to contain them.

**3. Heat.** An increase in the temperature of the tissue is due in part to the more rapid blood flow through the area. The warm blood from the interior of the body is brought to the extremity at a more rapid rate and therefore the temperature of the extremity rises and approaches that of the internal body temperature. In addition there is an increased rate of metabolism in the area of inflammation, and as a result an increased amount of heat is produced which causes a rise in temperature. Heat associated with inflamma-

tion is readily detected in the extremities. It is more difficult to detect it in the internal organs, and the only difference in temperature will be as the result of the increased metabolic rate. Within the interior of the body the heat is dissipated so quickly to the surrounding organs that a noticeable rise in temperature is seldom apparent.

**4. Pain.** Pain occurs in an area of inflammation as the result of injury to the nerve endings. Pain is also caused by the stretching of the tissues when exudate accumulates in the area of inflammation.

**5. Impaired function.** As a result of swelling, pain, and tissue destruction, the animal refuses or is unable to move the limb, or the specific functions (secretion, excretion, and motility) of the organ cannot take place. Impaired function is very apparent in the horse when injuries occur in a limb in the vicinity of a joint. The swelling alone causes so much tissue tension that the normal movement of the joint is prevented and the animal is lame.

### Tissue Alterations in Inflammation

The tissue alterations in inflammation can be placed into two groups — the circulatory changes and the cellular changes.

The circulatory or vascular changes were first described by Cohnheim in 1877. He spread the mesentery of a frog across the stage of a microscope and observed the flow of blood through the vessels. When he applied a drop of dilute acetic acid to the mesentery a remarkable change took place in the blood vessels. The capillaries, previously almost indistinguishable, dilated, and then there was a rush of blood into the dilated capillaries. Soon the flow through the capillaries slowed and was barely moving when compared with its former rapid rate. Then certain cellular components of the blood stream approached the wall of the vessel, attached to it, inserted a pseudopodium into the wall, and then followed the pseudopodium through the wall until the entire cell body was exterior to the blood vessel.

When free of the vessel the cell continued to migrate through the tissue towards the site where the irritant was applied. The conclusion was inevitable: The cells found in an area of inflammation were actually derived from the blood. This was a point the earlier pathologists, including Virchow, had never appreciated. They knew neutrophils were present at the site of inflammation but they were never able to determine how the neutrophils arrived there.

The cellular changes in inflammation were clarified by Metchnikoff in 1892. One evening he inserted rose thorns into the larvae of a starfish. The next morning when he observed the larvae he discovered a gray zone around each of the rose thorns. This attracted his attention and, examining the area more closely, he discovered this gray zone to be an accumulation of large cells which possessed considerable cytoplasm and contained a large single nucleus. He realized these cells had not been described by Cohnheim and were part of the body defense mechanism. Because the cells were large and possessed phagocytic properties he named them **macrophages** in contrast to the smaller phagocytic cell, the neutrophil, which was designated as the **microphage.** Additional work indicated the role of the various cells in inflammation and proved that the macrophage, instead of being brought to the area of inflammation by the blood stream, was actually produced at the site of inflammation from pre-existing macrophages already present in the tissue.

### Circulatory Changes in Inflammation

The circulatory changes in inflammation, as originally outlined by Cohnheim, had for their purpose the bringing of the body defenses to the site of injury so that the etiologic agent might be destroyed and the damaged tissue might be repaired or replaced. The circulatory changes in inflammation can be arranged into six major groups:

1. **Changes in the blood vessels.** Following the application of the irritant to the tissue there is a **momentary constriction** of the blood vessels. The blood vessels contract just as tissues do in general when stimulated by warm objects, ice, or a pin; the immediate response is to jump or contract. The momentary constriction of the vessel is followed very shortly by **dilatation.** Dilatation is caused by the vasodilatory nerve impulses and the local vasodilatory action of substances, such as histamine, which are formed at the site of irritation. If the irritant is mild to moderate in intensity, there will be a slight to moderate hyperemia. If the irritant is very severe, paralysis of the blood vessel walls and marked engorgement with blood may occur. The vasodilatation is first observed in the arteries, then in the veins, and finally in the capillaries. As paralysis of the vessel wall occurs, the engorgement of the vessels becomes most noticeable in the capillaries. Dilatation of the vessels is absolutely essential if healing is to be accomplished. If the vasoconstrictor fibers to a portion of the body are severed, the inflammatory reaction develops much more rapidly, is much more intense, and healing is accomplished in a shorter period of time. One of the purposes of hot applications to an area of injury is to increase the active hyperemia in the area and thereby aid the healing process. Because of hyperemia, several times the normal amount of blood may be contained in an area of inflammation. Along with the capillary dilatation there is also increased **endothelial permeability.** Because of this alteration in the wall of the vessel, plasma constituents, leukocytes, and erythrocytes can pass with comparative ease through the wall of the vessel into the surrounding tissue.

2. **Changes in the rate of flow.** The first alteration in the rate of flow of the blood is **acceleration.** When the arteries, veins, and capillaries in an area dilate, there is suddenly a large area into which the blood may flow. To fill this space there is a rush of blood into the vessels. It is much the same as when a dam is opened and the retained water rushes into the

relatively empty stream below. This acceleration, however, is only temporary and terminates when the dilated vessels are filled with blood. The next alteration in the rate of flow is **retardation.** It is absolutely essential that the rate of flow be retarded if diapedesis of the leukocytes is to be accomplished. It is extremely difficult for leukocytes to reach the wall of a vessel containing a rapidly flowing stream of blood. When the stream is slowed the current does not sweep the cells away and the leukocytes may approach the wall, attach, and migrate through it. Retardation in the rate of flow is accomplished in four ways: The first method of accomplishing retardation is by **increasing the capillary bed** in the area. The amount of blood entering the region through the major artery can only increase to a certain degree because of limitations in the diameter of the vessel. Since the size of the capillary bed has increased several times, there are many channels through which the blood may pass and the amount of blood flowing through any one channel is reduced. It is comparable to a plumbing system in a house. If a one-inch water main enters a house and one faucet is attached to the water line, the water pressure is high and the rate of flow through that faucet is rapid. However, if 50 faucets are placed on the same water line, the amount of water flowing through any one faucet is reduced to a trickle.

The second method of retardation is caused by the **swelling of the endothelial cells** lining the capillaries. As the endothelial cells swell and increase their diameter they protrude into the lumen of the capillary. This causes a rough endothelial surface of the blood vessel, which increases the peripheral friction to the flow of blood, thereby retarding the rate of flow. A comparison can be made with two iron water pipes of the same diameter. The interior surface of one of the pipes is allowed to rust, while the other pipe is coated with paraffin so that the surface is smooth. When the water passes through the pipes, the amount passing through the paraffined

pipe is much greater because the peripheral resistance to the flow of the fluid has been reduced to a minimum by the paraffin coating.

The third method of retardation is **hemoconcentration.** In the preceding paragraph it was indicated that the vessel wall became more permeable. As the result of this, the constituents of the plasma pass through the wall into the surrounding tissue, resulting in a concentration of the formed elements of the blood and the larger protein molecules retained within the lumen of the vessel. Because of this the blood becomes thicker and more viscid and therefore the rate of flow is slowed. This can be compared to the removal of water from maple sap. As water is removed, the more concentrated the sap becomes and the more difficult it is to pour the syrup.

The fourth method of retardation is the result of the **margination of the leukocytes.** When the rate of flow has been reduced enough that the leukocytes can approach the wall and attach, their presence on the vessel wall increases the roughness of the endothelial surface. This increases the peripheral resistance of the vessel wall and thereby retards the rate of flow.

Finally a state of near **stasis** is attained when the above factors have caused the rate of flow to be so reduced that the blood is barely moving through the vessel. In this state conditions are ideal for the diapedesis of the leukocytes. Complete stasis, however, is detrimental to diapedesis. If the major vessel to an area of inflammation is occluded, thus reducing the blood pressure to zero, diapedesis of the leukocytes stops immediately.

3. **Changes in the blood stream.** The principal alteration consists of a **redistribution of the cellular elements** of the blood stream. During the normal flow of blood through a vessel the stream of blood is divided into two distinct zones. In the center of the blood stream or in the vicinity of the axis of the blood vessel there is a concentration of the cellular elements (erythrocytes and leukocytes) of the

blood. This is known as the **axial stream.** Surrounding this axial stream, between the cellular elements and the vessel wall, there is a clear zone which consists primarily of plasma in which no or only a few cells are found. This zone is known as the **plasmatic stream.** The cellular, or the formed, elements of the blood are held in the center of the stream by the centripetal force of the flowing blood. As long as the stream is swift, the formed elements are unable to reach the wall of the vessel. Therefore, if diapedesis of the leukocytes is to be accomplished, the stream of blood must be slowed so that the centripetal force of the blood stream is overcome, thus obliterating the two distinct zones (axial and plasmatic) and allowing the cellular elements, especially the leukocytes, to come in contact with the vessel wall. How this slowing of the blood stream is accomplished has been indicated in preceding paragraphs.

The second change in the blood stream is **margination of the leukocytes.** In an area of injury a substance known as **leukotaxine** is formed in the tissue. This substance exerts a positive chemotaxis on the leukocytes and causes them to flow in the direction of the tissue injury or the site where the leukotaxine is being produced. Just how the leukotaxine exerts its influence on the leukocytes is not known. Perhaps it is merely a process of lowering the surface tension so that the cells flow in the direction of the leukotaxine. Since leukotaxine is very soluble in tissue fluids, it diffuses very readily through the walls of the blood vessels. As leukotaxine comes in contact with the leukocytes in the blood stream the leukocytes approach the vessel wall from where the leukotaxine is coming, attach to it, insert a pseudopodium into the vessel wall, follow the pseudopodium through the vessel wall, and then, when free of the vascular wall, continue their migration towards the site of the irritant. Once the leukotaxine enters the blood stream it is swept along in the current until it reaches the bone marrow. There it again attracts the leukocytes; they enter the blood stream and are swept away by the current. As the bone marrow liberates leukocytes into the blood the total number of leukocytes in the circulating blood increases. Since the total number of leukocytes per cubic millimeter in the circulating blood may have increased three, five, or even more times, the number of leukocytes available at the site of inflammation is greatly increased.

The veterinarian makes use of this flooding of the blood stream with leukocytes in making a diagnosis. For example, if an animal has a pain in the abdomen, the veterinarian may suspect there is an infection present. By making a total leukocyte count he observes the increase in the total number of leukocytes, which indicates the bone marrow is being stimulated by leukotaxine formed at the site of inflammation. He then feels justified in opening the abdomen and looking for the lesion which produced the leukotaxine.

4. **Exudation of plasma.** In an area of inflammation there is tissue acidosis as well as alterations in the protein, alterations in the tissue colloids and crystalloids, and accumulations of catabolic products in the area. All of these factors increase the osmotic pressure of the tissue. In addition to this, the capillary walls have become more permeable to plasma as the result of histamine and other products formed at the site of injury. When all of these factors are operating together they cause an accumulation of plasma constituents in the tissue in the region of inflammation.

The plasma has several functions in an area of inflammation. (1) It brings nutrient into the area which is needed for defense. (2) It dilutes the irritant. By dilution it may change the irritant to a stimulant, thereby reducing tissue injury, or it may disperse the irritant so that the leukocytes may engulf portions of it more easily. (3) It brings fibrin-forming constituents into the tissues. Clotting occurs, and the fibrin surrounds and entraps the irritant, forms a protective zone between the irritant and the tissue cells, and effectively seals lymphatics, thus preventing the entrance of bacteria and their extension to distant portions of the body. Finally it prepares a scaffold on which the angioblasts and fibroblasts may be supported as they grow into the area of inflammation in the process of organization and repair. (4) The plasma brings the humoral defenses of the body to the site of inflammation. These defenses consist of the globulin fractions of the plasma which contain the antibodies such as agglutinins, lysins, precipitins, and opsonins which aid the leukocytes in overcoming the irritant.

**5. Diapedesis or emigration of the leukocytes.** Leukocytes are needed in the area of inflammation to phagocytose the irritant (especially bacteria). The point at which the leukocytes pass through the vessel wall is quite sharply defined as the area where the capillary and the vein join. This area is known as the **zone of emigration.** The zone of emigration is located at this point because it is here that conditions are most suitable for diapedesis for the following reasons: (1) At this point blood pressure is at its lowest. (2) The rate of blood flow through the vessels is slowest in this area. (3) The greatest concentration of the cellular components of the blood has been achieved in this region. (4) It is at this point that the leukotaxine which has diffused through the capillary wall has had time to exert its action on the leukocytes as they passed through the capillaries and has finally caused them to approach the vessel wall. The leukocytes, with everything in their favor, are able to approach the vessel wall in this area, attach to the endothelium, migrate through the vessel wall, and proceed toward the irritant by amoeboid movement.

**6. Diapedesis of the erythrocytes.** In an area of inflammation the erythrocytes may enter the tissues by rhexis or diapedesis. Usually in an area of inflammation no actual rupture of a vessel can be demonstrated, but erythrocytes can be seen passing through the wall even though they do not possess amoeboid movement. The mechanism by which they pass through the wall of the blood vessel is not known but a number of theories have been proposed. It has been suggested that with the swelling of the endothelial cells the wall of the blood vessel can be compared with a net in which spaces appear between the endothelial cells through which the erythrocytes may pass. Others have suggested the swollen endothelial cells acquire phagocytic properties and, like an amoeba, ingest many of the objects which come in contact with them such as an erythrocyte. After ingesting it they find it is not suitable food material and extrude it on the other side of the endothelial cells, which in this case would be peripheral to the blood vessel. Still others have suggested there are alterations in the tissue tension of the endothelial cells in which they become quite permeable to all constituents of the blood stream and are therefore no longer able to contain the erythrocytes. Finally, others have suggested it is a physical-chemical phenomenon similar to that exhibited when a drop of mercury is placed on the surface of gelatin and the element flows through the column of gelatin. As desirable as it would be to know the exact reason why erythrocytes pass through the wall of a vessel, it is still more important to recognize that erythrocytes are found extravascularly in areas of inflammation where there is no apparent break in the vessel wall.

### The Cellular Changes in Inflammation

The cells primarily involved in the cellular changes in inflammation are the neutrophil, eosinophil, basophil, lymphocyte, plasma cell, macrophage, and giant cell.

#### NEUTROPHIL

The term neutrophil (Fig. 11.1) is an abbreviation of the complete term polymorphonuclear neutrophilic granulocyte. The polymorphonuclear characteristic is often difficult to observe in histological preparations since the dying cell contracts into the shape of a sphere and does not have the characteristic appearance the student has learned to recognize in blood

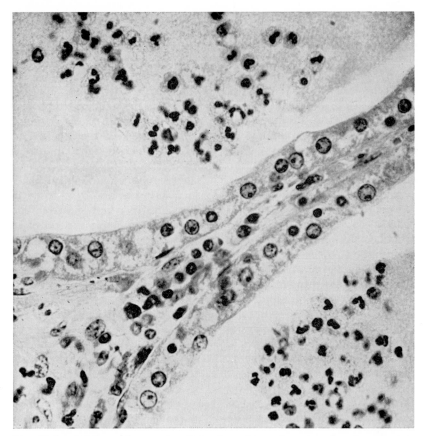

Fig. 11.1 — Portions of two alveoli in the udder of a cow showing exudate composed of neutrophils, lymphocytes, and macrophages. (Department of Veterinary Pathology, Michigan State University.)

smears. In the exudate any cell that has an irregularly shaped nucleus is probably a neutrophil. It should also be remembered that the autolytic enzymes of the cell may liquefy the cytoplasm of the cell, leaving only the nucleus visible in the exudate. As the cell digests itself, karyorrhexis occurs and then the exudate may contain multiple nuclear fragments with few intact cells. The eosinophilic granules in the cytoplasm of the neutrophil vary in both size and shape depending upon the species of animal. Unless this variation is recogized the cell may be confused with an eosinophil.

The neutrophil does not reproduce itself at the site of inflammation. Instead, it is formed in the hemopoietic centers (bone marrow) and is brought to the site of inflammation by the circulating blood stream.

In acute inflammation, not only do neutrophils appear in large numbers at the site of injury, but there is also a marked increase of them in the general circulation. The number of neutrophils in the circulating blood stream ranges from 4,000 to 10,000 per cubic millimeter, depending upon the species of animal. In most species they constitute approximately 60 to 75 per cent of the total number of leukocytes, but in a few species, such as the bovine, they comprise only 40 per cent. When inflammation is present and leukotaxine has stimulated the liberation of leukocytes into the blood stream, the total number of neutrophils in the circulating blood may increase to as much as 50,000, or even more, per cubic millimeter. This increase in the number of leukocytes in the circulating blood stream is known as **leukocytosis.**

Sometimes a **Schilling index** is made of the leukocytes in the circulating blood stream to determine the bone marrow response to the need for the production of neutrophils. The Shilling index is designed to give the clinician an indication of the maturity of the neutrophils released into the circulation. Under normal circumstances, when the bone marrow is able to meet the demands for neutrophils during the course of inflammation, the cell in the circulating blood stream is of a mature polymorphonuclear type. When the bone marrow is exhausted and is no longer able to meet the requirements of the body, immature forms of neutrophils are released into the circulating blood stream. The Schilling index differentiates the neutrophils into the various mature and immature types, thus giving the clinician some information as to the degree of stress that is being placed upon the bone marrow and the possible outcome of the disease. The appearance of large numbers of immature neutrophils in the circulating blood stream is serious and indicates the bone marrow is being depleted and is no longer able to meet the demands by the body for neutrophils.

While the rule is that in severe inflammation due to infection there is a general leukocytosis, this does not always hold true. For instance, in some very acute viral infections, as in hog cholera, there is a decrease in leukocytes — a **leukopenia** — instead of a leukocytosis. The leukopenia is probably the result of two factors. First, some viral diseases (hog cholera and viral feline enteritis) are extremely injurious to endothelium and hemopoietic tissue in general and therefore the injured cells are not able to reproduce. Secondly, the action of viral agents on the tissue is somewhat different than that produced by bacteria. Phagocytosis of viral particles probably does not occur and therefore cells capable of phagocytosis are not needed. The control of a viral agent appears to require a humoral defense mechanism rather than a cellular defense system.

Neutrophils are the principal constituent of the mobile cellular defense mechanism of the body and are rushed to the site of inflammation by the blood stream. Therefore they appear in an area of irritation very soon after the irritant has been applied. This is especially true if bacteria are present. Because of their early appearance at the site of irritation they are called the **first line of cellular defense** and are the main cellular defense of the body during the first three or four days following the application of an irritant. During this period the macrophages in the area are beginning to reproduce, and after about 72 hours the macrophages are numerous enough to assume the major defense role. When the irritation in the area is no longer severe, the pronounced circulatory changes in the area diminish in intensity, and then it is difficult for diapedesis of the leukocytes to occur. As a result, the total number of neutrophils in the area diminishes. However, as long as pyogenic bacteria are present, circulatory changes tend to persist and the disappearance of the neutrophils is delayed. The cells that survive the conflict at the site of inflammation are still amoeboid and therefore are able to return to the general circulation by means of the lymphatics and the blood vessels.

### EOSINOPHIL

Eosinophils (polymorphonuclear eosinophilic granulocytes) are normally found in the blood stream of domestic animals and comprise 1 to 7 per cent of the total differential leukocyte count. In certain diseases (allergy) the total number of eosinophils may increase considerably until 20 to 25 per cent of the total number of leukocytes in the circulating blood may consist of eosinophils. Eosinophils, along with the neutrophils, appear early in an area of inflammation. They are brought to the area by the circulating blood stream just as are the neutrophils. Since they have amoeboid movement they are able to leave the circulatory system quite easily and emigrate into the tissues. Apparently they do not regenerate as quickly as do the neutrophils and, as a result, in acute inflammation they may disappear entirely from the blood stream.

The function of these cells is not known. They are formed in the bone marrow and are distributed throughout the body by means of the circulatory system. They do not show mitosis nor multiply in an area of inflammation. They are not phagocytic, but it is suspected they contribute to the humoral defense system of the body. The eosinophils are particularly numerous in various allergic reactions such as occur when a animal has been sensitized by a previous exposure to a foreign protein. When an animal is affected with tuberculosis and tuberculin is injected into the caudal fold of the tail, an allergic reaction occurs at the site of injection. Histological preparations made of this area reveal large numbers of eosinophils. The eosinophils become a very prominent constituent of the cellular exudate in various allergic reactions of the respiratory system. This is especially prominent in asthma and hay fever in the human being and is also occasionally observed in animals. In the recovering stages of pneumonia eosinophils may be very numerous in the cellular exudate. The pulmonary protein has apparently sensitized the individual, and in response to this sensitivity eosinophils accumulate.

Eosinophils are also very numerous in parasitic infections. The tissue in the vicinity of a parasite becomes heavily infiltrated with eosinophils. Apparently a sensitizing infection must occur before eosinophilia is observed. The first infection of the animal with parasites results in little if any accumulation of eosinophils, but subsequent infections are characterized by large numbers of eosinophils in the exudate. Not only do large numbers of eosinophils accumulate in the tissues but there is also a sharp rise in the total number of eosinophils in the circulating blood stream. This is particularly prominent in *Trichinella spiralis* infections. The finding of an eosinophilia is an indication that parasitism or an allergy may be present.

### BASOPHIL OR MAST CELL

The basophil (polymorphonuclear basophilic granulocyte) has a slightly polymorphonuclear nucleus but the irregularity of the nucleus is not as distinct as that of the neutrophil. When the Giemsa stain is used to identify the cell, numerous blue granules are found in the cytoplasm. In the circulating blood stream this cell is known as the basophil. When it is found in the tissue it is known as the mast cell.

The basophils comprise 0.5 to 1.0 per cent of the total number of leukocytes in the circulating blood. When they make their appearance in disease processes they are associated with mild subacute inflammation. An increase of them in the blood of guinea pigs experimentally infected with swine lungworms has been reported. The proportion of basophils increased from a normal of less than 1 per cent to 47 per cent.

The function of the basophils is not known. They are very slowly amoeboid, are not phagocytic, and are capable of producing heparin. They show a marked tendency to disintegrate in hematological or histological preparations, and often only blue granules are found scattered through the tissue or blood smear. Basophils are formed in the bone marrow and are distributed through the body by the blood stream. Mast cells are scattered throughout the tissues of the body and are particularly numerous in the dermis and the tunica propria of the gastrointestinal tract. Whether all of the mast cells originate in the bone marrow or are produced in the tissue in which they are found is not always clear. If large numbers of mast cells are concentrated in a focal area, especially in the skin, it is well to suspect a myeloid tumor known as the mastocytoma (see Chapter 13), and in this case the cells are probably formed at the site.

## LYMPHOCYTE

The lymphocyte is a mononuclear cell that contains a spherical nucleus surrounded by varying amounts of pale blue cytoplasm. Occasionally a few red granules are observed in the cytoplasm.

Lymphocytes are found in the circulating blood stream in varying numbers. The total lymphocyte count ranges from 2,000 to 7,000 per cubic millimeter, comprising 40 to 60 per cent of the total number of leukocytes. Lymphocytes are formed in the lymph nodes and other lymphoid tissues and enter the blood primarily by way of the thoracic duct. The rate of turnover for lymphocytes is extremely great. In the cat, for instance, it has been estimated that the blood lymphocytes are replaced every 10 to 12 hours.

Lymphocytes possess limited amoeboid movement and are not phagocytic. The function of the lymphocytes appears to be primarily concerned with the humoral defense system and antibody-globulin production. The number of circulating lymphocytes is under the control of pituitary-adrenal cortical secretions. Excessive production of cortisone causes an atrophy of the lymphoid tissue and a consequent reduction in the number of lymphocytes in the circulating blood (lymphopenia). With the reduction in the number of lymphocytes there is obviously a reduction in antibody formation. This hormone therefore has an anti-inflammatory effect. It suppresses the inflammatory reaction but does not remove the cause.

At this point it is profitable to draw attention to the fact that some corticosteroids apparently have the ability to inhibit the formation of leukotaxine and leukocytosis-promoting factors by injured cells or else to suppress their activity after they are formed. Such a corticosteroid is called an anti-inflammatory steroid. With our present knowledge of the pathogenesis of the inflammatory process, it seems that the administration of such a steroid to an animal having an infectious lesion would be contraindicated. If a steroid such as cortisone blocks out the biochemical substances which are necessary to carry out the sequence of changes that remove the infection from the inflamed area, the end result may be disastrous. This would seem to mean, then, that the use of anti-inflammatory agents should be restricted chiefly to noninfectious forms of inflammation.

Lymphocytes are supposed to produce a lipase and probably also a protease. The former may be of service in the tubercles produced by *Mycobacterium tuberculosis*. At least lymphocytes are always numerous in the vicinity of these lesions. There is reason to believe that lymphocytes also synthesize, store, and transport nucleoproteins for use by other cells. The presence of large numbers of lymphocytes in areas of chronic inflammation and wound healing may be for the purpose of concentrating proteins in these areas for regeneration of cells and for the formation of fibroblasts.

Although lymphocytes are produced primarily in lymphatic tissue, mitosis and limited reproduction may occur in various regions of the body where they have accumulated as the result of inflammation. The lymphocytes usually appear rather late (after 48 to 72 hours) in the course of an inflammatory disease. They gradually increase in numbers as the inflammatory process continues and eventually become one of the main cellular components of chronic inflammation. They tend to occupy a perivascular location. Probably their perivascular location and their delayed appearance at the site of inflammation are a result of their rather limited amoeboid movement. They appear in a great variety of inflammations but usually only in moderate numbers. They tend to remain in the periphery of the lesion quite removed from the more active inflammatory areas where neutrophils are most abundant. The lymphocytes are quite numerous in lesions produced by viral diseases, particularly those which involve the central nervous system. This association with viral diseases is probably the result of their production of humoral substances that inactivate or destroy the invading virus. In viral infections of the central nervous system they are found in large numbers around blood vessels. This is known as cuffing or perivascular cuffing.

### PLASMA CELL

The plasma cell appears as a rather globular cell in tissue and possesses considerably more cytoplasm than the lymphocyte. The nucleus is excentrically placed in the cell, is spherical in shape, and the chromatin tends to be arranged along the nuclear membrane, giving the nucleus a clockface appearance. The cytoplasm of the cell, when stained with hematoxylin and eosin, has a purple color in contrast to the pale blue color of the lymphocyte.

Plasma cells are not found in the circulating blood stream. Neither mitotic figures nor dividing cells are ever observed, indicating they do not reproduce in the tissues. It is believed they are derived from lymphocytes when these cells are stimulated by certain injurious agents.

Although they have limited amoeboid movement and apparently at times have limited phagocytic properties, phagocytosis is not their main function in the tissues. It is believed they produce humoral defense substances similar to those produced by the lymphocytes. Although the plasma cells may be found anywhere in the body, they are particularly numerous in the tissue of the female reproductive tract, in the tunica propria of the intestinal tract, and in the interstitial tissue of the kidney affected with chronic interstitial nephritis. They are also numerous in some types of chronic inflammation, particularly in mild forms of long standing such as chronic mastitis, actinomycosis, and actinobacillosis.

### MACROPHAGE

The macrophage is a large mononuclear cell, globular in shape, and contains a single spherical nucleus. When stained with hematoxylin and eosin the cytoplasm is pink.

The macrophage has numerous synonyms such as endothelial leukocyte, polyblast, clasmatocyte, histiocyte, resting wandering cell, monocyte, large mononuclear, large mononuclear cell, and reticuloendothelial cell. The cell was first described by Metchnikoff, who indicated its large size in contrast to the neutrophil (the microphage). Because of its large size he gave it the name macrophage. Because of priority and because the term indicates the cell is large and capable of phagocytosis, the term macrophage is preferred.

The macrophages belong to a group of cellular components of the body which are brought together because of their physiological similarities rather than on an anatomical conception of a system which Aschoff named the reticuloendothelial system. The reticuloendothelial system can be demonstrated when India ink or carmine is injected intravenously. As the pigment circulates through the body certain cells in various organs (Kupffer cells of the liver and the cells of the sinusoids of the spleen, lymph nodes, and bone marrow) will phagocytose and contain the ingested material. These phagocytic cells having marked phagocytic properties comprise the reticuloendothelial system. Their production of pseudopodia, their movement, and their engulfment of foreign material can be easily observed in fresh tissue preparations or in tissue culture with the microscope. Macrophages generally are exceedingly pleomorphic. There is evidence to show their formation may be induced by the protein choline, which is liberated in the tissue under normal and pathological circumstances. A macrophage-promoting factor (M.P.F.) has been demonstrated in normal rabbit serum.

In the circulating blood stream the macrophages are known as the **monocytes.** They comprise from 1 to 5 per cent of the total number of leukocytes in the blood. Some of the macrophages (monocytes) are brought to the site of inflammation by the blood stream. The majority of the macrophages, however, are produced in the tissue at the site of inflammation and originate from members of the reticuloendothelial system that are already present in the tissues in the area. They do not appear early in the course of any inflammatory process but usually begin to appear in about 48 to 72 hours and eventually become more numerous than the neutrophils. The reason for this is that the neutrophils are brought to the site of inflammation in large numbers by the blood stream while the macrophages must be produced at the site of inflammation by the few macrophages normally present

in the tissue. After a few days the macrophages are present in large numbers and then may become more numerous than the neutrophils. They are the main phagocytic cells of the body and are the cells which eventually complete the destruction of the irritant and remove the necrotic tissue from the area. Because of their delayed appearance and their great phagocytic powers they are called the **second line of cellular defense.** The macrophages are particularly abundant in the persisting chronic inflammatory diseases (tuberculosis and paratuberculosis). When great phagocytic power is needed, the macrophages fuse together and form foreign-body giant cells (Figs. 11.2 and 11.3).

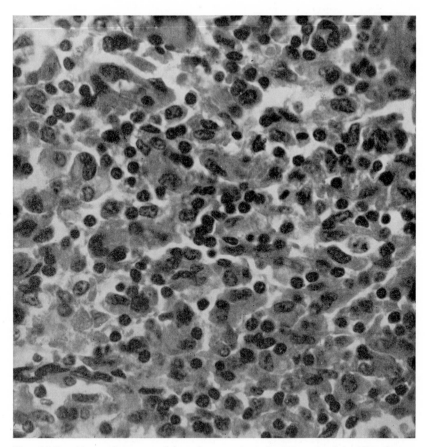

Fig. 11.2 — Macrophages and lymphocytes in a lesion caused by **Mycobacterium paratuberculosis** in the intestinal mucosa of a cow. There are indications of a feeble attempt to form giant cells. (Department of Veterinary Pathology, Michigan State University.)

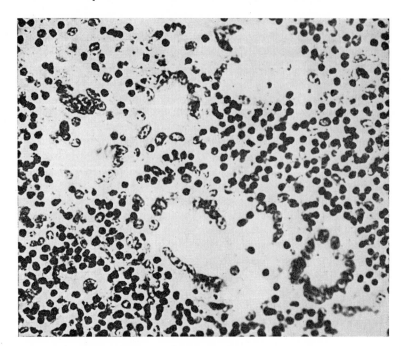

Fig. 11.3 — Macrophages arranged in groups which characterize the multinucleated giant cell of the Langhans' type. Mesenteric lymph node lesion caused by **Mycobacterium paratuberculosis.** (Hallman and Witter, Jour. A.V.M.A.)

GIANT CELL

When macrophages fuse together to form large phagocytic cells the combination is termed a giant cell. It contains multiple nuclei and an abundance of cytoplasm. There are two basic types of giant cells. The first is the **foreign-body giant cell** which must be differentiated from the second, the **tumor giant cell,** which is not associated with inflammation.

The term foreign-body giant cell is used to designate the cell produced by the fusion of macrophages because it is frequently associated with the presence of foreign material in the tissues. It is much larger than most body cells and contains multiple nuclei. Some cells will contain 50, 100, or even more nuclei. These nuclei are regular in size and shape, are not excessively large, are the size of the nuclei of the macrophage, and are normochromatic. The nuclei are arranged in three different ways: (1) They may be arranged around the periphery of the cell. This is the type of arrangement commonly observed in tuberculosis or when foreign bodies such as splinters or thorns have been inserted into the tissues. (2) The nuclei may be clustered at one or both poles of the cell. (3) Less commonly the nuclei are scattered throughout the cytoplasm of the giant cell.

Giant cells are observed in chronic infectious diseases such as tuberculosis, actinomycosis, blastomycosis, and paratuberculosis (Fig. 11.4). They are found surrounding foreign bodies such as splinters, thorns, beards, awns, and suture material which have been inserted into the tissues. They are frequently found in the periphery of necrotic tissue, particularly if fat necrosis is present. The altered tissue is actually foreign to the body. Great care should be exercised so as not to confuse necrotic tissue, particularly necrotic fat, with lesions of tuberculosis. Just because giant cells are present in the vicinity of necrotic tissue does not justify a diagnosis of tuberculosis. A diagnosis of tuberculosis cannot be made until the acid-fast organisms are demonstrated.

Foreign-body giant cells are frequently confused with tumor giant cells. Tumor giant cells are only found in tumors. The cells are large and possess multiple nuclei but the number of nuclei is usually relatively few (2, 4, 8, or 16). The nuclei vary considerably in size and shape, are much larger than the nuclei of normal cells, and are hyperchromatic (stain more intensely with nuclear stains). Tumor giant cells are neoplastic cells. Apparently nuclear division is not followed by cytoplasmic division, and as a result the cytoplasm contains several nuclei. They are not derived from the fusion of tumor cells. Tumor giant cells are particularly common in neoplasms involving bone and skeletal muscle.

## PHAGOCYTOSIS

**Definition.** Phagocytosis is the engulfing and digestion of degenerating, necrotic, or foreign material by certain cells of the body. A **phagocyte** is a cell which is capable of accomplishing phagocytosis.

Many cells within the body are capable of accomplishing phagocytosis. Under ordinary circumstances some cells show only limited phagocytosis, but properly stimulated by irritants they may become ac-

tively phagocytic. There are five major groups of cells which are most frequently associated with phagocytosis: (1) neutrophils, (2) macrophages, (3) endothelial cells in general but particularly those which are found in the capillaries, (4) simple squamous epithelium as is found on serous surfaces, and (5) the septal cells of the lung.

The phagocytic cell ingests and digests the engulfed object. If the object is not readily digested or if the cell is unable to accomplish digestion, it may be carried, within the cytoplasm of the phagocyte, away from the site where it was engulfed. Since the macropahges are the principal phagocytic cells and since they are present in large numbers within the medullary portions of the lymph nodes, a concentration of indigestible substances (anthacite pigment, hemosiderin, and silicon) accumulate in the regional lymph nodes. If the material is particularly insoluble, it can be found in the lymph nodes many years after it was deposited there. Anthracite pigment persists for many years in the bronchial and mediastinal lymph

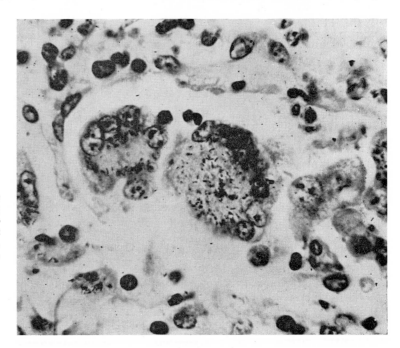

Fig. 11.4 — Foreign-body giant cells containing **Myobacterium paratuberculosis** in a mesenteric lymph node of a cow. (Hallman and Witter, Jour. A.V.M.A.)

nodes. Melanin pigments are found in the peripheral lymph nodes following chronic dermatitis or louse infestations. Sometimes the phagocytes are killed by the engulfed irritant. This is particularly true when very pathogenic bacteria are phagocytosed. The transportation of bacteria within phagocytes, from a site of infection to a distant lymph node or organ, is a common method of spread of microorganisms throughout the body. The cellular and humoral defense system of the body may have been quite successful in containing and enclosing the bacterial infection, but since the phagocyte containing bacteria is capable of amoeboid movement it may pass through the walls of defense formed around the irritant, and later in a distant organ the phagocyte is overcome by the bacteria and a new focus of infection is established.

Neutrophils and macrophages are the most active phagocytes. Neutrophils appear early in the course of inflammation while the macrophages begin to appear in about 48 to 72 hours and eventually may become more numerous than the neutrophil. Neutrophils are particularly abundant when pyogenic microorganisms are introduced into the tissues. The macrophages are the principal phagocytic cells of the body and eventually complete the destruction of the irritant and remove the degenerating and necrotic cells in the area of inflammation.

## The Exudate

**Definition.** The exudate is composed of the cellular and humoral substances which accumulate in an area of inflammation. The migration of cellular and humoral substances into an area of inflammation is known as **exudation.**

The exudate consists of five major components: (1) the irritant, (2) injured tissue cells, (3) leukocytes (neutrophils, macrophages, lymphocytes, plasma cells, eosinophils, and basophils), (4) plasma constituents (water, protein, fibrin, and antibodies), and (5) erythrocytes. These components give the exudate a very characteristic appearance and composition which differentiate it from a transudate.

## COMPARISON OF A TRANSUDATE AND AN EXUDATE

The clinician and pathologist must determine whether the fluid they are observing in tissues or body cavities is a transudate or an exudate. It is extremely important that a decision be made because the etiology, treatment, and prognosis vary considerably depending upon which it is. Usually this can be determined, but at times the fluid will have some of the characteristics of both, and then it may be impossible to arrive at a decision. Table 11.1 lists the principal characteristics of a transudate and an exudate and will aid in differentiating between them.

## FUNCTION OF THE EXUDATE

The various functions of the exudate have been mentioned from time to time and now are brought together to show the student that, contrary to popular belief, it is actually beneficial to the body and is not injurious. The functions of the exudate are as follows:

1. The irritant is diluted when the plasma constituents of the blood are poured into the area of inflammation. By dilution the irritant may be changed from a severe irritant to a mild irritant or even to a stimulant. In addition the particles of the irritant, such as bacteria, may be dispersed and then the leukocytes may phagocytose the irritant more easily.

2. The exudate acts mechanically by washing or carrying the irritant away. This is especially true on cutaneous or mucous surfaces where the constant flow of the exudate from the body sweeps the irritant, such as bacteria or dirt, to the exterior and away from the body, thus ridding the animal of the offending agent. The surgeon aids the body defense system by incising abscesses and inserting drainage tubes to facilitate the flow of exudate to the exterior.

3. It brings phagocytes to the area to phagocytose the irritant. Neutrophils and macrophages are the principal phagocytic cells.

TABLE 11.1
COMPARISON OF A TRANSUDATE AND AN EXUDATE

| Transudate | Exudate |
| --- | --- |
| 1. Clear. | 1. Cloudy. |
| 2. Thin, watery, resembles lymph, and contains no tissue fragments. | 2. Thick, creamy, and contains tissue fragments. |
| 3. No odor. | 3. May have an odor. |
| 4. Color — like water or pale yellow depending upon the normal plasma color of the animal. | 4. Color — white, yellow, or red. |
| 5. Alkaline. | 5. Acid. |
| 6. Specific gravity — 1.015 or lower. | 6. Specific gravity — 1.018 or higher. |
| 7. Low protein content — less than 3 per cent. | 7. High protein content — more than 4 per cent. |
| 8. Does not coagulate or contains only a few fibrin strands. | 8. Coagulates *in vivo* and *in vitro*. |
| 9. Low cell count — none or few leukocytes and erythrocytes. | 9. High cell count — many leukocytes and erythrocytes. |
| 10. Low enzyme content. | 10. High enzyme content. |
| 11. No bacteria are present. | 11. Bacteria may be present. |
| 12. No association with inflammation. | 12. Associated with inflammation. |

4. The exudate brings fibrin to the area. Fibrin has several functions. It entraps the irritant and thus retards its dissemination through the tissues until the phagocytes are able to phagocytose it. Fibrin provides protective sheets of protein between the irritant and the surrounding delicate tissue cells which might be damaged by the irritant. Fibrin effectively seals the lumen of the lymphatics, thus preventing the entrance of the irritant, such as bacteria, and thereby hindering the spread of the irritant to the regional lymph nodes or distant organs. Fibrin aids in healing and repair by forming a supporting scaffold on which the fibroblasts and angioblasts may invade the area of inflammation. Finally, fibrin has a stimulating effect on the proliferation of fibroblasts.

5. The exudate brings antibodies to the area of inflammation. Antibodies are serum proteins which have the chemical and physical properties of globulins. Observations have been made which indicate that they are formed in the liver, spleen, connective tissue, and especially in the lymph nodes. In these places they are formed by the reticuloendothelial cells and lymphocytes.

Antibodies are restricted in their effectiveness against the various types of irritants which cause inflammation. They are most effective against bacteria and viruses. Examples of antibodies that aid in the removal of bacteria are (1) agglutinins which cause the microorganisms to adhere to one another, forming clumps, (2) lysins which dissolve cells including bacteria, (3) antitoxins which neutralize exotoxins, (4) opsonins which in some way prepare bacteria for phagocytosis, and (5) precipitins which result in the precipitation of some antigens.

Little is known about antibodies for viruses except that they do exist. Just how they act has not been determined. If specific antibodies for viruses are brought in contact with the viruses before the latter enter body cells, disease does not result. The antibodies are said to neutralize the virus.

6. The exudate brings to the area of inflammation an increased amount of nutrient and oxygen which is needed for the defense mechanism, healing, and repair. There is also an increased rate of removal of catabolic products. By maintaining a constant flow of fluid into the area, the exudate tends to maintain a hydrogen-ion concentration which is most ideal for the phagocytosis of the irritant. It also furnishes a suitable fluid medium in which the phagocytes, enzymes, and antibodies may function under optimum conditions.

## Variations in the Inflammatory Reaction

The inflammatory reaction, like all other biological phenomena, is variable. Many classifications are employed to describe it and the terminology used is extremely loose, but the nomenclature does comprise a group of descriptive terms which effectively describe the tissue alterations.

The variations in the appearance of an area of inflammation are dependent upon three factors:

**1. The nature of the irritant.** Extremely concentrated agents cause necrosis of tissue, moderately severe substances irritate tissue, mildly injurious agents stimulate tissue, and extremely mild forms of injury may cause no alteration at all. The reaction of tissue to an obnoxious substance varies with the species of animal as well as with members within the species.

**2. The tissue involved.** There is great variation in the sensitivity of tissue to an irritant. The tissues of the central nervous system are easily injured. Columnar epithelium is much more susceptible to injury than is stratified squamous epithelium. The character of the exudate varies with the type of tissue affected. If mucous surfaces are involved, large amounts of mucin are found in the exudate. Serous surfaces produce an abundance of plasma and fibrin. When the skin or the mucous membranes of the gastrointestinal tract are involved, desquamation or sloughing of the superficial surfaces of the structure may occur.

**3. The duration of the application of the irritant.** The longer an irritant is applied the greater is the likelihood there will be injury to the tissue. When an irritant is applied over a long period of time there is excessive production of connective tissue and epithelium.

## Inflammation Classified According to Degree of Reaction

As has been previously pointed out, the reaction of the body and the course of the disease depends upon the intensity of the irritant and the response of the tissue to the irritant. It is extremely important for the veterinarian to recognize the degree of reaction so that the most desirable therapeutic measures for the well-being of the animal may be instituted.

According to the degree of reaction, inflammation may be classified into three major groups:

**1. An adequate reaction** occurs when the circulatory and cellular responses of the body are sufficient to bring about prompt destruction and removal of the irritant and healing occurs in a reasonably short period of time (e.g., rhinitis in the chicken, pink eye in the horse, or cow pox in cattle). This is the degree of reaction desired by the veterinarian, and his therapeutic measures should be directed so as to achieve it.

**2. An inadequate reaction** occurs when the irritant is not sufficiently severe to stimulate the body defenses enough to bring about the destruction and removal of the obnoxious agent and effect healing. This is observed in ring bone or quittor in the horse, brucellosis in cattle and swine, anaplasmosis in cattle, and tuberculosis, blastomycosis, actinomycosis, and staphylococcosis in many animals. The therapeutic efforts of the veterinarian must be directed in such a manner, by using hot packs, chemicals, or drugs, as to stimulate the tissues and increase the circulatory and cellular reactions in the area. Antibiotics may be used to aid the body defenses in overcoming bacteria. It is extremely important that the veterinarian recognize the probable outcome of the disease at its initiation so that proper therapeutic measures may be instituted as soon as possible to avoid delay in healing.

**3. An excessive reaction** occurs when the body responds to the irritant with violent circulatory and cellular reactions which may be of such magnitude that the body defenses themselves bring about the death of the animal. In pneumonia the pouring of exudate into the lungs may fill the alveoli and the animal will suffocate.

Sensitivity to protein may cause such a violent allergic reaction that a shocklike syndrome is produced and the individual dies from inadequate circulation of the blood. The veterinarian must realize the intensity of the reaction which has been initiated and control the extent of the reaction; otherwise the animal will die.

### Inflammation Classified According to Principal Constituent of Exudate

The classification is based upon the predominant constituent of the exudate. It is seldom that one constituent of the exudate does not predominate over the others. If two constituents of the exudate are in approximately equal amounts or if the pathologist wishes to indicate that both constituents are present, a combination of terms may be used.

#### SEROUS INFLAMMATION

**Definition.** A serous inflammation is present when the principal constituent of the exudate is lymph or plasma.

**Etiology.** Serous inflammation is the result of relatively mild irritants which cause the least amount of injury to the tissue. It may be produced by the rays of the sun when redness and blister formation occur. It results when chemicals of various types are applied to the skin and cause a blister. When traumatic injuries of a rubbing nature are applied to stratified squamous epithelium, swelling of the skin or the formation of a blister results. It occurs when various viral agents (vesicular stomatitis or foot-and-mouth disease) invade the skin or mucous membrane and produce blisters. It is a common type of inflammation involving serous surfaces (peritoneum and pleura) when mild irritants are present and large amounts of serous fluid accumulate in the cavity. Finally, it must be remembered that it is often the first stage in many inflammatory processes. If the irritant persists or becomes more severe, a more violent type of injury may occur in which more than just plasma is the principal constituent of the exudate, and then a different classification of the tissue alteration must be made.

**Macroscopic appearance.** The cardinal signs of inflammation are present. A watery type of exudate flows from the surface of the tissue or organ, or accumulates in tissue spaces and body cavities. The character of this watery fluid depends upon the permeability of the capillary wall. With slight permeability the exudate is very similar to lymph. With greater capillary permeability the exudate resembles blood plasma. Great care should be exercised so as not to confuse edema with serous inflammation. In edema the cardinal signs of inflammation are not present, while they must exist when serous inflammation occurs.

**Microscopic appearance.** The circulatory and cellular alterations characteristic of inflammation are present. The predominant constituent of the exudate is a fluid which resembles plasma in its characteristics. In hematoxylin- and eosin-stained preparations it appears as a homogeneous to finely granular material within the tissue spaces and body cavities and stains pink with eosin. The intensity of the eosin staining depends upon the amount of protein present. When the protein content is slight the eosin staining is barely visible, but when the protein content is great and approaches that of plasma the eosin staining becomes intense.

**Significance and result.** The presence of a serous inflammation indicates that a relatively mild irritant is present and that the outcome of the disease will probably be favorable as far as the life of the individual is concerned. Permanent injury or alteration in the area is not likely to occur because the serous fluid can be readily reabsorbed by the body. If, however, a serous inflammation is allowed to persist in the area for a long period of time, a permanent deposition of connective tissue may occur. If the irritant becomes more severe or persists for a long period of time, a more serious type of inflammation may result.

MUCOUS OR CATARRHAL INFLAMMATION

**Definition.** A mucous inflammation is present when the principal constituent of the exudate is mucin. Mucous inflammation only occurs in areas in which cuboidal or columnar epithelium capable of producing mucin is present. A diagnosis of mucous inflammation involving serous surfaces, connective tissue, muscle, or brain can never be made because mucin producing cells are not present.

**Etiology.** The various agents that may produce a mucous inflammation are all mild in nature. Mildly irritating chemicals (formaldehyde, phenol, cresol, and detergents) when applied to delicate mucous membranes, such as those of the nose and genital tract, produce a mucous inflammation. The student in anatomy is well aware of the mucous inflammation which he experiences in his respiratory passages while dissecting the cadaver. The veterinarian often produces a mucous inflammation of the genital passages of animals if he uses irritating disinfectants while performing examinations of these structures. Inhaled dust, cold air, or foreign protein irritates the mucous membranes of the respiratory passages, and inflammation of the respiratory tract occurs with the production of large amounts of mucin. Bacterial and viral diseases may irritate the mucous membranes and cause an excessive production of mucin as occurs in rhinitis and conjunctivitis. Ingested food containing irritating chemicals or decomposition products may irritate the gastrointestinal tract and cause excessive production of mucin. A mass of feces retained in the rectum or colon (constipation) will irritate the mucous membrane, and excessive amounts of mucin will be produced.

**Macroscopic appearance.** The cardinal signs of inflammation are present. The exudate flowing from or accumulating on the mucous surface consists of a clear transparent material, or it may be gray, yellow, or opaque depending upon what is entrapped within it. It is slimy and stringy in consistency and tends to cling to the mucous membrane or whatever it comes in contact with. The stringy slimy material flowing from the nose in rhinitis and the gray jelly-like material which covers equine fecal balls are good examples of the gross appearance of a mucous exudate. The student must always be cautious so as not to confuse mucous exudate with the slimy material found in the gastrointestinal tract as the result of the normal production of mucin during digestion and the disintegration of the mucous membrane and the ingesta by digestive enzymes and bacterial decomposition. The amount of mucin normally present in the gastrointestinal tract varies with the species. It is particularly abundant in the horse. In the dog the digestion of the mucous membrane produces a slimy gruel-like mass which is often erroneously called a mucous exudate.

**Microscopic appearance.** The circulatory and vascular alterations characteristic of inflammation are present. The principal constituent of the exudate on the mucous surface is mucin. The cuboidal or columnar epithelial cells contain globular masses which partially or completely fill the cell. When these cellular accumulations become large and fill the cell it becomes known as a goblet cell. Any mucous membrane, even though it does not normally have goblet cells, may contain an abundance of goblet cells when properly stimulated. The mucin within the cells or on the surface of the mucous membrane stains blue with hematoxylin. Specific stains such as thionine and mucicarmine stain the mucin red. It is extremely important that differential stains be used to accurately determine if the material on the mucous surface and within the cells is actually mucin. The columnar epithelial cells are hyperplastic and multiply rapidly. This is necessary because when a goblet cell is discharged it must be replaced by another cell; otherwise considerable loss of epithelium will occur.

**Significance and result.** The presence of a mucous inflammation indicates a mild irritant has been applied to the tissue. If the irritant is removed, recovery occurs very quickly because regeneration and repair of the epithelium is very rapid and complete. If the irritant persists or becomes more severe, a more serious type of inflammation may result. The production of mucin by injured epithelium entraps and contains the irritating substances so that they are removed by the normal flow of the secretion or excretion of the organ. It forms a barrier around the irritant, thus protecting the delicate mucous membrane. The mucin serves as a lubricant which facilitates the expulsion of the undesirable substance (masses of dry feces). If the mild irritant persists for a long period of time, the mucin-producing epithelium may become hypersensitive or hyperactive and excessive amounts of mucin may be produced. This is often referred to as catarrh and is commonly observed in the human family in those individuals who smoke excessively. Large amounts of mucin are eliminated, particularly in the morning when the individual first arises. Hyperactivity of the mucous glands is also observed in the gastrointestinal tract when irritating foods, particularly those partially decomposed by bacterial fermentation or injured by freezing, are consumed.

## FIBRINOUS INFLAMMATION

**Definition.** A fibrinous inflammation is present when the principal constituent of the exudate is fibrin.

**Etiology.** Fibrinous inflammation is caused by a more violent type of injury in which the permeability of the capillaries has been altered so that the larger protein constituents containing the precursors of fibrin have escaped into the surrounding tissue. It is observed in various viral diseases such as infectious feline enteritis in which masses of fibrin are found in the lumen of the intestine (Fig. 11.5). It is observed in sporadic bovine encephalitis which is characterized by the accumulation of large amounts of fibrin in the peritoneal and pleural cavities. A fibrinous inflammation often results when thermal agents or irritating chemicals are applied to the tissues. It is es-

pecially common when hot gases are inhaled by animals in barn fires. A fibrinous inflammation is very frequently observed when mucous membranes are invaded by *Corneybacterium diphtheriae*, various *Salmonella*, or *Spherophorus necrophorus*.

**Macroscopic appearance.** The cardinal signs of inflammation are present. If the fibrin has accumulated in the tissues, the organ is firmer and tenser than normal. This is well exemplified by the accumulation of fibrin in the alveoli of the lung. The lung becomes extremely firm and dense, resembling liver in both appearance and consistency. On serous or cutaneous surfaces the fibrin first appears as a stringy white or yellowish netlike material. The surface loses its shine and has a velvety appearance. As the fibrin accumulates on a mucous or cutaneous surface it forms a yellowish or grayish sheet and may entrap desquamated epithelium and foreign material (ingesta). When the fibrin accumulates on the surface of a tubular organ it may form a cast of the organ. These casts are frequently passed in the feces of the bovine and may be as much as 25 feet in length. Casts of the trachea and bronchi may be formed and, following violent coughing, a branching cast of the respiratory system may be coughed up.

Masses of fibrin on an epithelial surface are classified into two major groups: The first is known as a **pseudomembrane** or a **croupous membrane.** It may be peeled away from the surface quite easily and leaves an intact epithelial membrane. The second type is a **diphtheritic membrane** which is quite firmly attached to the underlying tissue. It cannot be removed without tearing the tissue and when removed no intact epithelial membrane remains. The epithelium has undergone coagulative necrosis, and because it is necrotic and infiltrated with fibrin it peels off with the exudate, leaving an exposed raw surface known as an ulcer. These membranes are frequently observed in the pharynx of calves with so-called calf diphtheria and in the intestinal tract of hogs affected with cholera.

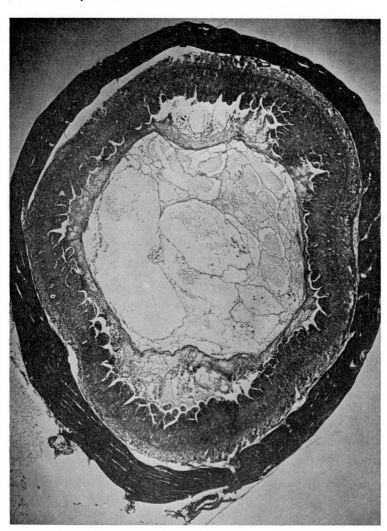

Fig. 11.5 — Acute fibri-nonecrotic jejunitis in a cat. Mucosa covered with a rather dense membrane of fibrin which is becoming detached from the mucosa to form a cast. Center of lumen filled with a looser network of fibrin. ×17. (Department of Veterinary Pathology, Iowa State University.)

**Microscopic appearance.** The circulatory and cellular alterations characteristic of inflammation are present. The major constituent of the exudate is fibrin, which may infiltrate the entire organ such as the lung or may accumulate on the surface of the organ in the form of a sheet, as a pseudomembrane or a diphtheritic membrane. The fibrin is recognized as finely beaded strands which stain a dirty pink with eosin. Specific fibrin stains can be used to identify the true nature of the strands. Since the irritant which produced the fibrinous inflammation is severe, there is often considerable coagulative necrosis in the area such as is observed in epithelium when a diphtheritic membrane is present.

Fibrin is frequently confused with a homogeneous protein precipitate in the tissue which is often referred to as fibrinoid (a most unfortunate term because it is not a specific structure). This protein precipitate is usually the result of an antigen-antibody reaction or of intense irritants which cause a firm coagulation of plasma protein (e.g., when egg white is exposed to extreme heat or strong acids).

**Significance and Result.** The presence of a fibrinous inflammation indicates the irritant has been severe. Often the tissue destruction is so great the animal will not survive. Fibrin on a cutaneous or mucous surface is desquamated, and the body rids itself of the exudate in this manner. When fibrin accumulates in a body cavity it must be removed by the phagocytes. Fibrin in the peritoneal cavity is extremely serious because it attaches to the various organs, and when it is organized and connective tissue is deposited in the area, **adhesions** are the result. These connective tissue bands extending through the peritoneal cavity are extremely serious because they interfere with the motility of the intestine or may impair the vascular circulation in an area. Adhesions frequently result from poor surgical technic in the peritoneal cavity.

## SUPPURATIVE OR PURULENT INFLAMMATION

**Definition.** A suppurative inflammation is present when the principal constituent of the exudate is the neutrophil. Many inflammatory reactions begin as a suppurative inflammation when the first line of cellular defense accumulates in the area.

**Etiology.** The most common cause of a suppurative inflammation is bacteria, particularly the pyogenic (pus producing) bacteria. Probably all bacteria produce a suppurative inflammation at some time during their sojourn in the tissues. Even *Mycobacterium tuberculosis*, not ordinarily thought of as a pyogenic organism, is characterized by a suppurative type of reaction when first introduced into the tissue. A suppurative inflammation is most frequently observed with a staphylococcic, streptococcic, or a corynebacterium infection. Viral diseases for the most part do not produce a suppurative inflammation. One of the exceptions is viral equine encephalomyelitis in which microabscesses are found in the brain in some cases. A few chemicals, such as turpentine, when injected into the tissues will produce a suppurative inflammation. Other chemicals may produce a transient suppurative inflammation shortly after the chemical is applied. Many chemicals and other eti-

ological agents produce tissue damage which is later invaded by bacteria, and then a complicating suppurative inflammation is present; but it was not the original etiological agent that produced the suppuration.

**Macroscopic appearance.** The cardinal signs of inflammation are present. The principal constituent of the exudate is pus. It may be white, yellow, green, red, black, or blue depending upon the species of animal and the etiological agent present. Streptococci and staphylococci usually produce a white or yellow pus. Corynebacteria, particularly if found in the bovine, produce a pus which has a greenish color. Red pus is present when erythrocytes exist in the exudate. Black pus is often observed in hoof injuries in the horse in which the sulfides from the manure combine with the iron in the hemoglobin of the blood and produce the black pigment iron sulfide. Some organisms produce a soluble pigment, and because of this a bluish-green pus may be observed when *Pseudomonas aeruginosa* is present in the exudate.

The consistency of the exudate may be thin and watery, creamy, thick, viscid, or granular depending upon the species of animal, the amount of necrotic material present, and the dehydration of the exudate. Pus is liquid because of the proteolytic enzymes of the neutrophil. Since the enzymes of the neutrophil of the dog are extremely proteolytic, canine pus tends to be thin and watery. Bovine pus is rather viscid. When pus has been dehydrated or contains numerous fragments of necrotic tissue it may be rather granular in consistency. An antitryptic enzyme is present in avian pus. Its presence probably explains why avian pus has a dry caseous consistency in the body cavities (peritoneal, pleural, pericardial, and nasal sinuses) and in abscesses such as bumblefoot.

There are a number of terms used to describe various alterations in tissue as the result of a suppurative inflammation. The first of these is **cellulitis**, or **phlegmon**, which is a diffuse suppurative inflammation of connective tissue in which the infection spreads rapidly through the loose connective tissue and frequently results in death of the animal.

An **abscess** is a focal suppurative inflammation involving any tissue or organ. Most abscesses are surrounded by a wall composed of connective tissue, proliferating capillaries, and leukocytes. This circumscribing structure is known as the **pyogenic membrane** (pus-producing membrane). Abscesses may be acute or chronic, focal or multiple (Fig. 11.6), depending upon how long they have existed in the tissue. Abscesses, unless enclosed in a very thick pyogenic membrane, tend to protrude into the surrounding tissue in the direction of least resistance. If they are located near a body surface, such as in the subcutaneous connective tissue, they tend to protrude to the exterior and eventually may rupture and discharge their content to the

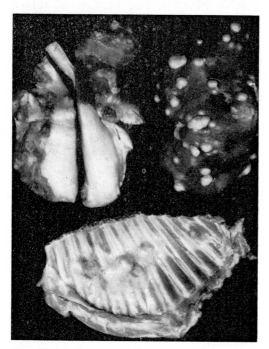

Fig. 11.6 – Metastatic abscesses in lung, liver, and costal pleura of a 15-day-old lamb. Primary infection of navel due to **Spherophorus necrophorus.** (Department of Veterinary Pathology, Michigan State University.)

exterior. This protrusion of an abscess to the exterior is known as **pointing.** The tract through which the content of the abscess is discharged to the exterior is known as the **sinus,** or **fistulous, tract.**

Specific names have been given to several types of abscesses, depending upon their location and size. A **pustule** is a small focal area of suppurative inflammation in the malpighian layer of the epidermis of the skin. A **furuncle (boil)** is a small focal area of suppurative inflammation in the skin which involves a hair follicle or a sebaceous gland. A **carbuncle** is a focal area of suppurative inflammation in the subcutaneous tissue which discharges pus to the exterior through several sinus tracts. Within some abscesses, especially the furuncle, there is often a central mass of necrotic inspissated exudate which is known as the core of the abscess.

An **erosion** is a defect in epithelium in which there has been a loss of the superficial cell layers but the basal cell layers are still intact. This type of lesion often results when a pustle ruptures to the exterior and leaves a defect in the stratified squamous epithelium.

An **ulcer** is a focal area of suppurative inflammation in the skin or mucous membrane (Fig. 11.7) in which there is loss of the entire epithelium and the base of the ulcer lies in the subcutaneous tissue, the submucosa, or has penetrated deeper into the underlying structures.

**Empyema** is the accumulation of pus in a preformed body cavity (peritoneal or pleural). **Pyorrhea** actually means a discharge of pus, but now has come to mean a purulent inflammation of the gum in the vicinity of an alveolus.

**Microscopic appearance.** The circulatory and cellular alterations characteristic of inflammation are present. The principal cell of the exudate is the neutrophil in various stages of disintegration (Fig. 11.8). The neutrophil contains very efficient proteolytic enzymes, and because of them the cell, after death, undergoes autolysis. As a result, depending upon the extent of the

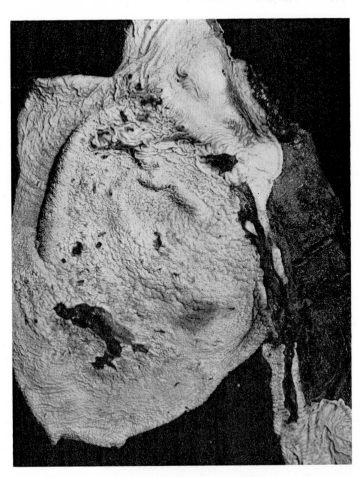

Fig. 11.7 — Ulcers in the mucous membrane of the stomach of a horse. (Schlotthauer, Jour. A.V.M.A.)

autolysis, cytoplasm may or may not be visible, and the nucleus may have undergone karyorrhexis with only fragments of the nucleus remaining. In some infections (listeriosis) only microscopically visible abscesses are present because the amount of pus accumulating in the vicinity of the bacteria is never great enough to be observed with the unaided eye.

**Significance and result.** The presence of pus in nearly every instance indicates bacteria are present in the area of inflammation. Some bacteria (streptococci, staphylococci, and corynebacteria) produce an abundance of pus, and these organisms are designated as the **pyogenic bacteria** (pus-producing bacteria).

Contrary to popular belief, the presence of pus in a wound is an extremely favorable sign because it indicates the first line of cellular defense has been brought to the area. When the defense mechanism of the body is in operation, the danger that the body will be invaded by bacteria is greatly reduced. Because of the favor with which the appearance of pus is looked upon by the clinician, and especially if the pus is of good consistency and free from odor, he calls it good, or laudable, pus.

If an abscess has persisted in the tissue for a period of time, it frequently happens that the bacteria are destroyed. When these abscesses are cultured on suitable media no microorganisms are isolated and the lesions are designated as **sterile abscesses.**

Toxic substances (bacterial toxins and products of protein disintegration) may

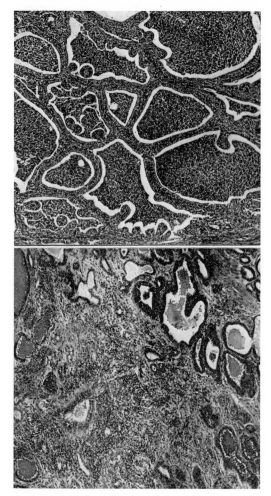

Fig. 11.8 — **Above,** purulent inflammation of the prostate of a dog. ×50. **Below,** chronic inflammation of the prostate of a dog. ×60. (Schlotthauer, Jour. A.V.M.A.)

diffuse out of abscesses, enter the vascular circulation, and cause a toxemia. The existence of confined pus has often been used to explain rather obscure illnesses, aches, and pains. Although toxemia from confined pus may occur, its importance in general debility is probably not as great as was formerly thought.

## HEMORRHAGIC INFLAMMATION

**Definition.** A hemorrhagic inflammation is present when the principal constituent of the exudate is the erythrocyte.

**Etiology.** A hemorrhagic inflammation is caused by a violent type of irritant which injures the blood vessels to such an extent that they are no longer able to contain the erythrocytes, and hemorrhage into the tissues occurs. It is observed when extremely injurious chemicals (phenol, arsenic, chloroform, and phosphorus) come in contact with the tissues. Bacterial and viral diseases (blackleg, anthrax, pasteurellosis, laryngotracheitis, and streptococcal infections) will cause such severe injury that hemorrhage occurs.

**Macroscopic appearance.** The cardinal signs of inflammation are present. The exudate in the area of inflammation will be pink or red in color according to the number of erythrocytes present. It may be fluid or clotted, depending upon the amount of fibrin present. If the hemorrhagic exudate originates in the stomach or the anterior portion of the intestinal tract, the feces will be brown or black in color due to the digestion of the blood and the formation of acid hematin. In the posterior portion of the digestive tract (colon and rectum) the blood will be bright red because it has not had time to undergo digestion, and acid hematin is not formed because hydrochloric acid is not present. If the blood comes in contact with hydrogen sulfide, as may occur when the infection involves the hoof of the horse, the exudate may be black in color because the sulfides combine with the iron in the hemoglobin to form black iron sulfide.

Great care should always be taken so as not to confuse a hemorrhagic inflammation with passive hyperemia. This error in diagnosis is frequently made, especially in the bovine, when passive hyperemia is present in the intestinal tract. The point of differentiation is that in passive hyperemia the cardinal signs of inflammation are not present.

A hemorrhagic inflammation must be differentiated from hemorrhage. In hemorrhagic inflammation the cardinal signs of inflammation are present, the escape of blood is primarily by diapedesis, and the hemorrhage does not appear to originate from any specific area. In hemorrhage the cardinal signs of inflammation are not present, and the blood escapes from one or a few local areas or wounds.

**Microscopic appearance.** The circulatory and cellular alterations characteristic of inflammation are present. The erythrocyte is the predominant cell in the exudate. Neutrophils are numerous in the area, and macrophages, lymphocytes, plasma cells, and giant cells have usually not had time to appear. By the time the latter cells appear, the animal will usually have died.

Hemorrhagic inflammation must be differentiated from hyperemia (physiological or passive). In hyperemia the erythrocytes are contained within the lumen of the vessel. In hemorrhagic inflammation they have escaped from the vessel into the surrounding tissue. A hemorrhagic inflammation must also be differentiated from hemorrhage. In a hemorrhagic inflammation, neutrophils are abundant in the area, and there is degeneration and necrosis of cells as the result of the injury.

**Significance and result.** The prognosis of hemorrhagic inflammation is extremely unfavorable. The irritant is very severe and extensive injury has usually taken place. In addition the hemorrhage from the area may be so extensive that the animal may die from anemia. This often occurs in coccidiosis in the chicken. If the animal survives, recovery is delayed because the tissue destruction has been great and extensive repair is necessary. There has been extensive damage to the blood vessels, and the body has difficulty in supplying the blood needed for healing and repair. In addition there is a mass of erythrocytes and fibrin in the area which must be removed by phagocytosis, and this requires an additional period of time.

## LYMPHOCYTIC INFLAMMATION

**Definition.** A lymphocytic inflammation is present when the predominant cell of the exudate is the lymphocyte. A lymphocytic inflammation is an arbitrary classification in that the cardinal signs of inflammation are not observed macroscopically, which is an exception to the general concept of the criteria for inflammation.

**Etiology.** A lymphocytic inflammation is associated with viral diseases in general. Apparently the antibodies produced by the lymphocytes are required to destroy the virus. It is observed in such diseases as canine distemper, rabies, and lymphocytic choriomeningitis. At times numerous lymphocytes are found in the tunica propria of the gastrointestinal tract. Since viruses are found in the tract, it has been suggested that the presence of the lymphocytes may be as the result of these ultramicroscopic organisms. Relatively mild toxins will also cause an increase in the number of lymphocytes in the tissues. This is observed in the hepatic triads as well as in the tunica propria of the intestinal tract when plant toxins (senecio and astragalus) are present.

**Macroscopic appearance.** A lymphocytic inflammation is not observed on gross examination of the organ, and the cardinal signs of inflammation are not present. In rabies, for example, even though the animal dies, no gross alterations are detectable in the brain or other organs.

**Microscopic appearance.** Circulatory and cellular alterations associated with inflammation are present. The exudate is rather scanty in amount as compared with other types of inflammation. The lymphocyte may be the only observable constituent of the exudate in the beginning of the disease. As degenerating and necrotic tissue is produced in the area, circulatory and cellular alterations may become more prominent and macrophages appear to remove the degenerating and necrotic tissue. The activity of the macrophage is directed primarily towards the altered tissue rather than at the virus. Lymphocytes tend to accumulate in the periphery of the blood vessels, assuming a perivascular arrangement. These accumulations are called lymphocytic cuffs and the process is known as cuffing. This is particularly prominent in the central nervous system. In the milder viral infections this may be the only alteration which is observed. In the brain the lymphocytes accumulate primarily in the Virchow-Robin space which surrounds the blood vessel and seldom migrate into the brain tissue proper.

In the tunica propria of the intestinal tract, lymphocytes are always present and their numbers fluctuate considerably. The fluctuation is probably due to mild viral infections as well as toxins associated with irritating feeds or constipation.

**Significance and result.** The presence of a lymphocytic inflammation indicates a viral disease or toxemia is present. If the viral agent can be overcome and if the toxin can be removed, healing is rapid and often complete. The lymphocytes return to the general vascular circulation, and since fibrin and extensive tissue destruction are not present, little or no permanent evidence of the existence of an inflammation remains in the area.

### ALLERGIC INFLAMMATION

**Definition.** An allergic inflammation is the reaction of the body to a protein to which it has been previously sensitized. It is a special type of body response in which the exudate may be serous, fibrinous, suppurative, or hemorrhagic.

Allergic inflammation occurs in animals which have been previously sensitized, either naturally or artificially, to foreign proteins, including those of bacterial origin. A subsequent subcutaneous or intradermic injection of a specific bacterial protein into a sensitized animal may result in a violent local acute inflammatory reaction. This allergic inflammation is the basis for the intradermic reactions used for the diagnosis of tuberculosis, paratuberculosis, glanders, and histoplasmosis.

The allergic inflammatory reaction has been studied thoroughly in the caudal folds of sensitized calves which have been injected intradermally with tuberculin. The reaction takes place in the dermis. Soon after the tuberculin is injected, a very acute suppurative inflammation begins. It is characterized by the formation of foci of edema containing many neutrophils. These foci form around small blood vessels and nerves and are said,

therefore, to be perivascular and perineural in location.

In the early stages the neutrophils steadily increase in numbers. As the perivascular infiltration increases, thrombi form in some of the involved veins and a proliferation of endothelial cells occurs in some of the small arteries.

As the course of the process extends into the third day, the amount of edema and the number of neutrophils gradually begin to diminish. The macrophages and the eosinophils begin to increase in number quite rapidly, but the macrophages become most numerous. The macrophages form giant cells but they are not produced in large numbers.

Seventy-two hours after the animals are injected with tuberculin they are examined for the existence of an allergic reaction. At this time the allergic reaction has usually reached its maximum intensity. If an allergic reaction is present at this time, it is an indication that the animal had become sensitized to the protein of *Mycobacterium tuberculosis*. A similar reaction is observed when johnin is injected into cattle sensitized by *Mycobacterium paratuberculosis*.

## Inflammation Classified According to Duration

Inflammation may be classified according to the length of time it persists. The shorter the period of time inflammation exists in an area, the less will be the permanent change in the tissue. In contrast, the longer it persists, the greater will be the extent of the local permanent alteration. The various inflammatory reactions may be classified as to duration into four groups.

### PERACUTE INFLAMMATION

In this type of inflammation the irritant is exceedingly severe or involves a very susceptible tissue or organ. The course of the disease is extremely rapid, lasting for only a few hours. In fact the course may be so rapid that the animal is not even observed to be ill until just a few minutes before it dies. Blackleg and malignant edema are examples of peracute inflammation. The cardinal signs of inflammation are present. The circulatory and cellular alterations have occurred, and an abundance of neutrophils may be present in the tissue. Macrophages, giant cells, lymphocytes, plasma cells, fibroblasts, and angioblasts are not present or are few in number. Peracute inflammation terminates in death because the irritant is so severe the body defenses are overwhelmed.

## ACUTE INFLAMMATION

In acute inflammation the irritant is not as severe as in peracute inflammation or a less critical tissue is involved. The inflammation persists over a period of several days and terminates in recovery or death. The cardinal signs of inflammation are present. Circulatory and cellular alterations have occurred in the area. Neutrophils are abundant. Macrophages and lymphocytes are beginning to make their appearance and their numbers will increase as the disease progresses. Immature fibroblasts, angioblasts, and epithelium are present but the amount is not in excess of that which is needed for repair and healing.

## SUBACUTE INFLAMMATION

Subacute inflammation is caused by an irritant of less intensity than that which produced an acute inflammation, It has persisted for a longer period of time or a less susceptible tissue is involved. Healing usually occurs but is delayed for several weeks. The cardinal signs of inflammation are present but they are not as pronounced as those observed when acute inflammation exists. Circulatory and cellular alterations have taken place but they are not as profuse as was observed in the two previous types of inflammation. Neutrophils are present, but macrophages, lymphocytes, plasma cells, and giant cells are quite numerous and may be present in greater numbers than the neutrophils. Immature connective tissue, angioblasts, and proliferating epithelium are present in the area in amounts in excess of that which is needed for healing and repair.

## CHRONIC INFLAMMATION

Chronic inflammation is caused by an irritant of low intensity. The tissues are not stimulated sufficiently to bring about the destruction and removal of the irritant. The course of the disease is extremely long and may never terminate. The cardinal signs of inflammation are present but they are not as obvious as in the preceding types of inflammation, and there may be some difficulty in demonstrating all of them. Circulatory and cellular alterations have occurred but they are not as intense. All of the cells of the exudate may be demonstrated in the area, but the macrophage predominates. There is an abundance of mature connective tissue and collagen, proliferating angioblasts are numerous, and there is an overproduction of epithelium. As a word of caution, do not confuse chronic inflammation with a scar. The presence of mature connective tissue in an area without the cardinal signs of inflammation is termed a scar or a healed lesion. All too frequently fibrosis of the kidney is diagnosed as nephritis when actually no inflammation is present.

Table 11.2 is presented to aid the student in remembering the most important characteristics of acute and chronic inflammation.

### Inflammation Classified According to Degenerative and Necrotic Changes

It must always be remembered that all of the changes studied previously under disturbances in circulation and cell metabolism and in necrosis are all observed in inflammation. The same etiologic agents which produced inflammation also produce these other tissue alterations. It must also be remembered that following tissue injury, as occurs in coagulative necrosis, the injured tissue must be removed, the altered body cells are now foreign to the animal, and to remove the dead tissue inflammation must occur.

At times the degenerative and necrotic alterations associated with inflammation are so prominent they can be conveniently used to describe the lesion. This is very desirable because by using these terms a

TABLE 11.2

COMPARISON OF ACUTE AND CHRONIC INFLAMMATION

| Acute Inflammation | Chronic Inflammation |
| --- | --- |
| 1. Short duration (comparative). | 1. Long duration (comparative). |
| 2. Irritant is severe. | 2. Irritant of low intensity. |
| 3. Marked vascular changes. | 3. Vascular changes are less prominent. |
| 4. Profuse exudation (as a rule). | 4. Exudation scanty (as a rule). |
| 5. Soft consistency (as a rule). | 5. Consistency more firm (as a rule). |
| 6. No, or only slight, proliferation of connective tissue, blood vessels, and epithelium. | 6. Proliferation of connective tissue, blood vessels, and epithelium. |

more accurate description of the alteration can be obtained. The term caseous lymphadenitis is used to describe an inflammation of the lymph nodes in which the most characteristic alteration is caseous necrosis. The term gangrenous metritis is used to describe an inflammation of the uterus in which gangrene is the most prominent alteration. Caseous tuberculosis indicates there is tuberculous inflammation in which the most characteristic alteration is caseous necrosis. Necrotic enteritis indicates necrosis is the principal alteration (Fig. 11.10).

### Inflammation Classified According to Sequelae

It is often convenient to use the various disturbances of growth to describe the reaction of tissue to the presence of an irritant. Some of the terminology which may be used is as follows:

**Hyperplastic inflammation** is a term used to describe an inflammation which is characterized by excessive hyperplasia. Paratuberculosis in the bovine is a disease in which there is a hyperplasia of the macrophages in the tunica propria of the large intestine. Hyperplastic dermatitis may occur when irritating chemicals are applied to the skin and there is an excessive production of epithelium.

**Hypertrophic inflammation** is a term used to describe the increased size of cells in an area of inflammation. This is observed in fowl pox when the affected cells in the epidermis become excessively large as the result of stimulation by the virus.

**Fibrous, or fibrosing, inflammation** is a term used to describe an excessive proliferation of white fibrous connective tissue in the area. This is observed in the pericardium in traumatic pericarditis or in the wounds of the legs of horses which have been prevented from healing by traumatic injury.

**Atrophic inflammation** is a term used to describe an inflammation which results in extensive atrophy of tissue. This is observed in the nose of swine when atrophy of the turbinates results from chronic rhinitis.

**An obliterative, or obliterating, inflammation** is present when certain structures (glomeruli of the kidney, blood vessels, and bronchi) in an area are destroyed by the inflammation.

**Adhesive inflammation** is a term used to describe the adherence of one structure to another by white fibrous connective tissue bands produced when the exudate was organized. This is frequently observed when the visceral and parietal pleura adhere to each other following pneumonia or when the epicardium and pericardium become adherent to each other as the result of traumatic pericarditis.

### The Terminology of Inflammation

To describe an inflammatory process in the most accurate manner and to use the fewest words possible, a definite arrangement of terms must be used. The series of terms used is terminated with **itis**, which signifies inflammation is present. Table 11.3 shows the proper order of descriptive terms when used to describe an inflammatory reaction in an animal.

Using this system of terminology, a descriptive series of words such as acute diffuse serofibrinous peritonitis signifies there is an acute inflammation of the entire peritoneum which is characterized by a serofibrinous exudate. The term chronic diffuse suppurative interstitial hepatitis indicates there is a chronic inflammation of the interstitial tissue of the liver in which the characteristic exudate is pus.

If a combination of descriptive terms is desired to better describe the exudate, the least important constituent of the exudate is placed first. For example, the term serofibrinous would indicate a serous fluid as well as fibrin in the exudate but that the fibrin was the predominant constituent. The term mucopurulent would indicate there was more pus in the exudate than mucin.

### Chronic Inflammation

Because so many diseases are characterized by chronic inflammation and because the tissue alterations are so great, additional discussion of this subject is needed.

**Definition.** Chronic inflammation is present when the irritant persists for a long period of time and the body responds by producing excessive amounts of connective tissue, reticuloendothelial tissue, and epithelium in the area.

**Etiology.** Chronic inflammation is found in any area where an irritant persists for a long period of time. Any tissue of the

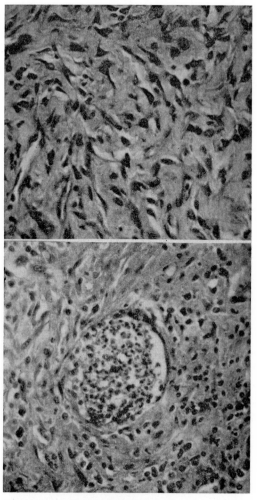

Fig. 11.9 — Chronic inflammation in the region of a castration wound in a barrow. Note fibroblasts and lymphocytes. (Howarth, Jour. A.V.M.A.)

TABLE 11.3
TERMINOLOGY OF INFLAMMATION

| Time | Extent | Exudate | Position in Organ | Anatomy | Suffix |
|------|--------|---------|-------------------|---------|--------|
| Acute | focal | serous | parenchymatous | pancreat- | itis |
| Chronic | diffuse | fibrinous | interstitial | hepat- | itis |
| | | suppurative | | periton- | itis |
| | | hemorrhagic | | dermat- | itis |
| | | gangrenous | | metr- | itis |

body may be involved; however, certain structures such as the skin, the mucous membrane of the gastrointestinal tract, and the lymph nodes are most frequently involved. Whatever the etiologic agent is, it must be remembered that the tissue must alter itself in some permanent manner to the presence of the irritant.

A chronic inflammation may follow an acute inflammation. The body is unable to remove and destroy the irritant, and because of its persistence in the body, healing does not occur and the constant irritation causes the proliferation of excessive amounts of tissue in the area. A chronic inflammation may follow an acute inflammation, even when the irritant has been destroyed, when there has been extensive destruction of tissue. The necrotic tissue in the area must be removed. Since its removal may require a considerable period of time and since the dead tissue is a foreign

body, chronic inflammation is the result.

Chronic inflammation also occurs when the irritant is of such low intensity that it fails to stimulate the body defenses sufficiently to cause its destruction and removal. This is observed in diseases such as tuberculosis, actinomycosis, actinobacillosis, paratuberculosis, blastomycosis, and coccidioidomycosis.

Chronic inflammation occurs when rather inert, difficult to phagocytose material (splinters, thorns, suture material, dead metazoa, and necrotic tissue) enters the tissue (Fig. 11.11). Because of the difficulty in accomplishing phagocytosis, these objects persist in the tissues for a long period of time, and a proliferative type of reaction occurs in the vicinity of them.

Plant poisons (senecio, astragalus, and crotalaria) may irritate the tissue over a long period of time, resulting in the deposition of connective tissue in the liver.

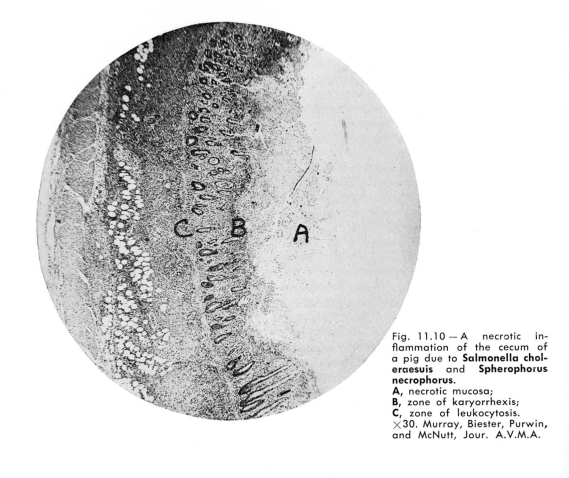

Fig. 11.10 — A necrotic inflammation of the cecum of a pig due to **Salmonella choleraesuis** and **Spherophorus necrophorus.**
**A,** necrotic mucosa;
**B,** zone of karyorrhexis;
**C,** zone of leukocytosis.
×30. Murray, Biester, Purwin, and McNutt, Jour. A.V.M.A.

Constant traumatic irritation to a wound will prevent or delay healing, and a chronic inflammation is the result. This is frequently observed when wounds, such as wire cuts, are present in the vicinity of an articulation. Each time the limb is moved the wound gapes and healing is prevented. Wounds in the legs of animals may be constantly traumatized by the bedding or vegetation so that healing is prevented.

**Macroscopic appearance.** The cardinal signs of inflammation are present but are not as easily distinguished as in acute inflammation, and some of them may not be observed unless careful examination is made. The exudate flowing from the area or accumulating in the tissue or body cavities is of the same type as is observed in acute inflammation but it is usually scanty in amount in contrast to the profuse outpouring of exudate observed in acute inflammation. There is a deposition of connective tissue and epithelium in the area in amounts in excess of what is needed for healing. The presence of connective tissue and excessive amounts of epithelium is the criterion used to determine whether chronic inflammation is present.

Connective tissue appears as a pearly white opalescent substance throughout the area or as a zone between the normal body tissues and the area of inflammation. When large amounts of it are present there may be great distortion of the region, and a leg, for example, may be several times its normal diameter. When the proliferating connective tissue protrudes above the surface of the wound it is frequently called proud flesh.

The presence of proliferating epithelium is best observed in the periphery of the lesion where the hyperplastic epithelium produces a raised border around the ulcer. In the liver the proliferating bile ducts can often be observed as cords or strands of glandular tissue, sometimes containing bile, extending through the excessive interlobular connective tissue.

Additional evidence which indicates the chronicity of the lesion is observed when the exudate, as it is discharged, pours over the skin of the animal. Whenever skin is macerated with exudate for a period of time the defense mechanism of the skin is impaired, bacteria in the exudate invade the skin, and inflammation occurs as a zone of dermatitis along the path taken by the exudate as it flows from the wound; along this path alopecia occurs. As the condition progresses, fibrosis of the skin occurs, the skin becomes thicker than normal, its ability to produce melanin is impaired, and hypopigmentation of the area is observed.

**Microscopic appearance.** The circulatory and cellular alterations characteristic of inflammation are present in the tissue, but they are not as prominent as in acute inflammation. Macrophages, giant cells, lymphocytes, and plasma cells predominate in the cellular exudate. Neutrophils may be abundant if bacteria are present. The area of inflammation is surrounded by a zone of proliferating white fibrous connective tissue and capillaries (Fig. 11.9). That portion of the connective tissue-capillary zone nearest to the irritant is extremely cellular. The predominating cells are the macrophages and the lymphocytes. Neutrophils may or may not be present, depending upon whether bacteria are present or not. This zone, because the cells in the exudate are coming from it and because it appears as if it were producing pus, is called the pyogenic membrane. The epithelial structures in the area show hyperplasia, hypertrophy, and may show metaplasia. The hypertrophy and hyperplasia of the epithelium of the skin or mucous membrane cause a raised border around the ulcer, and cords of proliferating epithelium may penetrate deep into the underlying tissue. Bile ducts may become exceedingly numerous and very prominent in the interstitial tissue of the liver when senecio or astragalus toxins damage the liver over a long period of time. Metaplasia is frequently observed in many organs. For example, the cuboidal epithelium of the bronchi may change to a stratified squamous type when parasites are present. In the lymph nodes the reticuloendothelial tissue of the medullary

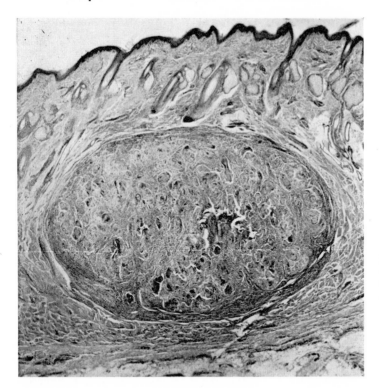

Fig. 11.11 — A chronic inflammatory process caused by foreign bodies (plant barbs) in the skin of a cow. ×25. (Runnells, Jour. A.V.M.A.)

portion in particular undergoes proliferation, and since reticuloendothelial tissue has a multipotent potential, metaplasia occurs, connective tissue is formed, and fibrosis of the lymph nodes is the result. In all of these alterations the criterion used to decide whether chronic inflammation is present or not is the proliferation and deposition of excessive amounts of connective tissue, reticuloendothelial tissue, and epithelium.

**Significance and result.** The presence of chronic inflammation indicates healing has been delayed for several weeks, months, or years. The deposition of tissue in the area (especially white fibrous connective tissue) is a permanent change and is an alteration which will persist for the remainder of the life of the animal. The hyperplastic and hypertrophic epithelial structures tend to diminish in amount, and in time the excessive epithelium may have disappeared. The proliferation of connective tissue and epithelium may re-

sult in considerable distortion and disfiguration of the part. The proliferating epithelium may cause obstruction of the lumen of ducts or organs, and retention of secretion or excretion may result. As white fibrous connective tissue shrinks and contracts with age the part may be unable to function, motility of organs may be hampered or prevented, or in the case of the limb it may become impossible to flex an articulation.

CHRONIC SYSTEMIC DISEASES

There are a number of chronic systemic diseases which affect many species of animals. They are all very similar as far as tissue reaction is concerned. All of them are examples of chronic inflammation, and their diagnosis is based on the demonstration of the etiologic agent rather than on any characteristic tissue alteration.

**Tuberculosis** is a chronic infectious disease of animals and man caused by *My-*

*cobacterium tuberculosis* and characterized by the formation of small nodules (tubercles) which have a tendency to undergo caseous necrosis in some species of animals.

The infection enters the body most frequently by way of the alimentary tract or the respiratory system. However, the infection may enter through any of the natural body openings or through wounds in the skin. Ordinarily the disease develops only after repeated infection. When the infection occurs only occasionally and is slight, local tubercles form which have a tendency to heal. Tubercles develop in this manner: After entering the body the organisms localize in the tissue. Their presence results in tissue necrosis and an infiltration with neutrophils. Later, macrophages begin to appear (Fig. 11.12) and these may form giant cells. The last to appear are the lymphocytes. This young tubercle then consists of a few neutrophils, macrophages, giant cells, and lymphocytes. Subsequently, it becomes encapsulated by fibroblasts which upon their maturity become adult connective tissue cells. As a result of the toxic action of the organism, central caseous necrosis occurs (Fig. 11.13). In the absence of the

proteolytic ferment elaborated by the neutrophils, the caseous necrotic tissue remains in a solid form.

There are some variations in the structure of tubercles in the different species of animals. In cattle, sheep, and goats, for instance, there is an abundant groundwork of connective tissue which usually contains giant cells but comparatively few lymphocytes. These tubercles usually become calcified (Fig. 9.11). They frequently coalesce to form large, firm, tumor-like masses (Fig. 11.14). In the horse the tubercle is more cellular and less fibrous and as a result undergoes central softening readily. Calcification is rare. In swine, lymphocytes are abundant and the connective tissue ground substance scarce when the infection is due to the bovine strain of the organism. Caseation occurs readily and calcification less frequently than in cattle. When the infection in swine is due to the avian strain of the mycobacterium, caseation and calcification are much less than when the infection is due to the bovine strain. The lesions, especially in the spleen, have a neoplastic-like appearance and can be mistaken for tumors. In dogs the tubercles undergo liquefactive necrosis. In fowls the cellular elements and

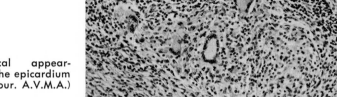

Fig. 11.12 — Histological appearance of a tubercle in the epicardium of a cow. (Feldman, Jour. A.V.M.A.)

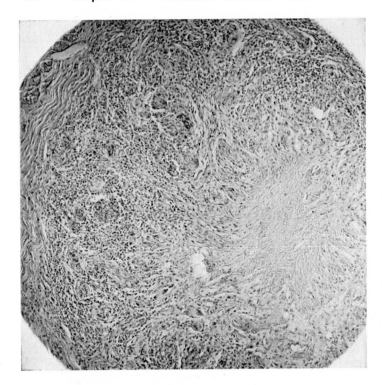

Fig. 11.13 — Portion of a tubercle in the subcutis of a cow. Note center of caseous necrosis at right center, next on the left a zone of macrophages with some attempt at giant-cell formation, then lymphocytes, and finally, at extreme left, the capsule. ×100. (Runnells, J o u r . A.V.M.A.)

connective tissue groundwork are deficient, but caseation without calcification is extensive.

In all animals, secondary, or daughter, tubercles may arise from the primary, or mother, tubercle. Phagocytes that have engulfed bacteria and have migrated to the tissue surrounding the primary tubercle, but which have failed to destroy the bacteria, are responsible for this spread of the infection. In this way the infection may

be carried to neighboring lymphatics and lymph nodes and eventually to the blood stream. If an organ becomes showered with bacteria by the blood stream, **miliary tuberculosis** develops. Wherever the organisms can establish themselves, new tubercles develop. Each new tubercle may become the source of other tubercles until **generalized tuberculosis** may result. Dissemination of the organisms in the body also occurs by means of infected secretions

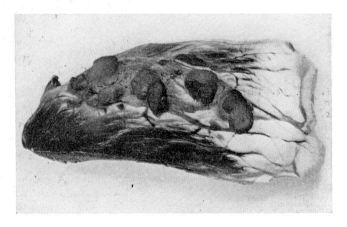

Fig. 11.14 — Multiple nodules on epicardium caused by **Mycobacterium tuberculosis** in a cow. (Feldman, Jour. A.V.M.A.)

and excretions. If the organisms in a tubercle die, healing occurs. Lesions of tuberculosis often furnish favorable sites for the localization of pyogenic microorganisms. The latter may so alter the specific inflammatory process that the original characteristic structure of the tubercle disappears. The period of incubation is variable but practically always of relatively long duration.

At first the tubercle is a barely visible, gray, transparent nodule. By the time it becomes plainly visible to the naked eye, it becomes yellow (cattle, sheep, goats, swine) or white (horses, carnivora) as the result of central caseous necrosis. Tubercles fuse and form large masses which are dry and cheesy (caseous lesions) and, if calcification is present, gritty (caseocalcareous lesions). On the serous surfaces tubercles appear as firm, dense, pearl-like nodules (pearl disease) having cheesy foci in their interior. They may have broad bases or be pedunculated They may attach to one another and produce bunches of tubercles resembling grapes or heads of cauliflower.

Lesions of tuberculosis may be found in all tissues of the body. The most frequent locations for food-producing animals are: **Cattle.** Lungs and pleura, liver, spleen, and peritoneum. Regional lymph nodes are frequently involved, the skin and bones occasionally. Feldman designates the skin

lesions found in otherwise "no-lesion reactors" as tuberculoid in nature. **Swine.** Several years ago, among 120,000 hogs affected with tuberculosis which were examined during a consecutive period by Federal Bureau of Animal Industry inspectors, the location and frequency of occurrence of the lesions were as follows: 93.3 per cent had lesions in the cervical, 27.2 per cent in the bronchial, 21.6 per cent in the portal, and 18.1 per cent in the mesenteric lymph nodes, 9.2 per cent in the liver, 7 per cent in the lungs, 3.8 per cent in the spleen (nodules located within the organ, not on the capsule as in cattle), and in the kidney only 3 cases of the 120,000. Federal meat inspectors in the Midwest state that these figures probably do not correspond with their present-day findings. They indicate that the percentage of lesions found in all the places listed above in swine apparently have decreased, except in the mesenteric lymph nodes where there has been a marked increase (Fig. 11.15).

**Fowls.** In the liver, spleen, intestine, lungs, bones, joints, peritoneum, kidneys, and ovaries. Lymph nodes are not numerous in fowls and consequently are unimportant as a site of lesions. The most frequent locations of lesions in **dogs** and **cats** are the lungs and pleura, and intestine, either with or without involvement of the regional lymph nodes.

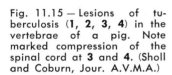

Fig. 11.15 — Lesions of tuberculosis (**1, 2, 3, 4**) in the vertebrae of a pig. Note marked compression of the spinal cord at **3** and **4**. (Sholl and Coburn, Jour. A.V.M.A.)

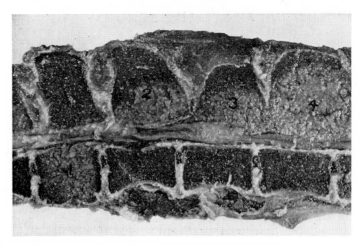

Actinomycosis and actinobacillosis are chronic infectious diseases of cattle and swine, rarely of dogs, characterized by the formation of connective tissue, tumor-like enlargements, or by chronic suppurative processes. The causative organisms are *Actinomyces bovis* and *Actinobacillus lignieresi*. Often combined with these organisms are *Corynebacterium pyogenes* and *Staphylococcus aureus*.

Clinically, and for the most part, pathologically, actinomycosis and actinobacillosis are quite similar. Their greatest dissimilarity is in their favored sites of localization. *Actinomyces bovis* usually involves osseous tissues of cattle (Fig. 11.16) and the udder of sows. *Actinobacillus lignieresi* affects soft tissues. In the head of cattle, then, the disease of the

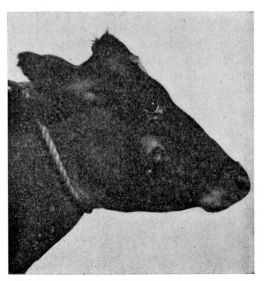

Fig. 11.16 — Actinomycosis of the maxilla. (Veterinary Practitioners' Bulletin, Iowa State University).

mandible and maxilla is actinomycosis, and of the tongue and soft tissues, actinobacillosis.

In bone *Actinomyces bovis* is often accompanied by *Corynebacterium pyogenes*. In the mammary gland of sows *Staphylococcus aureus* is a concomitant infection. In the udder of cows the staphylococcus alone often produces actinomycotic-like lesions.

One of the most probable avenues of entrance for the actinomyces into the bones of the jaws of cattle is between and around the teeth. Slivers of wood, and plant thorns, barbs, and awns may furnish the vehicle for the entrance of infection into the alveolus.

In sows, wounds in the mammary gland afford a place of entry. The most frequent place of entrance for the actinobacillus into the tongue is in the so-called food cavity just anterior to the dorsal eminence (Fig. 17.6). Here, too, sharp foreign bodies usually introduce the infection. The tonsils of cattle and also of swine become infected in a similar manner. Occasionally the actinobacillus reaches the lungs in dust-laden air.

Wherever the microorganisms locate, they act as an irritant, giving rise to a chronic inflammatory reaction. Macrophages, lymphocytes, and fibroblasts predominate in the exudate. The colonies of either the actinomyces or the actinobacilli are arranged in the form of rosettes. The macrophages are adjacent to the rosettes and may completely surround them by forming a huge foreign-body giant cell. In some instances the rosettes float in pus. At times a pyogenic organism may be present with the actinobacillus or actinomyces. Beyond the zone of neutrophils or of the macrophages there is a mixture of lymphocytes and macrophages, and outside this zone, a capsule of fibroblasts.

With continued growth of the organisms and the consequent proliferation of connective tissue and infiltration with leukocytes, large tumor-like masses form, which are either soft or hard, depending upon whether leukocytes or connective tissue predominates in their make-up. Upon incision, soft ones are homogenous, grayish white, and of lymph node consistency. Large ones are fibrous and reddish gray. Pale gray or yellow foci are often present in the ground substance. They feel like grains of sand and are called **sulfur granules**. In old cases, fistulous tracts permeate the tumor-like masses and drain to the surface. In the tongue the nodules may project above the surface, later rupture, and form ulcers. Production of bone lesions occurs in two ways: by the destruction of the bone lamellae on the one hand, and by the formation of new bone substance by the periosteum on the other. Occasionally the infection appears secondarily in other parts of the body as a result of metastasis.

The nature of the characteristic lesions is described under pathogenesis. The most frequent locations of lesions in the principal animals involved are: in cattle in the maxilla, mandible, tongue, pharynx, skin and subcutis of the head and neck, lymph nodes of the head, and rarely in other parts of the body. "**Lumpy jaw**" is practically always actinomycosis; "**wooden tongue**" is actinobacillosis. In swine the lesions appear in the tonsils, mammary glands, and castration wounds. As stated above, the mammary gland lesions of sows are almost always due to *Actinomyces bovis* and *Staphylococcus aureus*.

Federal meat inspectors occasionally encounter isolated cases of nodular lesions in the spleens of swine in which no lesions are observed in other organs or tissues. These nodules simulate those of tuberculosis, but Creech has evidence that they are actinomycotic. In view of recent researches these lesions may be caused by actinobacillus. In sheep in the Rocky Mountain area the lesions are confined to the lips and face.

The granules present in the pus in actinomycosis and actinobacillosis are gray or yellowish gray in color. They are usually soft, but those in actinomycosis have a tendency to undergo calcification more often than those of actinobacillosis. Consequently, the name "sulfur granules" probably is more often descriptive of the consistency of the colonies of the actinomyces than the actinobacillus. The granules of the actinomyces are larger than those of the actinobacillus. In stained preparations the centers of the granules of actinomyces contain Gram-positive filaments which radiate from a central point (ray-fungus pattern) and terminate in a fringed border of club-shaped processes. When the surface of a granule is viewed through a microscope, it has the appearance of a raspberry or mulberry (Fig. 11.17). A granule in actinobacillosis has the same outer appearance, but the center contains numerous, tiny, short bacilli which are Gram-negative.

**Staphylococcosis** is a chronic infectious disease, frequently a wound infection, mostly of horses, but occasionally of other animals, caused by *Staphylococcus aureus* and characterized by the formation of local tumor-like proliferations and occasionally by the occurrence of metastasis to the internal organs.

The infection usually enters through wounds in the skin. The two most common sites of infection are the shoulder region and the spermatic cord of geldings. The tumor-like enlargement of the cord is designated scirrhous cord. The microorganism constitutes a tissue irritant with an action similar to that of *Actinomyces bovis* and *Actinobacillus lignieresi*. Lymphocytes and macrophages migrate to and surround the colonies of organisms. Some of the macrophages form giant cells. Pus forms early around the colonies of bacteria. A thick capsule of connective tissue surrounds the abscess, forming a tumor-like mass. Occasionally, metastasis to the internal organs occurs. Primary internal staphylococcosis is rare.

**Macroscopic appearance.** The histological changes in general resemble those of actinomycosis and actinobacillosis. Characteristic colonies of *Staphylococcus aureus* are located in the pus in the center of the tumor-like formations (Fig. 11.18). The size of the colonies is about the same as that of *Actinomyces bovis* and *Actinobacillus lignieresi*. The contour of each subdivision of a colony is sharply defined and may be smooth or "clubbed." Clubs of this nature have also been observed in infections produced by a number of different fungi, bacteria, parasites, and even by certain inorganic substances. With hematoxylin and eosin staining, the substance of the colony has a finely stippled

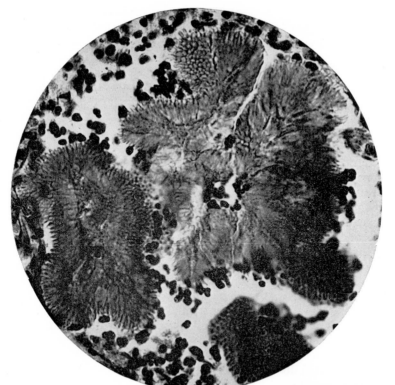

Fig. 11.17 — Sulfur granules, typical of either **Actinomyces bovis** or **Actinobacillus lignieresi,** in a subcutaneous lesion in the cervical region of a cow. ×600. (Department of Veterinary Pathology, Iowa State University.)

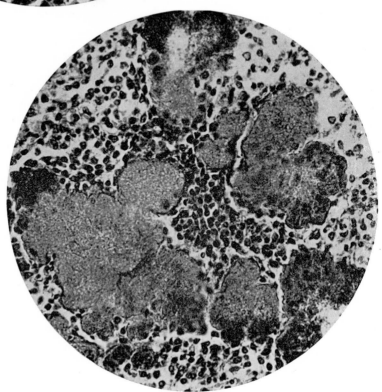

Fig. 11.18 — Colonies of **Staphylococcus aureus** in a lesion in the peritoneal cavity of a dog. ×410. (Section by W. H. Feldman; photo by E. A. Benbrook.)

appearance — the stippling consisting of myriads of tiny blue dots, the staphylococci. When the Gram stain is used, Gram-positive cocci can be demonstrated.

**Blastomycosis.** The majority of the reported cases are in dogs. The lungs have been the favored location for lesions. Because of the diffuse distribution of the lesions, the lungs have a grayish-white and pinkish mottled appearance (Fig. 11.19). At first the pulmonary lesions resemble miliary tuberculosis. The centers of the nodules are soft, not caseated, and not calcified. Later, as the nodules enlarge, they coalesce, and large areas of the lung become consolidated. At this stage the resemblance to tuberculosis is not so close because suppuration supervenes, leading to purulent bronchitis and empyema. Cutaneous abscesses are considered of secondary importance in the frequency of occurrence.

Microscopically, the lesions have the character of a chronic suppurative inflammation. The center of a nodule is composed of necrotic tissue infiltrated with neutrophils. Next comes a zone of macrophages and lymphocytes with an occasional foreign-body giant cell, some of which contain blastomyces (Fig. 11.20). Free parasites are also present. They are thick-walled, spherical, budding, yeastlike parasites easily recognized in sections. At the periphery of a nodule there is usually an attempt at encapsulation.

**Coccidioidomycosis.** This is generally a cattle disease in the Southwest, but an increasing number of canine cases are being reported. The parasites look like the oocysts of coccidia. These refractile, doubly contoured, non-budding, spherical fungi localize in the lungs and contiguous lymph nodes (Fig. 15.2) and cause a chronic inflammation. Alterations are less

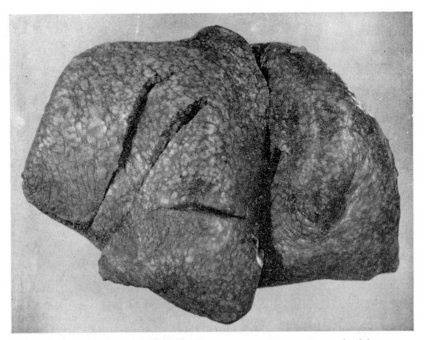

Fig. 11.19 — Pulmonary blastomycosis in a dog. The specimen had been preserved in fixing fluid prior to photographing; it therefore has a liver-like appearance. (Wayne H. Riser.)

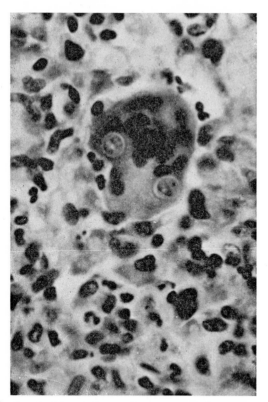

Fig. 11.20 — A foreign-body giant cell containing two blastomyces. (Wayne H. Riser.)

zone of liquefactive necrosis. This results in the microorganism floating in fluid in a tiny cystlike cavity. There are no giant cells, but numerous large macrophages with a foamy appearance phagocytize the cryptococci. Because of the constant attempt to wall off the lesions, the mammary gland becomes extensively fibrosed. The cut surface of such a gland is said to resemble that of a mammary gland carcinoma. The cut surface of an affected supramammary lymph node (Fig. 11.21) is reported to look like a node in leukemia or non-caseous bovine tuberculosis. The parasites sometimes metastasize to the lungs. They are not difficult to recognize in the lesions.

**Histoplasmosis.** Of the fungous diseases, histoplasmosis has become the most prevalent. Although it has been reported in cows and cats, its prevalence in dogs is prominent in the lungs than in the bronchial and mediastinal nodes. The lesions caused by coccidioides, like those caused by blastomyces, have a tendency to suppurate. The parasites are free or contained within giant cells in the lesions and are easy to detect.

**Cryptococcosis.** The number of reports of cryptococcosis (torulosis) which are appearing in the veterinary literature is either an indication that this fungous infection is on the increase or that it has been unrecognized in the past. The yeastlike microorganism, with a thick capsule and budding forms, apparently enters the body in most cases by way of the upper respiratory tract and localizes in the lung, where it produces pneumonia. In the mammary gland of cows the fungus has been introduced by careless use of teat tubes. The disease has been reported in dogs and cats.

Surrounding this parasite there is a

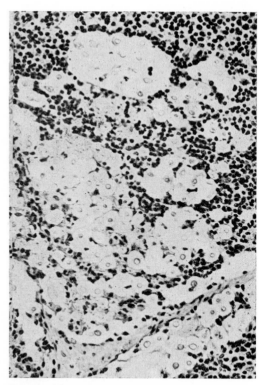

Fig. 11.21 — Cryptococcosis, supramammary lymph node. Showing dilated sinus containing many organisms, with invasion and destruction of cortical lymphoid tissue. (Innes, Seibold, and Arentzen, Amer. Jour. Vet. Res.)

most important because it presents a serious problem to dog breeders. Due to its slow development and its unrecognized existence among dogs in a kennel, the disease may become widespread before the owner is aware of its presence. In fact, individuals who have purchased pups may be the first to become aware that it is present.

Histoplasmata probably enter the digestive and respiratory tracts and metastasize by the blood and lymph to other organs since lesions may be found in almost any part of the body. Favored sites for primary localization are the liver and spleen. As a result of the chronic inflammation in these organs, hepatomegaly and splenomegaly become prominent lesions. To a lesser degree, the lungs (Fig. 11.22) and intestines become involved. Obviously when organs are infected, their lymph nodes soon become infected also. Histoplasmata which become free in the peritoneal cavity cause minute disseminated nodules that have much of the appearance of the "pearl disease" form of tuberculosis or of multiple tumor transplants on the serosa, especially on the omentum.

The histopathology of the lesions is that of a chronic inflammation with coagulative and caseous necrosis. Macrophages are extremely numerous and become engorged with the organisms, which are much smaller than the other fungi so far considered in this section. Giant cells may also be present and contain histoplasmata (Fig. 11.23). The central portion of each parasite takes the hematoxylin stain, but the thick capsule remains unstained. They are sometimes difficult to detect.

**Nocardiosis.** *Nocardia asteroides*, the cause of this infection in animals, is an inhabitant of the soil like the other fungi of this group. It enters the body through the skin or natural body openings. If it enters by way of the skin, the lesions may be entirely cutaneous, but if entrance is through the natural body openings, the

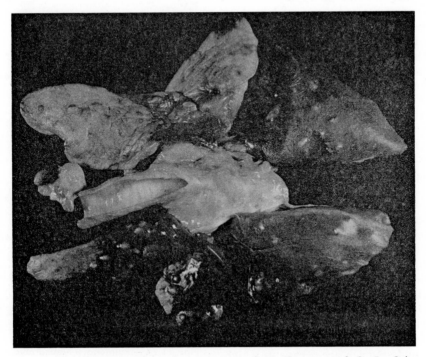

Fig. 11.22 — Pulmonary histoplasmosis in a dog. (Courtesy of C. R. Cole, Department of Veterinary Pathology, Ohio State University.)

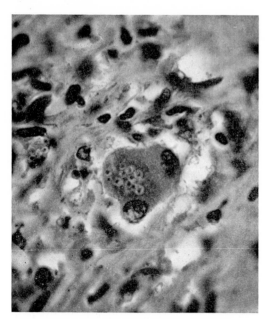

Fig. 11.23 — A foreign-body giant cell containing several histoplasmata. Free parasites also present. (Courtesy of C. R. Cole, Department of Veterinary Pathology, Ohio State University.)

infection may become generalized. About 30 per cent of the cases reported in dogs and cats have been cutaneous. In generalized infections the organs in either or both major body cavities become the seat of the lesions. In them the lesions have a tuberculosis-like appearance. Histologically, the nodules produced by this fungus present the appearance of a chronic suppurative inflammation. Granules (colonies of nocardia) present in the nodules resemble those of actinomycosis but have an acidophilic sheath instead of a fringe of clubs. The organism is partially Gram-positive.

**Mucormycosis** is a rather rare infection of animals caused by the mold *Mucor corymbifer*. The lesions caused by it have been found, for the most part, at necropsies of dogs when death was due to some other cause. They have also been discovered during routine post-mortem examination of cattle and hogs at abattoirs. Lymph nodes, lungs, bovine fetal membranes, kidneys, and stomach are organs in which they have been reported. By proper stain-

ing, the mold in the form of coarse, branching, nonseptate hyphae may be seen (Fig. 11.24). Portions of the fungus may be present in giant cells.

## HEALING

**Definition.** Healing is the process whereby the body destroys and removes the irritant and returns the part to as near a normal functional state as possible.

As has already been stated, healing is a process which is closely associated with inflammation. In fact, the two processes are so closely allied that one cannot be described without mentioning the other. In the foregoing discussion it has been noted that the two occur simultaneously.

In the process of healing, destroyed cells may be replaced by cells of their own kind — **repair by regeneration.** Much more often healing is accomplished by replacing

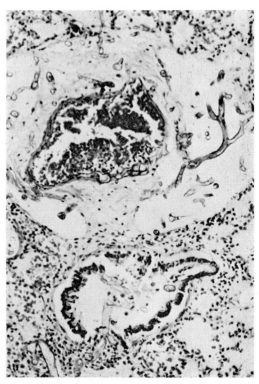

Fig. 11.24 — Pulmonary mucormycosis in the human. Typical branching mycelium. (Courtesy of Roger D. Baker, M. D.)

highly specialized cells with the less specialized connective tissue cells — **repair by substitution.** When cells with highly developed functions are destroyed, neighboring or distant cells of the same type may increase in number or size. This compensatory increase is also a part of repair.

### Repair by Regeneration

Healing is universal in nature and occurs in all animal and vegetable life. The lower an animal or plant is in its respective kingdom the more complete is the process of healing. The ability to achieve healing depends upon four factors.

1. **The genera, family, order, or phylum** to which the species belongs. When an earthworm is severed, a new part is formed quite quickly. If a salamander loses its tail, a new one is formed. In our larger domestic animals healing is often imperfect or incomplete. If a cow loses her tail, a new one will not form. Yet in young goats a remarkable regeneration of the rumen and reticulum after their complete removal has been reported. The power of regeneration is lost as an animal becomes more highly specialized and attains the more advanced evolutionary forms.

2. **The tissue or organ involved.** The more highly specialized a tissue or organ is the more difficult it is to bring about healing. Very limited regeneration of the brain and spinal cord occurs. When portions of glands such as the liver and kidneys are destroyed, regeneration of the highly specialized epithelial cells takes place to a limited extent. Regeneration of the less specialized epithelium of the ducts occurs more extensively. These less specialized cells are also more resistant to injury than the gland epithelium. They often survive when the same irritant completely destroys the gland epithelium. The surviving duct cells give rise to new cells. The new cells form like buds along the remaining ducts and then push out toward the areas of the gland parenchyma which are still alive. The newly formed ducts connect these areas of parenchyma with the surviving ducts and may produce gland epithelium. Sometimes, as in hepatic cirrhosis, when there is extensive destruction of the liver parenchyma followed by regeneration of the epithelium, the new cells are not able to arrange themselves into typical lobules but simply form nodules of liver cells lacking the usual pattern of cords of cells radiating from a central vein. When there has been slight destruction of the kidney, regeneration of the specialized secreting cells which remain may occur, but if all the cells of a convoluted tubule die the tubule collapses and disappears — there is no regeneration. Healthy remaining tubules undergo compensatory hypertrophy. After pregnancy the mammary gland displays regeneration of the acini from the lactiferous ducts.

Bone and cartilage regenerate from the periosteum and endosteum. In addition, cartilage can originate from perichondrium. Regeneration of cartilage, though, is slow because it is so avascular. Blood vessels take origin from pre-existing capillaries. The blood-forming tissues have exceptional capacity of regeneration which perhaps should simply be considered an increase in physiological activity.

3. **The degree of specialization of the cell.** Generally speaking, the more highly specialized a cell is in its function the less ability it has to regenerate. For instance, the highly specialized nerve cells cannot regenerate at all. When they die they are replaced in part by glia cells which regenerate readily. Peripheral nerves have a remarkable power of regeneration, but nerve fibers regenerate only if the body of the cell remains alive. Skeletal muscle cells have only a very limited ability to regenerate, and smooth and cardiac muscle cells do not regenerate at all. When the latter two disappear their places are filled by young connective tissue cells which lead all the cells in power of regeneration. In fact, they are always present to fill spaces caused by the death of cells of all tissues except those which form blood. When muscle cells of all kinds are required to compensate in function for destroyed cells, they hypertrophy.

The lining epithelial cells regenerate quickly — those on the surface from the basal layer of the epidermis and those lining tubular-shaped organs from remnants of the crypts (Fig. 11.25). Intact portions of accessory skin structures give origin to new structures of the same kind.

4. **The age of the animal.** The younger the animal the more rapid and complete is healing. In an older animal healing is slow and may not occur at all. A broken leg in a young animal heals quickly and often perfectly, while in an aged animal healing is delayed or the bone may never heal.

### Repair by Substitution

The essential feature of repair of this type is a replacement of the destroyed tissue with new tissue consisting principally of proliferating fibroblasts and angioblasts, the latter taking the form of young capillaries. The underlying changes of repair by substitution are the same regardless of whether they occur in a closed wound, an open wound, a deep-seated inflammation, an abscess, an ulcer, a surface exudate, a blood clot, a thrombus, or an infarct. The loss of substance is replaced with this new tissue and the part is restored to a semblance of its normal

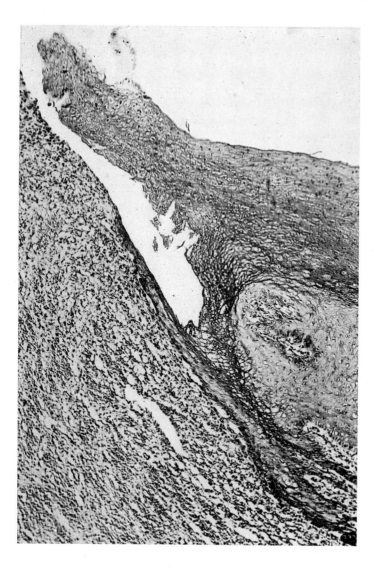

Fig. 11.25 — Regeneration of the epithelium in a gastric ulcer of a horse. In center of illustration note thin layer of epithelium growing out upon the granulation tissue at lower left.  ×100.  (Schlotthauer, Jour. A.V.M.A.)

shape. Without repair by substitution excessive disfiguration of an animal would occur following an injury.

## Cause of Healing

No one knows why healing occurs. Why does it start? Once initiated, what causes it to stop? When cells begin to grow why do they not keep on growing at the same accelerated rate? There are a number of theories which have been advanced but none of them entirely explain the situation. Until the cause of life is known — those properties of a cell which make it alive — the cause of healing will probably never be explained.

One of the first theories advanced was the **tissue tension theory of Ribbert,** often known as the conception of replacement fibrosis. In this theory it was thought that when cells in an area were destroyed the restraining pressure on the surrounding cells was removed. When this pressure was no longer present the cells began to proliferate and continued to proliferate until the former restraining pressure was reattained. This may explain some of the growth of cells but certainly does not explain all of the process of repair.

Later the **trephone theory of Carrel** was advanced. Carrel showed that lymphocytes, macrophages, and degenerating cells produced a growth-stimulating substance which he called a trephone. If all debris, blood, and bacteria were removed from a wound, healing was delayed and might not occur. If a chemical irritant or a few bacteria were added to the wound, healing began to occur almost immediately. This can be demonstrated in the healing of bone in the dog. If one femur is broken by a severe blow and this is followed by approximation of the ends of the bones and immobilization of the limb, healing occurs quickly and quite perfectly. If the other femur is exposed by sterile surgical technics and a portion of the bone removed with a minimum of trauma, using a rapidly oscillating surgical saw, the bones approximated, all of the blood and debris removed, and the limb immobilized, healing is greatly delayed, may not occur

for as long as 6 to 9 months, and even then healing may be imperfect. The excellent surgical manipulation in the area did not produce sufficient trauma to stimulate the tissues and produce enough exudate to bring about the production of the trephone of Carrel.

Later, another theory known as the **sulfydryl (SH) group of Hammet** was proposed. This compound appears to be the wound hormone previously described by Carrel. Sulfydryl is abundant in areas of rapid tissue growth. Mitosis appears to be associated with the re-arrangement of the sulfur in the molecules of the nucleus of the cell. When sulfydryl is applied to a wound the rate of healing and mitosis is greatly increased. It has also been observed that a number of ammonia compounds, such as urea and allantoin, have the power to stimulate healing. These compounds are placed in wounds to enhance the rate of healing. The realization that urea is beneficial in wound healing is nothing new. For centuries combat troops have placed human urine in wounds to aid healing. In the more backward areas of the world today it is common practice to place the urine of both man and animals in wounds to facilitate healing.

## Healing of a Closed Wound

The healing of a clean, closed wound is best illustrated by describing the changes which take place in an ovariectomy incision in a dog. This reparative process is called **healing by primary union** or **healing by first intention.** The skin, fascia, abdominal muscles, and peritoneum are cut and later pulled together by sutures. There is little loss of tissue and very slight bleeding. Infection is absent or nearly so. Soon a mild inflammatory reaction occurs. Repair begins in about 12 hours by a proliferation of young connective tissue cells (fibroblasts) and young blood-vascular endothelial cells (angioblasts). The fibroblasts literally sew the two cut surfaces together so that by the fourth day the sutures can be removed. At first the fibroblasts are simply large oval or fusiform cells consisting almost entirely of a nucleus. Soon, however, they begin to form collagen fibers and in the process become gradually smaller and separated from one another by the product of their own labor. As a result they appear to be nestled down in wavy bundles of fibers. The bundles of fibers become more and more prominent while the nuclei become less and less so. The fibers shrink, and the resultant tissue is called a **scar** or **cicatrix**. While the fibroblasts are busy proliferating, the angioblasts form buds along or at the ends of capillaries. The buds become hollow, blood is pushed into them, the angioblasts continue to proliferate and push out in columns among the fibroblasts. Thus new capillaries are formed. These connect with others to form a network. The new tissue is very vascular at first because young, rapidly growing cells need an abundance of nourishment. This vascularity imparts a red color to the new tissue. As the tissue matures its nutritive requirements are less and it becomes almost avascular. For this reason it looks white.

While these things are going on within the tissue, the surface epithelium regenerates from the margin of the wound and covers it by about the fourth day. By the end of three weeks the damage has been completely repaired. Viewed from the surface, the scar is white and puckered. It contains no hair follicles or sweat glands.

### Healing of an Open Wound

Healing of an open wound is known as **healing by second intention** or **healing by granulation**.

When an open wound occurs, the injury has caused an excessive loss of tissue and the gap must be filled in by substitution. The tissues in the area are not able to regenerate sufficiently to accomplish complete healing. Following injury an inflammatory reaction begins to appear in a very short period of time. Hemorrhage into the area has occurred and space normally occupied by the tissue has been filled in with a clotted mass of blood. In response to the irritant, neutrophils, the first line of cellular defense, begin to appear. Since bacteria, brought there by the etiologic agent or introduced by contamination from the surrounding skin or mucous membrane, are present in the wound, large numbers of neutrophils appear in the area in an attempt to control the bacterial invasion. By the second day pus should be visible in the wound. Its presence is desirable because it indicates the first line of cellular defense is present. In 48 to 72 hours macrophages and lymphocytes begin to appear in the area of inflammation and eventually may become more numerous than the neutrophils.

If, on the second day, the mass of blood filling the gap in the tissue is carefully removed, it will be noted that the surface of the wound is covered with tiny red granules, or buds, resembling the nap of red velvet and giving that surface a granular appearance. Because of its granular appearance this newly formed tissue is called **granulation tissue**. These little red buds consist of proliferating capillaries which are protruding into the exudate. If the surface of the wound is brushed, even lightly, these fragile capillaries rupture and hemorrhage occurs. Along with the budding capillaries there is a proliferation of fibroblasts, and soon the surface of the wound is covered with a layer of fibroblasts and proliferating capillaries. The fibrin in the gap aids the fibroblasts and capillaries by functioning as a scaffold on which they may grow and penetrate into the mass of exudate within the wound. The capillaries must invade the exudate if healing is to be accomplished, because the leukocytes in the area require nutrients. A leukocyte is not able to leave its blood supply for any great distance, otherwise the nutrient required by the phagocyte is no longer present. This mass of proliferating fibroblasts and capillaries continues to grow until the gap produced by the injury has been completely filled in. This newly formed tissue does not contain nerves and therefore is without sensation. Bits of it may be removed by surgical methods and the animal will have no sensation of pain.

The fibroblasts and the capillaries in

granulation tissue have a definite arrange-ment to each other. The capillaries grow at right angles to the base of the wound and continue to grow and protrude to-wards the surface of the wound. At the surface of the wound the fibroblasts are arranged parallel with the proliferating capillaries. They exert their tension at right angles to the wound surface so as to hold the tissues together and prevent them from bulging to the exterior. In the depths of the wound, fibroblasts are arranged at right angles to the capillaries and parallel with the wound surface (Fig. 11.26). In this position they exert their traction in a lateral direction, thereby pulling the tis-sues together in an attempt to reduce the gap to a minimum. This definite arrange-ment of fibroblasts to capillaries is ex-ceedingly important to recognize because it aids the pathologist in differentiating a fibrosarcoma from excessive granulation tissue. In a fibrosarcoma the fibroblasts and capillaries do not grow in an orderly manner and do not show this organiza-tion into a pattern designed to prevent ex-cessive distortion of tissue.

Since the neutrophils which appear in the wound are brought there by the capil-laries in the granulation tissue and since it appears as if the pus were originating from this membrane composed of fibro-blasts and capillaries, it has been called the pyogenic membrane. Because this membrane of granulation tissue contains an abundance of leukocytes (neutrophils, macrophages, and lymphocytes) it is ex-ceedingly resistant to bacterial invasion. The clinician is extremely pleased when granulation tissue appears in a wound because then he knows the danger of sep-ticemia is greatly reduced since bacteria will probably not be able to invade this cellular barrier. A few bacteria such as the spirochete, which are not ordinarily phagocytosed, are able to penetrate this membrane. Colloidal substances (tetanus toxin) if placed upon this membrane of granulation tissue will not penetrate it be-cause the colloidal particles are too large to pass through the semipermeable mem-brane represented by the endothelial wall of the capillaries. Crystalloids (morphine sulfate, strychnine sulfate, and mercuric chloride) will be absorbed by the pyogenic membrane.

While the process of granulation has been going on in the wound, the epi-thelium in the periphery of the wound has been undergoing hypertrophy and hyper-plasia. Newly formed epithelial cells can be observed on the second or third day. The epithelium regenerates and grows over the newly formed granulation tissue

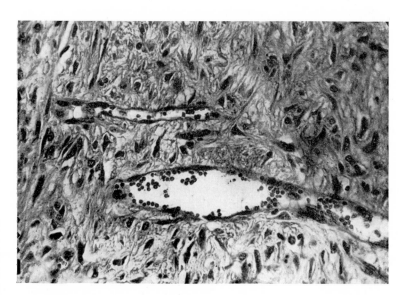

Fig. 11.26 — Granulation tissue with newly formed capillaries developing to-ward the surface and fi-broblasts parallel to the surface. (F. W. Schofield.)

but does not completely cover the wound until all of the exudate in the area has been removed. If the newly formed epithelium is cuboidal or columnar, it regenerates almost perfectly, but if it is squamous epithelium, regeneration may be imperfect. The more highly specialized skin structures (sweat glands, sebaceous glands, hair and hair follicles, and melanoblasts) do not regenerate. Therefore the new skin is not pigmented, and if hair does return to the area it likewise is not pigmented. The skin has a white, pearly-white, or bluish-white color. The bluish-white color is noted in the epithelium which is currently regenerating. With age the stratified squamous epithelium loses the bluish tinge and becomes white. The skin is dry because it lacks sweat and sebaceous glands and tends to have a shiny parchment-like appearance.

If the exudate cannot be removed from the wound, the area will not be covered with epithelium and an ulcer is the result. The presence of exudate, however, stimulates the surrounding epithelium, and excessive hyperplasia of the epithelium occurs. Long finger-like projections of epithelium extend into the underlying tissue at the edge of the wound. These protruding strands of epithelium are exceedingly dangerous because a disturbance in growth has been initiated, and quite frequently these invading strands of cells become neoplastic. At the same time, around the periphery of the ulcer the epithelium protrudes above the surrounding surface, giving the ulcer a crater-like appearance.

If the irritant persists in the area or if movement and trauma to the part prevent healing, granulation tissue continues to be produced and finally may be in excess of that which is needed to restore the normal conformity of the part. When it is present in abnormally large amounts it is called **excessive granulation tissue,** or proud flesh.

When the exudate is removed from the wound and the area becomes covered with epithelium, devascularization of the area occurs. Since inflammation in the area is no longer needed, there is no longer any necessity for the abundant blood supply.

As the capillaries gradually disappear from the granulation tissue a relatively avascular scar remains in the area. As the collagen of the connective tissue shrinks and contracts with age there may be considerable puckering, distortion, and disfiguration in the area. Sometimes a scar continues to grow even after the area has been covered with epithelium. This mass of proliferating connective tissue is known as a **keloid.** Although keloids are not true tumors, they may be confused with them since they continue to grow, and when surgical removal is attempted they may return.

In the healing of an open wound the primary object of the clinician is to cover the area with epithelium. To do this he may aid the healing process in several ways: (1) By aiding the body in overcoming the bacteria. This can be accomplished by cleansing the wound and by the use of antibiotics. (2) By debridement of the wound. Debridement is the removal of a thin layer of tissue, which will include the debris, necrotic tissue, and many of the contaminating bacteria, from the surface of the wound. This is of particular value when wounds have been contaminated with dirt, and is exceedingly important if malignant edema is to be prevented because clostridia flourish in necrotic tissue. (3) By using sterile maggots to remove the necrotic tissue. In the use of sterile maggots the larvae must be of a type which will feed only on dead tissue and will not invade the living flesh. Maggots are of great value since they may be used around tendons where surgical removal of the necrotic tissue is difficult. The maggots can crawl into the inaccessible areas and remove the necrotic tissue. Eventually, when the necrotic tissue has been removed, the maggots fall out of the wound. Urea compounds excreted by the maggots are quite valuable in stimulating wound healing. (4) By surgical removal of the entire ulcer when healing is slow or has not been accomplished. By removing the entire ulcer a new defense line must be formed, and the surgical removal stimulates the tissue. With a fresh start and a little more irritation the body defenses may be able to achieve healing. (5) By preventing additional trauma to the area. Bandages may be used to prevent the entrance of dirt and bacteria. A limb may be immobilized to restrict its movement, thus preventing excessive gaping of the wound as the animal moves about. (6) By placing skin grafts on the surface of the wound to hasten the spread of epithelium over the surface of the wound. This is of particular value in wounds having large surfaces; otherwise all of the epithelial regeneration will have to come from the periphery of the wound.

### Healing of an Abscess

The healing of an abscess is accomplished in the same manner as is the healing of an open wound. In the periphery of the lesion, capillaries and fibroblasts begin to grow into the mass of exudate, and soon a pyogenic membrane is formed. This granulation tissue is exceedingly desirable because it is quite impervious to the passage of bacteria, and thus the danger of septicemia is greatly reduced. If the abscess is small, the mass of exudate is eventually organized and the area will be converted into scar tissue. If the abscess is large, it may be impossible to remove all of the exudate. Then the granulation tissue forms a dense connective tissue wall around the mass of exudate, thus confining it and preventing it from escaping into the surrounding tissue (Fig. 11.27). With time the bacteria within the abscess are destroyed by the leukocytes. Later, especially if dehydration of the area occurs, calcification of the exudate takes place. This is particularly common in the bovine and the rabbit. If the abscess points to the exterior and the pus is discharged, healing is facilitated because the growing mass of granulation tissue pushes the mass of exudate ahead of it through the sinus tract to the exterior. When this occurs healing is more rapid and complete. Therefore the clinician can aid the defenses of the body by incising and draining abscesses. With age the collagen in the connective tissue begins to contract and shrink and this re-

sults in distortion of the part. If the abscess has occurred in the dermis of the skin or in the subcutaneous connective tissue, the shrinking of the scar results in a pit or depression in the skin. In the larger abscesses, in which complete organization of the exudate has not taken place, this shrinkage of the scar tissue results in considerable pressure upon the exudate, and when the abscess is incised the content will spurt.

### Healing of a Serous Surface

Healing of a serous surface occurs by organization of the exudate. The fibrinous exudate which is deposited upon the serosa is replaced by granulation tissue. Later the granulation tissue is transformed into cicatricial tissue, and the surface is said to have undergone fibrosis. Islands of intact mesothelial cells, or these cells at the margin of the inflamed area, regenerate and cover the fibrosed area. Sometimes two adjacent involved serous surfaces, the parietal and visceral surfaces, for instance, become adherent by strands of the newly formed tissue. These strands constitute **adhesions** and consist of bands of collagenous fibers which eventually become covered with mesothelium.

Adhesions between the parietal and visceral serous surfaces or between two visceral surfaces may break down, leaving fibrous tags on the two surfaces. This is especially the case when there is considerable movement of the organ whose serous surface is covered with the adhesions. Along the borders of the lungs such broken adhesions may have the appearance of a fibrous fringe on the pleura.

Fibrous bands uniting the synovial membranes of a joint either restrict the movements of the joint or completely immobilize it. This condition is called fibrous **ankylosis**.

### Healing of Bone

Bone is not as easily injured as tissue composed of masses of highly specialized cells having little intercellular substance. In postnatal life the source of new bone is not from the adult bone cells but from the specialized bone-forming cells, the osteo-blasts, which are found in the periosteum and endosteum, and are also formed from the capillary endothelium.

Under favorable conditions, that is, when the portions of broken bones are not too widely separated, when they are held immobile, and in the absence of infection, healing of bone occurs in the following manner:

Between the broken ends of the bone,

hemorrhage occurs immediately after the fracture. Fibroblasts, angioblasts, and osteoblasts from the periosteum, the endosteum, and the haversian canals begin to proliferate on the fourth or fifth day and form a vascular connective tissue not unlike the granulation tissue which appears in the reparative process in other parts of the body. The essential difference is that it contains osteoblasts which as yet have not begun to function. In a few days,

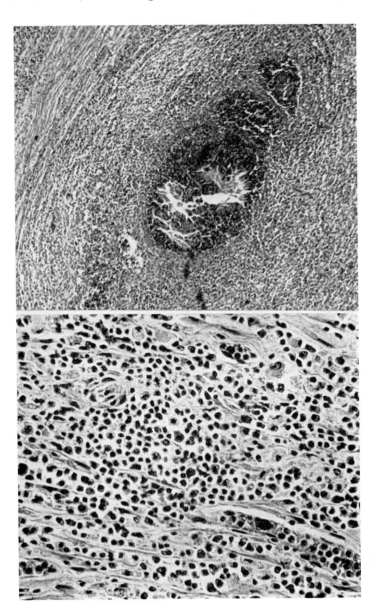

Fig. 11.27 — S m a l l chronic abscess of the brain of a hog due to **Brucella suis. Above,** note inflammatory cellular infiltration around the suppurating focus. ×70. **Below,** note inflammatory zone surrounding an abscess similar to the one above but larger. ×325. (Creech, Jour. A.V.M.A.)

however, they begin to align themselves around elongated strands of the newly formed connective tissue and to secrete a calcareous material which impregnates the bundles of collagenous fibers. The result is that a very irregular latticework of bone matrix is in the process of formation. The original strand of collagenous fibers serves as the core around which successive layers of bone matrix are formed, leaving some of the old osteoblasts (now osteocytes) incorporated in the bone matrix. In the early stages of the matrix formation, before calcium and phosphorus are deposited, the tissue is designated **osteoid,** but as soon as it is mineralized the designation is changed to **osseous tissue.**

The design of the bone matrix is like a very irregular latticework of anastomosing strands rather than of a regular pattern. The strands are designated **trabeculae.** Their thickness is variable. Between the trabeculae the newly formed connective tissue constitutes marrow. At this point a remodeling process begins by which the **spongy (cancellous) bone** becomes converted into **compact bone.**

The new bone at the site of the fracture, in its early stages of formation, that is, when it consists mostly of osteoid tissue, is designated a **soft callus.** In its later stages, when the osteoid tissue becomes true bone (osseous tissue), the name is changed from soft callus to **hard callus.**

The hard callus is prominent in three places: (1) outside of the bone around the fracture, (2) between the broken ends, and (3) inside, in the marrow cavity. At first the hard callus appears to be in excess of the amount actually necessary for the union of the broken bone. As time goes on, however, the excess newly formed bone on the outside around the fracture and that in the marrow cavity is absorbed. That part between the broken ends remains. When healing has been delayed, cartilage may appear between the broken ends of the bone. Later, endochondral ossification may occur.

As time goes on and the fractured bone is gradually brought back into use, the new bone is modified and adapted to withstand the stress and strain placed upon it. This is accomplished by a remodeling of the haversian systems.

There are a number of factors which interfere with the healing of bone: (1) Excessive movement between the ends of the broken bones causes repeated fractures of the newly formed osteoid tissue. Instead of bone a mass of connective tissue eventually appears in the area between the broken ends of the bone. Since the connective tissue lacks rigidity, movement is possible in this area and it becomes known as a **false joint.** (2) If the broken ends of the bone are too widely separated, or if muscle, fat, or fascia is present between the broken ends of the bone, it may be impossible for the growing osteoid tissue to unite the ends of the bone, and then restoration of the continuity of the bone is prevented. (3) Bacteria may be introduced into the site of injury when a compound fracture has occurred. The presence of bacteria causes an acute suppurative inflammation which destroys the newly formed osteoid tissue and prevents union of the broken bone. (4) When excessive splintering of the bone has occurred, as is often observed in the horse, fragments of bone may be without a blood supply and undergo necrosis. A mass of necrotic bone at the site of a fracture is known as a **sequester.** The necrotic tissue causes an inflammatory reaction which interferes with the healing of bone. (5) Old animals experience great difficulty in healing bone because their regenerative powers are lost. (6) The healing of bone is delayed or is prevented when chronic debilitating diseases or malnutrition is present. The tissue lacks the nutrient, vitality, and regenerative ability necessary for healing.

## FEVER

There is an increased metabolic rate (local or general) with all inflammatory diseases. If the increased metabolic rate is local, it may not be great enough to raise the temperature of the entire body. When the area of inflammation is large or when a septicemia exists, there is an increased rate of metabolic activity throughout the entire individual, and as a result the body temperature rises. Heat is normally lost by radiation, conduction, evaporation of sweat, pulmonary ventilation, and by the loss of heat when secretory (milk) or excretory (urine) substances are eliminated from the body. In very severe inflammatory processes the usual methods of heat dissipation are not able to keep up with the increased metabolic rate. At other times it would appear that the heat-regulating center, located in the hypothalamus, is injured by the disease and proper control of heat regulation is lost.

The entire process is called fever. It is characterized by a disturbance in metabolism, by an elevation of the body temperature (pyrexia), and by various functional disturbances such as increased pulse rate, anorexia, nausea, vomiting, constipation, increased thirst, scanty urine, and dehydration.

**Etiology.** Among the most common causes of fever are bacteria (*Erysipelothrix rhusiopathiae* and *Bacillus anthracis*). Protozoa such as some of the trypanosomes, anaplasmata, and piroplasmata also produce fever. The toxic products of some bacteria are additional etiologic agents. This can be demonstrated by injecting rabbits with sterile filtrates of cultures of *Pseudomonas aeruginosa*.

Products of cellular disintegration resulting from bacterial injury have an effect similar to the microbial toxins. Menkin has investigated two such pyrogenic factors in inflammatory exudate — **pyrexin** in alkaline exudate and **pyrogenic factor** in acid exudate. Both are biochemic substances derived from injured cells. Their exact chemical natures are still unknown. Menkin believes that they may have a direct effect on the heat-regulating centers in the hypothalamic region of the brain. Foreign proteins of various kinds injected subcutaneously or intravenously may have fever-producing characteristics.

Just how these various agencies operate to produce fever is not known. It is believed, however, that they disturb both the heat-producing and the heat-eliminating mechanisms but affect the latter more than the former. When only the work of the heat-producing apparatus is increased, fever does not occur even though the amount of heat generated is enormous. For instance, when a healthy track or draft horse, or a racing or hunting dog, is exercised violently, there is only a very temporary and insignificant increase in body temperature, although heat production may be increased 200 to 300 per cent. On the other hand, during fever when heat production is increased only 20 to 40 per cent, the body temperature may rise as much as 5 or 6 degrees. The trouble, then, apparently can be attributed to faulty heat dissipation.

**Chemical changes in fever.** Many chemical changes occur in the body during fever. First of all, there is increased oxidation of proteins, carbohydrates, and fats. The disturbance in protein metabolism is reflected in an increased output of urea. Acetonuria signifies the incomplete oxidation of fats, whereas their increased destruction results in acidosis which is compensated for in part by increased respiration which eliminates the excessive amount of carbon dioxide. There is a retention of sodium chloride, probably as a result of diminished urine formation and decreased vaporization from the skin. The loss of appetite may lead to vitamin deficiency.

**Functions of fever.** The function of fever is now believed to be defensive and protective in character. It has been shown that a moderate elevation of temperature improves phagocytosis by increasing the activity of leukocytes and by making them more permeable.

Not only does fever increase the activity of leukocytes but it also stimulates the bone marrow to produce more of them — chiefly neutrophils. They are reported to increase 200 to 300 per cent — principally the nonsegmented forms. Furthermore, the distribution of the leukocytes is accelerated because in fever blood velocity is reported to increase up to 400 per cent. Fever also aids in antibody production. Agglutinins and bacteriolysins appear to be formed more quickly and in larger amounts. The pyrexia may inhibit the growth of some kinds of bacteria, but heat sufficient for this is probably injurious to the cells of parenchymatous organs. The cloudy swelling and fatty degeneration of the parenchymal cells of the liver, kidneys, and heart may be attributed to this and also to the effect of toxins produced by the bacteria which cause the inflammation, and to toxic substances derived from disintegrating cells. Fever, however, has been shown to diminish the potency of these toxins. Of particular interest from the standpoint of clinical diagnosis is the fever which occurs in tuberculous, paratuberculous, and glanderous animals when small doses of a killed suspension of the respective causative organisms are injected subcutaneously into them.

## IMMUNITY

Production of immunity is still another complex response of the body to certain irritants. Special substances are formed by the cells and liberated into the body fluids — substances which aid in the destruction or the neutralization of the particular irritants. It is known that these substances (antibodies) are formed locally in several organs of the body when certain microorganisms cause inflammation in them. A detailed discussion of these substances belongs in the field of immunology. Mention has already been made of their functions in the inflammatory process. Here we need only to emphasize again their importance as co-workers with the phagocytes in the defense of the body against certain irritants.

CHAPTER 12 | # Concretions

Concretions are compact or solidified un-organized masses of material which may or may not originate within the body and which form in the hollow organs, in the secretory and excretory glands and their ducts, and sometimes in the tissues and body cavities. Those originating princi-pally from endogenous material are called **calculi.** They are stonelike bodies whose in-organic composition is chiefly the salts of calcium and phosphorus. They apparently are not due to disturbances in mineral metabolism. Two other types of concre-tions are common among animals. They are formed of either plant fiber or hair, or both, and are located in the gastrointes-tinal tract. Those consisting principally of plant fiber are called **phytoconcretions;** those made up of hair, **piliconcretions.**

## CALCULI

The formation of a calculus depends upon processes which alter the colloidal state of secretion and excretion fluids. In such fluids where the mineral salts exist normally in supersaturation, this state is maintained by the protective action of col-loids. Disturbances in the chemical and physical nature of the latter may reduce or completely remove their protective action and allow the salts to precipitate. It may be that the mere presence of the altered colloid favors the process because it fur-

nishes the nucleus for the adsorption of the salts. At other times the nucleus may be fibrin, mucus, desquamated epithelial cells, and clumps of bacteria. Once the process begins, the proper conditions for its continuance are provided because the resultant precipitated mass furnishes a surface for further adsorption of salts and concentration of coagulated colloids. Further, the calculus is a foreign body and as such incites an inflammatory reaction, the products of which contribute to the organic framework of the concrement. The alternate deposition of precipitated salts and coagulated colloids results in the rather artistic and uniform stratification which is a characteristic of many calculi.

In the laboratory, stones similar to uri-nary calculi have been produced by treat-ing blood plasma of the cow with calcium oxalate to prevent coagulation and then adding calcium chlorate, calcium phos-phate, and triple phosphate to it. The milky fluid containing fibrinogen then coagulates in a few minutes, and after several days or weeks the fibrinogen-inor-ganic salt mass becomes as hard as stone. When the process is carried out in a rubber sac, pressure favors the formation of the artificial calculus. If the calculus is allowed to remain in water or salt solution, it takes on, by a process of slow shrinkage, a rough superficial surface and an inner structural arrangement which is quite similar to that occurring in natural calculi. By gradual and repeated precipitation of the salts and coagulation of the fibrinogen, the calculus becomes laminated. Calculus formation does not occur when fibrin-free serum is used in the experiment unless other albuminous substances such as paraglobulin, nucleoalbumin, and mucin are added. Even clumps of bacteria can replace the fibrin in artificial calculus formation.

Microscopic concretions called **corpora amylacea** are concentrically laminated bodies occurring frequently in the alveoli of the mammary gland of cows, occasionally in the alveoli of the prostates of dogs, and in the brains of old animals. In sections stained with hematoxylin and eosin they are generally basophilic. In neural tissue they are composed of glycoprotein-like material. Their histogenesis has not been determined. In cats concretion-like calcified bodies occasionally occur at the junction of the cortex and medulla of the adrenals.

## Uroliths

Urinary calculi (uroliths) are formed in the uriniferous tubules, in the renal pelvis, and in the urinary bladder. Small concretions (microconcretions) formed in these places may be carried by the urine into the ureters and urethra.

Vitamin A deficiency appears to be favorable for the formation of uroliths. In vitamin A deficiency the transitional epithelium of the urinary tract may undergo keratinization, a metaplastic change. The exfoliated keratinized cells are believed to form the nuclei of calculi. Such an epithelium probably is more susceptible to infection also. In experiments set up to produce calculi it is necessary to establish a state of subclinical A avitaminosis and keep the animals in this condition for an extended period before calculi form. In field studies in Montana, however, urolithiasis was found to occur as frequently in range cattle which presumably received adequate supplies of vitamin A as it did among cattle on low vitamin A rations. The Montana researchers concluded that a vitamin A deficiency is neither a necessary nor, by itself, a sufficient condition to cause urinary calculi in range steers They suggest, though, that it may be a contributing factor in some cases.

Infection with *Escherichia coli*, micrococci, and streptococci is so common in urinary lithiasis that it is thought infection may be a primary cause of stone formation. In experimental lithiasis, however, all animals having calculi do not show evidence of infection. If infection does intervene, the development of lithiasis seems to be accelerated.

When the diet in vitamin A-deficient animals is regulated so that certain inorganic and organic salts are excreted in large amounts, uroliths composed of those salts are formed. By manipulating the diet in this manner all of the stones which have been described for both alkaline and acid urine have been reproduced. It seems, therefore, that three factors are possibly involved in urolith formation: (1) the deficiency of vitamin A in the diet; (2) the organic and inorganic salt content of the urine; and (3) the presence of infection in the urinary tract.

The first two factors apparently are of greater importance. Infection probably is a sequel to the initial calculus formation but once a stone begins to form, infection may speed up the process. Ammoniacal fermentation of the urine in the bladder by bacteria such as *E. coli* favors the formation of triple phosphate, a frequent constituent of calculi.

Another factor of importance in the causation of uroliths is medication with sulfonamides, especially if their use is not accompanied by the administration of sodium bicarbonate and the free-drinking of water. The procedure just mentioned is employed in therapeutics to prevent the precipitation and accumulation of the acetyl salt of the sulfonamides in the uriniferous tubules, renal pelvis, and ureters.

Still another factor in urinary stone formation may be the salt concentration of the urine. Some observers believe this plays a minor part in the process since calculi may occur in urine of low mineral concentration and not at all in urine of high concentration. On the other hand, other investigators point out that calculi in sheep and cattle, at least, occur most commonly in winter when water consumption is limited and the salt concentration of the urine is increased. Of course, one must remember also that in winter the vitamin A content of feed is much lower than in summer, and the deficiency of this vitamin and not the restricted intake of water may be the important factor.

In Colorado, in the experimental production of uroliths in steers by feeding, it was observed that the lithiasis was associated with shifting the ration from alfalfa hay to a fattening ration rich in concentrates. In this shift the ratio of concentrate to roughage was increased from 4:1 to 8:1. This shift appeared to have an important bearing on the formation of urinary calculi. It resulted in a significant increase in the urinary excretion of mucoproteins, which are known to form the matrix of uroliths. It is possible that the predisposition to urolithiasis can be measured by the amount of mucoproteins excreted in the urine.

Urolithiasis has been associated with the use of hormones or their analogs for stimulating growth in feed-lot lambs. Lambs which are fed diethylstilbestrol or have had implantations of this compound may develop urinary obstruction in several days. The obstruction is due to calculi forming in the bladder and subsequently lodging in the urethral process.

In man renal calculi are sometimes associated with parathyroid hyperactivity. Some pathologists believe that as many as 5 per cent of all kidney stones are due to overactivity of these endocrines. Whether a comparable relationship exists in animals is not known.

The size and shape of urinary calculi vary with the species of animal, place at which they are formed, and their composition. Renal concretions may be microscopic up to 1 or 2 mm. in diameter (Fig. 12.1). They are round and pearl-like. In sections even these tiny bodies are seen to be laminated. Pelvic calculi have a rough, knobby surface and often correspond in shape to the pelvis of the kidney (Fig. 12.2). Occasionally they become as much as 8 cm. in diameter. In the bladder they are either spherical or ovoid bodies. Their surface may be smooth and glistening or nodular like mulberries. Where adjacent surfaces rub upon one another facets develop. Some cystic calculi are laminated, others not. In size they range from that of a grain of sand to that of an indoor baseball (Figs. 12.2, 18.17, and 18.18). In the Iowa State University collection there is one, which was obtained from a mare, that is 17 x 13 x 10 cm. and weighs 2,620 grams.

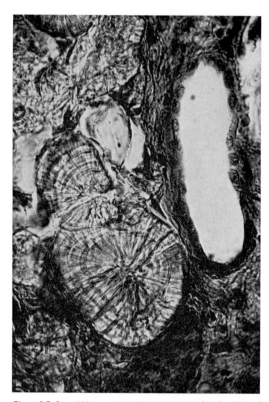

Fig. 12.1 — Microconcretions in renal tubules of a hog. Note lamination of the calculi and the atrophy of the renal epithelium around them. ×440. (Department of Veterinary Pathology, Iowa State University.)

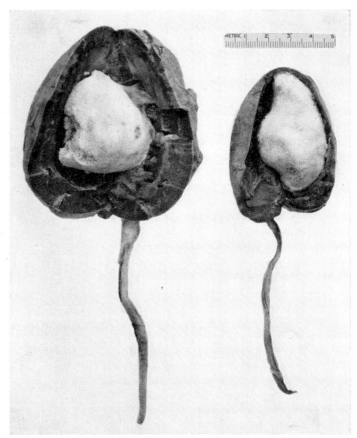

Fig. 12.2 — Bilateral p e l v i c uroliths in a dog. (Schlott-hauer, Jour. A.V.M.A.)

Urinary calculi are as variable in color as in size. Shades of brown, gray, and yellow are common. Occasionally a pure white chalky one is seen. The latter, when obtained from horses, retains the ammoniacal odor of fermented urine for years if kept in a stoppered jar.

Even more varied than their form and color is their chemical composition. Amorphous phosphates, carbonates, and triple phosphates are precipitated in urines of intense alkalinity, whereas the urates, oxalates, and crystalline phosphates and carbonates with occasional exceptions are thrown down from urines of relative neutrality or acidity. The more common calculi in the horse contain calcium carbonate and phosphate, and magnesium carbonate. In ruminants, calcium, magnesium, and aluminum salts of phosphoric acid are components. In Montana range steers all stones from 63 cases of occluding urinary calculi contained protein and silica. In addition, some contained calcium, oxalate, and occasionally magnesium. In swine there may be ammoniomagnesium phosphate, calcium and magnesium carbonate, magnesium phosphate, and oxalates. In carnivores uroliths usually consist of calcium carbonate, phosphate and urate, or sodium and ammonium urate, or ammoniomagnesium phosphate. Phosphatic calculi seem to be the most common and are thought to be secondary to cystitis. They often have a urate center. In England cystine stones, a type which is supposed to be very rare, appear to be quite common. They have smooth, rounded, cream- or buff-colored surfaces and are softer than phosphate calculi.

Urinary calculi are dangerous mainly for two reasons. They may incite an inflammatory reaction and they may occlude the urinary passages. The latter may result in grave conditions such as retention of the urine with its accompanying uremia, dilatation, and rupture of the bladder if the urethra is involved, or conversion of the kidney into a thin-walled sac (hydronephrosis) if the ureter is obstructed.

### Choleliths

Biliary concretions are rather common in man but rare in animals. While exact data on the occurrence of gallstones in many species of domestic mammals is lacking, it is stated in medical literature that in dogs, sheep, cats, and rabbits these calculi rarely form spontaneously but that they do develop in cattle and swine as they do in man. Among a large number of cattle examined in Minnesota and Colorado, the incidence was found to be 0.4 per cent in the former and 1 per cent in the latter state. Data on large numbers of animals of other species are not available for the United States.

More recently the explanation of the relative nonoccurrence of gallstones in the dog and sheep and the occurrence of them in man, cattle, and swine has been sought in the differences in the chemical constituents of bile in these two groups of animals. One of the important differences in the bile is that in the dog and sheep the saponifiable fatty acid fraction is relatively high, whereas in man, cattle, and swine it is low in comparison to the nonsaponifiable cholesterol fraction. The solvent action of the bile is dependent upon the saponifiable or fatty acid fraction. If the fatty acids cannot keep the cholesterol in solution, gallstones seem more likely to form.

Choleliths occur both in the gall bladder and bile ducts. They are often semisolid when fresh but become hard and brittle when air-dried. Some feel slightly fatty and soapy and float on water (cholesterin). In size they vary from 1 mm. to 3 cm. in diameter. Their usual shape is spherical or ovoid. Sometimes they are faceted. Cross sections of them often display concentric layers. Cholesterin, bilirubin, calcium carbonate, and coagulated colloids are their chief constituents. In large ones, foreign bodies such as particles of ingesta and grains of sand, which have been forced up the common bile duct from the duodenum by strong peristalsis, may form the nucleus. More often, however, the nucleus apparently consists of bacteria such as *Escherichia coli*, inflammatory exudate, and desquamated epithelium. It is now believed by some observers that if these elements are present when the hydrogen-ion concentration of bile fluctuates slowly back and forth past its iso-electric point, bile colloids may coagulate and condense around these nuclear elements.

These concretions may occlude the bile passages and cause bile stasis, which becomes apparent by symptoms of obstructive jaundice. Occasionally the stasis may be so great that rupture of the gall bladder results. If the calculi do not cause complete obstruction, their presence may incite a cholecystitis and cholangitis.

### Sialoliths

Concretions in the excretory ducts of the parotid, sublingual, and submaxillary salivary glands are usually hard, chalk-white in color, and cylindrical in shape, with facets at the ends. They are often 25 mm. or more in diameter. In the collection at Iowa State University there is an exceptionally large one which was removed from a horse. It looks much like an Irish Cobbler potato. It is 8 cm. in length and 6.5 cm. in diameter and weighs 368 grams. Chemically, sialoliths are made of calcium carbonate and phosphate or of magnesium, calcium, and sodium carbonate. In horses their nuclei are often pieces of plant fiber or oats. In the Iowa State University collection a pin forms the nucleus of one.

### Pancreoliths

Pancreatic concretions are pure white, grayish white, or yellowish white in color; spherical, cuboidal, or cylindrical in shape; varying in size from a millimeter to a centimeter in diameter; multiple in number and hard in consistency. They consist of calcium carbonate and phosphate, calcium oxalate, and various organic substances such as albumin, lecithin, fatty acids, and cholesterin. Pancreoliths are rare in animals. They have been reported mostly in cattle.

### Enteroliths

Enteroliths are sometimes found in the large intestines of horses and other domestic animals. In horses they are usually formed in the colon but may occasionally be found in the cecum. Their chief constituent is ammonium and magnesium phosphate. It is believed that they develop when wheat and rye bran are fed. Bran contains much magnesium phosphate. This salt is normally dissolved by the gastric juice and then absorbed to a great extent in the intestines. If an excessive amount is fed and especially if, at the same time, there happens to be a condition of chronic catarrhal gastroenteritis with diminished acid secretion, the material reaches the colon in an undissolved form. There it evidently combines with ammonia which is derived from protein decomposition. Even the high protein content of the bran may facilitate this reaction. The resultant triple phosphate crystalizes around such foreign and indigestible substances as pieces of metal and grains of sand. The deposition may be in layers so that the calculi are stratified. It is thought that the reason enteroliths do not form in the small intestines is that peristalsis is too rapid and that the conditions for the bacterial decomposition of protein and, therefore, for the formation of ammonia are not so favorable.

Enteroliths may attain the size of bowling balls. Usually they are spherical or irregular in shape, although there is one in the collection at Iowa State University that has the shape of a horseshoe. Their cut surface is grayish white, yellowish brown, or dark brown.

### Coproliths

In dogs, more rarely in cats, hard- dry, mortar-like, grayish or brownish cylindri-cal masses having a foul odor and containing pieces of undigested bone may be found in the colon and rectum, occasionally in the small intestine. Fecal concretions are observed once in a while in other animals, even in birds. While these are called coproliths they are not calculi in the same sense as those which have already been described. These coproliths are nothing more than hard masses of inspissated feces. They are most often associated with chronic constipation.

### Piliconcretions and Phytoconcretions

When cattle are lousy or mangy and lick their bodies to alleviate itchiness, or when calves penned together suck each other's ears, tails, and scrotums after being fed their milk, they usually swallow rather large amounts of hair. (See Chapter 17.) The muscular contractions of the forestomachs roll the hair up into balls which are designated piliconcretions or simply hair balls. Such balls are occasionally found also in the stomach and colon of

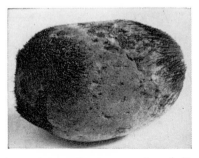

Fig. 12.3 — Piliconcretion (hair ball) from the stomach of a pig. (F. W. Schofield.)

swine (Fig. 12.3). They are usually encased within a smooth and glistening shell-like outer crust which is apparently mucus and other colloidal substances that have adsorbed mineral salts. In the large colon of horses, balls of plant fiber, often oat hulls, which become infiltrated with triple phosphate, occur. These are phytoconcretions, or food balls. Their outer surface is usually velvety. They are slightly spongy and soaked with fluid. They are light in weight, however, when compared to the stonelike concretions. In color they are brown. Their cut surface presents fissures and cavities filled with decomposing food particles and sand.

Even though hair and food concretions may become as large as bowling balls, they apparently cause little or no disturbance unless they occlude the funnel-shaped pyloric orifice of the stomach or the similarly shaped termination of the large colon (horse). Ordinarily they remain free in the stomach and intestines and move backward and forward with the peristaltic waves. Their surfaces are smooth, so they seldom cause trauma. However, when they completely occlude one of the funnel-shaped orifices, impaction and even rupture of the alimentary tube may result. Ruminants in the act of regurgitation, occasionally carry a food ball into the esophagus where it may cause obstruction.

## REFERENCES

Dolkart, R. E., Jones, K. K., and Brown, C. F. G.: 1938. Chemical factors concerned in the formation of gallstones. Arch. Int. Med., 62:618.

Fitch, C. P., Boyd, W. L., and Billings, W. A.: 1919. Pancreatic lithiasis of cattle. Cornell Vet., 9:68.

Graves, E. F.: 1937. Urinary calculi in furbearers. Jour. A.V.M.A., 43:665.

Higgins, C. C.: 1951. Experimental production of urinary calculi. Jour. A.V.M.A., 118:81.

Newsom, I. E.: 1937. Urinary calculi with special reference to cattle and sheep. Jour. A.V.M.A., 45:495.

Swingle, K. F.: 1953. The chemical composition of urinary calculi from range steers. Amer. Jour. Vet. Res., 14:493.

———, and Marsh, H.: 1956. Vitamin A deficiency and urolithiasis in range cattle. Amer. Jour. Vet. Res., 17:415.

Udall, R. H., Deem, A. W., and Maag, D. D.: 1958. Studies on urolithiasis. I. Experimental production associated with feeding steers. Amer. Jour. Vet. Res., 19:825.

———, and Jensen, R.: 1958. Studies on urolithiasis. II. The occurrence in feedlot lambs following implantation of diethylstilbestrol. Jour. A.V.M.A., 130:514.

White, E. G.: 1944. Urinary calculi in the dog with special reference to cystine stones. Jour. Comp. Path. and Therap., 54:16.

Whiting, F., Connell, R., and Forman, S. A.: 1958. Silica urolithiasis in beef cattle. Canad. Jour. Comp. Med., 22:332.

———, Connell, R., and Forman, S. A.: 1959. Silica urolithiasis in beef cattle. Canad. Jour. Comp. Med., 23:157.

CHAPTER 13    **Neoplasms**

**Definition.** A neoplasm (*neo,* new + *plasma,* thing formed) or tumor (swelling) is a growth of new cells that proliferates without control, serves no useful function, and has no orderly arrangement.

Although the word **tumor** means swelling, it does not follow that all swellings are tumors. Many swellings may be tumorlike, e.g., cold abscesses, chronic inflammation, hematocysts (hematomas), parasitic nodules, and masses of intra-abdominal fat necrosis. Most of these processes develop for a time and then subside. Tumors, on the contrary, continue to grow because the newly formed cells in them give rise to generation after generation of their own kind. The name **neoplasm** which is used synonymously for tumor is therefore quite appropriate.

The cells composing a tumor originate from pre-existing cells in the body. The cells usually resemble one another, but they are often quite unlike the normal adult cells from which they spring. Although most tumors have no definite pattern for the arrangement of their cells, some few attempt to reproduce the structure of the tissue from which they originate. The collection of aberrant cells which comprises a tumor is an independent growth and serves no useful purpose in the body. In most cases the cause is unknown.

The study or science of neoplastic growth constitutes **oncology.** In oncology most attention is paid to **cancers,** which are tumors that threaten the life of the individual and are therefore designated **malignant** in contrast to those which do not cause death unless their location interferes with an important body function and are consequently classified as **benign.**

## ETIOLOGY

The entire subject of neoplasia, and particularly the etiology of tumors, has long been associated with mystery, fantasy, and witchcraft. Many old wives' tales are still in existence today concerning the cause, meaning, and cure of cancer. According to some, the black spots that occur in tomatoes will cause tumors if they are eaten. Others maintain that if foods are prepared in certain types of containers (aluminum), a neoplasm will be the result.

The subject of neoplasia is of great concern to the veterinarian because much of his work deals with these new growths. He must be aware of the etiology, surgery, radiology, prognosis, and treatment of the tumors with which he comes in contact.

Each year vast sums of money are spent in an effort to determine the causes of tumors. The etiology of tumors is not known. It is true that much information is available as to the situations associated with the appearance of neoplasms, but exactly why certain cells begin to grow and multiply and eventually destroy the individual has not been determined.

The factors associated with the etiology of neoplasia can be divided into two main groups — the intrinsic factors and the extrinsic factors.

### Intrinsic (Predisposing) Factors

**Heredity.** A tremendous amount of work is being done in the field of genetics and its relation to neoplasia. Families of mice that are unusually susceptible or resistant to tumor growth can be produced. Maude Slye maintained a mouse colony for a number of years and showed that strains of mice could be reared that had an unusually high susceptibility or great resistance to tumors. She concluded tumor susceptibility was associated with a simple Mendelian recessive factor. She also demonstrated that by proper selection the incidence in various organs could be altered at will. Strains of mice could be produced that had a very high incidence of tumors of the skin, others with tumors of the mammary gland, and still others with tumors of the liver. Her work and the work of others has shown that, at least in some species of animals, heredity can be a factor in the appearance of a neoplasm.

It has been well demonstrated in the chicken that, in addition to the hereditary factor, an infectious agent also was associated with a neoplastic disease known as the leukosis complex. If both factors were present, leukosis might appear in a flock. As the result of this observation, the poultry industry has concentrated on selecting families of birds that have considerable resistance to the leukosis virus, and the incidence of leukosis has been greatly reduced.

It is difficult to apply the results of mouse and chicken experiments to the larger domestic animals. The genetic background of the animals becomes quite involved, and the number of generations of animals in the ordinary life span of a scientist is not great enough to allow him to draw conclusions. No one man will live long enough to know the entire answer, and it will require the compilation of the combined data of scientists for several generations before some of the questions can be answered. Even though the rate of reproduction is too slow to evaluate much of the complicated genetic patterns that do exist, there is information available to show that certain families of livestock, particularly on certain farms, have an unusually high incidence of tumors, while other families on neighboring farms will have very few neoplasms. It would appear that a few tumors, such as the lymphosarcoma in cattle and squamous-cell carcinoma of the eye in cattle, affecting our domestic mammals may have an etiology similar to leukosis in the chicken — that is, a tumor-susceptible family and a stimulating infectious agent.

**Cohnheim's theory of cell rests.** Cohnheim visualized that certain cells misplaced in the embryonic development of an individual might serve as a starting point for tumors. Cell rests (embryologically misplaced cells) are frequently found in the adrenal, kidney, testicle, thyroid, parathyroid, and pancreas. There is no doubt that some tumors do arise from these misplaced cells, but the majority of tumors arise from adult cells of the organ in which they are found. Cohnheim made the observation with inadequate data, and although it does apply in some cases (teratomas, dermoid cysts, embryonal nephromas, etc.), it does not explain the origin of most neoplasms.

**Age.** The incidence of tumors as well as the type is very closely associated with the age of the individual. Tumors are much more frequent in older individuals. The age factor suggests that a long incubation period is required for the production of tumors, particularly the carcinoma, and that perhaps multiple stimuli over a period of time are necessary if a disturbance of growth is to take place within a cell. The type of tumor varies somewhat with the age of the individual. Sarcomas are more frequently observed in younger individuals while carcinomas are found in older animals.

**Pigmentation.** Color is a factor in white-skinned animals, particularly in white and gray horses in which melanosarcomas are most common and in Hereford cattle which are subject to squamous-cell carcinoma of the eye (Fig. 13.1).

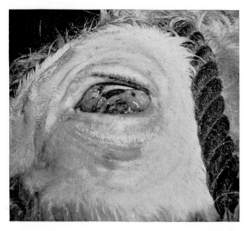

Fig. 13.1 — Squamous-cell carcinoma of the eye of a Hereford cow. (Iowa State University Veterinarian.)

**Sex.** Tumors are just as common in the male as in the female. There is, however, a difference between the male and the female in the incidence in various organs, especially the genital organs.

**Immunity.** Acquired immunity to artificially produced cancer in mice can be demonstrated. A tumor will result when certain tar compounds are applied to the skin of a mouse. If the new growth is removed and the area allowed to heal, further application of tar to this area does not result in the formation of another tumor, indicating a local immunity has been produced. The presence of one tumor appears to give some immunity against the appearance of another tumor. It is also uncommon to find multiple malignant growths of different types or the same type of tumor beginning at different locations in the same organ. Because of this, we search for the primary site of the tumor or the original tumor from which the metastases

were derived. The subject of immunity may become very important with certain types of tumors in the future if suitable immunizing agents can be developed for mass immunization of both human and animal populations.

**Extrinsic Factors**

Experimental evidence and clinical observation indicate an external stimulus is needed to bring about the appearance of a tumor. A neoplasm does not begin in normal tissue. Whenever a tumor appears in tissue, some disturbance of cell growth or metabolism has previously occurred in the area. An ulcer may have been present, hyperplasia or metaplasia may have occurred in the area, or a parasite may have been present in the tissue. In every case some alteration has occurred in the tissue prior to the appearance of the neoplasm.

As far back as the beginning of recorded history it is known that tumors have occurred in both man and animals. The theories as to the genesis of these tumors through the ages have varied, but as knowledge was amassed it became increasingly more obvious that the etiology of tumors was with us at all times. It is apparent that the industrial age has increased the hazards in our environment.

We can no longer say the entire etiology of tumors is unknown. The present question is which of the many stimuli in our modern environment will bring about an alteration in cell metabolism so that these stimulated cells will grow out of control and eventually bring about the death of the individual. With this newer concept, the definition of a tumor is beginning to change, and today it is being considered more as an abnormal mass of tissue, the growth of which exceeds and is uncoordinated with that of the normal tissue and persists in the same excessive manner after cessation of the stimuli which evoked the change.

The modern concepts of tumor etiology came with the observation that certain occupations were associated with an unusually high incidence of tumors in one or several organs. This initiated the search for specific agents that were capable of producing neoplasms. Many physical and chemical agents were found, and the literature was flooded with experimental data concerning the production of tumors with these cancerogenic factors.

In 1951 the Federal Security Agency of the United States Public Health Service published a volume entitled *Survey of Compounds Which Have Been Tested for Carcinogenic Activity.* This work lists 1,329 compounds of which 357 were shown to be capable of producing tumors. The work is out of date, as a tremendous number of new compounds have been introduced to the public since this volume was printed. No doubt many of these new agents are carcinogenic. Many of the compounds listed in this publication come in contract with our animal and human populations every day.

In 1775 Percival Scott pointed out that the chimney sweep had a very high incidence of tumors, particularly carcinoma of the scrotum. The men and boys in this trade were heavily contaminated with soot which contained a carcinogenic agent, and after many years of exposure, cancer developed. The incidence of tumors in these individuals varied with the type of fuel they came in contact with and was highest in the coal firing regions of England.

Later it was found there was a high incidence of skin tumors in those individuals employed in gas-producing plants, tar and pitch plants, and in other industries in which coal by-products were in abundance.

As oil came into use it was observed that men working with petroleum products were also afflicted with tumors. Coal or petroleum in the crude form as removed from nature was apparently not carcinogenic, but the products manufactured from these substances had definite carcinogenic properties. Examination of the various industrial plants and occupations has revealed that hazards are especially likely to exist under the circumstances given in detail by Hueper in his *Occupational Tu-*

*mors and Allied Diseases* (Thomas). In brief, the circumstances are as follows:

1. Operations associated with the production of tar (gas works, coke ovens, petroleum distilleries, and shale and lignite distillation plants).
2. Factories engaged in the fractionation of tar and in the production of pitch and asphalt.
3. Establishments employing tar, pitch, or asphalt for the manufacture of numerous products of diverse types or using materials containing these substances in a pure or mixed form.
   a. Patent fuel workers in the making of briquettes.
   b. The making of weather-proof bricks and foundations in which tar is used.
   c. The manufacture of corkstone and in the users of this material in building trades. (A mixture of cork and pitch used in the making of brick and tile sound-proofing, insulations, and floor tile.)
   d. Manufacture of roofing materials such as tar paper.
   e. Carpenters using creosote shingles, roofing, insulating, and sound-proofing materials.
   f. Road workers of all types who are using tars.
   g. Ship builders who use tars in caulking and preservation.
   h. Sailors and fishermen who use tar on nets, ropes, and cables.
   i. Electrical workers in the production of batteries, cables, and insulated electrical wire.
   j. Cobblers who use pitch-impregnated sewing threads.

Modern life and industry have exposed us to an entirely new series of agents in the form of oils, lubricants, and fuels. Even when the oil industry was in its infancy the users of certain oils were afflicted with neoplasms. One of the industries in which this occurred was in the cotton mills in those individuals operating spinning mules. A very fine grade of Scottish shale oil was used for lubricating these machines that run at a speed of 18,000 revolutions per minute. At this speed a fine mist of oil was thrown off. As the weaver leaned over the machine, the upper portion of his trousers became soiled with oil. The result was a very high incidence of tumors, particularly carcinoma of the scrotum. In England 20 per cent of all scrotal carcinomas occurred in the mule spinners.

In the early days of the oil industry it became apparent that tumors were very common in those individuals operating the presses which expressed oils from the waxes and hard paraffins used in industry. The pure paraffins apparently did not cause tumors but the impurities contained in the expressed oils were very carcinogenic. A tremendous amount of work was done in industry before the paraffin used in milk cartons was accepted. Impurities in the wax were extremely carcinogenic, as evidenced by the high incidence of skin cancer in the men engaged in its manufacture. The dairy industry must ever be on guard against the introduction of a wax that is carcinogenic.

The impure paraffins are used in many trades and industries, and carcinomas are occuring as the result of their use. It is an extreme hazard in the printing industry where impure paraffins are used. Waxed parchments are used in the manufacture of cartridges, explosives, water-proof wrappings, and similar products, and considerable danger is associated with them.

Evidence is rapidly accumulating to the effect that the oils sprayed on water for the control of mosquitoes are carcinogenic. Yet those engaged in mosquito control usually take little precaution, or if they wish to do so, the nature of the work is such that it is difficult for them to prevent contamination with oil.

Those individuals manufacturing or handling creosote-treated products such as railroad ties, fence posts, and telephone posts are exposing themselves to a known carcinogenic agent, and tumors are occurring as the result of this exposure.

Anthracene, a product obtained from tar, is used in the preparation of grease, diesel engine fuel, carbolineum, and wood preservatives. This is a vicious carcinogenic agent, and most of us come in contact with it every day in the form of grease and diesel engine exhaust fumes. Carbolineum is recommended as an agent to be painted on the inside of chicken houses in the control of certain parasites. Wood preservatives containing this very dangerous chemical are being recommended for use around livestock.

The casual observer is apt to think the amount of material livestock would come in contact with in the form of wood preservatives is so slight that no danger could be associated with it. However, only a very slight amount is needed to bring about alterations in the growth of epithelium.

Several years ago it was shown that a chlorinated naphthalene found in oils, greases, fly sprays, and wood preservatives caused epithelial hyperplasia in the bovine. The disease was known as hyperkeratosis. Many thousands of animals were killed by this toxic agent. The substance was so toxic that cattle placed in the center of a barn, the walls of which had been treated with a wood preservative several years previously, would develop the disease. Feed mills and feed mixers greased with this agent would leave enough residue in the feed to kill cattle. Cattle coming in contact with machinery left in the barnyard died from hyperkeratosis. Even the vehicle in some fly sprays contained it, and it was sprayed on the backs of cattle.

This gives a clear insight as to how infinitestimal the amount was that produced an abnormal tissue growth. Hyperkeratosis was studied for more than ten years before the cause was discovered when a similar disease was observed in men working with this material. No doubt many of us as well as our animals were also exposed. It may require ten to thirty years before we know what this agent might have done to us, but any agent capable of bringing about such a tremendous growth of epithelial tissue should certainly be considered capable of causing the appearance of tumors in years to come.

The relation of aniline dyes and aromatic chemicals to carcinogenesis is an interesting one. The aniline dyes, such as butter yellow, scarlet red, Sudan I, II, and III, methyl red, and many others, have long been known to be agents capable of producing tumors of the urinary bladder and liver. A dye used in the leather industry is one of the more carcinogenic agents. We are exposed daily to the coloring matter in our foodstuffs (candies, pastries, fruit juices, fruit preserves, butter, oleo, fresh fruit coloring as found on oranges, and many others). They are found in drugs, cosmetics, and deodorants of various types. They are used in the clothing industry for dyeing cloth. Aniline itself is used as a rubber preservative, as a vulcanizing agent, and as an acid-resistant surfacing agent on laboratory tables. Their use is so widespread that none of us can escape them. The Food and Drug Administration has attempted to enact legislation that will control the use of these substances, but activities of this group have been seriously hampered by influential people who sway legislative opinion even though the use of these products may result in death to their users.

The Mississippi River Valley, the tropical ocean, and parts of Africa and Australia have an extremely high incidence of skin cancer due to the effect of solar radiation. This has been observed in the eyes and adjacent structures of cattle, particularly in the Hereford breed, where it seems to be associated with the amount of protective pigmentation present. Chronic sunburn over a period of months or years results in alterations in skin growth that eventually become neoplastic in nature. The fad of sunburning may bring about the appearance of tumors in areas of the body other than the face and hands of the human. Every time an individual drives through the countryside during the summer he cannot help but shudder when he thinks of the damage that is being done by this modern fad of working in the field without a shirt. No doubt there will be an increase in the incidence of skin tumors of the back in twenty to thirty years as the result of this exposure. Still more serious is the exposure to other carcinogenic agents at the same time. When carcinogenic oils are applied to the skin, their ability to produce a carcinoma is increased if sunlight is applied at the same time. So today we have the farmer exposed excessively to the sun, smeared with oil and grease, and contaminated with various chemicals. Carcinogens are at work and the incidence of skin cancer will increase.

The etiology of squamous-cell carcinoma of the eye of Hereford cattle (Fig. 13.1) has been made a problem for special study in western United States. This tumor quite frequently develops on the lower eyelid, occasionally on the nictitating membrane. It begins as a wartlike growth covered with a waxy exudate. Quite often the wartlike growths become ulcers which become gradually more extensive in summer but often heal in winter. Eventually the ulcers may become converted into malignant epithelial tumors and in the course of two or three months involve the entire lower lid and extend onto the surrounding tissues. Cattle over three years of age are most subject to this tumor. In California 10.5 per cent of the animals in two Hereford herds developed these eye tumors, and 4.4 per cent of the tumors became malignant. The two chief etiologic factors incriminated are lack of pigment in the eyelid and direct exposure to strong sunlight. It is believed by some that a photosensitizing agent in some plant consumed by the animals may also play a part in producing this tumor.

A cutaneous carcinoma is observed in light-colored Australian cattle that have developed photosensitization after eating certain plants. The so-called brand cancer of cattle is observed in range animals where pigmentation is lacking at the site of the brand and the chronic irritation from the sunlight on the nonpigmented skin results in a carcinoma.

Ultraviolet light is one of the more dangerous rays as far as the production of carcinoma of the skin is concerned. The modern fad of using the sun lamp is not without danger. Tumors of the skin are produced in experimental animals with exposures not too dissimilar from those used in acquiring the so-called tan of health.

Radium, radio active materials, and the X-ray will produce tumors when the individual is exposed to excessive radiation. This group of agents is extensively used in the experimental production of tumors. Veterinarians working with any of these radioactive substances should use great caution to prevent overexposure to these rays. The atomic bomb with its resulting atom cloud has attracted a great deal of attention because of its death-dealing power and its cancerogenic potentialities.

There is another cloud that has not received a great deal of publicity and yet it is of more immediate concern to us than the fallout from the atomic bomb, and that is the arsenic cloud. We all are aware that arsenic is a poison, but the general public does not realize the great cancerogenic properties of this element.

Many years ago it was noted that individuals engaged in the mining, smelting, and refining of arsenic-containing ores had an extremely high incidence of tumors, especially neoplasms of the skin. Experimental work has shown that arsenic was responsible for these tumors. Yet, in spite of this work, the general public is not aware of the extreme danger associated with the handling of these substances. Those individuals manufacturing sheep dip frequently become afflicted with cancer. Vineyard workers, orchard workers, and vegetable growers who are constantly in contact with arsenic have an exceptionally high incidence of tumors. Yet, anyone who watches arsenic sprayers and dusters at work cannot help but be impressed by the extreme carelessness with which they handle the material. Apparently they are not aware of the danger.

In Silesia, Africa, and Argentina there are areas that are notorious for an exceptionally high incidence of tumors. Investigation of these regions has revealed the drinking water to be contaminated with arsenic. Improved water supplies have led to a great reduction in the incidence of neoplasms in these areas, indicating the importance of preventing chronic arsenic poisoning.

Domestic animals that feed on vegetation covered with arsenic dust are known to be afflicted with chronic skin disease, tumors, and may even die from arsenic poisoning. Sheep develop tumors of the nasal passages when they graze on vegetation heavily contaminated with arsenic dust from near-by smelters.

Arsenic is recommended for the control of plant and animal parasites. This results in an arsenic cloud that settles on our population far removed from the smelter. The vegetables and fruit we eat, the water we consume, and the air we breath are frequently contaminated with arsenic. Every year more and more cases of chronic arsenic poisoning are appearing in fruit growers, vegetable growers, farmers, the general public, and in our livestock. Isolated cases have been found in which the food and water consumed by individuals in this country contain the amount of arsenic found in the drinking water of Argentina and Silesia where tumors were so prevalent. What is the arsenic cloud doing to the American public and the livestock population? We can only speculate, but probably tumors are resulting from its presence.

The mining of ores other than arsenic, or the refining of these minerals, has also been associated with an exceptionally high incidence of neoplasms. This has been particularly true with nickel, chromate, radium, and cobalt. In some of these mines there has also been a high arsenic content of the ore. The most notorious example of the hazard associated with mining is the pulmonary tumors found in the Schneeberg and Joachimsthal miners in Europe. Over a period of years, 75 to 80 per cent of the miners died with lung cancer, and during the period from 1869 to 1877, 150 out of 650 miners died with lung tumors.

Chronic irritation of various types has

long been known to produce tumors. Burns often result in skin tumors. This is best exemplified with the tumors of the skin of the abdomen in the natives of Kashmir. It is the habit of these natives to carry warming pans containing hot coals under their robes during the winter to keep themselves warm. Frequent burning of the abdominal wall occurs and after a period of years a skin tumor develops at the site.

Tumors of the lips and tongue are common in man as the result of chronic irritation from smoking tobacco. It is the habit of pipe or cigarette smokers to hold the smoking device at one particular place in the mouth and as a result a specific area of the lips and tongue receives considerable irritation from the hot gases and the irritating chemicals in the smoke. It is at this point of excessive irritation that the tumor appears. Considerable evidence indicates the increased incidence of lung tumors in the human may be associated with the excessive use of tobacco.

A high incidence of mouth tumors is observed in those individuals who consume large amounts of alcohol. Usually these individuals smoke excessively as well, and the two factors operating together may be responsible for the neoplasms.

Carcinomas are very common in the natives of the South Sea Islands and the Orient, particularly India and the Philippines, who chew the betel nut obtained from the betel palm. It has been reported that more than 90 per cent of the tumors in these countries occur in the chewers of betel nut, and these neoplasms are found in the mouth.

The chronic irritation from parasite infections has long been known to produce tumors. *Gongylonema neoplasticum* will produce tumors in the stomach of the rat. *Cysticercus fasciolaris* invasion of the liver of the rat will result in a hepatic neoplasm. Gastric adenomas are found in horses and mules when *Habronema megastoma* is present. *Eimeria stiedae* invasion of the liver of the rabbit results in multiple adenomas of the bile ducts.

The many insecticides on the market have been tested for their ability to kill insects but, other than this, little is known about them. Their carcinogenic activities have not, for the most part, been examined, nor has much consideration been given to the vehicle in which they have been administered. Some insecticides and the vehicles with which they are administered are carcinogenic for experimental animals.

Hormones and related substances have been definitely associated with the production of tumors in the genital organs, adrenal, and pituitary. High estrogen levels associated with retention of milk in the mammary gland will produce mammary tumors in mice. The dog has a very high incidence of mammary tumors associated with disturbances of hormone balance. Drugs such as stilbestrol are proven carcinogenic agents in experimental animals.

Hormones may be purchased and used by anyone. Usually little is known about their mode of action or the dangers associated with their use. These hormones are normally produced by the endocrine glands, sometimes in excessive amounts. If they are produced in excess they may be placing the individual near the danger point in the production of an endocrine disorder or a tumor. Some of these substances are found in foods, but, in addition to this, foods may be fortified with these drugs or they may be given to the plants or animals from which human food is prepared. They are placed in animal feeds in an attempt to increase the rate of growth. This increased amount of hormone in the ration or environment may be just enough to bring about an endocrine disorder or produce a tumor. If a drug is administered and a tumor is the result, is not the administrator guilty of mammalicide?

Modern science has created a new group of substances known as plastics. It is too early to state with certainty the amount of carcinogenic activity they produce. Tumors have been produced in rodents with cellophane, Dacron, polyethylene, polyvinylchloride, Silastic, Pliofilm, nylon, polymethyl methacylate, polystyrene, Saran, Ivalon, Kel-F, and Teflon. Additional research needs to be done to determine the carcinogenic properties of these substances, but it should be remembered they may be dangerous.

Leukemia is found in both animals and man. The cause of this disease is not clear, but evidence is accumulating both experimentally and occupationally that some of these cases are associated with the use of certain chemical agents such as benzol, arsphenamine, quinine, sulfanilamide, indol, benpyrene, phenylhydrazine, and many others.

Brain tumors can easily be produced in experimental animals by injecting dibenzanthracene, methylcholanthrene, or styryl 430 into the brain.

There is ample evidence to indicate that certain carcinogenic agents are formed within the body. Bile acids, sex hormones, cholesterol, and vitamin D are very similar in structure to known carcinogenic agents. Carcinogenic agents capable of producing tumors in other animals have been isolated from man and animals. It is quite probable in certain diseases that substances found normally within the body may be altered and the result will be a carcinogenic agent. It is suspected that bile acids are changed in chronic inflammation of the gall bladder, as is associated with gallstones, and that in the process an agent is produced that will bring about the production of a tumor in the wall of the gall bladder.

At present the infection theory is receiving much attention. Arguments against it are that neoplasms do not occur in epizootics, that it is almost unbelievable that there is a great enough variety of organisms to cause such a multiplicity of growths in so many species of animals, that for the most part tumors remain localized, and that with few exceptions no specific antibodies are produced. These arguments are less valid now, for some animal tumors at least, than formerly.

Among animals there is a rather exten-

sive list of neoplasms caused by filtrable viruses. In this list belong infectious cutaneous papillomas of cattle and wild rabbits, infectious oral papillomas of puppies, transmissible venereal tumors of dogs, leukotic tumors and Rous sarcoma of chickens, and myxomas of rabbits (Fig. 13.2).

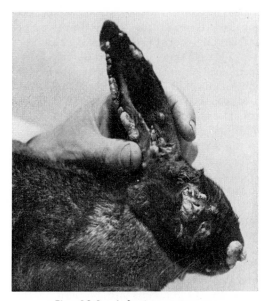

Fig. 13.2 — Infectious myxomas of a rabbit. (McKenney and Shillinger, Jour. A.V.M.A.)

Proponents of virus infections as the cause of many neoplasms suggest that the healthy body may have a virus population comparable to that of its bacterial population but that the types of viruses may be more considerable and diverse. They contend that since there is a variety of cells in the body, there may also be a variety of viruses but that the problem is simplified because it has already been demonstrated that one virus can produce varied changes in the same type of cell. An example is the rabbit papilloma virus which can stimulate the epidermal cells to form cystic tumors, papillomas, and squamous-cell carcinomas. The contention that specific antibodies are not produced in neoplastic conditions is likewise refuted in the case of most of the transmissible tumors named above. Several of these eventually disappear and leave in the animal a high degree of protection against recurrence of the particular tumor.

**Single traumatic factor.** The question often arises as to whether a single traumatic factor will produce a tumor. Frequently, when a tumor appears there is a history of injury having occurred at some previous time in the area. However, an individual receives so many injuries during life that there is little difficulty in remembering some injury to the tissues in the region of the tumor. Because of this, a single traumatic factor can hardly be considered as the cause of a tumor. In addition, the tumor may have been present in the area before the injury occurred. In the case of bone, perhaps it was the presence of the tumor that caused the bone to fracture. Furthermore, following an injury there is hyperemia and other circulatory changes in the area of inflammation. Because of the increased volume of blood flow into the area, it is quite easy for tumor cells, if present in the circulation, to find their way to the area of inflammation. Once the tumor cells are brought to the area, the vascular phenomena associated with inflammation enable them to lodge in the vessels since the speed of circulation has been retarded by capillary dilatation, increased peripheral resistance, and hemoconcentration.

**Association of intrinsic and extrinsic factors.** In the study of neoplasia it is apparent that in many instances both intrinsic and extrinsic factors operate together in the production of a tumor. These observations can best be observed in identical twins, triplets, or quadruplets. Warthin describes a family of four brothers. Three brothers were heavy smokers and died with cancer of the lip between the ages of 40 to 45 years. The fourth was a nonsmoker, and he died at the age of 63 with cancer of the lip, indicating that his nonsmoking habits increased his life span by twenty years.

Another example of the relation of intrinsic and extrinsic factors is the case of two identical twins. One was struck in the right testicle and died shortly thereafter with a tumor of that testicle at the age of 26 years. The other twin died at 31 years of age with the same type of tumor in the right testicle, indicating both twins had the intrinsic factor but the extrinsic factor, trauma, caused the tumor to appear in one twin five years earlier.

In summing up we can say that the appearance of a tumor depends on the sum total of the cell stimuli received by an individual during life. It is our duty to substitute non-carcinogenic agents for carcinogenic substances whenever they come in contract with man or animals. It is only in this way that we can reduce the incidence of neoplasms in man and domestic animals.

## MACROSCOPIC APPEARANCE

It is well to remember that neoplasms have no definite size, shape, color, or consistency. Several factors, such as location, the type of tumor, blood supply, rate of growth, and length of time the tumor has been present, influence the macroscopic appearance of the neoplasm.

In **size,** neoplasms measure from one or two millimeters to those that are several centimeters in diameter. As to **weight,** they vary from a few milligrams to as much as 60 kilograms or even more. The tumor may be larger than the host in the smaller animals such as mice.

The **shape** of a tumor is quite variable. It may be round, spherical, elliptical, or multilobulated (Fig. 13.3). It may protrude above the surrounding tissue or infiltrate deeply into underlying structures. A slowly growing tumor tends to be spherical or pedunculated. A rapidly growing neoplasm is usually irregular in shape and is multilobulated.

The **color** of a neoplasm is usually grayish white but may be yellow, red, brown, or black. Areas of necrosis within a tumor often appear as white or yellow areas. A tumor composed of fat pigmented with lipochromes is yellow in color. Hemorrhage

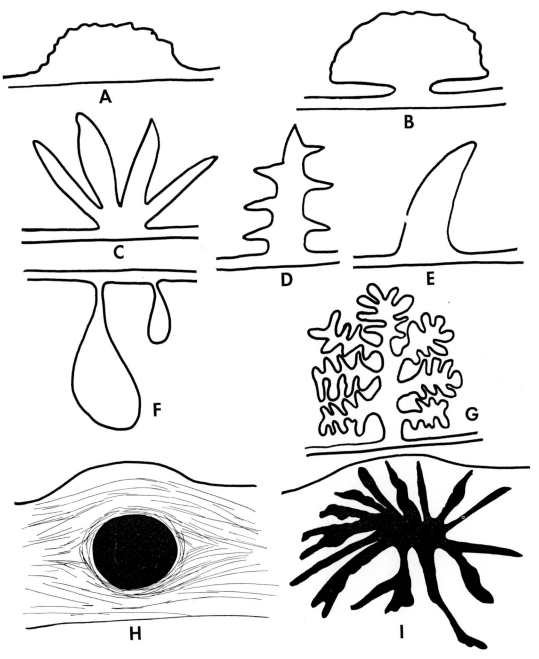

Fig. 13.3 — Classification of tumors according to shape.

**A**, wartlike;

**B**, fungoid;

**C**, villous;

**D**, spinous;

**E**, hornlike;

**F**, polypoid;

**G**, papillomatous;

**H**, expansive;

**I**, infiltrative.

or hyperemia gives the tumor a pink or red color, depending on the number of erythrocytes present. The presence of melanin results in gray or black tumor tissue. A brown color is frequently associated with the disintegration of hemoglobin and the presence of hemosiderin in the neoplastic tissue.

The **consistency** of the tumor varies with the type of tissue contained within the neoplasm. Tumors of bone are very hard because they are composed of osteoid or osseous tissue. If tumors of connective tissue contain considerable amounts of collagen, they are dense and firm. Tumors of this type are said to be **sclerotic** or **fibrotic** in consistency. Some tumors are very soft and friable and are designated as

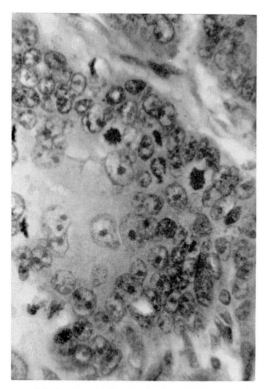

Fig. 13.4 — Signs of anaplasia in a highly malignant carcinoma: large nuclei with large nucleoli; in some instances two nucleoli; increased mitosis; atypical mitosis with figures resembling pyknotic nuclei. X540. (Department of Veterinary Pathology, Michigan State University.)

encephaloid in consistency because they resemble brain tissue. Tumors may be soft and liquefied if degeneration, suppuration, and necrosis are present. Some tumors are watery in consistency because of edema. Tumors that contain mucin are slimy in consistency.

## MICROSCOPIC APPEARANCE OF TUMORS

Tumors are composed of cells just as is any other tissue or organ. These cells resemble the cells of the tissue from which the tumor was derived. The appearance of these cells varies with the degree of malignancy of the tumor. The more benign the tumor the more the cells resemble the adult cell type. The more malignant the tumor the more the cells resemble the immature or the embryonal cell type. The histological recognition of the tumor depends upon the identification of the cell type in its various morphological variations from the adult cells to the extremely embryonal forms. When a tumor cell becomes malignant, it reverts back to the more embryonal type and this reversion is called **anaplasia** or the cell is said to be **anaplastic.** The more anaplasia a tumor cell shows, the more malignant is the neoplasm.

There are several factors that indicate the degree of anaplasia present:

1. **Enlargement of the nucleus.** Enlargement of the nucleus is an indication of rapid cell growth and an embryonal cell type.

2. **Multiple nuclei in a cell.** This is another indication of a rapidly growing embryonal cell type. The nucleus is dividing more rapidly than is the cytoplasm, and as a result multiple nuclei are found within the cell. Such cells are called *tumor giant cells.*

3. **Enlargement of the nucleolus.** Enlargement of the nucleolus is associated with rapid cell growth. The nucleolus may become two or three times its normal size (Fig. 13.4).

4. **Increased number of mitotic figures.** This is indicated by an increase in the

number of mitotic figures above the normal few that can be found in the tissue. The more rapidly the cells are multiplying the greater is the chance the mitotic figures will be found. When mitotic figures are abundant it is an indication the cells are growing and multiplying rapidly (Figs. 13.4 and 13.16).

**5. Hyperchromasia of the cell.** The more embryonal the cell the more intensely the cell stains with hematoxylin, especially the nucleus. The intensity of the hematoxylin staining of the cell compared with the normal adult cell gives an indication as to the maturity of the cell (Fig. 13.5).

**6. Embryonal type cells.** The cell loses its resemblance to the cells from which it originated and approaches the undifferentiated embryonal cell type. This indicates cell growth is no longer under the control of growth regulating and maturating factors.

## SPREAD OF TUMORS THROUGH THE BODY

There are three important ways by which malignant cells may spread through the body. They are (1) infiltration, (2) metastasis, and (3) implantation.

**Infiltration.** The most common method

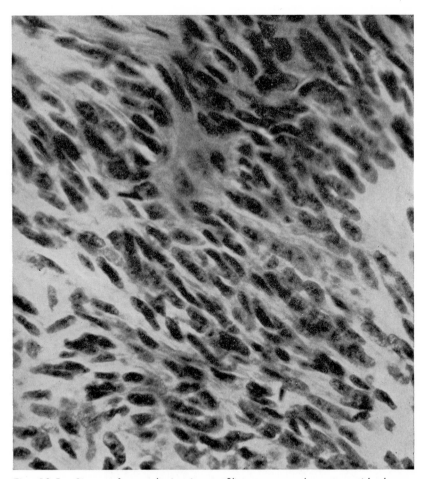

Fig. 13.5 — Signs of anaplasia in a fibrosarcoma: large, ovoid, hyperchromatic nuclei. X780. (Department of Veterinary Pathology, Michigan State University. )

of spread of malignant cells is by infiltration. There is a tendency for the cells to grow along the line of least resistance, and therefore they tend to spread through the loose connective tissue and become interwoven with the parenchymatous and interstitial tissue of the part. The tumor may also invade lymphatics and blood vessels and extend for great distances by growth along the lumen of the vessel. Infiltration is a great problem to the surgeon who must determine how much tissue to remove at the time of surgery. At times the tumor cells have extended for a considerable distance into the adjacent tissue, and it is extremely difficult to detect small cords or nests of tumor cells. For this reason tumor surgery tends to be rather radical, and the surgeon must remove considerable tissue in the vicinity of the neoplasm to assure himself that all tumor cells have been removed.

Metastasis. The spread of malignant cells from one part of the body to another by way of the lymphatics or the blood vessels as an embolus is called metastasis (Fig. 13.6). If multiple tumor emboli spread to distant tissues or organs, they are designated as metastases (Fig. 13.7). The term metastasize is the verb used to indicate that metastasis has or will occur. The term metastatic is the adjective indicating the tumor has metastasized. Tumor cells that invade the lumen of a blood vessel are swept away by the current and are carried to distant organs. The site of deposition depends on the diameter of the blood vessel. As a result, most tumor cells lodge in the capillaries, and since the lung contains the most central capillary bed, it is in this organ that most of the metastatic tumors are found. The tumor cells that enter the lymphatics are carried to the regional lymph nodes where the reduced diameter of the sinuses of the lymph node serves as a filter and retains the metastatic cells. Carcinomas are more prone to metastasize by way of the lymphatics, and sarcomas by way of the blood vessels; however, metastasis may take place by either route in both types of tumors.

The majority of metastatic tumor cells die and do not produce tumors in the tissue or organ in which they have been deposited. The tumor cells must lodge in a suitable environment if continued growth is to occur. Muscle, for example, is apparently not a suitable medium for the growth of most tumor cells. Metastatic

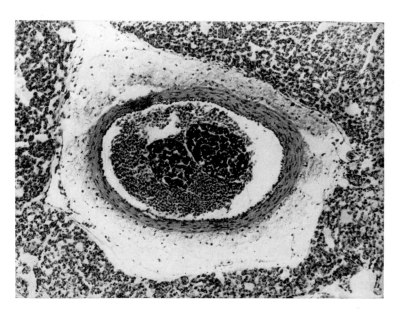

Fig. 13.6 — Two masses of tumor cells, constituting two emboli, being carried from the primary site to a secondary site in the artery of a chicken. (Carl Olson, Jr.)

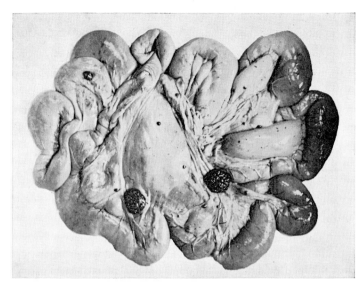

Fig. 13.7 — Metastases of a melanosarcoma from the brisket to the mesentery of an aged mule. (Mathews, Jour. A.V.M.A.)

tumors are uncommon in muscle, yet this tissue in many instances must be showered with emboli.

**Transplantation.** The transplantation of a neoplasm is the transfer of tumor cells from one serous or mucous surface to another by direct contact (Figs. 13.8 and 17.43). For example, the tumor cells of an adenocarcinoma of the ovary come in contact with the serous surface of the intestine (Fig. 13.9). Some of the cells are dislodged and are transplanted on the serous surface of the intestine. These transplanted cells grow and multiply, and as the intestinal motility moves the viscera about, the entire visceral and parietal peritoneum soon becomes covered with tumor cells. Another example of transplantation is observed with the histiocytoma in the dog where tumor cells are spread by coitus.

## CLASSIFICATION AND NOMENCLATURE

Neoplasms are divided into two major groups — benign tumors and malignant tumors. A **benign** tumor usually does not

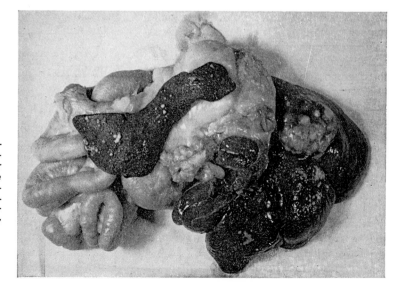

Fig. 13.8 — Transplantation of a secondary adenocarcinoma of the liver to the peritoneum of the liver and spleen in a 14-year-old female fox terrier. The primary tumor was in the mammary gland. (W. H. Riser.)

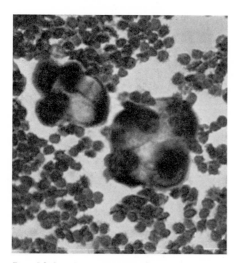

Fig. 13.9 — Free tumor cells among erythrocytes in the ascitic fluid of a dog with carcinoma of the ovary. Such cells gave rise to transplants on the visceral peritoneum. (Department of Veterinary Pathology, Michigan State University.)

kill the individual, grows slowly, and does not spread to distant organs. A **malignant** tumor is a new growth that will kill the individual by progressive invasion unless completely removed. It may spread to distant organs.

Benign tumors are harmless unless their location interferes with the function of an important organ. They grow slowly, frequently become encapsulated, are often pedunculated if located on a surface, do not metastasize, and do not recur when removed. Malignant neoplasms are harmful because they infiltrate vital organs, grow rapidly, are not encapsulated, spread to other parts of the body by metastasis, and recur after excision, cautery, or irradiation unless every infiltrating cell is removed or destroyed in the surrounding tissues.

## Tumor Classification

A. **Epithelial:** Tumors derived from epithelial surfaces, either squamous or glandular.
  1. **Benign**
    a. Papilloma, involving the squamous epithelial surface.
    b. Adenoma, involving glandular epithelium.

  2. **Malignant**
    a. Carcinoma, involving either squamous or glandular epithelium.
B. **Non-epithelial:** Tumors derived from connective tissue in general (bone, cartilage, white fibrous connective tissue, muscle).
  1. **Benign:** The name of the tissue plus "oma" (fibroma, osteoma, chondroma).
  2. **Malignant:** Indicated by the term sarcoma (fibrosarcoma, osteosarcoma, chondrosarcoma).
C. **Dermoid cyst:** A tumor arising from an embryonic defect in growth that is composed of one germ layer, the skin, and contains teeth, hair, and other dermal structures.
D. **Teratoma:** A tumor arising from an embryonic defect and composed of two or more germ layers.

The pathologist classifies tumors on a histogenetic basis (Table 13.1), that is, according to the origin of the cells in them. This is often difficult, however, because it is not always possible to identify the type of cell present and associate it with its parent. This means that the more undifferentiated (anaplastic) the cells are, the more difficult the tumor is to classify. Variations in differentiation as well as the tissue origin of the cells are two exceedingly important elements taken into consideration in a histogenetic classification.

## MACROSCOPIC COMPARISON OF BENIGN AND MALIGNANT NEOPLASMS

### Benign

**1. They occur singly.** The majority of tumors originate in one single area, and since the tumor is benign and does not spread, only the single original tumor will be found.

**2. The shape is round, elliptical, wartlike, or pedunculated.** Since the tumor grows slowly, the tissues of the body have ample time to adjust themselves to the increased pressure. Since the pressure is equal in all directions, the tumor masses tend to be round or elliptical. If the benign tumor

TABLE 13.1

HISTOGENIC CLASSIFICATION OF NEOPLASMS

| Parent Cell | Benign Neoplasms | Malignant Neoplasms |
|---|---|---|
| White fibrous connective tissue cell | fibroma[c] | fibrosarcoma[b] |
| Embryonal white fibrous connective tissue cell that produces mucin | myxoma[a] | myxosarcoma[a] |
| Adipose tissue cell | lipoma[b] | liposarcoma[a] |
| Chondrocyte | chondroma[b] | chondrosarcoma[b] |
| Osteocyte | osteoma[b] | osteosarcoma[c] |
| Striated muscle cell | rhabdomyoma[a] | rhabdomyosarcoma[a] |
| Smooth muscle cell | leiomyoma[b] | leiomyosarcoma[a] |
| Neuron | neuroma[a] | neurosarcoma[a] |
| Glia | glioma[b] | gliosarcoma[b] |
| Blood vascular endothelial cell | hemangioma[b] | hemangiosarcoma[a] |
| Lymph vascular endothelial cell | lymphangioma[a] | lymphangiosarcoma[a] |
| Lymphocyte | lymphoma[a] | lymphosarcoma[c] |
| Melanoblast | melanoma[a] | melanosarcoma[b] |
| Squamous epithelial cell | papilloma[c] | squamous-cell carcinoma[c] |
| Glandular epithelial cell | adenoma[c] | adenocarcinoma[c] |

[a] = uncommon.
[b] = common.
[c] = very common.

occurs on an epithelial or mucous surface, it grows as a pedunculated or wartlike mass projecting to the exterior or into the lumen of the organ. This occurs because the exterior of the individual or the lumen of the organ has little or no resistance to the tumor growth.

**3. Encapsulation is present.** Since the tumor is mildly irritating and grows slowly, the tissues surrounding the tumor respond to the mild stimulation or irritation produced by the tumor, and as a result a connective tissue capsule is deposited around the new growth.

**4. The rate of growth is slow.** A regulating force still influences the rapidity and extent of cell growth.

**5. Degenerative and necrotic changes** within the tumor are slight. Since the tumor grows slowly, the blood vascular system within the tumor is able to grow in sufficient amounts to supply the need of the neoplasm.

**6. Removal is not difficult.** The tumor grows slowly and does not infiltrate the surrounding tissue. The entire tumor is contained within the connective tissue capsule. Since the limiting capsule is easily discerned, the borders of the tumor are quite evident and the tumor can be removed in its entirety.

**7. The tumor is not toxic to the patient.** Toxicity is not present because the degenerative and necrotic changes that liberate toxic materials do not occur in the benign form of the tumor.

**8. Metastases are lacking.** The tumor does not invade the blood vessels and lymphatics and therefore metastasis does not occur.

**9. There is no recurrence of the tumor once it is removed.** The entire mass retained within the capsule can be removed quite easily by the surgeon. Islands and cords of infiltrating tumor cells are not present in the tissues.

**10. Death of the individual does not occur.** Unless the tumor is found in a vital organ such as the heart, brain, or spinal cord, where volume and pressure alone may interfere with the function of the part, death does not occur.

## Malignant

**1. Malignant neoplasms are usually multiple.** The reason for this is that the tumor infiltrates the surrounding tissue, and daughter tumors appear in the vicinity of the primary growth. Metastasis to distant organs takes place. In the case of serous surfaces, transplantation of tumor cells may occur. As the result of these three methods of spread, multiple tumors are found.

**2. The shape is irregular.** Since the tumor grows rapidly and extends in all directions, following the paths of least resistance through the tissues, and the rate of tumor growth varies with the different portions of the neoplasm, the tumor is not sharply demarked from the surrounding tissue and its appearance is irregular.

**3. Encapsulation is not present.** The tumor grows so rapidly that the surrounding tissue is not able to respond to the stimulation and irritation sufficiently rapidly enough to enclose the tumor mass with a connective tissue capsule. In addition, the malignant tumor destroys the blood supply of the surrounding tissue, thus making it more difficult for a connective tissue capsule to be formed.

**4. The rate of growth is rapid.** The normal regulating force that controls the rapidity and extent of cellular growth is not present.

**5. Degenerative and necrotic changes within the tumor are extensive.** The tumor grows so rapidly that the blood vascular system is not capable of supplying the nutritive requirements of the new growth, and, as a result, portions of the tumor undergo degeneration and necrosis. In addition, the infiltrating tumor has no respect for its own blood supply. By invading the arteries that supply its nutrient, thrombosis and occlusion of the vessels occur which result in infarction of portions of the neoplasm.

**6. Removal of the tumor is difficult.** The neoplasm grows rapidly, and columns of infiltrating neoplastic cells follow the path of least resistance through the tissue. They may also be extending along the lumen of the blood vessels or lymph vessels. As a result, tumor cells are found at a considerable distance from the primary lesion. Because of this widespread infiltration of the tissue, it is extremely difficult for the surgeon to remove all of the cords or islands of tumor cells that may be present in the tissue adjacent to the neoplasm.

**7. The tumor is toxic to the patient.** Extensive degeneration and necrosis is present within the tumor, and the toxic products absorbed from these areas by the host are extremely deleterious to his well-being.

**8. Infiltration, metastasis, and transplantation are present.** One or all of these methods of tumor spread through the tissues are present.

**9. The tumor tends to recur after apparent removal.** Unless the entire tumor mass is removed, the cells remaining in the tissue continue to grow and multiply and the tumor is again observed in the area.

**10. Death of the individual occurs.** The tumor continues to grow and spread through the tissue until tissue destruction is so great as to bring about the death of the individual.

## MICROSCOPIC COMPARISON OF BENIGN AND MALIGNANT NEOPLASMS

### Benign

1. The morphology of the tumor is approximately normal. The parenchyma approaches the normal arrangement of the tissue or organ. Interstitial tissue is present and has a normal relation to the parenchyma.

2. The tumor does not extend beyond the basement membrane or the basal layer of cells. When the tumor involves a mucous membrane, all of the growth is to the exterior into the lumen of the organ. The same is true of skin tumors; all of the growth is to the exterior of the body. The tumor does not infiltrate the tissues below the line of epithelium.

3. The tumor does not penetrate the connective tissue capsule.

4. The tumor does not grow beyond the blood supply. The slow rate of growth allows the vascular system to develop sufficiently to keep up with the growth of the new tissue.

5. Degenerative and necrotic changes within the tumor are slight.

6. There is no invasion of the vascular system (lymph and blood).

7. The cells comprising the tumor are mature.

8. Mitotic figures are few in number or are not present.

### Malignant

1. The morphology of the tumor is abnormal. The parenchyma has an abnormal arrangement or is foreign to the tissue or organ in which it is found. The normal arrangement of the interstitial tissue and parenchyma is lacking.

2. The tumor extends beyond the basement membrane or the basal layer of cells. The neoplastic cells infiltrate the tissue underlying the epithelium from which the tumor originated.

3. The neoplasm is not enclosed with a connective tissue capsule. The rapid, infiltrating character of the growth prevents the formation of a distinct enclosing capsule.

4. The tumor grows beyond its blood supply. The growth of the neoplasm is so profuse the vascular system is not able to develop rapidly enough to meet the requirements of the new growth.

5. Degenerative and necrotic changes within the tumor are extensive. Because the tumor grows beyond its blood supply, the nutritive requirements cannot be supplied, and as a result the tissue undergoes degeneration and necrosis. In addition, the tumor may invade and destroy the blood supply, and infarction is the result.

6. Invasion of the vascular system occurs (lymph and blood). The tumor cells invade the wall of the blood vessel, and thrombosis of the vessel may occur. If the neoplasm invades the lumen of the vessel, the cells can be observed in the blood within the vessel. These masses of cells may result in obstruction of the vessel or they may float away as emboli and initiate metastatic foci in other tissues or organs.

7. The cells comprising the tumor are embryonal.

8. Mitotic figures are present and may be abundant.

## RESULTS OF NEOPLASIA

The effect of a tumor upon the body depends upon (1) location, (2) the tissue from which it was derived, and (3) whether it is malignant or benign. The methods by which a tumor injures an individual are as follows:

1. Pressure atrophy of the surrounding cells. As the tumor enlarges peripherally, more and more pressure is placed upon the adjacent cells. Since the growing tumor cells are more vigorous than the cells of the organ in which the neoplasm is found, the pressure exerted on the tissue cells interferes with the metabolic

fluid exchanges of the cell and, as a result, atrophy occurs. In addition, there is compression of the blood vessels and lymphatics in the area, and again the nutrition of the tissue cells is interfered with.

**2. Obstruction of the lumen of organs.** The obstruction may occur as the result of growth that fills the lumen within the organ or pressure from without that compresses the organ until the lumen is stenosed. This obstruction prevents the passage of ingesta, secretion, or excretion.

**3. Destruction of the blood or lymph vessels.** The tumor invades and penetrates the wall of the vessel, and when the endothelium of the vessel is damaged, thrombosis of the blood vessel takes place. If the lumen of the vessel is invaded by the tumor, the growing tumor mass within the lumen of the vessel will cause obstruction.

**4. Destruction of the nerve supply.** Pressure upon the nerve by the growing tumor results in pressure atrophy. In addition, the tumor infiltrates the nerve and brings about its destruction.

**5. Bacterial invasion of the tumor and the tissue in its vicinity.** The disintegration of the tumor as well as of the normal tissue interferes with the defense mechanism. directed against bacteria in the area. Quite often, degenerating and necrotic tissue, which is a suitable medium for bacterial growth, is present in the region. As a result, bacteria are able to invade and multiply within the tissue and may extend to other portions of the body.

**6. Emaciation.** The emaciation is due to starvation when the tumor involves the gastrointestinal tract. The emaciation may be the result of a toxemia. These toxins may be derived from the degenerating and necrotic tissue contained within the tumor, or the toxin may be elaborated by the bacteria that have invaded the site of the neoplasm. At times a septicemia will result when bacteria have gained entrance to the body through the tumor, and as a result of the bacterial invasion and the resulting complications, emaciation occurs.

**7. Anemia.** Anemia may occur as the result of hemorrhage when vessels have been eroded by the tumor. Tumors of the gastrointestinal tract, particularly tumors of the stomach, interfere with digestion, and a nutritional anemia may be the result when certain essential substances necessary for blood formation, such as folic acid and hydrochloric acid, are no longer present. If the tumor invades the bone marrow, the expanding tumor may cause pressure atrophy of the hemopoietic tissue and the production of erythrocytes and leukocytes will be prevented. Atrophy of the hemopoietic centers may occur when toxins liberated by the neoplasm exert an inhibitory effect on hematopoiesis and, as a result, erythrocytes and leukocytes are not produced.

**8. Excessive production of hormones elaborated by the endocrine system.** If the tumor involves an endocrine gland and excessive hormone is produced, the effect of this hormone is often manifested by an abnormality in growth and metabolism. Tumors of the parathyroid gland result in decalcification of the skeleton. Neoplasms of the Sertoli cells of the testicle result in a feminization of the male.

**9. Death of the individual.** When the tumor is found in a vital organ or when many tumors are found throughout the individual, the destruction of tissue is so great the vital functions of the body can no longer be maintained and death is the result.

**10. Spontaneous regression and recovery from neoplasia.** Occasionally individuals with extensive neoplasia experience regression of the tumor, its eventual disappearance, and healing of the involved tissue. One explanation for such cases is that neoplastic tissue is also susceptible to toxic and infectious diseases. At times the toxic or infectious disease is more injurious to the neoplasm than it is to the host, and when this occurs the neoplasm is destroyed. Several of these agents are utilized in the treatment of tumors. X-ray, radium, and radioactive isotopes are much more toxic to tumor tissue in general than they are to the normal tissue. As a result, proper application of these substances may result in the destruction of a tumor. Certain viral diseases are more injurious to embryonal tumor tissue than they are to the host, and when the host becomes infected with these viral agents, complete destruction of the tumor may take place. The viral treatment of tumors, although yet in its experimental state, may some day offer a method by which neoplastic growth may be destroyed. The viral agents selected must be capable of destroying tumor cells without producing undue injury to the host.

## METHODS USED IN DIAGNOSIS OF TUMORS

The most accurate and reliable method of tumor diagnosis depends upon the macroscopic and microscopic identification of the tumor tissue. Since the identification of tissue is accomplished by histological observation of the component cells, microscopic examination is the most useful method. Considerable skill and experience are required for accurate identification of neoplasms.

In the clinic, radiologic methods may be used to locate tumors in various organs. In addition, the use of radiology as a therapeutic tool may give some indication as to the identity of the tumor as judged by its response to radiation.

Biopsy may be employed by the clinician to aid him in identifying the growth. Exfoliate cytology may be employed for the identification of tumor cells. The tumor cells are obtained from the secretions and excretions of the individual or are obtained by scraping the surface of suspected growths and then examining the cells that have been obtained in this manner. The diagnosis depends upon the recognition of the cytological changes occurring in the cells.

Serological methods of tumor identification are unsatisfactory. It is true that certain tissues may be identified by serological methods, but they are of little value in estimating the degree of malignancy or the exact nature of the tissue.

Chemical analysis has been attempted in tumor identification. Certain tumors may be recognized by some of their tinctorial staining properties (mastosarcoma), but, for the most part, chemical analysis is not satisfactory for tumor identification because the chemical constituents of tissue are similar, making specific identification as to tissue, organ, and degree of malignancy almost impossible.

## THE COMPOUNDING OF TERMS USED IN THE DESCRIPTION OF NEOPLASMS

Frequently tumors are composed of more than one tissue. This is particularly true of neoplasms of the mammary gland of the dog. In describing these types of neoplasms, there are two alternative methods that may be followed. The tumor may be called a mixed tumor, for example a mixed mammary gland tumor, and the term may be followed by a list of types of neoplastic tissue present — for example, mixed mammary gland tumor composed of white fibrous connective tissue, cartilage, and bone.

The other alternative method is to list the constituents of the tumor in a compound word. In doing this, the least important or the least malignant portion of the tumor is placed first. The predominating tissue or the most malignant tissue is placed last — for example, fibro-chondrosarcoma, osteo-fibro-chondrosarcoma, fibro-chondro-osteosarcoma, myxo-fibrosarcoma, and fibro-osteo-chondrosarcoma.

## THE INCIDENCE OF NEOPLASMS IN DOMESTIC ANIMALS

It is extremely difficult to arrive at figures indicating the incidence of neoplasms in domestic animals because so much of the livestock population does not come under the observation of individuals who have the facilities to arrive at a correct tumor identification. Also, a large number of animals are not examined for the presence of a neoplasm. In addition, the incidence of neoplasia varies greatly with the type, breed, and species of animal. The small-animal practitioner, if supported by suitable laboratory service, can probably present the most accurate appraisal of the incidence and type of neoplasms found in small animals. The same is true with the poultry inspector. If suitable laboratory facilities are available, he is able to arrive at an estimate of incidence of the number and types of neoplasms in the domestic fowl. The large-animal clinician is quite familiar with the cutaneous types of tumors, but, since many of our large animals are submitted for slaughter rather than post-mortem examination when no longer suitable for profitable animal husbandry production, the tumors within the animals are usually not known. The meat inspection service of the U. S. Department of Agriculture probably gives the best over-all picture of the incidence of tumors in our larger domestic animals. However, it is recognized that many of the cutaneous neoplasms have been removed by practicing veterinarians. In addition, many of the neoplasms encountered in meat inspection are not submitted for histological examination because the number of tumors is so great that it is economically not feasible to carry out these extensive investigations.

Tables 13.2, 13.3, 13.4, and 13.5, presented by Monlux, Anderson, and Davis from a survey of tumors occurring in cattle, sheep, and swine, give some indication as to the number and relative importance of neoplasms in domestic animals in the United States as they appeared in a group of animals slaughtered in Denver abattoirs for a period of one year. It should be remembered that many of the affected animals were sent to slaughter because of failing health and that perhaps no more than half were in apparent good health.

## RELATIVE IMPORTANCE OF NEOPLASMS

Lymphoid tumors are the only neoplasms that are of common occurrence in all species of domestic animals. Their appearance at any age and their rapid transformation into malignant tumors make them extremely important. One should not consider the possibility of an early appearance unusual for the malignant lymphomas and other neoplasms of the non-epithelial group. If histiocytoma in

TABLE 13.2

The Occurrence of Tumors in Three Species of Animals Slaughtered at All Federally Inspected Abattoirs in 1953*

| Species | Number of Animals Inspected | Number of Carcasses Condemned at Ante- or Post-Mortem Inspection | | | | | Number of Parts of Carcasses Condemned at Post-Mortem Inspection | | |
|---|---|---|---|---|---|---|---|---|---|
| | | Carcinoma | Epithelioma | Leukemia or Lymphoma | Sarcoma | Misc. | Carcinoma | Epithelioma | Misc. |
| Cattle..... | 15,208,023 | 1,538 | 4,402 | 1,518 | 540 | 2,247 | 40 | 25,608 | 87 |
| Calves .... | 6,027,449 | 14 | 2 | 100 | 15 | 89 | | 64 | 5 |
| Sheep and lambs... | 13,623,394 | 51 | 4 | 34 | 26 | 131 | | | 2 |
| Swine..... | 57,395,484 | 241 | | 529 | 234 | 624 | | 3 | 13 |

* Compiled from the annual report of the Chief of the Bureau of Animal Industry, U. S. Department of Agriculture.

Blank spaces indicate no condemnations.

the dog is a true tumor, it would be another good example of a non-epithelial tumor common in young dogs but unique in its rarity of appearance in older animals. The common embryonal nephromas of swine seldom metastasize although they may be seen at an early age.

Squamous-cell carcinomas of the eyes of Hereford cattle in the United States cause great economic loss in older breeding animals. Adenocarcinomas of the uterus are apt to produce terminal metastases in older cows while the fairly common Schwann cell and adrenal-cortical tumors of cattle will seldom metastasize. Mammary gland tumors and the skin tu-

mors discussed in the following pages, in addition to the lymphoid tumors, cause the most concern in dogs and cats.

## IS THE INCIDENCE OF NEOPLASMS INCREASING?

Whether there is an increased incidence of tumors is a very difficult question to answer. Actually more neoplasms are being diagnosed today than ever before, but when one considers the greater number of animals, the better understanding of tumors, the greater number of necropsies, and the better diagnostic facilities now available, it is quite possible the increase in tumors is more apparent than real.

TABLE 13.3

THE NUMBER AND TYPE OF BOVINE TUMORS
COLLECTED IN 1953 AND 1954 IN DENVER ABATTOIRS

| Type | 1953 | 1954 | Total |
|---|---|---|---|
| Epithelial Tumors | | | |
|   Ocular squamous-cell ....... | 722* | | 722 |
|   Adenocarcinoma of uterus ... | 9 | 4 | 13 |
|   Metastatic adenocarcinoma | | | |
|     (probable uterine origin) .. | 7 | 6 | 13 |
|   Carcinoma of the lung ...... | 3 | | 3 |
|   Adenocarcinoma of the | | | |
|     intestine ................ | | 1 | 1 |
|   Ovary .................... | 3 | 4 | 7 |
|   Kidney ................... | 1 | 3 | 4 |
|   Gall bladder .............. | 3 | 7 | 10 |
|   Liver .................... | 5 | 3 | 8 |
|   Metastatic adenocarcinomas | | | |
|     (not of uterine origin) .... | 2 | 1 | 3 |
|   Adrenal cortical ........... | 8 | 15 | 23 |
|   Squamous-cell carcinoma of | | | |
|     skin ..................... | 1 | 2 | 3 |
|   Metastatic squamous-cell | | | |
|     carcinoma (not primary | | | |
|     ocular tumor) ........... | 1 | | 1 |
|   Squamous-cell carcinoma of | | | |
|     vulva .................. | | 1 | 1 |
|   Multiple papillomas of oral | | | |
|     cavity .................. | | 1 | 1 |
| Non-epithelial Tumors | | | |
|   Lymphoid ................. | 10 | 10 | 20 |
|   Schwann's cell ............. | 20 | 23 | 43 |
|   Adrenal medullary ......... | 2 | 3 | 5 |
|   Smooth muscle ............. | 6 | 2 | 8 |
|   Angioid .................. | 3 | 3 | 6 |
|   Fibrous connective tissue .... | 5 | 2 | 7 |
|   Mesothelioma ............. | 1 | 1 | 2 |
|   Melanoma ................. | 1 | 1 | 2 |
|   Lipoma .................. | | 1 | 1 |
|   Meningioma .............. | | 1 | 1 |
| Totals ..................... | 813 | 95 | 908 |

*Partial collection for only the calendar year 1953.
Blank spaces indicate no tumors collected.

A similar situation is observed in the human population. The increase in the length of the life span of man has resulted in a marked increase in the incidence of neoplasms. The longer life span of the individual may explain part, if not all, of this apparent increase since neoplasms are much more common in older individuals than they are in the young.

In final conclusion it can be said that not enough data is available to prove without doubt that tumors are more common now than formerly. The accumulation of data from several generations may show a significant trend.

## CONNECTIVE TISSUE TUMORS

### Fibroma

A fibroma is a tumor composed of mature fibrous connective tissue cells. According to the amount of collagenous fibers and their arrangement into dense or loose bundles, a fibroma is either hard or soft. Soft fibromas often have a high

TABLE 13.4

THE NUMBER AND TYPE OF OVINE TUMORS
COLLECTED IN DENVER ABATTOIRS IN 1953 AND 1954

| Type | 1953 | 1954 | Total |
|---|---|---|---|
| Epithelial Tumors | | | |
| Metastatic adenocarcinoma (primary site undetermined) | 1 | 4 | 5 |
| Adenocarcinoma of kidney ... | | 1 | 1 |
| Adenocarcinoma of thyroid ... | 1 | | 1 |
| Liver ...................... | 3 | 5 | 8 |
| Adrenal cortical ............ | | 5 | 5 |
| Squamous-cell carcinoma of skin ................... | 1 | 1 | 2 |
| Squamous-cell carcinoma of vulva ................. | | 1 | 1 |
| Squamous-cell carcinoma of eyelid ................ | 1 | | 1 |
| Non-epithelial Tumors | | | |
| Lymphoid ................... | 8 | 12 | 20 |
| Myeloid ................... | | 2 | 2 |
| Adrenal medullary .......... | 3 | 6 | 9 |
| Leiomyoma ................ | | 1 | 1 |
| Angioid ................... | 1 | 2 | 3 |
| Fibrosarcoma ............... | 2 | | 2 |
| Chondrosarcomas ........... | 2 | 1 | 3 |
| Lipoid ..................... | 1 | 1 | 2 |
| Totals ..................... | 24 | 42 | 66 |

Blank spaces indicate no tumors collected.

TABLE 13.5

THE NUMBER AND TYPE OF PORCINE TUMORS
COLLECTED IN DENVER ABATTOIRS IN 1953 AND 1954

| Type | 1953 | 1954 | Total |
|---|---|---|---|
| Embryonal nephroma .......... | 4 | 9 | 13 |
| Embryonic sarcoma of vagina ... | | 1 | 1 |
| Lymphoid ................... | 3 | 6 | 9 |
| Ganglioneuroma .............. | 1 | | 1 |
| Fibroma .................... | | 1 | 1 |
| Melanoma ................... | 3 | | 3 |
| Totals ..................... | 11 | 17 | 28 |

Blank spaces indicate no tumors collected.

lymph content and are quite vascular. They do not recur or metastasize.

**Macroscopic appearance.** Hard fibromas are round and firm. Sometimes they are as firm as tendon. The new growth does not infiltrate the surrounding tissue and is encapsulated and sharply circumscribed. Their cut surface is dry and white or yellowish white. Close inspection of the cut surface reveals that the tumor is made up of bundles of connective tissue, some cut in cross section and others longitudinally.

Soft fibromas are spongy, more vascular, and often edematous. The lymph may coagulate into a jelly-like mass. These tumors, when involving a mucous membrane are often pedunculated and are called **polyps** (Fig. 17.9). The cut surface of soft fibromas may be pink due to their rich blood supply.

Fibromas grow slowly, usually occur singly, and vary in size from tiny nodules to masses weighing more than 100 pounds. They must be distinguished from chronic inflammation (tuberculosis, staphylococcosis, actinomycosis) in which large amounts of connective tissue are deposited in the area of infection.

**Microscopic appearance.** The **hard fibromas** are composed of adult-type white fibrous connective tissue cells. Both the cells and their nuclei are spindle-shaped. Long collagenous fibers extend from either end of the cells and are interspersed between other connective tissue cells. As these fibers are produced by the cells, more and more collagen is deposited in the tumor, and the amount of collagen determines the firmness of the fibroma. These collagenous fibers arrange themselves in compact bundles of wavy fibers and tend to be laid down in a concentric manner around blood vessels. The reason for the concentric arrangement is that the nutrient for the tumor cells must diffuse from the blood vessels, and for that reason the growing cells will be arranged around the nutrient vessels. The **soft fibromas** contain very little collagen. The connective tissue cells are very loosely arranged, are distinctly stellate in form and are separated from each other by a transudate. The blood vessels may be quite numerous in the tumor mass.

**Location.** Naturally, fibromas may occur wherever there is connective tissue. Since connective tissue is abundant in all parts of the body, one may expect to find fibromas a l m o s t anywhere. Statistics, though, indicate that fibromas most often occur in the skin and subcutis. However, these statistics may not be entirely reliable because some of these masses are undoubtedly the reaction to chronic inflammation and injury and not true neoplastic growth. Since the skin is most subject to trauma, it is logical that these reactions to irritation would be most frequent in the skin. The soft fibromas called polyps are common in the nasal passages, especially of the horse and sheep.

Some fibromas, particularly those of the skin, may actually be nerve sheath tumors. Morphologically, the cells of the sheath of Schwann and white fibrous connective tissue cells are quite similar in appearance. In many instances careful methods of dissection to demonstrate the entrance of a nerve into the tumor mass is necessary if a correct differentiation is to be made. A group of tumors resembling fibromas, and in which the unit cellular structure is arranged concentrically around the blood vessels, is known as hemangiopericytomas.

Gingival fibromas are extremely common in the dog. They are usually found along the gum line near the canine and incisor teeth. Quite frequently they are referred to as an epulis or as epuli. The gingival fibroma is usually covered with stratified squamous epithelium, although areas of ulceration resulting from trauma may be present. The white fibrous connective tissue within the new growth is extremely firm and dense. At times bone, which may represent metaplasia of the white fibrous connective tissue or hyperplasia of the bone of the mandible or premaxilla, will be found in the area of attachment of the tumor. It is believed that many of these are not true fibromas but rather are the reaction of tissue to trauma and alveolar periostitis. These tumors are quite easily removed. They may be multiple, and new tumors may form, but this does not represent malignancy since in these animals the tissues appear to be particularly responsive to injury and react by proliferation and the formation of gingival gum-line growths.

**Combinations.** If more or less mature adipose, osseous, cartilaginous, or mucoid connective tissue is present with the fibrous connective tissue in an amount less than one-half of the total bulk of the tumor, the designation becomes lipofibroma, osteofibroma, chondrofibroma, or myxofibroma.

**Prognosis.** The prognosis of a fibroma is good if it is in an area that lends itself to surgical removal. When fibromas are exceedingly large or when they occur in vital organs, the surgery required for removal may be so drastic that the animal is permanently incapacitated.

### Myxoma

A myxoma is a benign tumor of white fibrous connective tissue that is capable of producing mucin. The production of mucin is a characteristic of embryonal connective tissue as is observed in embryology in Wharton's jelly of the umbilical cord. Any tumor that produces mucin should be regarded with suspicion because mucin production is an indication of an embryonal type of cell, and an embryonal cell is one of the characteristics of malignancy.

**Macroscopic appearance.** The myxomas resemble soft fibromas in appearance and consistency. Their size is variable but they are usually not large. Their cut surface is moist, gelatinous, and slimy because of the mucin that is present. They are rather transparent and have a pale yellow or grayish color (Fig. 13.10).

**Microscopic appearance.** This tumor consists of spindle-shaped and stellate connective tissue cells possessing long branching fibrils which are suspended in an abundance of intercellular mucin. Extreme care should be exercised in identi-

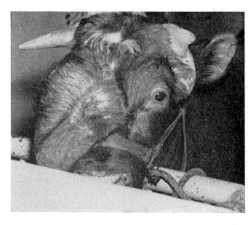

Fig. 13.10 — Myxofibromas on the head of an 18-month-old Shorthorn bull. The large tumor on the frontal region covered the right eye. The other tumor was on the temporal region below the left horn. (Iowa State University Veterinarian.)

fying this intercellular substance as mucin. The majority of so-called myxomas are nothing more than soft fibromas that have been over-stained with hematoxylin. A diagnosis of myxoma should not be made unless histochemical methods reveal that the intercellular substance is actually mucin. Blood vessels are prominent.

**Location.** Although nasal polyps have been reported to be myxomas rather than soft fibromas, most of these diagnoses are in error because histochemical identification reveals that the intercellular fluid is a transudate and not mucin. Myxomas have also been reported occasionally in the heart and uterus. They are not common in animals.

**Combinations.** Often only parts of the tumor contain mucin-producing connective tissue. The remainder may be fibrous connective tissue, fat, cartilage, or bone, so that the tumor may be called a fibromyxoma, lipomyxoma, chondromyxoma, or osteomyxoma. At times, too, the tumor may consist of a mixture of three or more members of the connective tissue group of cells.

**Prognosis.** The prognosis of a myxoma is good. However, the tumor site should be observed frequently since the embryonal nature of the cell is indicated by its tendency to produce mucin.

### Lipoma

A benign tumor made up of adult adipose tissue is a lipoma. Like other benign tumors it grows slowly, does not recur when completely extirpated, and does not metastasize. This tumor may or may not be encapsulated.

**Macroscopic appearance.** Lipomas are either single or multiple. They are variable in size. One reported in the abdominal cavity of an aged mare weighed 120 pounds. The outer surface of a lipoma is smooth, its consistency soft, and its cut surface has a greasy or oily translucent appearance, white to yellow in color. Calcification of the tumor may take place. Occasionally, when metaplasia occurs, bone will be found in the tumor.

**Microscopic appearance.** Most of the lipomas have a simple structure made up of cells each of which contains one large fat globule or several smaller ones. The nucleus is usually pushed to the periphery and may even be obliterated. Interspersed between the fat cells are strands of collagenous fibers.

Occasionally lipomas of a more immature type are found. These are characterized by the presence of numerous immature lipoblasts in clumps or patches. These cells have a spherical nucleus, with abundant fine chromatin granules, and a small eccentric nucleolus. The nucleus stains intensely with hematoxylin. The cytoplasm is finely granular and acidophilic. Special fat stains, such as scarlet red used on formalin-fixed tissue, will demonstrate the early formation of fat in these immature cells.

Great care should be taken not to confuse the chronic inflammation associated with fat necrosis with a lipoma. Phagocytic cells containing an abundance of fat droplets resemble the lipoblasts. The traumatic fat necrosis that occurs in the vagina of cattle is frequently diagnosed as a vaginal lipoma when actually it represents the herniation of perivaginal fat into the lumen of the vagina through rents or defects in the musculature of the vaginal wall.

**Location.** This neoplasm occurs in places where fat is physiologically abundant such as in the mesentery, peritoneum, subcutis, and submucosa. It is rather frequent in the abdominal cavity, where it often becomes pedunculated and sometimes detached.

The pedunculated lipoma hanging into the peritoneal cavity may be as much as 18 inches or more in length. The pendulous mass of fat attached to the peritoneal surface by a long narrow stalk may become entwined around loops of the intestine, and strangulation of the intestine may occur.

**Prognosis.** The prognosis is good as far as the life of the individual is concerned. Quite often lipomas are so large that the extensive surgery required for removal may seriously injure the host.

### Chondroma

A chondroma is a benign neoplasm consisting of cartilage.

**Macroscopic appearance.** It is a hard, lobulated, well-encapsulated tumor. On the outer surface it is gray in color, but the cut surface is a translucent bluish white. The capsule is so well developed that it resembles a shuck around a nut. Chondromas sometimes attain a weight of over 20 pounds in cattle and 10 pounds in dogs.

**Microscopic appearance.** Some chondromas are very cellular; others are not. The cells are arranged singly and not in groups as in normal cartilage. They vary much in size and shape. At the periphery they are usually small, at the center large. Between the cells there is usually a hyaline matrix. As in normal cartilage there are no vessels, but nourishment is brought to the cells by blood vessels in the capsule. Circulation, however, is often so poor that the tumor undergoes degeneration, calcification, and ossification.

**Location.** Chondromas occur in places

where cartilage is normally present, e.g., at the epiphyses of long bones of the extremities, the costochondral and the chondrosternal articulations, and in the cartilages of the larynx, trachea, and bronchi. Chondromas appear to be most common in the larger breeds of dogs such as the German shepherd.

Developmental tumors containing cartilage, such as those occurring in the testicles, ovaries, and the mammary, thyroid, and parotid glands, should not be called chondromas — they are teratomas. They originate from misplaced embryonic cells.

**Combinations.** Chondromas are frequently combined with other connective tissue elements and are reported as osteochondromas, chondro-osteomas, or fibrochondromas.

**Prognosis.** The prognosis of chondromas is good. Usually they are located in areas where surgical removal can be accomplished, and since they are well encapsulated, it is quite easy to remove them from the tissue in their entirety.

### Osteoma

An osteoma is a benign bony growth which is often hard to differentiate from inflammatory new formation of bone such as the exostoses which so frequently occur on the limbs of horses or on the mandible of the horse in the region receiving trauma from the manger or breaker bits. The latter are not true neoplasms.

**Macroscopic appearance.** Osteomas are generally small, slow-growing tumors attached to the skeleton. These tumors are sharply circumscribed and encapsulated. They are round or elliptical in shape. If they have a tendency to show irregularities, they probably are injury-caused exostoses rather than neoplasms.

**Microscopic appearance.** The arrangement of lamellae is like that of normal bone. The Haversian canals are not so regular and run at right angle to the bone axis. Marrow may be seen in the large canals. The capsule of the tumor is similar to the bone periosteum.

**Location.** The bones of the head, particularly those of the nasal passages of horses and cattle and those in the orbital region are the principal locations of osteomas. Osteoma-like masses are occasionally found in the lungs, diaphragm, mesentery, mammary gland, testicle, ovary, and in the right cardiac atrium. Some of these are examples of metaplasia; others originate from misplaced embryonic cells; that is, they are teratomas and not true osteomas.

**Combinations.** At times osteomas will contain considerable white fibrous connective tissue or cartilage. This is observed most frequently in the nasal passages of the horse.

**Prognosis.** The prognosis of an osteoma is good if the tumor exists in an area where surgical removal can be performed.

### Leiomyoma

A benign of tumor of smooth muscle is called a leiomyoma.

**Macroscopic appearance.** The leiomyomas vary considerably in size from a few millimeters to as much as 18 centimeters in diameter. They are usually spherical or elliptical in shape and tend to be rather demarked from the surrounding tissue. They are located in areas where smooth muscle is usually found. They are usually pink in color. The tumor tends to be firm in consistency, and in those in which considerable connective tissue is deposited, the texture is exceedingly dense and sclerotic. Areas of degeneration, necrosis, and hemorrhages are usually not contained within the tumor. Those tumors that protrude into the lumen of an organ may have an ulcerated surface (vaginal leiomyoma). On cross section the tumor is made up of interlacing fibers and strands of tissue that tend to have somewhat of a whorled appearance, and the surface tends to have a glassy, rather dry appearance in contrast to the fibroma.

**Microscopic appearance.** The basic cell type is a long spindle-shaped cell containing an elliptically shaped nucleus. The nuclei are rather rich in chromatin, and the nucleoli are not prominent. At times the muscle cells are interspersed with white fibrous connective tissue cells, and it is difficult to determine whether the cells are fibroblasts or myoblasts. For this reason connective tissue stains, such as Van Gieson's stain, should be used to determine accurately whether the tissue is muscle or connective tissue. The collagen of connective tissue stains red with Van Gieson's stain while muscle tissue stains yellow.

Histological examination reveals the cells to be arranged in bundles, strands, and bands that interlace and form somewhat of a whorled pattern. Usually the muscle cells merge with the normal musculature of the organ, showing the origin of the cells.

**Location.** Leiomyomas are most frequently encountered in the musculature of the tubular and hollow organs such as the digestive tract, urinary tract, and genital tract. In the horse they are usually located in the wall of the small intestine. In the dog they are quite frequently encountered in the walls of the uterus and the vagina. Those attached to the wall of the vagina are often pedunculated and may protrude through the vulva. A leiomyoma is commonly located in the mesosalpinx of the chicken where it is found as a firm globular mass measuring one to three centimeters in diameter.

**Prognosis.** Leiomyomas located in areas where surgery can be performed are quite easily removed. Many of the leiomyomas are not discovered until after the death of the animal. This is particularly true when they are located in the wall of a hollow organ, such as the intestine, where their size causes an obstruction to the passage of secretion, excretion, or ingesta, and death of the animal occurs as the result of this obstruction.

## Rhabdomyoma

The rhabdomyoma is a benign tumor of skeletal or cardiac muscle. Rhabdomyomas are uncommon. Most of those that have been described have occurred in the myocardium, the lateral thoracic wall or the muscles of the limbs.

**Macroscopic appearance.** These tumors are most easily observed in the myocardium where they appear as a globular mass one to three centimeters in diameter. In consistency and color they resemble heart muscle. Probably many of these striated muscle tumors in the skeletal musculature are overlooked unless they become exceedingly large.

**Microscopic examination.** The basic cell of the rhabdomyoma is the cardiac muscle cell or the striated muscle cell. The cells resemble the parent tissue, and exact identification of their nature depends upon the demonstration of the cross striations with special staining technics (silver stains).

**Prognosis.** Most rhabdomyomas are found at necropsy when the heart or skeletal musculature is examined. They apparently do not contribute to the death of the individual.

### Sarcoma

A sarcoma is a malignant tumor of all tissue other than epithelium. The five principal types of connective tissue sarcomas are fibrosarcoma, myxosarcoma, liposarcoma, chondrosarcoma, and osteosarcoma.

**Macroscopic appearance.** Sarcomas vary much in appearance, but they have some characteristics in common (Figs. 13.11, 13.12, 13.13, and 19.14). All of them are fleshy in appearance, hence the name sarcoma from *sarko* in Greek meaning flesh.

Slowly growing sarcomas are white or grayish white in color and relatively firm in consistency. Rapidly growing sarcomas are white, gray, or pink in color and are encephaloid in consistency. Examination of the cut surface reveals that the tumor consists of interlacing bands or strands of tumor tissue. Areas of degeneration, necrosis, and hemorrhage are scattered throughout the tumor, particularly in the more central areas. These retrogressive

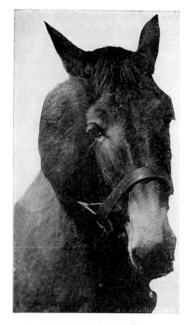

Fig. 13.11 — Fibrosarcoma involving lower mandibular and upper cervical region of a 4-year-old mule. Weight of tumor — 14.5 kg. (32 pounds avoir). (G. R. Fowler.)

primary. These metastatic tumors spread most frequently by way of the blood vascular system and eventually reach the lungs. They then become widely disseminated throughout the body. The sarcomas may also metastasize by way of the lymphatic system and then follow the lymph node chain draining the area in which the tumor is found.

The macroscopic recognition of a connective tissue sarcoma depends first of all on determining if the tumor is composed of connective tissue and secondly, whether fat, muscle, cartilage, or bone can be found within the tumor.

**Microscopic appearance.** The basic cell of the sarcoma is the primitive connective tissue cell. The more malignant the sarcoma, the closer it resembles this primitive connective tissue cell; the more differentiated the cell is, the easier it is to establish the identity of the tissue. Since all sarcomas basically come from this primitive connective tissue cell, difficulty is experienced with the more malignant types in determining just exactly the nomenclature to be applied to the tumor. If osteoid or osseous tissue is detected in the tumor, it is called an osteosarcoma (Figs. 13.15 and 17.8). If cartilage is found, it is designated as a chondrosarcoma. If fat is present, it is a liposarcoma. If muscle is present, it is called a leiomyosarcoma or a rhabdomyosarcoma. If no differentiated

changes occur most often in very rapidly growing tumors where the blood supply becomes insufficient for the large mass of young tissue. At the periphery of the neoplasm a distinct capsule is lacking. The macroscopic appearance of secondary or metastatic sarcomas is the same as the

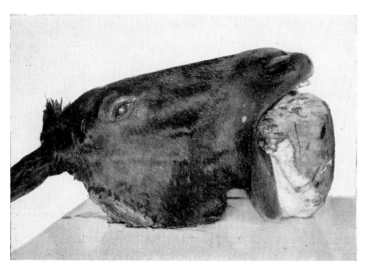

Fig. 13.12 — Osteosarcoma of the mandible of a horse. (Thorp and Graham, Jour. A.V.M.A.)

tissue can be found, it is called a fibrosarcoma (Fig. 13.14). The degree of tissue differentiation within a sarcoma varies greatly from extremely embryonal or primitive connective tissue cells to cells that are quite adult and well differentiated types. For this reason it is very important to examine representative portions of tissue from all parts of the neoplasm. Unless this is done, errors in diagnosis may be made.

Many sarcomas contain numerous blood vessels. Frequently they are thin walled, and the endothelial cells are large. At times these capillaries have an extremely large lumen resembling sinusoids. It is a common error to consider these as blood vessel tumors and to designate them as hemangiosarcomas when actually they are vascular fibrosarcomas. No diagnosis of hemangiosarcoma should be made without extremely careful consideration of the primary and secondary tumor sites, the history, and the breed of animal involved.

Retrogressive changes occur most often in very rapidly growing tumors where the blood supply becomes insufficient for the large mass of young tissue. At the

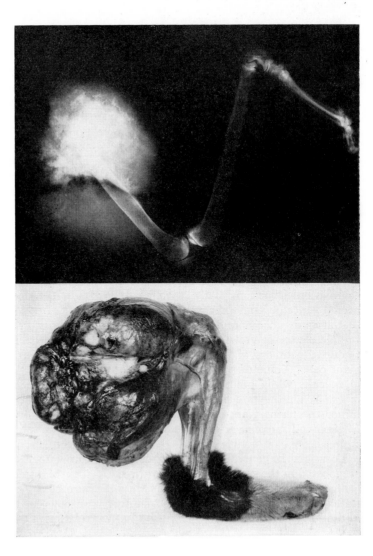

Fig. 13.13 — **Above:** X-ray of osteochondrosarcoma of left hind leg of 13-year-old cat. **Below:** Dissection showing tumor mass. (Stubbs, Jour. A.V.M.A.)

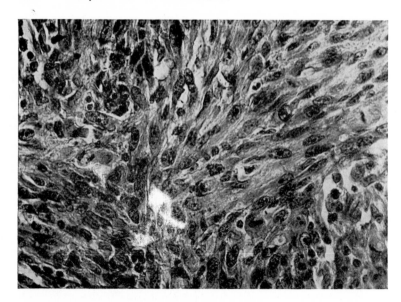

Fig. 13.14 — Fibrosarcoma from hind leg of a dog. Note spindle-shaped cells, hyperchromatic n u c l e i , and mitotic figures denoting malignancy. X400. (Department of Veterinary Pathology, Iowa State University.)

periphery of the neoplasm a distinct capsule is lacking. The macroscopic appearance of secondary or metastatic sarcomas is the same as the primary.

The cells of the osteosarcomas tend to have very distinct outlines, giving the cellular component a rather hard appearance much the same as if the cells had been printed on very highly differentiating photographic paper (Fig. 13.15). Even though osteoid or osseous tissue is not observed in the neoplasm, this characteristic of the cells is quite reliable in establishing a diagnosis of osteosarcoma. The bone in the vicinity of an osteosarcoma usually shows extensive destruction. This is to be expected since a characteristic of bone is that it undergoes demineralization whenever active tissue growth is present. Quite frequently tumors of bone contain many giant cells. Some of these are true tumor giant cells while others are fused osteocytes. When they are numerous in a bone tumor the terms **giant-cell tumor of bone** or **giant-cell sarcoma** are used.

**Location.** In general, primary sarcomas are located in the same sites as the various benign connective tissue tumors. Metastatic sarcomas are found most frequently in the lungs.

Fibrosarcomas, chondrosarcomas, and osteosarcomas are extremely common in the mammary gland of the dog and are associated with the proliferation of glandular epithelium. The tumor growth in the mammary gland of the dog is associated with hormonal stimulation. The hormone stimulates both glandular and connective tissue elements. In the case of the connective tissue elements, metaplasia occurs and all connective tissue types of tumors may be found. Since these neoplasms contain so many different tissues, they are frequently diagnosed as **mixed mammary gland tumors.**

In the dog osteosarcomas are observed most frequently involving the scapula, humerus, radius, tibia, and fibula. They tend to be located near the ends of the bone; a common site is the distal end of the radius. They are more frequent in the larger breeds of dogs such as the German shepherd. Quite often the tumor appears in a bone in which fracture has occurred at some previous time. The importance of the fracture in the appearance of the tumor is still open to debate, but the history of osteosarcoma following the fracture of a long bone in the heavier breeds of dogs is so common that an etiologic relation must be present.

In the equine, osteosarcomas frequently involve the bones enclosing the nasal cavity and sinuses.

Leiomyosarcomas are occasionally encountered. They are most frequently seen along with fibrous connective tissue, cartilage, bone, and glandular elements in the mammary gland of the dog.

Rhabdomyosarcomas are extremely uncommon. Those that have been described have involved the lateral thoracic wall or the muscles of the thighs.

**Prognosis.** The prognosis of all sarcomas is unfavorable. Since they represent malignant tumors that can eventually destroy the animal, prompt and radical surgery is usually required if death is to be prevented.

There is considerable variation in the degree of malignancy of sarcomas as well as variation in type. The fibrosarcoma is the most serious because it is most frequently encountered and is usually quite malignant.

Osteosarcomas tend to metastasize rather late — a fact which is of importance to the clinician because early removal of the primary growth may save the life of the animal. In the horse, extensive involvement of the head may be present, yet no metastases will be found in other organs.

## MASTOSARCOMA

This is a tumor chiefly of dogs, but occasionally of cats. The parent cells are the mast cells of the connective tissue of the skin. The tumor may develop anywhere in the skin, but the favored sites are the thighs and external genitals. Mast cell tumors usually appear at a later age than histiosarcomas. The majority occur in the age range of 6 to 15 years. Sex seems to have no relationship to incidence, but breed does. The tumor is reported most often in Boston terriers, fox terriers, boxers, and English setters.

**Macroscopic appearance.** The mastosarcoma usually originates as a small, solitary swelling in the corium of the skin but may have a multicentric origin. It gradually infiltrates the surrounding tissues so that the demarcation between tumor and normal tissue becomes lost. Most mastosarcomas vary in size from 1 cm. up to 20 cm. in diameter. There is a tendency for about 30 per cent of them to ulcerate. It is believed that the ulceration is brought

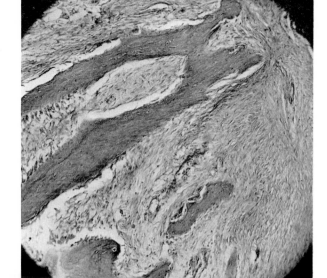

Fig. 13.15 — A photomicrograph of a section of the osteosarcoma shown in Fig. 13.12. ×80. (Thorp and Graham, Jour. A.V.M.A.)

about in two ways: (1) by tumor cell invasion of the epidermis which, as a result of pressure and ischemia, destroys the epithelium, and (2) by mechanical rubbing.

On section the cut surface is gray, pink-gray, or white, and has a lobulated or whorled appearance. The consistency varies according to the rapidity of growth. Slowly growing tumors are often soft and spongy while the rapidly growing ones are firm. Encapsulation or pedunculation is lacking. Metastasis and recurrence take place quite often.

**Microscopic appearance.** The majority of the tumor cells are round, oval, or polyhedral. The borders of these cells are often indistinct or fuzzy. The nuclei are round or oval with a distinct nuclear membrane. The chromatin granules are medium to coarse, and usually more prominent at the periphery of the nucleus. One or more nucleoli may be observed. In hematoxylin- and eosin-stained sections, the metachromatic cytoplasmic granules that characterize this tumor are not usually apparent. Therefore it is necessary to use Giemsa's or Nissl's staining methods to demonstrate the granules.

Even though metachromatic granules are not found in the mastosarcoma, that does not mean a diagnosis of mastosarcoma cannot be made. There is a tendency to call all mastosarcomas in which metachromatic granules are not numerous or cannot be found histiosarcomas without any consideration being given to the other characteristics of the two neoplasms.

Bundles of collagenous fibers surrounding large numbers of tumor cells may give the tumor a lobulated or whorled appearance. A predominant feature in this tumor is the occurrence of numerous leukocytes such as neutrophils and eosinophils.

In the slowly growing tumors, mitotic figures are not very obvious but tend to increase with the degree of malignancy.

### HISTIOSARCOMA

A histiosarcoma is a tumor composed of histiocytes. It is located in the skin, vulva, vagina, penis, or prepuce of dogs.

In the literature this tumor is also referred to as canine condyloma, venereal granuloma, infectious sarcoma, infectious lymphosarcoma, and transmissible lymphosarcoma.

**Macroscopic appearance.** These tumors are single or multiple, small or large, soft or friable, sessile or pedunculated, nodular or papillary masses, and gray to red in color. In the vaginal mucosa the nodules are often red and vary in size from nodules of several millimeters to large ulcerating masses that may protrude from the vulva. Ulceration, necrosis, and hemorrhage of the tumor may occur. If metastasis takes place, it usually involves only the regional lymph nodes.

**Microscopic appearance.** The histiosarcoma is characterized by round, oval, or polyhedral cells which often have indistinct boundaries and poorly stained cytoplasm when stained with hematoxylin and eosin (Fig. 13.16). The nucleus is large, round, or oval with fine chromatin granules and an eccentrically situated nucleolus. The cytoplasm stains pale pink with eosin unless overstained with hematoxylin. Then it may be slightly bluish. Metachromatic granules are not observed when a special stain such as Giemsa's is used. Mitotic figures are quite numerous.

The cells usually appear in compact masses which are surrounded by a connective tissue stroma. This tends to give the tumor an alveolar arrangement. In some instances the cells are arranged in rows or columns with a well-defined stroma. If ulceration and necrosis have occurred, inflammatory cells and hemorrhage will be seen throughout the neoplasm.

Great care should be taken not to diagnose mastosarcomas as histiosarcomas. Just because metachromatic granules are not found in a tumor of the skin of the dog, that does not mean the tumor is a histiosarcoma. The other morphological characteristics of the tumor must also be considered, particularly the staining characteristics of the cell with hematoxylin and eosin, the presence of mitotic figures,

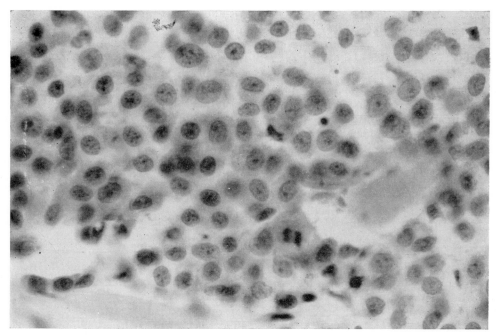

Fig. 13.16 — Signs of anaplasia in a histiosarcoma of a dog: large nuclei, some with large nucleoli; nucleoli often eccentrically placed; hyperchromatism of some nuclei; prominent mitotic figures. ×780. (Department of Veterinary Pathology, Michigan State University.)

and the alveolar arrangement of the tumor. Particular caution should be exercised if involvement of the genital organs is not observed in the local dog population. If tumors of the genital organs are never encountered, one is probably observing mastosarcomas rather than histiosarcomas. The histiosarcoma is a tumor of young dogs while the mastosarcoma is found in older animals.

**Location.** Viable cells are transmitted from dog to dog by coitus. Most of the tumors are confined to the genitalia but occasionally may appear in the skin on other parts of the body. It is a tumor of younger dogs — one to six years of age — and is more common in the female.

**Prognosis.** The surgery associated with the removal of these tumors must be done with great care because the cells of the histiosarcoma can be easily transplanted in the wound of surgery or may contaminate other portions of the body. Because of the ease with which these cells are transplanted, recurrence of the tumor is quite frequent. The tumor seldom extends to the regional lymph nodes or distant organs. The neoplasm can be of considerable concern if it is present in a kennel or a stud because of the ease with which it is transmitted to other dogs.

Occasionally dogs will have an extensive involvement of the turbinate bones resulting in considerable destruction of the skull. The skull deformity that results as well as the copious nasal exudate usually results in a request for euthanasia. It is believed that infection occurs as the result of the inhalation of tumor cells during the process of social introduction as practiced by dogs.

Because of the unsightly nature of the neoplasm and its tendency to ulcerate and recur, many owners request the affected dog be euthanized. However, if the owner can tolerate the unpleasantness associated with the neoplasm, he will find that these neoplasms will spontaneously regress, and when they do, the dogs appear to be immune to further transplants.

## NERVOUS TISSUE TUMORS

Tumors composed of nerve cells and fibers (neuromas) and of neuroglia (gliomas) are common. Tumor-like masses of coiled, regenerating axis cylinders covered with connective tissue, which develop at the ends of nerves following neurectomy in horses, are called **amputation neuromas.** They are not true neoplasms.

The incidence of neoplasms of the central nervous system depends upon the interest one has in looking for these new growths and the time he will devote to careful examination of brain, spinal cord, and the peripheral nervous system.

The **primary tumors** of the brain and spinal cord are particularly common in the brachiocephalic type of dog, in fact they are so common in the boxer breed that the brain and spinal cord of every boxer coming to necropsy should be examined for the presence of a neoplasm even though clinical symptoms of neoplasia were not present.

**Secondary tumors** of the central nervous system that reach the brain by metastasis are exceedingly common. The reason they are seldom found is that the brain is not routinely examined for the presence of neoplasms when malignancies are found in other organs.

These brain tumors are present in about 2 per cent of canines submitted for post-mortem examination. The incidence is lower in the other domestic mammals, probably because the meat-producing breeds are usually slaughtered at a very early age. Next to the dog, the neoplasms are most frequently observed in the bovine. Tumors of the leukosis complex are very common in the chicken.

The examination of the brain and spinal cord for neoplasms must be done with the fixed specimen. The brain and spinal cord must be fixed in 25 per cent formalin until thoroughly hardened, which requires approximately one week. Fixation should be accomplished in the refrigerator so as to prevent putrefaction within the brain. If this is not done, particularly in warm weather, numerous gas bubbles will be found within the brain, giving the organ a "Swiss cheese" appearance. When this occurs the brain is not suitable for histological examination. Following fixation, the entire brain and cord is cut with a brain knife at intervals of not more than 5 mm. at right angles to the long axis of the brain and cord. Careful examination of the cut surface of all sections should be made for any abnormal color or distortion of tracts and nuclei.

The histological identification of brain tumors is based upon the identification of the cell composing them, whether they are glia, ependymal cells, neurones, or those arising from the meninges or the blood vascular system. The **primary brain tumors** are usually single and do not metastasize to distant organs. Since they are single and do not metastasize, they are often described by using a benign tumor nomenclature such as **glioma** or **glioblastoma,** but since they are progressively invasive and eventually bring about the death of the individual, the use of the term **gliosarcoma** is appropriate.

Tumors of the glia are most common and are designated as **gliomas.** If the cell type is differentiated enough, additional terms such as **astrocytoma** or **oligodendroglioma** may be used. If the astroglioma is sufficiently differentiated so that it can be determined whether they are protoplasmic or fibrous astrocytes, the terms **protoplasmic astrocytoma** or **fibrous astrocytoma** may be used. If the neoplastic growth consists of ganglion cells, it is designated as a **ganglio-neuroma.** Tumors involving the ependymal cells of the ventricles are called **ependynomas.** These tumors usually can be recognized by their location in the vicinity of the ependyma, and frequently they protrude into the lumen of the ventricular system. Tumors involving the meninges are designated as **meningiomas.** A fairly common tumor involving the acoustic nerve is known as the acoustic nerve sheath tumor. The **acoustic nerve sheath tumors** are most common in the bovine. Careful consideration of the basic cell type within the neoplasm will usually indicate the type of tumor present. Since the classification of tumors of the central nervous system is so simple, it is regrettable that the average student unfamiliar with neurocytology becomes so confused by the very thought of neuroanatomy that he makes little if any attempt to classify these neoplasms.

The primary brain tumors in the domestic animals are usually found within the thalamus, pons, medulla oblongata, and cerebellum. Their location is such that it is impossible to remove them surgically. The meningiomas, so common in the human being, are much less frequent in the domestic animals. Likewise, the vascular hemartia, found in the brain of the human being, are very uncommon in domestic animals. Since these last two tumors are found primarily in the meninges, they can be removed with relative ease as compared to the tumors contained within the brain stem.

The secondary brain tumors are most frequently observed in the cerebral hemispheres. Quite often they are multiple, which in itself indicates they are metastatic. The majority of these metastatic tumors have their primary site in the lung or they represent metastasis from some other organ to the lung and later extension from the lung to the brain. In the dog the original tumor is most frequently located in the mammary gland or the thyroid gland.

## Nerve Sheath Tumors

The nerve sheath tumor is quite common in cattle. It is also present in other domestic animals. These tumors arise from the sheath of Schwann and are most frequently observed in the heart, brachial plexus, coeliac plexus, and along the intercostal nerves. In most instances, except where lesions involve the heart or the mediastinum, the tumors are found adjacent to or incorporated in one or more nerves, ganglia, or plexuses. Careful dissection is necessary if the association with nervous tissue is to be demonstrated. The tumors are usually found in several lo-

cations within the animal, indicating they have multicentric origin. They are usually benign and involve animals of all age groups.

**Macroscopic appearance.** Because of their benign progressive growth, lesions are generally overlooked until the tumors are large and the animal is considered to be in an older age group. The lesions in the brachial plexus are frequently bilateral and easily recognized by the extensive involvement of one or more nerves. The involved nerve is enlarged diffusely or has nodular masses within the nerve. The involved portion of the nerve is shiny and glistening, white to gray in color, often lobulated, slightly gelatinous in consistency, and at times contains areas of degeneration, necrosis, and hemorrhage. The highest incidence of the neoplasm is found in the heart. However, in routine meat inspection a thorough examination of the heart for tapeworm cysts is made, and it is quite likely that a higher percentage of cases involving other organs would be found if similar careful and detailed examinations were made. European literature indicates the highest incidence is found in the brachial plexus and this is probably correct.

**Microscopic appearance.** The tumor cells derived from the sheath of Schwann are elongated and spindle-shaped with oval or long cylindrical nuclei. The cells tend to arrange themselves parallel with each other, and this arrangement is called palisading. Distinct palisading of the cells is found in each tumor, and equally as characteristic is the alignment of cells in interlacing fasciculi and whorls. Intercellular fibers similar to a fine reticulum, or, in the more solid or compactly organized tumors, connective tissue collagen is present. The orderly arrangement in bundles of parallel cells and intercellular fibers and the whorling of the tissue into structures resembling Meissner's corpuscles is quite characteristic. The tendency to regard connective tissue tumors as neurofibrosarcomas on the basis of nuclear palisading alone may lead to confusion in diagnosis. Therefore, it is highly important to consider the location of the neoplasm and its relation to nerves in establishing it as a nerve sheath tumor.

**Prognosis.** The prognosis of nerve sheath tumors is usually good. Occasionally the involvement of a spinal nerve may cause pressure on the spinal cord, or involvement of a major nerve such as one of those of the brachial plexus may interfere with locomotion. Since the tumors appear to have a multicentric origin, little hope can be expected in removing all of the tumors by surgical procedures.

## ENDOTHELIAL TUMORS

Tumors may arise from endothelial cells of capillaries or lymphatics. The benign ones are called hemangiomas and lymphangiomas. The malignant ones are designated hemangiosarcomas and lymphangiosarcomas. Primary malignant hemangiosarcomas have been reported in the liver and spleen of dogs. Hemangiosarcomas are most frequently observed in the German shepherd dog. In the Michigan State University collection, three were primary in the subcutis of dogs. This tumor has also been reported in horses and cattle. Lymphangiomas and lymphangiosarcomas are of such rare occurrence that they will not be described.

Extreme caution should be exercised when observing tumors composed of blood vessels before a diagnosis of hemangioma or hemangiosarcoma is made. The majority of tumors consisting primarily of blood vessels are not hemangiomas or hemangiosarcomas. Quite frequently they are merely vascular fibrosarcomas. The majority of so-called hemangiomas and hemangiosarcomas are actually blood vascular hemartia, or developmental defects in the blood vascular system. The common red birthmark of man is actually a vascular hemartia and not an angioma or a true tumor as it is often diagnosed.

Using the common red birthmark of man as an example, it is to be remembered that the birthmark is present at the time of birth or shortly thereafter. It has no power of progressive disproportionate growth but grows and enlarges as the individual grows and matures. If subjected to trauma, it may bleed profusely. There may be thrombosis, edema, and inflammation which give the growth the false clinical appearance of being a neoplasm. Frequently it will be noted that the hemartia are multiple. This in itself indicates it is probably a disturbance in growth and development rather than a neoplastic alteration, since true neoplasms, almost without exception, arise in one specific area. It is recognized that in many instances it is quite difficult to draw a line of distinction between vascular hemartia and hemangiomas or hemangiosarcomas, but simple observation of the case and careful evaluation of the history as to the length of time the tumor has been present, whether it has enlarged, if metastasis has occurred, and if the lesions are multiple will usually reveal whether the new growth is a hemartia or a neoplasm.

Care should be taken not to confuse hemangiomas or hemangiosarcomas with telangiectasis. Telangiectasis is the dilatation of pre-existing vessels. The telangiectatic alterations are most commonly observed in the liver of cattle. The pathogenesis for the vascular dilatation is apparently hepatic cell death and disintegration. The sinusoids within the liver, when no longer supported by the adjacent hepatic cells, undergo dilatation and when then observed, consist of greatly dilated channels within the liver. The endothelium lining these telangiectatic cavities is adult in type and shows none of the cellular characteristics of neoplasia. In addition, the telangiectasis usually occurs as multiple areas throughout the liver; and finally there is no invasion of the regional lymph nodes nor is there any evidence of metastasis to the lungs or other organs.

Quite frequently the circulatory changes associated with inflammation in which large numbers of capillaries are produced are confused with a hemangioma. Here again, history, location, and the ability to recognize the connective tissue and vascular arrangement of chronic inflammation are necessary if an error in diagnosis is to be prevented.

Hemartia are especially common in the skin and occasionally in the internal organs of White Leghorn chickens. The presence of these tumors in the skin is often detected when birds are submitted for post-mortem examination after fatal hemorrhage or when they are plucked during the process of slaughter for food. There may be multiple tumor growths in the skin, shanks, and occasionally in a feather follicle. When hemorrhage from the skin tumors occurs, it may initiate the vice of picking in a flock of birds. Then the basic lesion may be overlooked because the loss will be blamed on cannibalism.

The number of tumors varies greatly with the individual. At times only one tumor is observed but as many as twenty tumors have been found in the skin of some birds. The tumors vary in size from just visible reddish-blue patches in the skin to round bulging purple protrusions that measure as much as 3 cm. in diameter. As the hemartia increase in size, they project above the surrounding skin surface and become increasingly more susceptible to trauma. Massive hemorrhage occurs when the skin is broken and the walls of the capillaries and cavernous spaces are ruptured by trauma. Repeated hemorrhage from the same site is frequent, often leading to the death of the bird. The tendency of the birds to pick at blood-soiled areas favors the recurrence of hemorrhage.

Histological examination of these skin hemartia reveals they consist of small capillary nests and large masses of interlacing capillaries in the subcutaneous tissue and occasionally in the dermis. The neoplasms are covered with a thin layer of epidermis. Some of the tumors contain cavernous spaces and others contain hematocysts, which explains the sudden increase in size of some of the tumors. There is no indication that metastasis of the tumor occurs. The occasional bird in which involvement of the internal organs is observed probably represents defects in development rather than metastasis from the skin lesions.

Rigdon has produced similar hemartia in the skin of ducks following the application of irritating chemicals.

Hemangiomas may be divided into solid, capillary, and cavernous types. The capillary type consists of capillaries more or less uniform in size. The cavernous type is composed of capillaries that are greatly dilated. In contrast, the solid type consists of masses of endothelial cells in which little or no vascular lumen is discernible.

**Macroscopic appearance.** Hemangiomas are dark red or purple in color and soft in consistency. They bleed profusely when traumatized. In size they are variable, up to 15 or more cm. in diameter. Some have weighed as much as 2,000 grams.

While the color is generally red or purple, it should be said that this characteristic is variable depending upon how vascular the tumor really is. That is, the color varies with the proportion of endothelial cells to the number of lumina. This variation in composition of the hemangioma also affects the consistency. The more vascular type is red and soft; the more cellular type looks like a sarcoma and is more firm or solid. See Figures 13.17 and 17.39 for illustrations of each type.

**Microscopic appearance.** The more vascular type of hemangioma consists of newly formed capillaries lined usually by a single layer of endothelial cells. Occasionally two or three layers are present. The capillaries are surrounded by varying amounts of collagenous fibers. The more solid type of hemangioma may have relatively few lumina, but each lumen is lined with several layers of endothelial cells. In a hepatic hemangioma these cells appear to arise from the reticuloendothelial cells lining the sinusoids.

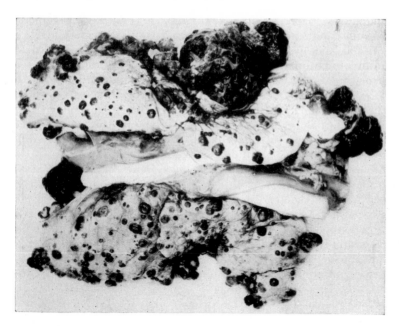

Fig. 13.17 — Hemangiosarcomas of the lungs of a dog. Soft, vascular type. (Department of Veterinary Pathology, Michigan State University.)

The nuclei of hemangiosarcomas are round, oval, or ellipsoidal, and have fine to medium chromatin granules. One or more nuclei may be present in a cell. Both normal and atypical mitotic figures are present. The cytoplasm is not conspicuously stained and the cell boundaries tend to fuse. Connective tissue fibrils make up the stroma.

Location. Hemangiomas and hemangiosarcomas are most frequently observed in the extremities, thorax, perianal region, and in the liver and spleen. The majority of these tumors are found in the German shepherd dog.

Prognosis. The prognosis of the hemartia and hemangiomas is good, as there is no recurrence after adequate surgery. The prognosis of the hemangiosarcoma is very unfavorable. Since it is a malignant tumor of blood vessels, metastasis occurs early and with relative ease because the malignant cells are in contact with the blood stream. Usually, by the time a hemangiosarcoma is recognized, the metastases are already so extensive that death is the result.

## TUMORS OF THE HEMATOPOIETIC TISSUES

Tumors of the hematopoietic tissues consist of two basic cell types, lymphocytes and myelocytes.

### Tumors Composed of Lymphocytes

A benign tumor composed of lymphocytes is known as a **lymphoma**. However, diagnosis of a lymphoma is seldom made because it is extremely difficult to decide whether the enlargement composed of lymphocytes represents hyperplasia of the lymphocytes as the result of irritation or whether it is a benign neoplastic growth.

The malignant form is called a lymphosarcoma. Immature lymphocytes comprise its parenchyma. There is little stroma. Rapid growth and easy and extensive metastasis are among its outstanding characteristics. Cattle, dogs, swine, and chickens are most commonly affected (Figs. 14.6, 14.7, 17.42, and 18.12).

Etiology. Lymphosarcomas possess a few outstanding characteristics which raise two questions about their etiology:

Why is metastasis confined principally to organs or parts consisting of lymphoid tissue, and why is there often intermittent fever in connection with their development? While this condition is to some degree transmissible, it has not yet been absolutely proven to be infectious except perhaps in the domestic fowl. Some of the transmission experiments have actually been transplantation experiments. In other experiments the irritants causing the condition appear to be nonspecific.

Lymphoid tissues throughout the body, whether contained in lymph nodes, the wall of the uterus, wall of the stomach, or in the lung, simultaneously show this neoplastic alteration. This suggests that some infectious agent, probably viral in nature, has existed or is existing as a septicemia and that all the lymphoid structures of the body coming in contact with this inciting agent undergo neoplasia.

A strikingly similar hyperplasia of the lymphatic system is observed in East Coast Fever in which there is a viremia and the lymphatic tissues in general are stimulated and proliferate. The uninitiated will probably diagnose their first case of East Coast Fever as a lymphosarcoma because of the similarity in lymphoid tissue hyperplasia.

The high incidence of lymphosarcoma in certain areas, on certain farms, and even within certain families of animals suggests that, just as in the chicken, a hereditary factor as well as an infectious agent is necessary if a lymphosarcoma is to occur. Probably, if the correct strains of animals, such as cattle, are obtained, transmission experiments with cell-free filtrates will be successful in transmitting the disease.

**Macroscopic appearance.** Lymphosarcomas may appear as solitary tumors, more or less sharply defined in organs composed of lymphatic tissue. They have the grayish-white color and appearance of the lymphoid tissue. In chickens, however, they may have a yellowish hue much like the nodules of tuberculosis. Because they become progressively larger while the surrounding tissue remains at a constant volume, their cut surface bulges. Lymphosarcomas are usually multiple.

When the tumor involves the lymphoid tissue in general, all of the lymphoid organs become greatly enlarged. As a result there is splenomegaly (Fig. 15.8), hepatomegaly, and enlargement of the lymph nodes (Figs. 15.7 and 15.8), tonsils, thymus, and Peyer's patches. The bone marrow is also involved and is grayish red or brownish red in color.

**Microscopic appearance.** The normal architecture of the involved lymphoid structure disappears. Normal lymphocytes are present, but their arrangement into follicles with germ centers, corpuscles with central arteries, cortex and medulla, sinuses and cords, cell-rich and cell-poor areas is gone. Besides the normal adult lymphocytes, there are myriads of embryonic cells quite variable in size (Fig. 13.18).

The total leukocyte count may show increases up to 5 times the normal number for horses, up to 15 for cattle and swine, and up to 60 for dogs. The predominating cells are lymphocytes and lymphoblasts. The total erythrocyte shows a marked decrease because the infiltrating lymphocytes cause atrophy of the erythropoietic tissue of the marrow. For the same reason there is a decrease in the number of granulocytes and platelets.

According to the degree of maturity of the lymphocytes comprising the tumor, they may be classified as follows: (1) Lymphosarcoma, lymphocyte type — meaning the lymphosarcoma is composed primarily of cells that resemble mature lymphocytes. (2) Lymphosarcoma, lymphoblast type — indicating the cells comprising the tumor are more immature and resemble lymphoblasts. (3) Lymphosarcoma, clasmatocyte type — signifying the lymphocytes are still more immature and resemble clasmatocytes in size, shape, and appearance. (4) Lymphosarcoma, stem-cell type — representing the most

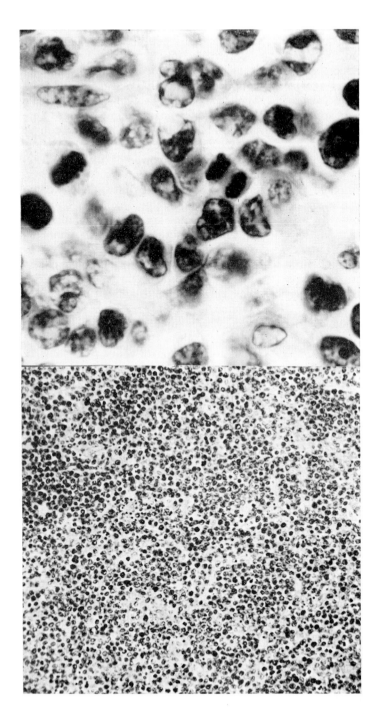

Fig. 13.18 — Lymphosarcoma of the abomasum of a cow. **Above:** Immature tumor cells with several cells in different phases of mitosis. X1,400. **Below:** Diffuse distribution of the tumor cells with scant stroma e v i d e n t . (Feldman, Jour. A.V.M.A.)

embryonic type of cell in which the primitive hematopoietic tissue cell is the primary constituent.

When the neoplastic cells are found circulating in the blood vascular system, the term **leukemia** is used. If the circulating cells are lymphocytic in origin, it is called a lymphocytic leukemia; likewise, if the cells consist of myeloid cells — those cells that mature into granulocytes — the leukemia is designated as myelocytic in type. Because of the irregularity with which the immature blood forms are found in the circulating blood stream, a great deal of confusion has arisen and many inappropriate terms have been coined. Of these terms, only the term leukemia, preceded by an adjective such as lymphocytic or myelocytic, should ever be used. This is particularly true in the domestic animals since the occurrence of immature cells in the circulatory system is much less frequently observed than in the human being. Likewise, it must be remembered that the appearance of these cells in the blood stream varies from day to day. They will be found for several days and then they may disappear for a number of days and then again recur. This appearance and disappearance of neoplastic cells in the circulatory system has only added to the confusion. Why the circulatory system is invaded on some occasions and not on others or why this invasion of the blood stream is variable from day to day has never been entirely explained. On the other hand, even the discharge of fully developed leukocytes and erythrocytes from the bone marrow into the circulatory system in the normal individual is likewise not clearly understood.

The term chronic leukemia should not be used, because the term chronic indicates connective tissue is being deposited and this is not true. The term chronic is reserved for a specific alteration in inflammation. Likewise the term acute leukemia should not be used because the term acute is reserved for certain vascular changes devoid of connective tissue proliferation under the subject of inflammation. Subleukemic and aleukemic should never be used, and the term aleukemic leukemia is even more undesirable. If cells are not circulating in the blood stream, the term leukemia cannot be used at all because the term signifies that leukocytes are present in the blood stream. In the growth and development of these neoplastic alterations, certain periods may exist in which the immature cells will invade the circulating blood stream, and when this occurs, the hematological alteration is designated as a leukemia.

**Location.** Lymphosarcomas are located first of all in pre-existing lymphoid tissue. In the very malignant generalized types the tumor cells invade the systemic circulation and collect in and around the vessels in various organs. In cattle a rather frequent location is the wall of the forestomachs and heart.

### Tumors Composed of Myelocytes

Tumors arising from myeloid tissues are not as common as those arising from lymphocytes. The benign tumor composed of myeloid cells is known as a **myeloma.** This diagnosis is seldom made, and before the term is used, very careful consideration of the neoplastic alteration must be made. A myelosarcoma is a malignant tumor of myeloid cells. In general it can be said that all tumors of myeloid cells are myelosarcomas, and according to their differentiation they are designated as neutrophilic, eosinophilic, or basophilic in type. The basophilic type has been more popularly designated as a mastosarcoma. In the domestic fowl the very important disease, leukosis, which is caused by a virus, assumes forms which can properly be considered as neoplasms of myeloid cells.

**Macroscopic appearance.** Myelosarcomas involve the hemopoietic tissues in general. As would be expected, the lesions are found most frequently in the bone marrow. In addition, involvement of the lymph nodes, liver, and spleen occurs. The tumor may also be found in other organs.

In mammals there is a tendency for the tumor to have a bright pale-green color which tends to fade when exposed to air. This color may be restored temporarily if a solution of hydrogen peroxide is applied to the tumor tissue.

The tumor is most commonly found in the domestic fowl, but in this species it does not have a green color. It is white to grayish white in color, and the masses are rather friable in consistency. They are most frequently encountered in the chicken, other than in the bone marrow, adjacent to the periosteum, particularly on the visceral surface of the sternum and the posteriomedial surface of the ribs.

In cattle this tumor may be easily confused with eosinophilic myositis. Eosinophilic myositis, believed to be a parasitic invasion of muscle, is usually confined to skeletal and cardiac muscle. The reason it is confused with the myelosarcoma is that the lesions are green in color and the predominent cell is the eosinophil. Examination of the bovine reveals that in the true myelosarcoma there will also be involvement of the regional lymph nodes, bone marrow, spleen, and other tissues.

**Microscopic appearance.** The basic cell constituent of the myelosarcoma is the myelocyte in its various stages or various degrees of differentiation. According to the differentiation that is present, they are classified as neutrophilic, eosinophilic, or basophilic. The cells vary greatly in morphology from rather large cells with prominent nuclei, which is the primitive myelocyte, to those cells that possess an irregular, indented, or lobulated nucleus and contain basophilic or eosinophilic granules in their cytoplasm. Mitotic figures are numerous. A typical myelosarcoma usually contains primitive myelocytes, neutrophils, eosinophils, basophils and even lymphocytes. The myelosarcoma of the fowl is the most constant in its histological appearance. This tumor is composed of roughly spherical cells containing oval-shaped nuclei and the cytoplasm of the cell is filled with large eosinophilic granules.

A sample of blood drawn from a case of granulocytic leukemia coagulates slowly, is pale red or light brown in color, and after coagulating presents a thick grayish-white layer of leukocytes on top of the red cell layer which may have less than the normal thickness. The delayed clotting is the result of a deficiency in platelets, and the thinner red layer is the result of the crowding-out effect of the proliferating granulocytes in the bone marrow.

The total count of leukocytes shows an increase which may reach 20,000 to 40,000 in dogs, the animals whose blood is most frequently examined in this disease. More than 100,000 have been reported in dogs, however.

In differential counts, neutrophils make up 80 to 90 per cent of the number; myelocytes and myeloblasts up to 4 to 6 per cent. Eosinophils increase in the early stages but decrease later. Monocytes increase about 10 per cent. The lymphocyte count remains normal or only slightly decreased. There is a falling off of erythrocytes and platelets because the cells which form them are crowded out by the proliferating granulocytes. The erythrocytes which are present frequently are variable in size (anisocytosis), irregular in shape and size (poikilocytosis), and stain atypically (polychromasia) because they are being formed under stress. Associated with this decrease in erythrocytes there is a diminution in the total hemoglobin.

**Location.** The tumor is most frequently found in the bone marrow, then in the liver, spleen, lymph nodes, and other organs throughout the body. In the chicken it is especially common adjacent to the periosteum of the sternum and the ribs.

**Prognosis.** The prognosis is extremely unfavorable. Surgical removal is impossible because the tumor is found throughout the body. In the chicken where the infectious nature together with the hereditary susceptibility to the neoplasm has been demonstrated, the selection of birds from flocks in which the tumor does not occur is the best method of controlling the disease. In domestic mammals, hereditary and infectious factors have not been demonstrated.

The anemia which accompanies granulocytic leukemia results in hypoxia which causes degeneration (cloudy swelling and fatty degeneration) of the heart, liver, and kidneys. The capillary endothelium is also affected by the hypoxia and becomes more permeable. This permits petechial (purpuric) hemorrhages to form which are made more numerous by the deficiency in platelets (thrombocytopenia). The functions of the enlarged organs are upset, and pressure exerted by these organs upon other organs disturbs their functions. The termination is practically always death.

## AVIAN LEUKOSIS COMPLEX

In the domestic fowl there is a disease or a disease complex that is variously designated as fowl leukemia, fowl leukosis, range paralysis, fowl paralysis, iritis, lymphomatosis, lymphocytoma, neurolymphomatosis, leukotic tumors, and leukemoid disease. In order to facilitate uniformity in terminology and in the interpretation of data with reference to these diseases most of the above terms should be eliminated and in their place the simple classification listed below should be used.

1. Lymphocytic leukosis
   a. Neural
   b. Visceral
   c. Ocular
   d. Osteopetrotic

2. Myelocytic leukosis
   a. Erythrocytic
   b. Granulocytic

From the economic standpoint this disease is of great importance. Experiments seem to indicate that the various manifestations of leukosis are caused by a single etiologic agent, *Trifur gallinarum*, which is filtrable, transplantable, and has the properties of a virus.

The forms of lymphocytic leukosis are:

1. **Neural,** also called range or fowl paralysis, in which the spinal and cranial nerves are attacked. Involvement of the brachial and lumbrosacral plexuses or the nerves originating from them results in partial or complete paralysis of the wings and legs (Figs. 13.19 and 13.20). Involvement of the vagus nerve in young chicks is indicated by the appearance of respiratory symptoms unaccompanied by a mucoid or purulent exudate in the air passages. Involvement of the splanchnic plexus is shown by obscure digestive disturbances.

2. **Visceral,** characterized by a diffuse or localized infiltration of lymphoid cells in any visceral organ.

3. **Ocular,** in which the iris becomes gray and the pupil distorted, resulting in blindness (Fig. 13.21).

4. **Osteopetrotic,** characterized by alterations in the shaft and marrow cavity of the long bones of the wings and legs so that they become thickened and very hard.

The forms of myelocytic leukosis are:

1. **Erythrocytic,** in which excessive numbers of immature red cells appear in the circulating blood and other organs, such as the liver and spleen (Fig. 13.22).

2. **Granulocytic,** which is similar to the

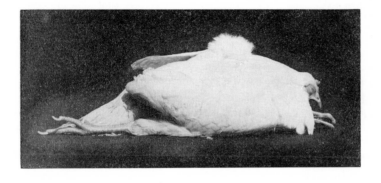

Fig. 13.19 — A characteristic position of a bird in an advanced stage of neural lymphocytic leukosis. (Doyle, Jour. A.V.M.A.)

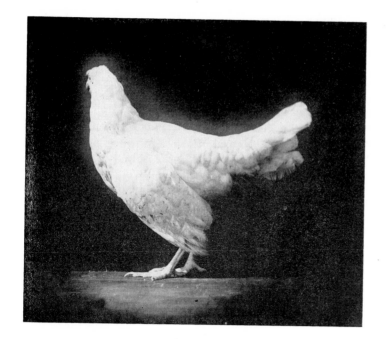

Fig. 13.20 — A drooping wing due to involvement of the nerves of the brachial plexus in neural leukosis. (Doyle, Jour. A.V.M.A.)

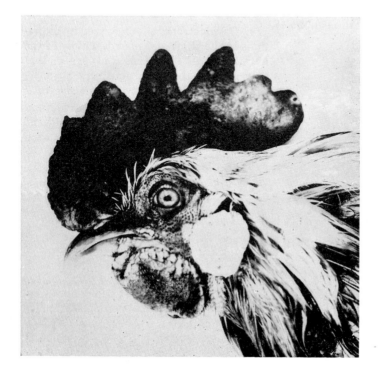

Fig. 13.21 — A mature cock bird, showing the peculiar "white eye" frequently associated with ocular leukosis. (Doyle, Jour. A.V.M.A.)

erythrocytic form except that the cells undergoing the increase in numbers are immature granulocytes instead of immature erythrocytes.

**Susceptibility and period of incubation.** The knowledge concerning susceptibility, period of incubation, and course of leukosis is far from complete. Information available relative to these factors is based mostly on experimental birds and is often confusing and contradictory. Apparently birds of all ages are susceptible. In farm flocks the effects of the disease are noticed most when birds are from three to eleven months of age. The course depends upon the parts of the body affected and is therefore quite variable. Obviously a bird with paralysis of the wings or even of its legs can survive longer than one which is blind or one with paralysis of the splanchnic or the vagus nerve or with involvement of the liver.

**Pathogenesis.** The pathogenesis of the avian leukosis complex lacks much of having been completely determined. The manner in which the transmissible agent enters the body under natural conditions is not known. Even the results of experimental transmission are not uniform.

It is apparent that leukosis spreads by contact and that it is transmitted through the egg. After a variable period of incubation, depending upon the stock and its genetic constitution, the lymphocytic form makes its appearance by symptoms which are traceable to abnormal, extravascular accumulations of lymphoid cells. These infiltrations can occur in any part of the body.

It has been surmised that the viral agent may be introduced into susceptible birds by the bites of certain ectoparasites such as mites, ticks, and mosquitoes, but experiments to prove this have not been of absolute conclusiveness. Transmisson through the egg has been demonstrated.

Experimentally, leukosis can be transmitted by the inoculation of various body fluids and tissue emulsions of diseased birds into susceptible ones. It appears that it also can be transmitted by immunizing chickens for fowl pox with a vaccine prepared from pox nodules removed from chickens affected with leukosis. Follow-

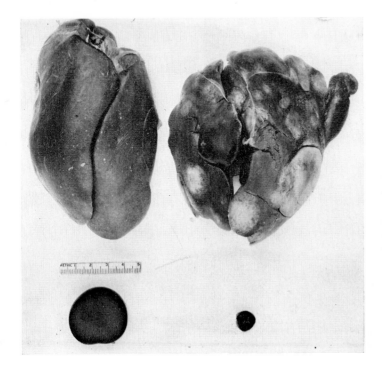

Fig. 13.22 — The liver and spleen on the left are from a chicken affected with spontaneous erythroleukosis. Specimens on the right were obtained from a chicken affected with lymphocytic leukosis. (Feldman and Olson, Jour. A.V.M.A.)

ing successful inoculation, the blood stream becomes so burdened with immature erythrocytes or granulocytes that highly vascular organs like the liver and spleen become packed with them (Fig. 13.23).

The pathogenesis of the bone form (osteopetrosis) is very complex. The process seems to begin in the connective tissue of the periosteum and endosteum, or in the epiphyseal cartilage. A diffuse thickening occurs in these places, accompanied by an excessive calcification. As a result, the compact bone on the outside of the shaft as well as the spongy bone next to the marrow cavity becomes exceedingly thick and marble-like. The marrow cavity becomes constricted while the diaphysis in general becomes thicker.

Lesions. In the neural form there may be no macroscopic changes. Frequently, though, the lumbosacral plexus, the brachial plexus, and their branches are enlarged, grayish instead of white in color, and entirely opaque instead of partially transparent, so that the normal zigzag course of the bundles of nerve fibers in the nerve trunk cannot be distinguished. The splanchnic plexus and its branches to the viscera often display the same changes. These latter alterations probably account for sickness and death of some affected birds that do not show the usual paralytic symptoms of the legs and wings which

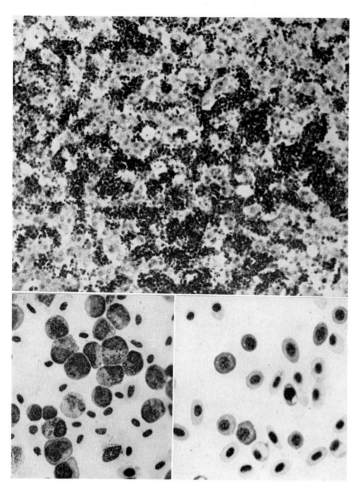

Fig. 13.23 — **Above:** Liver of a chicken with erythrocytic leukosis. The marked engorgement of the blood sinusoids with erythroblasts is characteristic. X220. **Below, left:** Blood-film of chicken with myelocytic leukosis. **Below, right:** Erythrocytic leukosis. X540. (Feldman and Olson, Jour. A.V.M.A.)

characterize fowl paralysis. Other nerves which are visibly involved are the vagus and the intercostals. Microscopically, the affected nerves show focal infiltrations of large and small lymphoid cells (Fig. 13.24). Degeneration and edema of the nerves accompany the lymphoid cell infiltration.

In the ocular form the optic nerve and the iris are frequently infiltrated with lymphoid cells. When the iris is involved, it becomes grayish white and the pupil small. This lesion constitutes the "white eye" of fowl paralysis. Birds may have this lesion without showing signs of other anatomical alterations. This form must not be confused with alterations in the color of the iris resulting from dietary constituents, the productive cycle, and certain genetic factors.

In the visceral form, any organ, but especially the ovary, liver, kidneys, spleen — and less often the heart, lungs, and digestive tract — may contain grayish tu-

mors composed of densely packed collections of lymphoid cells having the appearances of immature lymphocytes (Fig. 13.25). Occasionally the bursa of Fabricius and the thymus are involved.

In the myelocytic type the blood is pale, watery, and of poor coagulability. The liver is usually enlarged; its color is light brown to cherry red. The spleen is always enlarged four, five, or more times (Fig. 13.22). Its consistency is softer than normal, its color reddish violet, and it bulges on the cut surface. The bone marrow varies in color from light yellowish red to dark purplish red, and its consistency is pasty, with a relative absence of bony lamellae. It may not, however, deviate from the normal in appearance. The kidney is not constantly the seat of lesions. Its color varies from light yellowish to reddish brown. It may be enlarged, and it is occasionally sprinkled with foci similar to those in the liver.

Microscopically, in the myelocytic type,

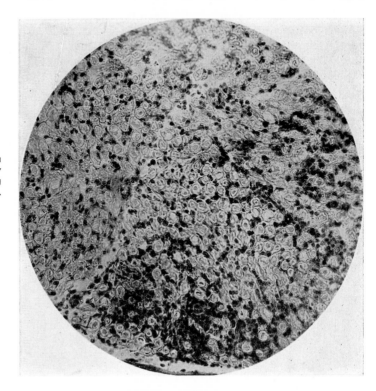

Fig. 13.24 — Cross section of a sciatic nerve showing a patchy distribution of the infiltrating lymphocytes. (Doyle, Jour. A.V.M.A.)

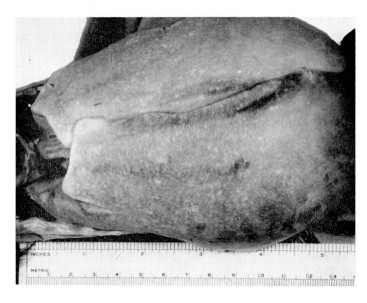

Fig. 13.25 — The enlarged liver of a chicken affected with visceral leukosis. (Patterson, Jour. A.V.M.A.)

the essential histopathology consists of an intravascular accumulation of immature granulocytes or immature erythrocytes, with consequent pressure atrophy upon the adjacent tissues (Fig. 13.23). The capillaries in the areas where the accumulations occur are gorged with the immature cells, and as a result, their walls rupture. Organs having an enormous supply of blood vascular channels, such as the liver, spleen, lungs, and kidneys, usually display the most severe lesions.

## TUMORS COMPOSED OF MELANOBLASTS

A benign tumor composed of specialized pigment-producing cells called melanoblasts is a **melanoma**. The malignant tumor composed of melanoblasts is known as a **melanosarcoma** (Figs. 9.12, 9.13, 13.26, 13.27). In man many of these tumors

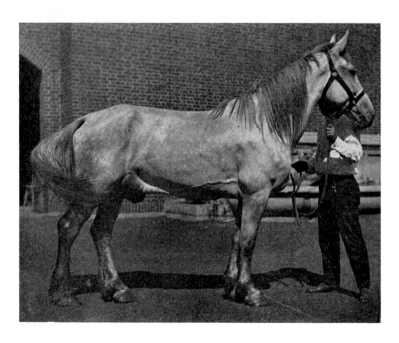

Fig. 13.26 — Melanosarcoma of the inguinal region of a gray gelding. Metastases in the lungs, liver, spleen, and adjacent lymph nodes. (Department of Veterinary Pathology, Iowa State University.)

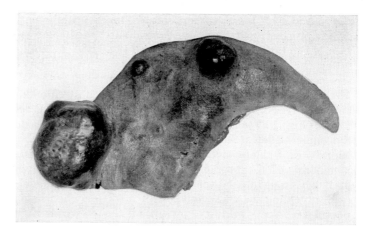

Fig. 13.27 — The spleen of an aged mule showing three metastatic melanosarcomas. The spleen weighed 17 pounds. (Mathews, Jour. A.V.M.A.)

originate from benign cutaneous melanomas called pigmented moles or nevi. These seldom if ever occur in domestic animals.

Melanosis of the skin, particularly in dogs and swine, may complicate the study of melanomas. The concept that non-elevated pigmented cutaneous areas can usually be considered as melanosis is well established; however, difficulties in differential diagnosis between melanosis and melanomas of the skin are encountered. A histological diagnosis of melanosis is made when encapsulated, free, or phagocytosed pigment, but not melanoblasts, is seen in these lesions. Melanosis occurs in areas of variable size in the subcutaneous tissue of the abdomen of the dog. At the same time, deposits of pigment may be found in other organs within the body. Since these foci represent nothing more than groups of macrophages loaded with melanin, they are not true tumors.

**Macroscopic appearance.** The most outstanding gross characteristic of a melanotic tumor is the brown, black, or gray color. The intensity of pigmentation depends upon the amount of melanin contained within the tumor. Occasionally tumors, particularly those that are exceedingly malignant, will have little and at times no pigment within them. The size of the tumor is exceedingly variable. They may be barely visible or as much as 60 centimeters in diameter. With the size there is a variation in weight from a few milligrams to as much as 20 kilograms and

even more. The shape of the melanotic tumor is also variable depending upon the degree of malignancy. The majority of equine and bovine melanotic tumors are roughly globular in shape and, when present in the skin, protrude as nodules. In swine and dogs, the tumors of the skin are more flattened and irregular and have a wartlike appearance. In consistency they may be extremely soft or encephaloid or they may be dense and firm, depending upon the amount of connective tissue and necrosis present and how malignant and invasive the tumor is. Tumors involving the skin may contain cutaneous ulcers.

**Microscopic appearance.** The most conspicuous objects in sections are rather sharply circumscribed clumps of brownish-black pigment granules (Fig. 9.12). Most of these are in cells — either melanoblasts or macrophages. The melanoblasts are irregularly round, spindle shaped, or stellate. The phagocytes are round. Most of the cells are so distended with pigment that no cytoplasm or nuclei can be seen. Often these pigmented cells are so closely packed together that nothing but pigment is discernible. The more malignant tumors composed of the more embryonal cells may contain little if any pigment. The lack of pigment indicates the tumor is probably quite malignant. In these tumors devoid of pigment, the spindle-shaped cells containing prominent chromatin-rich nuclei resemble cells of the nervous system.

**Location.** In gray and white horses,

where most of these tumors occur, the common primary sites are the ventral surface of the tail, the rectoanal region (Fig. 9.13), the external genitals of both sexes, the perineum, the head, and shoulders. Metastases are common in the lungs, spleen (Fig. 13.27), liver, kidneys, lymph nodes (Fig. 13.7), and bone marrow. In the clinic at Iowa State University a 43-pound (19.5 kg.) metastatic malignant melanoma of the bronchial lymph node and right lung in a 10-year-old white Percheron gelding was associated with a 15-pound (6.8 kg.) primary growth of the left shoulder region.

In swine the tumors are most common in the jowl, flank, and the anterolateral surface of the hind leg. Melanotic tumors are not common in cattle. There is reason to believe that tumors are more common in cattle with more lightly pigmented skin. The location of the tumors in cattle is apparently not confined to any particular area. In the dog, tumors are most frequently observed in the skin of the head, thorax, and extremities. They are especially common in the eyelids, along the gum line, and in the cheeks and lips. An occasional melanotic tumor is observed in the canine eye.

**Prognosis.** Areas of melanosis and melanomas can be removed quite easily by surgical procedures. The melanosarcoma is extremely serious and metastasizes early. As a result, by the time the animal is presented for removal of the tumor, metastasis with involvement of many organs has already taken place.

## EPITHELIAL TUMORS

On the surface of the body, epithelial tumors spring from the epidermis and hair follicles. Within the body they originate from the mucous membranes, glands, and gland tubules and ducts.

A benign tumor of the stratified squamous epithelium of the skin or a mucous membrane is a **papilloma** or wart. This is a very common tumor of domestic mammals of all ages. An infectious type of papilloma occurs most often in the young of some species (puppies and calves).

A malignant tumor of the stratified squamous epithelium of either the skin or a mucous membrane is a **squamous-cell carcinoma.** A malignant tumor composed of basal cells of the skin or of hair-follicle cells is a **basal-cell carcinoma.** Squamous-cell carcinomas are relatively common, especially in older animals.

An epithelial tumor stemming from simple cuboidal or columnar epithelium, when benign, is designated **adenoma,** and when malignant, **adenocarcinoma.** This designation is given because these tumors, for the most part, are derived from the cells of glands or the tubules and ducts of glands.

### Papilloma

**Macroscopic appearance.** A papilloma is more or less wartlike in shape. An extremely large one may become as large as a fist. Its surface is smooth, tufted, or nodular (Fig. 13.28). Occasionally a papilloma takes the form of a hornlike process projecting from the skin. The base of a papilloma may be broad or so small that the growth is pedunculated (Fig. 13.29). An incision from the surface downward shows the epithelium to be thickened.

**Microscopic appearance.** In most respects a section of a papilloma looks like normal skin. The major differences are centered around the finger-like processes of stratified squamous epithelium that protrude above the surrounding epithelial surface and contain a connective tissue core.

A very important observation to make in connection with a papilloma is that the epidermis is intact. There are no breaks in the basal layer through which epithelial cells infiltrate into the corium and subcutis as they do in the malignant form of this tumor — the squamous-cell carcinoma. The characteristics of a papilloma on a stratified squamous mucous membrane are similar to those on the skin. The cells of a papilloma are of an adult type.

Mitotic figures are not present. With routine staining, normochromasia is evident, which indicates that the tumor is of a benign type.

Location. In cattle, dogs, and rabbits infectious papillomas are common (see Fig. 13.28). Cattle are subject also to esophageal and omasal papillomas. In horses, papillomas are located mostly on the skin of the pre-pectoral and shoulder regions, ears, eyelids, upper lip and external genital organs.

## INFECTIOUS ORAL PAPILLOMA OF DOGS

This is a viral disease of puppies, characterized by the formation on the oral mucosa of papillomas which disappear spontaneously and leave the animal with a high degree of immunity. It is caused by a filtrable virus, *Molitor buccalis*, which has a specificity for the oral mucosa and which will pass through a Berkefeld filter. The period of incubation in healthy puppies is 30 to 33 days and 10 days longer

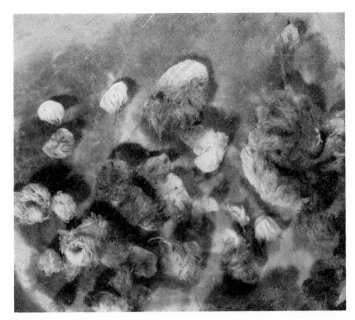

Fig. 13.28 — Multiple papillomas of the esophagus of a cow. (Davis, Jour. A.V.M.A.)

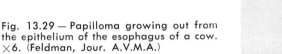

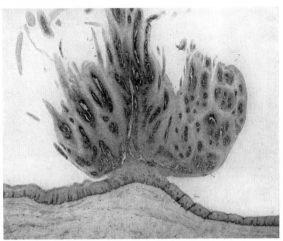

Fig. 13.29 — Papilloma growing out from the epithelium of the esophagus of a cow. ×6. (Feldman, Jour. A.V.M.A.)

in malnourished, sickly puppies. It is believed that the chemical reaction of the tissues in malnourished puppies may exert an inhibiting influence on the virus. Usually there are multiple pedunculated warts on all parts of the oral mucosa. In the larger wart-cells there are basophilic, intranuclear bodies, similar to the Lipschütz bodies in human warts. They have not been proven to have a connection with the etiological agent.

### INFECTIOUS PAPILLOMA OF CATTLE

This is a cutaneous viral disease of cattle caused by *Molitor bovis* and characterized by the appearance of warts on various parts of the body. One large abattoir in this country estimated that 15 to 25 per cent of the hides during certain seasons, particularly in the summer, showed some warts. According to the work of Creech, it appears that the warts are due to a filtrable virus. He got 15 "takes" in 22 artificially inoculated cattle. Transmission is easiest in cattle under 1 year of age. Warts appear on various parts of the body. On cows they occur principally on the teats and udder; on yearlings, mostly on the head, sides of the neck, and shoulders. In calves the warts may become large and pendulous. Sometimes they have a very offensive odor, like that of a large squamous-cell carcinoma of a horse or cow. Often they disappear spontaneously.

## Squamous-Cell Carcinoma

**Definition.** A squamous-cell carcinoma is a malignant tumor of stratified squamous epithelium.

**Macroscopic appearance.** One way to describe a squamous-cell carcinoma is to state how it differs from a papilloma. It grows more rapidly. In rate of growth a squamous-cell carcinoma often outstrips a papilloma several times within a few weeks. The most alarming thing about its growth is that it seems to have no limit. This neoplasm, therefore, is very destructive — in fact the most destructive of the external ones. The surface of a cutaneous carcinoma is not so densely

keratinized as that of a papilloma. This characteristic, however, varies with the rate of growth. Rapid growth and slight keratinization go hand in hand. The surface of a rapidly growing carcinoma is usually inflamed and often ulcerated. Slowly growing ones may have the appearance of a cauliflower head. Because of the surface necrosis and the action of putrefactive bacteria in filth accumulations in crevices on the surface, a skin carcinoma frequently has a distinctive, offensive odor. Its consistency is softer than that of a papilloma. On the cut surface it can be seen to have a parenchyma and stroma. The contrast between them is noticeable. The parenchyma is in the form of nodules of white or gray, soft, homogeneous tissue. White fibrous bands of connective tissue, the stroma, separate these nodules. There are often foci of hemorrhage and necrosis. The regional lymph nodes are frequently swollen because they become the seat of secondary growths. When squamous-cell carcinomas are removed incompletely, they recur within a few weeks or months.

**Microscopic appearance.** A squamous-cell carcinoma has many of the microscopic characteristics of a papilloma. Outstanding differences are:

1. The epithelial cells of a carcinoma are more embryonic as determined by their larger size, the apparent deficiency of nuclear chromatin, the large nucleolus, and the presence of numerous mitotic figures (Figs. 13.30 and 13.31).

2. The tumor cells are not confined within the epidermis or mucosa. They infiltrate the underlying tissues.

3. The infiltrating cells grow at random in directions of least resistance, i.e., into soft tissues, thin-walled blood vessels, and lymphatics. Penetration into these vessels favors metastasis into the venous circulation and to the lymph nodes. Tumor-cell emboli are often noticed in lymphatics and veins adjacent to the main tumor mass.

4. The proliferating cells appear in large groups without an admixture of

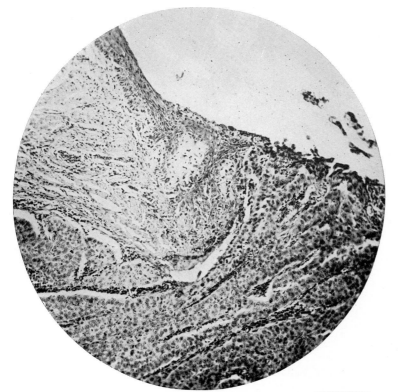

Fig. 13.30 — Squamous-cell carcinoma of the membrana nictitans of a horse. At upper left the normal epithelium is confined within the basement membrane. At lower right it has broken through the membrane and is deeply infiltrating the underlying tissue. X100. (Department of Veterinary Pathology, Iowa State University.)

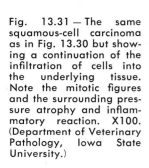

Fig. 13.31 — The same squamous-cell carcinoma as in Fig. 13.30 but showing a continuation of the infiltration of cells into the underlying tissue. Note the mitotic figures and the surrounding pressure atrophy and inflammatory reaction. X100. (Department of Veterinary Pathology, Iowa State University.)

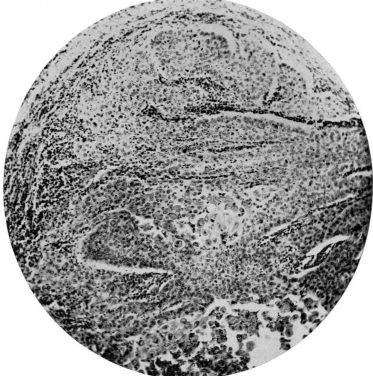

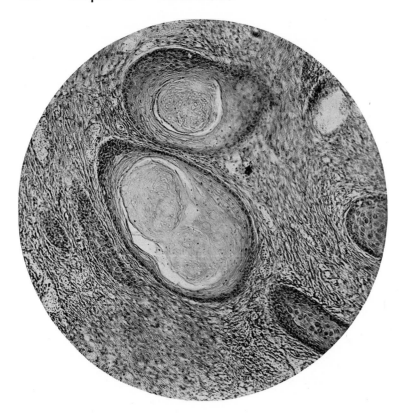

Fig. 13.32 — Epithelial pearls in a squamous-cell carcinoma of the glans penis of a gelding. X90. (Department of Veterinary Pathology, Iowa State University.)

stroma, but individual groups are separated from one another by strands of the stroma. This is a different arrangement than occurs in sarcomas in which the parenchyma and stroma are uniformly mixed.

5. In cutaneous carcinomas, round masses of keratinized epithelial cells arranged concentrically may be numerous (Fig. 13.32). These are called **epithelial pearls.**

6. The underlying tissue usually displays signs of a chronic inflammatory reaction.

**Location.** The skin and places where the skin passes over into a mucous membrane are the more common sites of primary squamous-cell carcinomas. Three very common sites in horses are the membrana nictitans (Fig. 13.33), the eyelid, and the external genitals. In cattle, particularly in Herefords, the lower eyelid and

the membrana nictitans are the most usual initial locations (Figs. 13.1 and 17.7). Squamous-cell carcinomas are particularly common in areas of the skin in which there is a deficiency in melanin either partially or completely. The deficiency of melanin probably explains in part why the occurrence of squamous-cell carcinoma of the eye of the Hereford is more common than in those breeds in which pigment is more abundant. The pigment acts as a screening agent that prevents part of the rays of the sun from penetrating into the skin. This reduction in the intensity of the rays reduces the amount of injury to the skin.

One of the examples of defective pigmentation can be demonstrated in Ayrshire cattle in which tumors of the vulva are quite common. A deficiency of pigment exists in the skin of the vulva. When the vulva has been exposed to sunlight for a considerable period of time, a papilloma appears which later becomes malignant and then is a squamous-cell carcinoma.

Squamous-cell carcinomas of the skin of the Angora goat are quite common. The tumors are most frequently encountered in the perineum and involve primarily the anus and vulva. Tumors of this type are quite common in the frontal-parietal region of sheep. The location of the tumors is quite specific.

Squamous-cell carcinomas are often observed in cattle in the vicinity of brands. Following the healing of a brand,

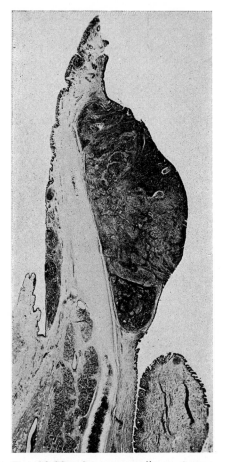

Fig. 13.33 — Squamous-cell carcinoma of the membrana nictitans of a horse. X6. (Department of Veterinary Pathology, Iowa State University.)

a deficiency of pigment will be found in this area and is apparently the reason why carcinomas appear. Metastases to the regional lymph nodes by way of the lymphatics and to the lungs by way of the veins, right side of the heart, and pulmonary artery are frequent. Further metastasis to still other organs may follow.

## SQUAMOUS-CELL CARCINOMA OF THE BOVINE EYE

Squamous-cell carcinoma of the eye is the most common malignancy in cattle in the United States. Monlux, Anderson, and Davis reported in a study of 722 ocular squamous-cell tumors removed from 532 cattle that 52 had bilateral squamous-cell tumors. These tumors were collected during a twelve-month survey of bovine eye tumors from three Denver abattoirs.

A detailed study was made of 613 of the ocular tumors, using the most malignant neoplasm or group of neoplasms from each eye studied. The other 109 tumors were independent tumors of a more benign classification, occurring as one or more additional growths on the affected eyes; they were not used as a source of data in the evaluation of the behavior of the individual ocular tumors.

Of the 613 tumors, 471 were diagnosed as squamous-cell carcinomas, 30 as early squamous-cell carcinomas, 38 as epidermal papillomas, and 74 as epidermal plaques.

Of the 471 carcinomas, 22 had metastasized to the parotid lymph nodes and four of these had additional metastatic lesions.

There were 199 carcinomas which had ulcerated surfaces and would have been a source of contamination of meat removed from the head if the lesions had not been detected in the inspection procedures.

Of 335 carcinomas involving the eyeball, 67 had penetrated into the anterior chamber of that structure.

The probable inherited susceptibility of certain families of cattle to carcinoma of the eye and the questionable value of salvaging an afflicted animal for additional use as a member of a breeding herd are problems of importance to the breeder, geneticist, and veterinarian. No attempt was made to identify the herd origin of the above cases, so these problems will only be mentioned. Investigators are conducting long-term studies on individual herds, and their preliminary reports indicate a higher hereditary predisposition to the development of bovine ocular carcinoma in some bloodlines.

A histological examination is often necessary in the study of inflammatory and neoplastic conditions of the eye to confirm or refute the clinical or post-mortem impressions. The adoption of elaborate classifications of the ocular neoplasms based on clinical or pathological features should be avoided. Errors in diagnosis are easily made if improper specimens are submitted for histological examination. All too frequently only a small biopsy specimen of the superficial portions of the neoplasm is submitted. Examination of this specimen reveals it to be composed almost entirely of squamous cells. If the biopsy is not adequate, a correct evaluation of the neoplasm is made more difficult.

Monlux, Anderson, and Davis divided the epidermal eye tumors into four types according to the degree of malignancy.

1. **Epidermal plaque.** This is a thickening of epithelium which is at least two times the normal and is a result of proliferation of the prickle cell layers so that they exceed the average height of the remainder of the tumefied epithelium. The growths do not have a papillary surface, but occasional inward growths of the tumor may cause islands of connective tissue resembling the connective tissue cores of a papilloma to be included in histological sections. Although Bowman's membrane of the cornea may appear thin and even disappear where there are corneal plaques, there is always an acceptable basal line to the tumefied epithelium of either the cornea, conjunctiva, or skin. Dyskeratotic changes such as hyper-

chromatism may occur in the thickened epithelium but usually are limited to individual cells. Formation of anaplastic nests of epithelial cells within the growths is rare. Subepithelial inflammatory reactions may be marked and there may be a pseudo-epitheliomatous hyperplasia with great enlargement of rete pegs.

2. **Epidermal papilloma.** Included are all benign, papillary, epithelial outgrowths which have stalks, spines, or rounded protuberances represented by a central connective tissue core covered to a variable depth by a tumefied epithelium. In addition, benign tumors having a marked hyperkeratosis or parakeratosis of the stratum corneum are designated as papillomas. At least one projection of this cornified eipthelium equals or exceeds the average height of the remainder of tumefied epithelium in these growths. Again, the Bowman's membrane of the cornea may appear thin and even disappear in places where there are corneal papillomas, but there is always an acceptable basal line to the tumefied epithelium of either the cornea, conjunctiva, or skin. Dyskeratotic changes such as hyperchromatism may occur in the epithelium and are more common than in plaques. Small, intradermal nests of anaplastic cells (carcinomas *in situ*), including such cellular phenomena as increased numbers of mitotic figures, enlargement of nuclei and nucleoli to form giant or sometimes double nuclei, great variation in size and shape of individual cells, and small, isolated cornified bodies (epithelial pearls) may appear singly in the tumors, be found in several areas, or be absent. Subepithelial inflammatory reactions may be marked, and there may be a pseudo-epitheliomatous hyperplasia with great enlargement of rete pegs.

3. **Early squamous-cell carcinoma.** Nests of tumor cells at the base of an epithelial eye tumor appear to break through the basal cell layer of the tumefied epithelium and invade the subcutaneous tissues. If the tumor is on the cornea, the underlying Bowman's membrane is no longer intact or may have completely disappeared. On

section, the nests usually appear as rounded subconjunctival groups of rather anaplastic cells and often have a central cornified center (sometimes advanced enough to be a classic epithelial pearl). The tumor, except for the carcinomatous changes in its basal area, may resemble a plaque or papilloma. However, as a group and compared with papillomas, there is a much greater tendency for the early carcinomas to form intradermal nests of anaplastic cells (carcinoma *in situ* described under epidermal papillomas). In addition, it is not uncommon for large portions of the basal cell layer of the tumefied epithelium to be replaced by these nests of anaplastic cells. Most of the invasive carcinomatous groups of cells still maintain intercellular bridges (prickles), particularly when there is cornification of their centers.

Occasional spindling of small groups of neoplastic cells is seen. In these areas the cytoplasmic bridges are absent and the cells may be difficult to differentiate from those of a reticulum-cell sarcoma or from epithelioid inflammatory cells invariably present as a component of a secondary tissue reaction. There may be marked pseudo-epitheliomatous hyperplasia with greatly enlarged or elongated rete pegs in basal portions of the growths adjacent to the invasive areas. Usually the rete pegs have slender and tapering projections in contrast to the rounded invasive neoplastic masses of cells which most characteristically distinguish an early carcinoma. The hyperplastic rete pegs may have a distinctive basal cell perimeter which can often be recognized even if the plane of the section results in rete pegs appearing as a single or several isolated groups of cells in addition to the portion continuous with the epithelium. Subepithelial inflammatory reactions are prominent and include infiltrations of lymphocytes, plasma cells, fibroblasts, and epithelioid cells and increased vascularization and fibrosis of the substantia propria of the cornea and conjunctiva. Although the substantia propria of the cornea is normally almost devoid of blood vessels and lymphatics, such vessels do increase rapidly in number in the subepithelial tissues in apparent direct relation to the degree of irritation produced by the growing tumor.

4. **Squamous-cell carcinoma.** While the tumors classed as early squamous-cell carcinomas are distinguished by what is considered to be one or more initial carcinomatous invasive growths into the substantia propria, the full-fledged carcinomas include all eye tumors which have secondary or more advanced outgrowths from the invaded areas. There may be deep invasion through the substantia propria of the cornea to Descemet's membrane; lateral invasion under intact corneal, conjunctival, or cutaneous epithelium; or there may be a reversed invasion through the tumefied epithelium (probably responsible for many of the ulcerating, necrotic surfaces). In the more differentiated carcinomas, multiple epithelial pearls may be found, and it is not unusual for individual pearls to reach a size large enough to replace one half of the normal depth of the cornea. Anaplasia and other malignant changes are much more advanced than those seen in carcinoma *in situ*. Sometimes groups of epithelial tumor cells appear either fusiform or in extremely cellular arrangements in which cytoplasmic boundaries may be indistinct. Mitotic activity and formation of giant, double, or lobed nuclei usually increase in crude proportion to the malignancy of the tumor. A few tumors show definite neoplastic glandular formation in parts of their growths and an origin in or near glands associated with the eye is postulated. Scattered areas of necrosis are common in the larger tumors. In the more malignant tumors, invasions of veins or lymphatics may be demonstrable as well as metastasis to lymph nodes or body organs.

**Prognosis.** The prognosis of squamous-cell carcinoma of the eye is good if proper treatment is instituted early. Surgery, beta radiation, radioactive cobalt, and randon are used by practitioners. Squamous-cell carcinoma of the bovine eye is a tumor which usually metastasizes only after a long period of progressive growth. Those originating on the eyeball metastasize only in the most advanced stages. There is only meager recorded data on the follow-ups of cattle afflicted with eye tumors in respect to local recurrence of the growths after treatment. Correlated information on the clinical and microscopic appearance of the neoplasms, and the method and result of treatment, would be valuable data.

As the name indicates, the papillomas and plaques represent benign squamous-cell tumors and have a very favorable prognosis. These tumors may be removed by relatively minor surgery and do not necessitate the enucleation of the eyeball. If allowed to remain, they may eventually become malignant.

### Basal-Cell Carcinoma

The basal-cell carcinoma is sometimes called rodent ulcer, basal-cell epithelioma, and hair-matrix carcinoma. The cells originate from hair follicles. Most of the reported tumors have been on the heads of horses, dogs, and cats, although they may occur in the skin of other areas. No favored sex or age has been established.

**Macroscopic appearance.** These tumors are slow growing, firm, nodular, and usually attached by a broad base. The skin over the tumor may be devoid of hair. There is a great tendency for ulceration to occur and for the cells to infiltrate the surrounding tissues. Metastasis seldom occurs.

**Microscopic appearance.** The cells tend to resemble the basal cells of the Malpighian layer and retain the relatively small size of the basal cell rather than becoming large and squamous-like as is the case with squamous-cell carcinomas. They are cuboidal or columnar and stain deeply with basic stains. The cells tend to form columns that are often vertical to the surface. Eventually large numbers fuse and have a concentric or alveolar arrangement. There are no lumina in the centers of these cells. One or two nucleoli may be seen in the nucleus. Mitotic figures are not abundant. The stroma is variable in the same tumor; that is, the collagenous fibers may be abundant in one part but scanty in another.

**Prognosis.** The prognosis of basal-cell carcinomas is good. Although there is local destruction and invasion of the tissue, they seldom metastasize to the regional lymph nodes or to other organs. The clinical appearance of the tumor — ulceration, secondary bacterial infection, and extension into the surrounding tissue — makes them seem much more malignant than they really are.

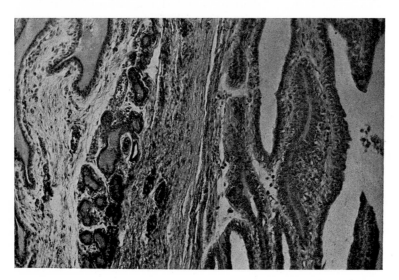

Fig. 13.34 — Adenoma of mammary gland of a dog. Normal gland at left center is separated from the neoplastic gland at the right by a capsule of connective tissue. X130. (Department of Veterinary Pathology, Iowa State University.)

## Adenoma

**Definition.** An adenoma is a benign tumor of glandular epithelium.

**Location.** There seems to be no particularly favored location for adenomas in most species of domestic animals except in the dog. In this animal sebaceous, mammary, and prostate gland adenomas seem to be fairly common. In swine in the vicinity of Iowa State University polypoid adenomatosis of the large intestine has been seen several times. In south-eastern Minnesota thyroid adenomas in horses have been reported by Schlotthauer.

**Macroscopic and microscopic appearances.** The gross appearance of adenomas varies considerably depending upon their location and the tissue from which they spring. In general they are sharply circumscribed and encapsulated (Figs. 13.34 and 19.1). In the stomach and intestine it is common for them to become polypoid in shape. They are then spoken of as **polypoid adenomas** or **adenomatous polyps.**

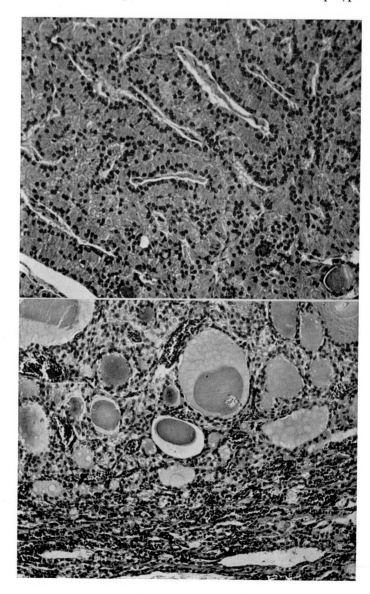

Fig. 13.35 — **Above:** Adenoma of the thyroid of a horse showing a papillary arrangement of cells. **Below:** Fetal and colloid adenoma of a horse. (Schlotthauer, Jour. A.V.M.A.)

Microscopically, adenomas often look so much like the gland from which they originate that the difference between them can scarcely be distinguished. While the amount of gland tissue is far in excess of normal, and while the acini may be lined with more than one layer of cells, it is important to note that the epithelium remains held in bounds by its basement membrane. Sometimes the secretions of an adenoma are retained in the acini, causing them to become extremely distended and their epithelium to undergo atrophy. **Cystadenoma** is the name given to this neoplasm. Cystadenomas are frequently found in the thyroid gland of elderly dogs and horses (Fig. 19.15). Occasionally, too, the proliferating epithelium may push into the lumen of the acini and take the form of branching papillae (Fig. 13.35). **Papillary adenoma** is the name given to this form. Its best example is furnished by the prostate adenoma of aged dogs. There is a question as to whether this is a true neoplasm or an example of hyperplasia.

**Prognosis.** The prognosis of adenoma is good. If they are in a position where surgical methods can be used to remove them, there is little danger of recurrence. Some adenomas, if allowed to remain in the tissues, become malignant, which is indicated by infiltration, transplantation, metastasis, and extensive local tissue destruction.

### SEBACEOUS GLAND ADENOMAS OF DOGS

These adenomas originate in the specialized sebaceous glands of the perianal region, the prepuce, and the skin of the back, loin, and tail. The majority of these tumors occur in aged male dogs.

**Macroscopic appearance.** These tumors are usually circumscribed, yellowish brown in color, single or multiple, and on section have a slightly lobulated appearance. In some cases the overlying skin may be ulcerated and hemorrhagic. The neoplasm then appears much darker. The size varies from 0.5 cm. to 6 cm. in diameter.

**Microscopic appearance.** The neoplastic cells appear very much like the perianal gland tissue. Their arrangement, however, is not that of a normal gland. The cells are in cords, bundles, or irregular masses which often have the appearance of lobules.

The neoplastic cells are large, polyhedral, and have a finely granular, acidophilic cytoplasm. The nuclei are centrally located, contain fine chromatin granules, and have one or two nucleoli. Mitotic figures are not usually seen. Rounded bodies resembling epithelial pearls may be found. Typical ducts are usually scattered through the growth. There may be voluntary muscle deep in the tumor, but this does not indicate invasiveness as this muscle is a feature of the normal gland.

### Adenocarcinoma

**Definition.** An adenocarcinoma is a malignant tumor of glandular epithelium.

**Macroscopic appearance.** The gross appearance of an adenocarcinoma varies with its location, the gland tissue of which it consists, and the age of the growth. On mucous surfaces it may simply be a well-defined, rather flat, undulating, thickened area which has the characteristics of chronic focal inflammation. At the other extreme it may be much more conspicuous and take the form of a head of cauliflower. The extent of growth of a primary adenocarcinoma in an internal organ follows no set rule. It may be round and sharply defined; or it may so diffusely permeate the organ that it becomes completely lost in it. Between these two extremes come metastatic adenocarcinomas which may consist of several sharply defined nodules quite uniformly distributed throughout the organ. Metastasis in these cases occurs by way of the venous circulation to the right heart, and from it to the lungs, and eventually to other organs by way of the arterial circulation. Similar metastasis to lymph nodes takes place by way of the lymphatics. Miliary foci on the serous surfaces of the thoracic and abdominal cavities arise from transplantations resulting from respiratory and peristaltic movements. The cut surface of adenocarcinomas is homogeneous and somewhat milky. Accumulations of glandular secretion are denoted by the presence of cysts. Some adenocarcinomas have considerable stroma and are firm. Others have a minimum of stroma and are soft.

**Microscopic appearance.** In sections it can be seen that the adenocarcinoma grows differently than an adenoma. Whereas in the adenoma there is an increase in mature glandular epithelial cells of the acini or alveoli, in the adenocarcinoma there is an alarming proliferation of an embryonic type of epithelial cells of the acini or alveoli and an infiltration of these cells into the tunica propria of the mucosa and into the interstitial tissue of the gland (Fig. 13.36). The epithelium has gone on a growth rampage and has no respect for the normal boundary line, the membrana propria. In this respect it is much like a hostile army invading the territory of a nonaggressive neighboring country. The invading cells take the line of least resistance — into loose connective tissue, lymph spaces, and thin-walled blood vessels. In pushing out into these structures, the infiltrating cells may take the form of cords or of gland ducts. The epithelium may be single or multiple layered. These processes branch in all directions and then rebranch. The infiltrated tunica propria and interstitial tissue display some resistance to the invasion in the form of a mild chronic inflammatory reaction. The cells possess the usual characteristics of malignancy, i.e., large, rather vesicular nuclei with large nucleoli and mitotic figures. The cells often retain the special characters of the cells from which they originate. This is especially true with reference to their secretory function and is even true in the metastatic growths. Sometimes, when a secondary carcinoma is examined before its primary, the character of its cells reveals the nature of the primary tumor. In rapidly growing adenocarcinomas, retrogressive changes may be so extensive that the true nature of the neoplasm can be determined only in its most recently formed parts.

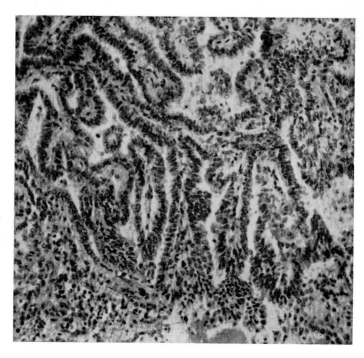

Fig. 13.36 — Papillary adenocarcinoma of the lung of a dog. X150. (Feldman, Jour. A.V.M.A.)

Incidence and location. Since the adenocarcinoma is a tumor of middle and late life, it is apparent that in domestic animals it is found mostly in the species and types that are raised for purposes other than meat production. Horses, dairy cattle, and dogs, therefore, furnish us with the majority of these tumors. In horses there appears to be no particularly favored location for them. In Colorado the adrenal gland was found to be the most common site in cattle and sheep. In dogs in the clinic at Iowa State University, adenocarcinomas of the mammary, thyroid, and prostate glands and of the liver have been the most common ones. Ovarian tumors of this type are frequently encountered in hens.

Metastatic adenocarcinomas originating by way of the lymphatics are of frequent occurrence in regional lymph nodes. Metastasis by the venous circulation involves first of all the lungs and later other viscera.

Prognosis. The prognosis of an adenocarcinoma is always serious. Unless the tumor is removed in its early stages, infiltration, metastasis, and transplantation to other tissue and organs become so extensive that surgical removal of all of the tumor masses is impossible. The rapidity with which adenocarcinomas spread varies with the species of animal as well as the type of tumor.

### ADENOCARCINOMA OF THE UTERUS OF THE COW

Adenocarcinoma of the uterus is the most common malignant glandular tumor of the bovine. Of the epithelial tumors in general, it is second only to squamous-cell carcinoma of the eye. Unfortunately, incomplete clinical and post-mortem examinations fail to demonstrate the primary of the neoplasm. How frequently sterility is associated with the uterine carcinoma is not known since clinical data are lacking. Likewise, it is not known if an endocrine imbalance is associated with the appearance of these tumors. Uterine carcinoma is most common in cattle that are 7 to 12 years of age.

Macroscopic appearance. The tumor may occur in either horn of the uterus or in the area that is sometimes referred to as the body of the uterus. The tendency of the lesions to form a sclerotic, annular constriction without perforation of the serosa and little or no extension onto the surface of the endometrium is its most constant feature. The uterine growth as well as its metastases and transplants is yellow to gray in color and is quite firm and dense because of the connective tissue that is present. One characteristic of this tumor is that tumor cells from the serosal surface of the uterus are transplanted on the abdominal viscera. As a result, tumor nodules are found in the broad ligaments of the uterus, and other nodules are scattered throughout the visceral and parietal peritoneum. Tumor nodules are also found involving the spleen and the liver, but careful examination reveals the majority of these tumors involve the serosa of the spleen and the liver. Metastatic tumor masses are found in the internal iliac and sublumbar lymph nodes and in the lung.

Microscopic appearance. A significant finding in the examination of this tumor is the observation that, in the metastases of the bovine uterine adenocarcinoma, there is maintained a degree of differentiation and a limit to anaplastic changes. Even in the transplanted and metastatic nodules, the glandular pattern is maintained. This is particularly important because many adenocarcinomas of other organs lose this glandular pattern and form anaplastic masses in both the primary and secondary tumor sites. Within these glandular structures, both in the primary and secondary sites, there are masses of cellular, often necrotic, debris. Most of the growth has a very fibrous stroma. There is little evidence that progressive growth occurs through and on the surface epithelium of the uterus. The tumor is usually centered deep in the endometrium and spreads laterally under an intact surface epithelium. The growing uterine tumor apparently at some stage in its development is able to spread through the muscular layers of the myometrium. Where the tumor has broken through into the myometrium, groups of tumor cells are found in the perimeter of the thick-walled blood vessels forming vascular channels through the myometrium. Sometimes these tumor cells appear to be in thin-walled vessels, probably lymphatics or dilated veins. They are also seen as clumps of cells near the adventitia of the vessel. The general route of both blood vessels and lymphatics through the myometrium is from the endometrium to the serosa. The extension of the neoplastic tissue to the serosal surface suggests that tumors on the surface of the uterine serosa are brushed off and transplanted on the visceral and parietal peritoneum. The regional lymph node involvement comes from lymphatic metastasis.

Since the primary site of uterine carcinoma is often overlooked, it is important to remember the characteristics of this tumor, especially in differentiating it from primary lung neoplasms. (1) Uterine adenocarcinomas maintain a degree of differentiation both in primary and secondary sites. (2) The lumen of the glands comprising the neoplasm contains an abundance of cellular debris. (3) Uterine carcinomas display extreme fibrosis in both the primary and secondary sites. (4) Parietal and visceral peritoneal transplants are numerous. (5) If the uterus is available, an annular ring is usually present in the wall at the site of the neoplasm. In most instances, the primary site will be small and the uterus will not show much increase in size or weight.

### Tumors of the Adrenal Gland

Epithelial cortical tumors represent one of the most frequently diagnosed primary neoplasms of an individual bovine organ. It occurs as the third most frequently encountered epithelial tumor, being exceeded by adenocarcinoma of the uterus and squamous-cell carcinoma of the eye. Just as in the thyroid gland, it is difficult if not impossible to draw a sharp line of demarcation between adrenal hyperplasias, adrenal adenomas, and adrenal adenocarcinomas. This is particularly true when small areas of adrenal hyperplasia are found in a great number of domestic animals, particularly the dog. Likewise, with the adenocarcinoma, it is difficult to tell just when an adenoma becomes an adenocarcinoma, because the majority of these tumors do not metastasize. Of 78 adrenal carcinomas in the Monlux, Anderson, and Davis collection, only two had metastases in other organs. In an attempt to establish a basis for diagnosis of adrenal cortical carcinoma in cattle, it is concluded that the factors of invasiveness and actual size are most important in the absence of metastasis. Otherwise, except for variable deposition of fibrous connective tissue and calcium and areas undergoing necrotic and cystic changes, the tumors are remarkably similar in appearance. The actual size of the cortical tumors is consistently large. Nearly all are more than 5 cm. in diameter, and 25 cm. in diameter is about their maximum size. All of the cortical tumors, except a few of the smaller growths, have a thick, fibrous capsule. It is noted that if the tumor contacts rather firm adjacent tissue (liver, kidney, or aorta) the capsule covering the contact surface of the neoplasm is often very thin. The tumor pressing upon the wall of the aorta produces pressure atrophy and a thinning of the aortic wall, resulting in an encapsulated protrusion of the tumor into the lumen of the aorta. The penetration of the tumor into the aorta rather than into the vena cava is of particular interest as it is the vena cava that is most commonly invaded by these tumors in the human being.

Adrenal tumors are found in old animals. In the bovine they usually occur in animals more than 6 years of age. No endocrine disturbances are observed.

**Microscopic appearance.** The cells of the tumor resemble those of the adrenal cortex. In selected portions of adrenal cortical tumors it may be difficult to see any appreciable alteration from the normal adrenal cell. The tumors are encapsulated, are usually yellow or orange in color because of the abundance of fat contained within them. They are usually lobulated, frequently cystic, and at times contain areas of calcification, hemorrhage, and hemosiderosis.

The **adrenal medullary tumors** are pheochromocytomas, neuroblastomas, and ganglioneuromas. Pheochromocytomas are apparently most common in the adrenals of old ewes. While chromaffin granules are reported within the cells when fixed with chromate salts, in most cases they are not demonstrable. The tumors are firm, grayish, lobulated, thinly encapsulated, and on gross examination resemble adrenal cortical tumors. They usually vary from 1 to 12 cm. in diameter. Protrusion into the lumen of the vena cava and the aorta is observed with some of these malignancies. Excessive production of adrenalin has not been observed.

**Prognosis.** The prognosis of adrenal tumors is good as far as the life of the animal is concerned since metastasis to other organs is uncommon.

### Neoplasms of the Thyroid Gland

The incidence of neoplasms of the thyroid gland varies greatly throughout the country depending upon the incidence of goiter or the iodine deficiency in an area. The greater the iodine deficiency and the more goiter present, the greater is the incidence of thyroid tumors. With the use of iodized salt, the incidence of goiter and thyroid tumors has been on the decrease.

It is extremely difficult to differentiate between hyperplasias of the thyroid (goiter), adenomas, and adenocarcinomas, since one blends imperceptibly into the other. The extremes, such as the diffuse hyperplasia of the thyroid, are easily recognized; and the infiltrating, metastasizing, and destructive adenocarcinoma is likewise readily recognized. However, no sharp line of differentiation exists between hyperplasia and the neoplasia of the thyroid gland.

The **adenoma** is usually considered as a focal encapsulated thyroid growth, sharply demarked from the surrounding tissue. It usually has a more yellow or gray color than the surrounding glandular tissue. These growths are frequently called nodular goiter. The adenomas are most commonly observed in old horses.

Microscopically, the cells of the thyroid adenoma resemble the normal cells of the thyroid gland very closely; in fact, it is sometimes difficult to detect any difference in the cells of the adenoma and the cells of the normal thyroid. Usually the adenoma has smaller follicles than the normal gland and contains little or no colloid. The entire mass is enclosed with a connective tissue capsule, and the adjacent thyroid tissue shows pressure atrophy.

The **adenocarcinoma** of the thyroid is most frequently observed in old dogs. It is not common in other domestic animals. In old dogs, particularly in goiter areas, it is extremely important that the thyroid be carefully examined when any neoplasm is found in other organs, particularly the lungs. In old dogs the most common source of metastatic tumors in the lung is the thyroid gland.

The size of the carcinoma varies from just visible foci to masses measuring 10 to 15 cm. in diameter. They are usually gray or grayish white in color, but frequently they contain areas of hemorrhage and necrosis. The necrotic areas are usually yellow, and the areas of hemorrhage are red or brown depending upon the amount of blood decomposition that has taken place. Cystic cavities are frequently found within the carcinoma. There may be infiltration of the surrounding tissue, compression of the trachea so that stenosis occurs, and metastasis to the regional lymph nodes and the lungs. The consistency may be firm or soft depending on the amount of connective tissue and necrosis present. Calcification of the tumor may occur.

Microscopically, the cells are typical of an adenocarcinoma and may be cylindrical or cuboidal in shape. The more malignant portions of the tumor appear as solid masses of cells. Other portions of the tumor produce follicles which may or may not contain colloid. The nuclei of the cells are large and contain hypertrophic necleoli. The nuclei are hyperchromatic and stain quite distinctly. Mitotic figures are quite numerous.

It is particularly important to remember that thyroid tissue may be found anywhere from the larynx to the heart and at times even approaching the diaphragm. Any tumor in this general region should be considered first of all as a thyroid tumor. Thyroid tumors in the vicinity of the base of the heart are frequently erroneously diagnosed as heart-base tumors.

The metastatic thyroid tumors are the most anaplastic portion of the tumor, and if only the metastatic tumors are examined, the similarity to the thyroid tissue may be overlooked. However, if the thyroid gland tumor is examined along with any metastatic nodule that is found in other organs, the similarity of the cellular structure is usually apparent. This is particularly important when attempting to decide whether neoplasms in the lung are of thyroid origin or primary pulmonary neoplasms.

**Prognosis.** Adenomas of the thyroid are usually not serious, but, as with all disturbances of growth, they may become malignant. Since the majority of adenomas are found in the horse, and malignancies of the thyroid are seldom encountered in the horse, the prognosis in general is good. If the tumors become excessively large, surgical removal is usually successful.

Adenocarcinomas of the thyroid are always serious and they metastasize to the lungs very early. It is frequently noted that the lung metastases are multiple and involve a great share of the lung, while the primary tumor in the thyroid is relatively small. Usually, by the time the thyroid carcinoma is observed, metastasis to the lung has already taken place. Bone metastasis from thyroid carcinomas is uncommon in domestic animals.

**Mammary Gland Neoplasms**

Mammary gland tumors in domestic animals are most frequently observed in the dog. In other animals they are relatively uncommon, and hyperactivity of the mammary gland apparently does not bring about the appearance of a neoplasm. The bovine with a highly developed mammary gland has the lowest incidence of mammary tumors.

Mammary gland tumors are of great concern to the small animal practitioner because they represent one of the more common neoplastic diseases of older dogs in which rather extensive and radical surgery must be carried out. The tumors for the most part are associated with endocrine stimulation, and multiple tumors arising in several mammae of the mammary gland may be found occuring at the same time. The neoplasms are most frequently observed in dogs that are 10 to 14 years of age.

**Macroscopic appearance.** The tumors in the mammary gland of the dog may be single or multiple. The majority of the neoplasms will be found in the posterior pair of mammary glands, fewer in the first two mammary glands, and the least in the central glands of the mammary line. It has been suggested that trauma from the legs as the animal moves about may exert an influence on the location of the mammary tumors. Usually the tumors are observed for some time before surgical intervention is attempted, and in most instances the tumors show periods of particularly active growth associated with the period of estrus. Sometimes periods of extremely rapid growth occur which may indicate a very invasive tumor, extensive hemorrhage into the neoplasm, or the accumulation of secretion within the tumor. The size varies greatly from just palpable nodules of a centimeter or less in diameter up to those that may be 8 or 10 inches in diameter. In consistency they may be quite soft and edematous and at other times may be firm and sclerotic and may contain bone and cartilage. They may be solid and rather homogeneous, or they may contain numerous cysts filled with secretion or may contain hematocysts. The color is quite variable. The majority are gray or white, but shades of red, yellow, orange, and brown are found, depending on the amount of hemorrhage and necrosis that has taken place. Ulceration of the surface of the tumor may occur.

**Microscopic appearance.** The microscopic appearance of the tumor varies greatly, and one of the reasons for this variation is that the hormonal stimulation causes both glandular and connective tissue elements to proliferate. The amount of glandular or connective tissue elements that proliferates varies with the individual tumor. At times the tumor will consist primarily of glandular epithelium of relatively benign adenomatous tissue or it may consist of extremely anaplastic tissue. The connective tissue proliferation may consist of white fibrous connective tissue, cartilage, bone, and even muscle. The appearance of cartilage and bone is the result of metaplasia. Areas of necrosis are very common within the tumor, and because dead and degenerating tissue is present, calcification is common.

Because these tumors are composed of glandular and connective tissue elements in varying proportions, it is best to designate them as **mixed mammary gland tumors** and then indicate the type of tissue that is contained within them (e.g. mixed mammary gland tumor composed of glandular elements, connective tissue, cartilage, bone, and muscle).

**Prognosis.** Mammary gland tumors in the dog are definitely not as malignant as those found in the human family. Attempts to compare the neoplasms of the domestic animals with those of the human being have led to many errors both in diagnosis and in prognosis. The majority of mammary gland tumors in the dog will not have metastasized at the time they are first noted, and if removed at that time, the chances of recovery are very good. However, at the time of removal, hormonal treatment or ovarectomy should be used in the attempt to prevent additional tumors from occurring in the mammary tissue. These new tumors do not represent metastasis or extension from the first neoplasm that was removed. If the tumor or tumors are allowed to remain in the mammary gland and thus allowed to develop until they achieve considerable size, metastasis will probably occur to the regional lymph nodes and to the lungs. Attempts to classify the mammary tumors of domestic animals according to more elaborate classifications used in the human being are not justified. Likewise, the radical surgery and extensive radiation recommended in human treatment are not necessary nor desirable in the dog.

## Sweat Gland Neoplasms

The sweat gland neoplasms are derived from the epithelium of the sweat glands. They are most frequently located on the anterior portions of the body such as the face, neck, and shoulders. Most of these tumors are adenomas.

**Macroscopic appearance.** The usual sweat gland tumor measures 1 to 2 cm. in diameter. It is grayish white in color, firm in consistency, uniform in structure, and contains no visible cysts.

**Microscopic appearance.** The tumor resembles the basal-cell carcinoma. The individual cells are small, retain the normal small size of sweat gland epithelium, do not become large and irregular as is the case with the squamous-cell carcinoma, and tend to arrange themselves in columns or tortuous strands simulating the normal arrangement of a sweat gland. The nuclei of the cells are oval, the nucleoli are small, and the nuclei are rich in chromatin. Since the mammary gland is actually a modified sweat gland, some of these tumors resemble the mammary gland or mammary gland tumors. Cysts are found within the tumor, and many of the glandular structures will have secretion within their lumen.

**Prognosis.** The prognosis is usually good. The majority of the tumors are benign, and early removal is sufficient to prevent a recurrence. Conservative early surgical removal is usually adequate to prevent a recurrence.

## Testicular Neoplasms

Testicular neoplasms of the dog consist of three tumors: (1) adenocarcinoma (seminoma), (2) sustentacular-cell tumor (Sertoli-cell tumor), and (3) interstitial-cell tumor. These neoplasms are very common, particularly in those animals that are cryptorchids, and the neoplasm is usually observed in the cryptorchid testicle. Many of these tumors are overlooked merely because the testicles are not incised and examined.

### ADENOCARCINOMA (SEMINOMA)

The adenocarcinoma of the testicle varies from 1 or 2 cm. up to 3 cm. in diameter. Most of the tumors are soft in consistency and gray in color. Areas of necrosis and hemorrhage may give the tumor a yellow or red appearance.

**Microscopic appearance.** Various stages in cell development are present, duplicating most of the cell forms found in spermatogenesis. The cells may be small and rather compact to very large cells with large nuclei. Multiple nuclei may be found within the cell. Mitotic figures are numerous. The tumor is not arranged within tubules as is the case with the sustentacular-cell tumor. The cytoplasm of the cell does not contain much fat.

**Prognosis.** This is the most malignant of the testicular neoplasms, and metastases will be found in the regional lymph nodes and other organs. Surgical removal of both testicles is advised. Estrogen is not produced by this tumor and, as a result, alterations in secondary sex characteristics are not present. Estrogen determinations may be made as an aid to diagnosis, but usually clinical examination of the individual as to alterations in the secondary sex characteristics will give as much information as will the various techniques of hormone assay.

### SUSTENTACULAR-CELL TUMOR (SERTOLI-CELL TUMOR)

This tumor is composed of sustentacular cells (Sertoli cells). It varies in size from just visible to 3 cm. in diameter. Bilateral involvement of the testicles is occasionally observed. The tumors are gray or grayish white in color, round in shape, firm in consistency, and may contain areas of hemorrhage and necrosis.

**Microscopic appearance.** The tumor cells grow within the lumen of the seminiferous tubules. In the more malignant types, portions of the tumor may lose this intratubular arrangement because the cells destroy the wall and expand diffusely into the tissue. The cells tend to be rather long, extending from the wall of the tubule toward the center, mimicing to some extent the normal position and arrangement of the sustentacular cells. As a result, the oval-shaped nuclei are arranged parallel with each other, giving a palisaded appearance. The luminal end of the cell has a rather irregular or feathered appearance as is characteristic of this cell in the normal testicular tubule. Fat is contained within the cytoplasm of the cell but usually it is not as abundant as in the interstitial-cell tumor.

**Prognosis.** This tumor is less serious than the adenocarcinoma but more dangerous than the interstitial-cell tumor since some of these tumors will metastasize and spread to other organs. The sustentacular-cell tumor elaborates estrogen, and, as a result, the effects of estrogen can be seen on other organs. The testicular tissue undergoes atrophy of the spermatogenic cells. There is atrophy and squamous-cell metaplasia of the prostate. Hyperplasia of the mammary gland and hyperpigmentation of the ventral abdominal wall are observed. Other male dogs are attracted to the dog with the testicular tumor, and quite frequently this dog becomes involved in many fights. Apparently he resents the advances of his former male companions.

INTERSTITIAL-CELL TUMOR

**Macroscopic appearance.** The interstitial-cell tumor is the most common of the testicular tumors. The majority of these tumors measure 2 to 5 mm. in diameter, but a few tumors will measure as much as 5 cm. in diameter. The smaller tumors are usually yellow in color and solid in consistency, while the larger tumors frequently contain cysts and areas of hemorrhage.

**Microscopic appearance.** The cells are rather large, polyhedral in shape, have acidophilic cytoplasm, and contain numerous fat droplets. They resemble the normal interstitial cells of the testicle. The nuclei are small and the nucleoli are usually not prominent. Mitotic figures are uncommon.

**Prognosis.** The prognosis of the interstitial-cell tumor is good. Interstitial-cell tumors seldom become malignant and metastasize. Surgical removal of the testicle is usually sufficient to prevent the spread of the neoplasm since it has seldom metastasized or invaded other organs or tissues at the time of removal. Endocrine disturbances are not associated with this tumor.

## Primary Pulmonary Neoplasms

A survey of the literature prepared by the authors in 1952 revealed a total of 155 primary pulmonary neoplasms — 64 in the canine, 8 in the feline, 33 in the equine, 32 in the bovine, 12 in the ovine, and 6 in miscellaneous species of animals. No pulmonary neoplasms were reported in swine. Numerous references were found concerning pulmonary neoplasms in guinea pigs, rabbits, mice, and birds. Many of the reports lacked adequate information to substantiate the diagnoses, and probably a number of them did not describe primary lung tumors. A number of primary pulmonary neoplasms have been reported since this survey was published.

**Etiology.** In man it has been shown that the occurrence of pulmonary carcinoma is in many cases associated with certain occupational groups such as miners, artisans, and laborers. The most notable example is the Schneeberg cobalt miners. Members of the learned professions are relatively immune in respect to carcinoma of the lung. No occupational examples can be cited in animals. Adequate data are not available to show that there is a higher incidence in city animals than in those found in the country. Many horses have been used for years in mines, especially coal mines, but not a single case has been reported among them. It has been stated that the continuous inhalation of plant dust appears to be the cause of the frequent occurrence of carcinoma in the respiratory tract of the cow, sheep, and horse. There is no information or data to support this statement, and it does not appear that there is any justification for it.

Chronic irritation of a mechanical, chemical, or infectious nature has received most attention in the search for the etiological agent of pulmonary neoplasia. The irritations from the inhalation of fumes or particulate matter from such substances as coal tar, road oil, tobacco, coal dust, and motor vehicle exhaust gases have all been advanced as suspected etiological factors, but none has been backed by sufficiently sound evidence to establish a carcinogenic role.

At present the role that coal tar, road oil, and motor vehicle exhaust fumes may play in the production of pulmonary neoplasms is receiving great attention in the field of human medicine. The city dog's lungs and bronchial lymph nodes usually contain varying amounts of anthracotic pigment. These canines are exposed to many of the suspected etiological agents, but adequate information is not available to prove that they have a higher incidence of pulmonary neoplasms than rural animals. Farm horses and ruminants which have been exposed only slightly, if at all, to these agents also have lung tumors. Pneumonkoniosis is much more frequently observed in the dog than in the horse and cow, yet the incidence of lung neoplasms is approximately the same in all species.

These data tend to indicate that pneumokoniosis plays little or no role in pulmonary tumors in animals.

Tobacco has received considerable attention as an etiological agent in pulmonary neoplasms. It is true that animals, especially dogs, are exposed to tobacco smoke but, when the intensity of their exposure is compared to that of the human, it does not appear that tobacco is of any importance in domestic animals.

Sufficient evidence for the establishment of a mechanical or chemical agent as an etiological factor in the production of pulmonary neoplasms in domestic animals is lacking.

Pneumonia has been suggested as a cause of some pulmonary neoplasms. A case has been reported in a dog in which pneumonia was present six weeks prior to the appearance of a tumor.

The human pathologist attaches much significance to the role of tuberculosis as a possible etiological agent in human lung neoplasms. One of the cases reported by Monlux was in a dog that had tuberculosis. In this case there was no histological evidence of tuberculosis in the tumor. The anatomical location of the tuberculous lesions in relation to the tumor suggests that the bacilli were not an etiological factor in the occurrence of the neoplasm.

The possible role of an infectious agent is well exemplified by a peculiar disease of sheep occurring in Africa known as jaagziekte and the same or a similar disease known in the United States as Montana progressive pneumonia. This disease is characterized by a chronic pneumonia and a proliferation of the lung tissue. Sections of these lung lesions can resemble a carcinoma so closely that they cannot be differentiated. There are never metastases to the regional lymph nodes or other organs. The etiology has not been established but it is thought to be some infectious agent. A similar disease has been described in Iceland and in several areas in Europe. The condition is probably more widespread than reports would indicate.

Jaagziekte in the horses of South Africa is characterized by chronic pneumonia and bronchial epithelial proliferation. It is found in horses that have eaten *Crotalaria dura*, a plant growing in that region. Since the plant's eradication, no more cases of the disease have occurred. There is speculation as to how many other plants might produce a similar condition. This disease could be confused with primary pulmonary neoplasms.

Chronic parasitic irritation has been advanced as a possible etiological factor. A case of pulmonary carcinoma in a tiger which had *Paragonimus westermani* in its lungs has been reported in Germany. The sheep lung, in response to parasitic pulmonary infections, develops multiple adenoma-like lesions. Although the sheep lung responds to this chronic irritation with tumor-like proliferations, there is no evidence to indicate that the new growth goes beyond this point and develops into a metastasizing carcinoma. However, sheep are killed at an early age, and perhaps if they were allowed to live an entire normal life-span, some cases of carcinoma would develop among them. Available data do not indicate that parasites play a role in the production of pulmonary neoplasms.

Summing up the evidence on lung tumor etiology, it appears that pulmonary neoplasms are probably caused by the irritation produced by a multitude of diverse agents on the lung of an animal having a predisposition for pulmonary neoplasia, and that they are not due to any single etiological factor.

There is an increase in the total number of pulmonary neoplasms reported in domestic animals but this does not necessarily indicate that there is an increased incidence per thousand animals. The lung tumors grouped as to decade of occurrence are given in Table 13.6

It is true that the incidence of lung tumors in the dog showed a sharp rise in the 1940's and 1950's, but during this period canine veterinary practice grew tremendously. There has been a great increase in the number of cases reported

TABLE 13.6

LUNG TUMORS ARRANGED ACCORDING TO DECADE OF OCCURRENCE

| Decade | Canine | Feline | Equine | Bovine | Ovine | Total |
|--------|--------|--------|--------|--------|-------|-------|
| 1870–79 | 0 | 0 | 2 | 0 | 1 | 3 |
| 1880–89 | 3 | 1 | 6 | 1 | 0 | 11 |
| 1890–99 | 2 | 1 | 7 | 0 | 5 | 15 |
| 1900–09 | 6 | 0 | 1 | 1 | 0 | 8 |
| 1910–19 | 5 | 1 | 6 | 9 | 0 | 21 |
| 1920–29 | 6 | 1 | 2 | 2 | 2 | 13 |
| 1930–39 | 17 | 3 | 4 | 14 | 4 | 42 |
| 1940–49 | 20 | 1 | 3 | 1 | 0 | 25 |

in the bovine, but dairying has become a major industry, and because of this, many more old cows exist. In addition, the value of the individual animals has increased, and for this reason more animals are being observed by veterinarians. The number of pulmonary neoplasms in the equine has decreased. This can probably be explained by the decline of the horse population as compared to the greater number existing in previous years.

The number of reported cases of pulmonary neoplasms is so small that it can hardly be considered as having statistical significance in proving that the incidence of pulmonary tumors has been increasing. Due to the increase in animal population and the greater number of livestock being examined by veterinarians, the increased tumor incidence is probably more apparent than real. The trend of pulmonary tumor incidence in the future should give us some data on which we can base more definite conclusions.

It is apparent that the sex incidence of pulmonary tumors in animals has little statistical significance, as the sex predominance of the species varies with its economic use. In the bovine, all but one of the tumors occurred in the female, but when one considers the large number of cows, especially old cows, as compared with the smaller number of bulls and steers permitted to live long enough to reach a tumor age, the probable reason for the high incidence is obvious.

Part of the very high sex incidence in the cow can be explained as a result of the tuberculosis eradication program. As cases of bovine tuberculosis become less frequent, lung lesions are subjected to a more intense examination and, as a result, an abnormally high pulmonary tumor incidence becomes evident. This was especially true in the cases reported in Norway where bovine tuberculosis has been eradicated. Since pulmonary tumors in the bovine closely resemble the lesions of tuberculosis, it is not possible to differentiate them with certainty by gross examination. When the incidence of bovine tuberculosis became low and later absent, all suspected lung lesions found in routine meat inspection were submitted to a central laboratory for further examination. As a result, the incidence of pulmonary tumors in the bovine was high in Norway. In those countries where bovine tuberculosis exists, it appears that most of the pulmonary carcinomas encountered in routine meat inspection and post-mortem examination, based on a macroscopic examination, are erroneously diagnosed as pulmonary tuberculosis. Therefore the reports of pulmonary tumors in the literature do not give a true picture of the incidence of pulmonary carcinoma in the bovine.

It has not been shown that there is a sex predominance of pulmonary carcinomas in the canine. In a series of cases observed in the dog at the Royal Veterinary College, 9 occurred in males and 10 in females. Of 5,607 canine post-mortem specimens at this college 52 per cent were male and 48 per cent female. These figures show that there is no significant pulmonary tumor sex predominance in the Stockholm dogs. In Denmark, reports indicate there are about 2 male dogs examined post-mortem to 1 female and, in accordance with this, the tumor incidence is approximately the same in both sexes ( 6 in males to 4 in females).

The incidence of pulmonary tumors is dependent upon the age to which the species is allowed to live. Swine, which seldom reach an age of more than 2 years and are usually killed at less than 1 year of age, had no neoplasms reported among them. The dog, horse, and cow, which attain an old age, show the highest incidence. The average age for pulmonary neoplasms in the domestic animals is: dog 9 years, horse 16, cow 10, and cat 11. Two sheep were listed as old, a third as 4 to 5 months, and another as 4 years.

**Macroscopic appearance.** The right lung of domestic animals has a higher incidence of primary pulmonary neoplasms than does the left. In man the right lung shows a slightly higher frequency. The occurrence in animals is given in Table 13.7.

TABLE 13.7

INCIDENCE OF TUMORS ACCORDING TO LUNG INVOLVED

| Species | Left Lung | Right Lung |
|---|---|---|
| Canine | 9 | 13 |
| Feline | 1 | 0 |
| Equine | 4 | 6 |
| Bovine | 2 | 9 |
| Ovine | 0 | 2 |
| Total | 16 | 30 |

Some of the right lung tumor predominance can be explained by the size of the lungs. In all species the right lung is larger than the left. The horse lungs have a ratio of 4:3 and the cow lungs a ratio of 1.4:1. This does not explain all of the greater right lung frequency and therefore it appears that the right lung has a greater tendency for tumor development.

The diaphragmatic lobe is the most frequent site of the primary pulmonary tumors. Malignant lung neoplasms in the human are most frequently encountered in

TABLE 13.8

LOBE LOCATION OF MALIGNANT PULMONARY NEOPLASMS

| Species | Apical Lobe | Cardiac Lobe | Diaphragmatic Lobe |
|---|---|---|---|
| Canine | 2 | 1 | 16 |
| Feline | 0 | 0 | 0 |
| Equine | 2 | 0 | 4 |
| Bovine | 2 | 1 | 4 |
| Ovine | 1 | 0 | 0 |
| Total | 7 | 2 | 24 |

the right upper lobe. The lobe location in animals is given in Table 13.8.

Probably most of this difference can be explained by the variation in size of lobes. The diaphragmatic lobe is considerably larger than any of the other lobes and the tumor incidence is also greatest in this lobe. The location of the neoplasm is reported in so few instances that a definite lobe incidence cannot be established.

The primary lung carcinoma in man is usually located at the hilus. Only in seven instances among the 155 described primary lung neoplasms in domestic animals was the primary lesion located at the hilus of the lung. It may be that the hilar origin was overlooked in some instances, but massive tumors as described at the hilus of the human lung would not have been overlooked. Apparently the primary hilar location of pulmonary neoplasms is not as common in animals as it is in man. A preceding table showed that the primary lesion was most frequently found in the body of the diaphragmatic lobe.

Multiple focal neoplasms involving one or more lobes and one or both lungs are the most frequently described lung lesions. Data concerning their incidence are given in Tables 13.7 and 13.9. A multiple tumor origin is always regarded with suspicion as it is probable that there was an overlooked primary lesion in the lung or some other organ. Probably in some of these cases the primary location of the carcinoma in the lung was overlooked because the metastases resembled the primary lesion so closely that they could not be differentiated from each other.

A massive diffuse-invading lung tumor may involve one or both lungs and one or more lobes. The condition may resemble chronic pneumonia or tuberculosis. Jaagziekte lung lesions may have a similar gross appearance.

Many of the reported lung tumors have not given rise to metastases in the regional lymph nodes or in other organs. Pulmonary carcinomas in the human usually produce metastases. It is possible that some metastases were overlooked. Many of the animals were destroyed when they no longer had economic value, and perhaps if the disease had been allowed to run its course, a greater incidence of metastatic tumors would have been found.

**Microscopic apperance.** The cell origin of a pulmonary neoplasm may be a difficult question to answer. Theoretically, tumors can arise from the alveolar wall, the bronchial epithelium, the bronchial glands, and the supporting connective tissue. Many of the authors who have described lung malignancies in animals have expressed opinions as to which cells their cases probably originated from.

The general opinion of human pathologists is that most pulmonary tumors originate from the bronchial epithelium. A number of writers have described tumors originating from alveolar epithelium. The existence of alveolar epithelium has been claimed by many anatomists and pathologists. The trend of thought tends to be that expressed by E. T. Bell when he states in the *American Journal of Pathology* (19:901, 1943): "It seems well established that in the postnatal lung the alveolar walls are largely bare of epithelium but that occasional epithelial cells may be found." Later on he states, "Although lining epithelial cells are inconspicuous in the normal lung, there are numerous pulmonary diseases in which they become prominent and form a continuous epithelial layer." Others concur with Bell when they state that no evidence of continuous alveolar epithelium is observed in normal adult lungs, and only occasional scattered septal cells are seen. Epithelium-like lining cells are found under various spontaneous pathological conditions. In animals, although isolated septal cells are present, no definite alveolar lining is evident in the lungs. As a result, an alveolar tumor must originate from the septal cells. Several who have described alveolar carcinomas seem to have based their diagnoses on the presence of a squamous-type cell. This is not acceptable as the septal cells, when they do proliferate, do so as cuboidal cells — the cell type considered as being the component of most alveolar neoplasms in the human lung.

The various lung components have a common embryological origin. There is no sharp demarkation in the gradation of tissue differentiation from bronchi, through bronchioles to alveoli, but rather a gradual change from one to the other. Scientists engaged in pathological anatomy are well aware of the ability of the cells lining the alveoli and bronchi to change their epithelial type as well as their great metaplastic potentialities when acted upon by various irritants. Since the lung has such great potentialities for variable differentiation, it may be very difficult to say from which cells a tumor originated. If the first neoplastic change were accidentally encountered, the definite origin might be established. Once a neoplasm begins to grow it acts as a chronic irritant, and the lung tissue components are stimulated to proliferate and may undergo metaplastic changes. Unless these changes in the lung are carefully considered, they are likely to be interpreted falsely as an indication of a change from normal to neoplastic cells, thereby being established as the ones from which the tumor originated. The neoplasm itself frequently shows considerable variation in its cytological structure, with squamous cells, cuboidal cells, tall columnar cells, and undifferentiated cells all mingled together in the same tumor.

Some investigators have attached significance to the peribronchial extension of lung carcinomas as an indication that they are of bronchial gland origin. This may or may not be valid reasoning. The peribronchial tissue contains numerous lymphatics and these seem to be the path of least resistance in the spread and extension of bacterial and viral diseases such as pasteurellosis and contagious pleural pneumonia throughout the lung. If the peribronchial tissue is the path of least resistance for infectious agents, perhaps such is also the case with lung carcinomas, which would account for their frequent peribronchial arrangement. At times the presence of cords of tumor cells extending for a considerable distance from the primary tumor in a peribronchial arrangement would lend support to the assumption that the peribronchial tissue is the path of least resistance in tumor extension in the lung. Tumor cells in the peribronchial tissue may act as a chronic irritant, causing a hypertrophy of the bronchial glands which may give the false impression that these cells are showing neoplastic tendencies.

Álveolar cell tumors have been reported in animals, but there is some question if these diagnoses were correct, as the supporting evidence does not seem adequate. There is also considerable doubt if it can be determined whether a tumor originated from bronchial gland cells or bronchial epithelial cells, as the epithelium is quite capable, under various pathological conditions, of changing from one cell type to another.

**Classification of Pulmonary Neoplasms.** Considering present information and evidence, it does not seem possible to state from which histological element pulmonary carcinomas in animals originate, and therefore it seems more suitable to classify them on a general anatomical basis. On this basis the malignant pulmonary tumors can be divided into three large groups: (1) primary-focal, (2) multiple-focal, and (3) diffuse-infiltrating.

The primary-focal group contains those carcinomas in which the primary location in the lung is determined and from which there may or may not be metastases throughout the lungs. The primary lesion is usually sharply circumscribed but generally is not encapsulated and, if encapsulated, the capsule is very thin. Small daughter neoplasms are commonly found in the lung tissue surrounding the primary lesion. Within the muliple-focal group are included those tumors in which there are multiple neoplasms in one or both lungs and in which the tumor has a multiple origin or the primary lesion cannot be distinguished from the metastases. These multiple neoplasms are usually sharply circumscribed and are generally not encapsulated or have only a very thin capsule. The diffuse-infiltrating group contains those cases in which there is a general involvement of one or more lobes of one or both lungs.

Employing this method, the described pulmonary carcinomas can be classified according to group as shown in Table 13.9.

TABLE 13.9

CLASSIFICATION OF PULMONARY CARCINOMAS ACCORDING TO GROUP

| Species | Primary-Focal | Multiple-Focal | Diffuse-Infiltrating |
|---|---|---|---|
| Canine ....... | 24 | 11 | 9 |
| Feline ........ | 0 | 1 | 3 |
| Equine ....... | 8 | 10 | 0 |
| Bovine ....... | 11 | 13 | 1 |
| Ovine ........ | 2 | 2 | 2 |
| Total ..... | 45 | 37 | 15 |

Employing a microscopic anatomical classification, each of these above groups can be subdivided into 4 types: (1) squamous-cell, (2) columnar-cell, (3) mixed-cell, and (4) undifferentiated-cell.

According to type, the described lung carcinomas can be classified as shown in Table 13.10.

TABLE 13.10

CLASSIFICATION OF PULMONARY CARCINOMAS ACCORDING TO TYPE

| Species | Squamous-Cell | Columnar-Cell | Mixed-Cell | Undifferentiated-Cell |
|---|---|---|---|---|
| Canine ..... | 3 | 33 | 5 | 3 |
| Feline ..... | 0 | 3 | 0 | 0 |
| Equine .... | 3 | 13 | 0 | 2 |
| Bovine .... | 4 | 10 | 1 | 9 |
| Ovine ...... | 0 | 6 | 0 | 0 |
| Total .... | 10 | 65 | 6 | 14 |

The squamous-cell type is composed of squamous cells and the columnar-cell type of columnar cells. The columnar cells vary in shape from cuboidal to high columnar. They are arranged as solid masses or cords, as alveoli, or as tubules. A combination of all three types is at times seen in the same neoplasm. The squamous cells vary greatly in the amount of keratinization. Epithelial pearls are occasionally encountered. A large number of tumors are composed of cells occurring loosely or in compact masses or cords which cannot be called squamous or columnar cells. These are called undifferentiated epithelial cells, and the tumor containing them is known as the undifferentiated-cell type. The tumor may be composed of only one type of cell but quite often it contains two or even all three types, and when this occurs it is known as a mixed-cell type.

The character of the stroma of the pulmonary carcinomas varies greatly. In some, the stroma is scanty, while in others it is very abundant and may make up the bulk of the tumor. The structure of the stroma may be loose and open, or firm, compact, and even hyalinized, and may contain islands of cartilage and bone. Tumors containing bone are most frequently encountered in the horse. Bone formation is quite common in the equine in areas of chronic inflammation or necrosis.

Some of the carcinomas observed by the authors contained large amounts of mucin occurring extracellularly and as intracellular globules. The presence of mucin cannot be used as a criterion for establishing a bronchial gland origin of the neoplasm.

Mitotic figures are occasionally encountered. Mitotic figures in a tumor do not have much reliable significance unless sections are made from fresh biopsy material or from the tumor immediately after the death of the host. Otherwise the number of mitotic figures will be too low. This was not done in the cases reported in domestic animals by the authors, and for this reason the total number of mitotic figures

present has little diagnostic significance.

Ciliated epithelial cells are occasionally reported. Since the normal epithelium of the bronchi is ciliated, care must be taken that these ciliated normal cells in the cancerous lung are not mistaken for ciliated neoplastic cells.

Intranuclear bodies — apparently large, swollen, altered nucleoli — are quite numerous in the neoplastic cells. These are probably the bodies mentioned by Jackson and others as intranuclear inclusion bodies. They do resemble the usual inclusion body seen in various viral diseases. In general, the greater the amount of retrogressive change, the more numerous are these bodies. Apparently they are an indication of necrobiotic changes within the cell nuclei.

**Prognosis.** The prognosis of primary pulmonary neoplasms is very unfavorable.

### Epidermal Inclusion Cysts

The epidermal inclusion cysts are tumor-like structures in the skin of animals, particularly dogs, that arise primarily from the hair follicle and sometimes from the adjacent skin glands. Because the desquamated cells and secretion cannot escape, they gradually accumulate, forming cystic structures lined with stratified squamous or glandular epithelium.

Epidermal cysts may result from developmental defects in which epidermal cell rests are located deep in the skin. In the Rhodesian ridgeback dog they are very common along the dorsal mid-line where there is an imperfect closure of the neural groove in the developing embryo. Epidermal inclusion cysts may be the result of injury in which fragments of epithelium are carried into the underlying tissue where growth, with secretion and desquamation, continues to take place. Occasionally, following gunshot wounds, epidermal structures and even epidermal inclusion cysts may be found in the internal organs such as the liver. The shot carries fragments of epithelium deep into the interior of the body. The fact that many of the cysts are found in the skin of the head, neck, thorax, forelegs, and between the toes of dogs suggests that trauma plays a very important role in the appearance of inclusion cysts.

**Macroscopic appearance.** The cysts are usually seen in older canines and appear to be most common in the boxer dog. The majority of the tumors are single, but occasionally multiple cysts are found. The average cyst is about 1 cm. in diameter, although larger and smaller cysts are encountered. The contents of the cysts are white or gray, occasionally yellow in color, and may be dry, fluid, or greasy in consistency.

**Microscopic appearance.** The cysts consist of a thin wall of stratified squamous or glandular epithelium, and the lumen is filled with secretion, desquamated epithelial cells, and remnants of hair. If trauma causes rupture of the cyst or if bacteria are able to invade the cyst, particularly after trauma, the contents of the cyst and the bacteria cause a chronic inflammation. The neutrophil and the macrophage are the predominant cells in the exudate. This complicating chronic inflammation often gives the tumor a much more serious clinical appearance than those not infected.

**Prognosis.** The cysts are benign, and surgical removal is usually quite successful. In the case of the Rhodesian ridgeback dog, very radical and extensive surgery must be performed to remove all of the cystic structures.

## Hyperpasia of Special Epithelial Structures

The hyperplasias of special epithelial structures, which are about to be described briefly, can be considered along with tumors, but they are actually disturbances of development. These tumor-like structures are developed from one germinal layer. One such growth is the **dermoid cyst,** which consists of skin and accessory skin structures. It usually occurs in the subcutaneous connective tissue at places where fetal clefts or fissures occurred and in the testicles and ovaries. An unusual location for dermoids in Hereford cattle is in the eyelid and on the cornea. The wall of the cyst is thin and is lined with epidermis containing hair in the case of mammals and feathers in that of birds. The cyst cavity is filled with masses of loose hair or feathers. Rarely teeth are present.

Another growth in this group is the **odontoma** of the mandible and maxilla. Dental enamel and cement give origin to the tumor-like structure. At the place where an odontoma develops, a tooth is absent. The growth may be a single, large dental crown formed mostly of dentin or more rarely a dental root. In many cases it is formed by a mass of cement. Still other odontomas may consist of many rudimentary teeth in a connective tissue stroma (Fig. 13.37).

The third important tumor-like growth in this class in the **dentigerous cyst.** It is a

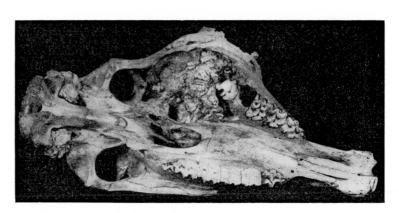

Fig. 13.37 — Odontoma, composed of more or less perfectly formed teeth. (F. W. Schofield.)

cystic odontoma which contains one or more imperfectly formed teeth. It originates from a tooth follicle, is lined with epithelium, grows slowly, but may cause marked enlargement of the mandible or maxilla. Occasionally in young horses a cyst occurs at the base of the ear over the temporal bone. The cyst contains one or two teeth and usually communicates with the exterior through a fistulous canal lined with epithelium. This congenital tumor-like structure has its origin in a branchial cleft and is called a branchial dentigerous cyst.

### Teratomas

A teratoma is a tumor-like mass of tissues which arises from fetal remains that persist in post-natal life. It is derived from more than one germinal layer and is thought to be an abortive fetus included within a normal individual — an included twin so-to-speak. As a result several tissues are often present in the growth at the onset, but the rate of growth of the individual tissues may be so variable that one eventually predominates over the others and may even cause them to undergo pressure atrophy. Occasionally the cells of a teratoma become malignant.

The most important teratoma of animals is the **embryonal nephroma.** It is apparently the result of a congenital displacement of tissues in the kidney. Feldman states that it is the most common tumor of swine. It has also been reported in cattle and poultry. In the Iowa State University collection there is one which was obtained from an 18-year-old stallion. The kidney of the stallion, in addition to possessing the embryonal nephroma, showed distinct persistent fetal lobulation. The embryonal nephroma is usually well encapsulated and made up of a heterogeneous mixture of tissue elements among which epithelial and connective tissue cells predominate. For this reason it is often designated an adenosarcoma (an undesirable term).

Ovarian and testicular teratomas are also occasionally encountered. Usually they consist of an admixture of fragments of all the tissues of the body but show very little or no tendency to become arranged into organs. Sometimes one tissue grows at the expense of all the others, in which case a teratoma comes to look exactly like a true tumor composed of one tissue. The line of demarcation, therefore, between teratomas and true neoplasms is sometimes not well defined.

Part IV

# SPECIAL PATHOLOGY
## OF THE SYSTEMS

# CHAPTER 14

# Cardiovascular System

## FUNCTIONAL DISTURBANCES

The function of the cardiovascular system can be summarized as follows: to assist in maintaining life and health by supplying the lungs and tissues of the body with blood adequate for respiration and nutrition. This system may function properly insofar as the quantity of blood transported is concerned, yet the health of the animal may be impaired because the quality of blood is poor. It must be remembered that, while this system is usually responsible for the quality of blood that it carries, it is dependent upon other systems for its supply of materials.

The normal heart possesses a wonderful ability to withstand the strain which changing body conditions place upon it. It accommodates itself immediately to the quantity of blood passing through it, to the resistance the blood meets in the vessels, and to the needs of the organs. The strength and elasticity of its muscular walls, the perfect seating of its valves, and the efficiency of its pace-setting mechanism function harmoniously under all sorts of conditions.

It is also remarkable how the heart can accommodate itself to the changes which arise in disease — conditions that affect the passing of blood through the heart itself, and through the vessels and organs. This ability to maintain circulation under pathological conditions is referred to as compensation. When there is a slowly developing, continuous hindrance to circulation or to the heart's action, the myocardium hypertrophies in order to maintain adequate circulation. If the time comes when the organ becomes fatigued and compensation can no longer occur, **decompensation,** or failure of compensation, is said to be the result.

A decrease in heart force is designated as heart weakness or **cardiac insufficiency.** Such a decrease of cardiac function is caused by various influences injuring the myocardium or its ganglia. These agencies are responsible for the cardiac weakness because they may cause heart strain or fatigue, a diminished blood supply to the heart muscle, myocarditis and myocardial degeneration, fatty degeneration of the heart, and myocardial atrophy.

All pathological changes which lead to cardiac insufficiency result in disturbances in the movement and distribution of blood in the body. Two opposing forces are needed for the maintenance of blood pressure. One force is myocardial contraction and the other is the elasticity of the arteries. The heart, to force blood into the vessels, must overcome the elasticity of the arteries. The contraction of the arteries maintains blood pressure when the aortic valve is closed. When the heart cannot overcome the elasticity of the arteries, the cardiac blood cannot enter the arteries, and the blood within the arteries is forced into the venous side of the circulatory system. Blood accumulates in the venous side of the circulatory system and passive hyperemia is the result. This interferes with internal respiration in all the tissues, resulting in air hunger (hypoxia) and abnormal fatigue. The heart's aspirating force which normally draws blood from the large veins is diminished in the weakened heart so that blood collects in the veins. Insufficiency of the heart has a further damaging effect upon the organ itself because its own blood supply becomes deficient. During this weakened state, blood accumulates in the heart, and the myocardium stretches (cardiac dilatation). Because of cardiac dilatation the right and left atrioventricular valves can no longer span the lumen of the heart, and valvular insufficiency is the result. There is a backflow of blood through the incompletely closed valve and a further accumulation of blood in the heart chamber into which the blood regurgitates. If the condition causing the cardiac weakness subsides or disappears, the injured myocardium undergoes fibrosis which renders the chamber wall less elastic. The cardiac insufficiency then becomes chronic. Cardiac fatigue may increase to the point of exhaustion and, finally, to complete loss of function. Death from asphyxia is the termination.

Lesions of various kinds along the cardiac impulse conduction system (pacemaking mechanism) may cause a disturbance in the transmission of impulses. The disturbance is characterized by a grave upset of the rhythmic beating of the heart and is designated **heart block**. Indications of such disturbed function are prolongation of one phase of a beat, skipping of beats, and loss of coordination between the beats of the atria and the ventricles.

Heart block, complete or partial, is observed in domestic animals and is probably most frequently encountered in the horse and dog. It is one of the causes of so-called fainting in horses. Horses so afflicted will stagger, stumble, and even fall when being worked. A saddle horse that stumbles and falls is an exceedingly dangerous animal.

Lesions responsible for cardiac block are hemorrhages, infarcts, deposits of calcium, focal inflammatory reactions, tumors, abscesses, areas of necrosis, and foci of replacement fibrosis. The foci of replacement fibrosis are in areas where degenerated and necrotic cardiac muscle are replaced with connective tissue. To cause heart block, these lesions must be close to and impinge upon the main parts of the conduction system (the ventricular bundle or its right and left branches). The most crucial location for such lesions therefore is in the dorsal aspect of the ventricular septum where the ventricular bundle has its origin. At this point the bundle may or may not originate in a node of modified muscle fibers. In cattle and sheep the node is present. In the horse, the pig, and the dog it is absent. Whether the node is present or not, the bundle of modified muscle fibers forms and extends down the septum for a very short distance before it is joined by amyelinated nerve fibers from cytons located in the epicardium of the circular coronary groove. The modified muscle fibers together with these amyelinated nerve fibers constitute the ventricular bundle. The bundle is separated from the myocardium by a fibrous sheath. In the horse the bundle is more fibrous than in the ruminants and swine. In the dog the bundle is absent but is replaced by an insignificant muscle fasciculus. The bundle (or its homologue in the dog) divides in the septum of the ventricles into right and left branches. At the origins of the papillary muscles the two branches subdivide to form a network of subendocardial and intramyocardial Purkinje fibers. In the dog the muscle fibers of the special fasciculus are distributed much like Purkinje fibers.

Anatomical changes in the arteries and veins result in an unequal distribution and movement of blood similarly as do cardiac disturbances. Constrictions of various kinds in the arteries increase the blood pressure in the heart and give rise to cardiac dilatation and hypertrophy. An organ supplied by a constricted artery receives less blood than normal (ischemia). Reduction in the elasticity of the vessel wall leads to a local distension of the the vessel (aneurysm).

A reduction in the muscular tone of the blood vessels of the splanchnic region, as the result of bacterial and other intoxications, results in a hyperemia and fall of blood pressure in that area. This is probably the result of a paralysis of the vasomotor nerves. The diversion of blood to the abdominal cavity may terminate in fatal collapse.

In the veins the movement of blood is hindered by heart weakness which lessens the aspirating force in the vena cava. Venous flow is also obstructed by valvular lesions, by pulmonary diseases, venous thrombosis, and constriction due to pressure upon the thin-walled vessels. The nearer the venous obstruction is to the heart, the more damaging are its effects.

Lymph flow in the body is dependent upon blood flow. With disorders in blood circulation, abnormal collections of lymph in the tissues and body cavities are also quite likely to occur.

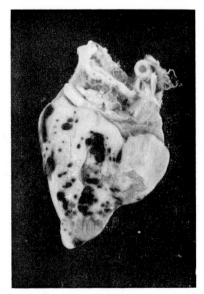

Fig. 14.1 — Hemorrhages of the epicardium and myocardium in acute **Crotalaria spectabilis** seed poisoning in a chicken. (Emmel, Jour. A.V.M.A.)

## CARDIAC MALFORMATIONS

The two most important and most frequently occurring cardiac malformations of domestic animals are **persistent foramen ovale** and **persistent common atrioventricular canal.** To understand the origin of these defects it is necessary to review briefly the embryonic development of the heart.

The first indication of the partitioning of the heart into two chambers — a common atrium and a common ventricle — is the appearance of a rather elongated constriction midway in the heart tube. This muscular constriction forms the atrioventricular canal. The first indication of partitioning the common atrium and the common ventricle into right and left

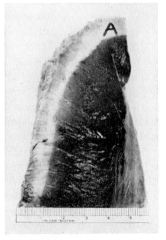

Fig. 14.2 — Cross section of the heart shown in Figure 14.3. **A,** thick outer layer of granulation a n d cicatrial tissue. (Witter, Jour. A.V.M.A.)

chambers appears at points on opposite sides of this newly formed atrioventricular canal. These two foci are the endocardial cushions (dorsal and ventral). They grow towards each other, meet, and fuse (a part of the septum), dividing the common atrioventricular canal into a right and left atrioventricular canal. The right canal becomes the orifice of the tricuspid valve and the left canal becomes the orifice of the mitral valve.

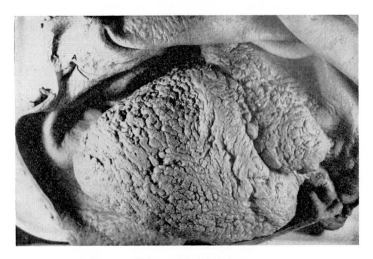

Fig. 14.3 — Chronic suppurative pericarditis in a cow due to wire shown at **A**. Note thickening of the pericardial sac and the roughened surface of the epicardium. (Witter, Jour. A.V.M.A.)

The fused dorsal and ventral atrioventricular cushions furnish tissue for parts of the two atrioventricular valves. The right side of the fused cushions forms the medial or septal leaflet of the tricuspid, and the left side of the fused cushions forms the aortic leaflet of the mitral.

In this discussion we are not concerned with the other leaflets of the two atrioventricular valves because they are formed by the parietal portions of the atrioventricular canal.

At the time the atrioventricular canal is being divided by the two atrioventricular endocardial cushions, the common atrium itself is also being partitioned into a right and left chamber. This is done by the formation of septum I (interatrial septum), which develops from the dorsocephalic wall of the common atrium. This septum grows towards the atrioventricular endocardial cushions and divides the common atrium into a right and left atrium. The gradually closing opening between the developing septum I and the fusing atrioventricular endocardial cushions is the interatrial foramen I primary foramen. This foramen is completely closed when the fused atrioventricular cushions and interatrial septum I are completely joined to form a septum.

Before interatrial foramen I disappears, a second opening develops in septum I. It is designated interatrial foramen II (secondary foramen) and is the opening through which fetal blood passes from the right atrium to the left atrium after interatrial foramen I disappears.

A little later septum I has a companion septum develop on its right, close to it and almost parallel with it. It is called septum II (interatrial). This septum does not develop from the atrioventricular cushions but from the ventral wall of the right atrium. It does not develop as a solid membrane but in two portions — an upper and a lower — leaving an opening between but subsequently joining and fusing. The opening between the two portions of septum II is the foramen ovale.

Within a month or so after birth of the fetus of most domestic animals the blood should be completely diverted from the right side of the heart to the lungs. There is then no further need for the foramen ovale. By this time septa I and II have fused, and as a consequence the foramen is closed and only a scar remains to mark its former location. Occasionally, however, septum I atrophies before fusion occurs with septum II so that the openings of interatrial foramen II and foramen ovale coincide. This leaves foramen ovale partially or completely open. This consti-

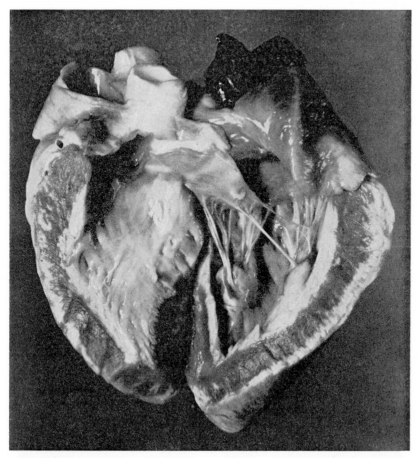

Fig. 14.4 — Coagulative necrosis of the heart of a 3½-week-old calf with white muscle disease. The white discoloration indicates the presence of necrosis. (Department of Veterinary Pathology, Michigan State University.)

tutes the condition of persistent foramen ovale, which may or may not be serious. If it leads to a circulatory disturbance or permits harmful emboli to pass directly from the venous circulation into the arterial circulation, the life of the animal may be terminated early; otherwise the condition may not be discovered until the animal is slaughtered or necropsied at some future time.

With the union of the fused atrioventricular endocardial cushions with the duplex atrial septum, the partitioning of the common atrium is complete. Simultaneously, partitioning of the common ventricle is occurring. To aid in this the fused atrioventricular endocardial c u s h i o n s make a contribution. They supply the tissue ventrally which joins the muscular part of the interventicular septum that springs from the wall of the ventricle. This membrane of tissue closes the interventricular opening which thus far has been present below the fused atrioventricular endocardial cushions.

From this review of the embryonic development of the heart it becomes apparent that a defect can arise either from lack of growth of tissue or failure of structures to fuse. Both of these occur in the condition of persistent common atrioventricular canal. Deficient development of the interatrial septum or failure of union of this septum with the fused atrioventricular endocardial cushions results in persistence of foramen I (foramen ovale). Lack of growth ventrally from the fused atrioventricular endocardial cushions or failure of this tissue to unite with the interventricular septum leaves persistent interventricular foramen. These are considered as partial forms of persistent common atrioventricular canal. Incomplete development of the atrioventricular endocardial cushions or failure of them to fuse results in a more complete form of this same condition. The partial forms, especially the one involving the interventricular septum, are seen more often in domestic animals, and while they usually go unrecognized during life, they create considerable interest when discovered at necropsy or in an abattoir. Obviously, even lesions such as those classed as partial forms of persistent atrioventricular canal can be serious in work

and race horses, and in racing and hunting dogs.

## PERICARDIUM, EPICARDIUM, AND PERICARDIAL SAC

### Abnormal Contents of the Pericardial Sac

The pericardial sac normally contains a small amount of clear serous fluid. If it is increased, the condition is designated **hydropericardium** (a transudate, not an exudate). This constitutes edema in the pericardial sac. The amount of fluid may be increased from 100 to 200 times. It contains very little or no fibrin. If it contains any, it becomes gelatinous upon exposure to air. Hydropericardium is associated (1) with conditions which increase the blood pressure in the coronary circulation, (2) with conditions in which there is a decrease in the colloidal osmotic pressure of the blood plasma, and (3) with increased capillary permeability.

Lesions which increase the blood pressure in the coronary circulation may be intracardial or extracardial. Two good

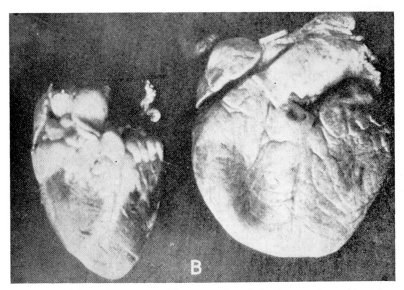

Fig. 14.5 — **Right:** Dilatation and hypertrophy of the heart of a calf with so-called brisket disease. **Left:** Normal heart of a calf of same age. (Glover and Newsom, Colo. Agr. Exp. Sta.)

examples of intracardial conditions which may raise the venous coronary pressure are stenosis and insufficiency of the right atrioventricular valve. Extracardial lesions which may result in the same venous disturbance are chronic diffuse pulmonary alveolar emphysema (heaves of horses) and the diffuse interstitial fibrosis which may follow incomplete recovery of the lung after pneumonia. As a result of any of these processes the capillaries of the coronary circulation become dilated and the capillary blood pressure is raised. These are conditions which render the capillary wall more permeable to plasma proteins and therefore pave the way for edema to occur. The fluid obviously can readily appear in the pericardial sac.

Stomach worm infestations of sheep cause a decrease in colloidal osmotic pressure of the blood plasma which may result in hydropericardium. The anticoagulant produced by the stomach worms delays clotting at the points where the worms puncture the mucosa so that there is constant hemorrhage into the stomach. This bleeding reduces the plasma protein more rapidly than it can be replenished. In stomach worm parasitism the loss of blood protein decreases the colloidal osmotic pressure in the coronary circulation as well as elsewhere in the circulation and permits pericardial edema to occur.

The occurrence of blood in the sac is called **hemopericardium.** It is caused by trauma (foreign bodies), spontaneous rupture (degeneration), and dilatation (aneurysm) and rupture of the coronary artery.

The most common cause of hemopericardium in the horse is transverse rupture of the aorta through one of the dorsal attachments of the aortic valve. The blood escapes into the pericardial sac, resulting in peripheral pressure on the heart that prevents diastole, and death is the result.

The sudden accumulation of a transudate, an exudate, or blood in the pericardial sac in large amounts will so compress the heart that cardiac failure results. If the foreign material accumulates gradu-

ally, the heart and circulatory system have time to compensate for the alteration, and tremendous amounts of material may collect in the pericardial sac before death occurs. Death is due to pressure upon the heart, not from loss of blood, and is possibly also due to hindrance to the return of venous blood. Gas in the sac (**pneumopericardium**) and likewise, pus (**pyopericardium**) are seen in traumatic pericarditis of cattle.

## Local Disturbances of Cell Metabolism

In chickens a disturbance of **protein** metabolism sometimes occurs in which uric acid salts are deposited in and upon the serous surfaces (visceral gout), especially on the surfaces of the heart sac. The heart has a frosty appearance. Microscopic examination reveals the urates imbedded in a cellular fibrinous network upon the epicardium. An inflammatory process often involves the subepicardium. At times the uratic fibrinous exudate becomes organized.

A serous atrophy of the subepicardial **fat** occurs in cachetic animals. Fat normally found in the coronary grooves is changed to a reddish-yellow gelatinous substance and should be differentiated from edema. An increased amount of epicardial and pericardial fat occurs in excessively fat animals.

**Pigment** (melanin), in sheep and calves appears as focal subepicardial deposits.

## Circulatory Disturbances

### HYPEREMIA

**Active hyperemia** occurs in association with generalized infectious diseases and with inflammatory diseases of the pericardium and epicardium. **Passive hyperemia** occurs when there is a general accumulation of blood in the veins due to lesions in the heart and lungs.

### HEMORRHAGES

Hemorrhages of the parietal and visceral pericardium occur frequently. Their size may vary from petechiae to suffusions. They are caused by hypoxemia and various toxic agents. Hemorrhages are most frequently associated with the agony of dying (**agonal hemorrhages**) in which the lack of oxygen and spasmotic contraction of tissues cause rupture of the vessels. Bacterial and viral toxins are also of importance and, consequently, pericardial hemorrhages are often an indication of a septicemia.

It is **impossible to differentiate** hemorrhages as toxic, hypoxic, bacterial, or viral on gross appearance alone. When blood escapes from a vessel it accumulates in the tissues in a pattern dictated by tissue pressures and not according to the type of etiologic agent.

In horses a post-infection bacterial intoxication called purpura hemorrhagica or petechial fever may have as one of its lesions small hemorrhages in the epicardium. This intoxication most frequently is a sequel to streptococcic infections. The hemorrhages appear to result from damage to the capillary endothelium and the destruction of blood platelets.

Intoxications of plant origin may produce similar hemorrhages on the heart. White snake root (*Eupatrium urticaefolium*) may cause them in cattle and sheep, the seeds of *Crotalaria spectabilis* in chickens (Fig. 14.1), and the toxic agent, dicoumarin, in damaged sweet clover (*Melilotus albus, Melilotus officinalis*). In the so-called sweet clover disease, the hemorrhages are associated with a low prothrombin content of the blood. A low concentration of blood calcium may be a contributing factor. A similar condition occurs in chicks fed on a vitamin K-deficient diet, but the marked reduction of prothrombin in sweet clover disease does not appear to be related to vitamin K deficiency. It is believed that the dicoumarin either destroys or inactivates prothrombin, or interferes with the mechanism which is responsible for its production.

Cardiac hemorrhages may also be an indication of a sapremia. This condition is the result of absorption of products of protein autolysis or of the bacterial destruction of body tissues by saprophytes. It is an intoxication quite similar in appearance to a septicemia or a toxemia. In domestic mammals it occurs most often in female animals that have retained dead fetuses or retained fetal membranes.

Thrifty calves, lambs and kids nursing well-fed dams, and feeder lambs that are supplied a heavy grain ration sometimes die of an **enterotoxemia**. Death comes suddenly, and among the lesions present are petechial and ecchymotic hemorrhages of the epicardium. The lesions are due to the toxin of *Clostridium perfringens*, usually type C or D. The organism is found in the ingesta of affected animals. Filtrates obtained by washing the ingesta are toxic for healthy animals when injected intravenously. The relationship between heavy feeding and the intoxication seems to be that an abundance of milk or other highly nutritious food in the stomach and intestine furnishes an excellent medium for the growth of the toxin-producing clostridium. The toxin which is absorbed into the blood stream from the intestine damages the capillary endothelium of the epicardium and other parts of the body.

## Pericarditis

Inflammation of the pericardium is due to (1) trauma (foreign bodies penetrating from the reticulum) and (2) infection. The origin of the latter is either (*a*) hematogenous or (*b*) by extension from the myocardium, pleura, or bronchial or mediastinal lymph nodes.

Pericarditis is observed in several infectious diseases (pasteurellosis, sporadic bovine encephalitis, pleuropneumonia-like disease (PPLO) of swine, pullorum disease, and pneumonia). The classification of pericarditis is based upon the character of the exudate: (1) serous, (2) fibrinous, (3) suppurative, or (4) gangrenous.

### SEROUS AND FIBRINOUS PERICARDITIS

Serous, fibrinous, and serofibrinous pericarditis are most frequent in cows, calves, and swine. Macroscopically, the pericardial fluid is increased in amount. The maximum amounts of fluid reported are:

horse, 36 to 40 liters; cow, 18½ liters; dog, ½ liter. The epicardium at first is simply dull (not glistening) in appearance. Later, a fine, pale yellow, fibrinous exudate appears which is easily removed. The exudate becomes laminated. If the fibrin is abundant, the heart's action may whip it into tufts. The exudate may increase until the two serous surfaces stick together, and if the exudate is removed, a raw, bleeding surface is exposed. Microscopically, at first, there is hyperemia with a slight serofibrinous exudate, like fibrinous inflammation of any serous surface. The serous covering is intact. Later, degeneration and desquamation of the serous membrane occur. Leukocytes appear in the fibrinous exudate.

**Common terminations are:** (1) Liquefaction of the fibrinous exudate by proteolytic enzymes of the leukocytes followed by absorption. Regeneration of the serous coat then occurs. This kind of termination is probably rare, occurring only in low-grade irritation. (2) The usual termination is organization of the exudate (Fig. 14.2). Capillaries which are derived from the capillary bed of the epicardium grow vertically to the surface. Fibroblasts grow parallel to the surface. Later, the capillaries decrease in number; the connective tissue matures and contracts, becoming dense connective tissue (cicatrical tissue). This new tissue may have focal or diffuse distribution. It may extend across the sac joining the two serous surfaces (adhesions). (3) If the exudate is extensive, all of it may not be absorbed or organized. Caseous necrosis with calcification may then occur, especially in cattle with traumatic pericarditis.

### SUPPURATIVE PERICARDITIS

Suppurative pericarditis is seen most frequently in cattle afflicted with traumatic pericarditis (Fig. 14.3). The bacteria are carried into the pericardium from the reticulum on the penetrating foreign body (nail or wire). The exudate contains pus in addition to the elements already named above. The termination is usually a combination of the latter two just described.

### Tumors

Tumors are fairly common. Primary ones are lipoma, fibroma, endothelioma, fibrosarcoma, and nerve sheath tumors. Secondary tumors occur either by metastasis (lymphosarcoma, fibrosarcoma, carcinoma) or by extension (lymphosarcoma).

## MYOCARDIUM

### Disturbances of Cell Metabolism

#### CLOUDY SWELLING

Cloudy swelling is observed in the course of various intoxications (bacterial, plant, mineral). It occurs in practically all septicemic diseases. Microscopically, the cytoplasm of the muscle fibers becomes granular. The cells are swollen slightly. The cross striations are less prominent than normal. The nuclei may be indistinct. Cloudy swelling must be differentiated from post-mortem changes which are similar. Macroscopically, the heart is slightly enlarged as determined by incising the myocardium, and the cut surface has a parboiled appearance. Within 6 to 8 hours after death, even when the carcass of the animal is kept cold, post-mortem autolytic changes develop which simulate cloudy swelling.

#### FATTY DEGENERATION

The etiology is the same as that for cloudy swelling, but the irritant is more intense. Only a relatively slight irritation is necessary to disturb protein metabolism (cloudy swelling). A more drastic one also disturbs fat metabolism (fatty degeneration). Macroscopically, it is much like cloudy swelling except the color is slightly yellowish brown instead of grayish brown. It is hard to differentiate except in severe cases. In such cases the heart is soft and flabby. Microscopically, in mild cases fat droplets appear in parallel rows between the myofibrils. In severe cases the droplets are more diffuse with no regular arrangement. The nuclei are poorly stained or pyknotic.

The effects of cardiac degeneration are not apparent unless the changes are quite severe. The damaged myocardium may lose its ability to contract to its normal extent, and cardiac dilatation is the result. This is sometimes a terminal condition in severe acute septicemic diseases. The dilatation may lead to cardiac rupture. If the heart withstands the acute condition, and repair by substitution occurs, the newly formed connective tissue may encroach upon the conduction system of the organ and disturb the rhythm of the heart beats (heart-block).

### FATTY INFILTRATION

A subepicardial increase of adipose tissue is common in fat animals, but it seldom penetrates into the myocardium. When it does, the wall of the right ventricle is most frequently involved, especially toward the apex. Wherever it occurs, the increased adipose tissue crowds out the muscle fibers. At times the infiltration extends from the epicardium through the myocardium to the endocardium. When this happens, the heart becomes weakened and may rupture at this point. Even if the heart does not rupture, the animal may die as a result of slow or sudden cardiac failure. Fat foci are often found in old myocardial cicatricial tissue.

### CALCIFICATION

Calcification occurs in the epi-, myo-, and endocardium, and is most common in the wall of the left ventricle. The calcium appears as gray, white, or green streaks or masses in the involved tissue. For calcification to appear there must first be necrotic or degenerating tissue. As a result, it is observed following coagulative necrosis of the myocardium and in elastic tissue degeneration of the endocardium.

### PIGMENTATION

**Melanosis.** Melanosis of the heart is frequently observed in normal calves and sheep upon slaughter and is thought to be due to faulty distribution of the melanoblasts during fetal development. It may be accompanied by melanosis of the lungs, liver, and meninges. The melanin appears as brown or black foci and streaks in the endocardium, less frequently in the epicardium, and occasionally in the myocardium. It is most frequently observed in heavily pigmented animals such as Angus cattle and Hampshire sheep. As the animal ages the pigment tends to disappear.

**Brown pigmentation** occurs mostly in old cows, especially in chronic cachectic diseases. Macroscopically, there is a disappearance of subepicardial fat. The color of the myocardium is brownish gray or bronze. Brown pigmentation is seen also in the masseter muscles, muscles of the cervical region, and may extend to the whole musculature. Microscopically, at the poles of the nuclei of the muscle cells there are accumulations of granular, brown pigment combined with a lipochrome.

## Necrosis

### COAGULATIVE NECROSIS

Myocardial coagulative necrosis is a lesion of vitamin E and selenium deficiencies in lambs and calves. If the necrosis is extensive, sudden death from cardiac failure is the result.

**Macroscopically,** the myocardium has the same white or cooked appearance as is seen in coagulative necrosis of skeletal muscle (Fig. 14.4). The necrotic areas appear as foci or streaks in the myocardium and are most numerous in the papillary muscles and under the epicardium. If the animal survives, scarring of the myocardium occurs.

**Microscopically,** the muscle fibers have the usual appearance of coagulative necrosis. After several days, leukocytes, primarily macrophages, appear in the areas of necrosis, and phagocytosis of the necrotic muscle occurs. At the same time fibroblasts proliferate in the area. If the sarcolemma is not destroyed, the cytoplasm of the damaged muscle cell will regenerate. When the muscle damage is so extensive that the cells do not regenerate, the area is partially filled in with connective tissue.

Myocardial coagulative necrosis is also

found to be associated with thiamine deficiency in swine. The myocardial damage is usually not as prominent as in vitamin E deficiency in lambs. This lesion explains many of the sudden deaths in swine.

Myocardial coagulative necrosis in swine is frequently associated with the feeding of excessive amounts of cottonseed meal. Cottonseed meal is practically devoid of vitamin E, and in addition the gossypol it contains is toxic.

## Disturbances of Circulation

**Active hyperemia** is seen in infectious diseases and other injuries to the heart. **Passive hyperemia** is associated with obstructing vascular diseases of the heart and lungs.

**Infarction** of the myocardium is due to occlusion of a branch of the coronary artery by a thrombus. This is a common pathological condition in man but is uncommon in animals since the latter do not have a high incidence of arteriosclerotic diseases. In dogs it has been shown that it is difficult to experimentally produce a cardiac infarct comparable to one in man. When the major coronary artery in a dog is ligated, a large infarct results, but it contains islands of normal tissue. It is not an area of complete necrosis as in man. Extensive collateral coronary circulation in the dog apparently is sufficient to prevent necrosis of all the tissue in the area. As a consequence the effects are not as serious and repair can occur quickly. The gross and microscopic appearance of the infarcts is similar to that observed in infarcts of other organs. Large infarcts may so weaken the myocardium that the wall can no longer withstand the high intracardial blood pressure and a rupture or aneurysm at the site occurs. Large infarcts may give rise to heart aneurysms or may even rupture. Small ones may become organized so that scars result.

In cardiac infarction the membranes of the injured cells become more permeable to the intracellular enzymes, glutamic oxaloacetic transaminase and glutamic pyruvic transaminase, particularly to the former. This permits the enzymes to escape into the blood plasma. Their presence there can be detected by the clinical pathologist and can be used as an aid in diagnosing the cardiac injury.

**Petechial hemorrhages** of the myocardium are very common. They occur in various intoxications, particularly bacterial and plant. Their etiology, therefore, is similiar to that of epicardial and pericardial hemorrhages.

## Disturbances of Continuity
RUPTURE

Favored places of rupture are the right auricle and ventricle. The etiology is a combination of factors: a weakened area in the myocardium plus hindrance to the outflow of blood plus consequent increase in blood pressure. Primary weakening is due to various causes: heart aneurysm, myocardial degenerative changes in intoxications, infarction from coronary thrombosis, and parasitic cysts.

The causes of traumatic perforation or rupture are bullets, cannulas, syringe needles, foreign bodies from the reticulum, and violent injury such as being run over by a vehicle. In the latter case the heart shows a ragged tear with a hemorrhagic border. Death results quickly because blood in the pericardial sac prevents diastolic movement. Foreign bodies from the reticulum seldom produce fatal hemorrhage because they penetrate the thick muscle wall of the ventricles. Cannula wounds of the thin-walled auricles are frequently fatal.

## Myocarditis

Opportunities for the development of myocarditis among animals would seem to be abundant, and while the condition frequently does occur, it is surprising that its occurrence is not much greater than it is.

A nonsuppurative myocarditis is associated with various toxemias. These irritants reach the myocardium by way of the coronary circulation. The irritant may be a mineral poison such as thallium sulfate, toxins from bacterial or parasitic infections, or necrotic tissue as occurs in coagulative necrosis of the myocardium.

Suppurative myocarditis is associated with the presence of bacteria. The inflammation is usually localized and is characterized by the formation of abscesses, thus differing from a nonsuppurative myocarditis which tends to be a diffuse involvement of the myocardium.

The bacteria reach the myocardium by way of the blood stream or extension from adjacent organs. As a result, focal suppurative myocarditis is associated with septicemias or bacteremias when the organisms are carried to the heart from suppurative processes in other organs. Septic emboli may lodge in a coronary artery and produce an abscess.

Another way that the myocardium can become involved in a suppurative inflammation is by extension of the process from a near-by inflamed organ or part, e.g., from t h e pericardium, endocardium, pleura, lungs, and bronchial and mediastinal lymph nodes. Lastly, the irritant giving rise to the inflammation may be a foreign body penetrating the myocardium.

**Macroscopic appearance.** Macroscopically, **acute nonsuppurative myocarditis** presents numerous, irregularly shaped foci and streaks which may vary in color from dull grayish red to a pale yellowish red. Occasionally these discolored areas have a tigroid appearance. The heart is soft and flabby. In **suppurative myocarditis** the myocardium presents either a few or many abscesses (Fig. 21.2). Recently formed abscesses have a red border as the result of hyperemia and hemorrhage; older ones may be encapsulated. Character and color of the pus in the abscesses vary depending upon the etiology. Most characteristic is the pale greenish-yellow pus produced by *Corynebacterium pyogenes*. *Spherophorus necrophorus* infection of the myocardium is usually characterized by formation of irregular-shaped areas of coagulative necrosis rather than by abscesses.

**Microscopic appearance.** Microscopically, the changes in nonsuppurative myocarditis are even more variable than the gross changes. In very acute cases, degenerative alterations of the muscle cells predominate over the strictly inflammatory vascular and exudative changes. In such cases one may recognize cloudy swelling, fatty degeneration, hyaline degeneration, myolysis, and atrophy of the muscle cells. In less acute cases, the vascular and exudative changes predominate; and in the chronic cases, proliferative changes. The microscopic picture of the abscesses in suppurative myocarditis is that usually seen in abscesses in any tissue. In necrophorus infection of the myocardium, areas of coagulative necrosis are surrounded by a margin of hyperemia, hemorrhage, and leukocytes.

**Termination.** The terminations of nonsuppurative myocarditis are practically the same as for myocardial degeneration. This is because this form of myocarditis is a combination of myocardial degenerative changes and the purely inflammatory process. The end result then may be heart aneurysm, dilatation of one or more chambers, cardiac rupture, or a gradual repair of the damage done to the myocardium by fibroplasia. If regeneration of the myocardium does not occur, the area occupied by the destroyed muscle cells is filled in with white fibrous connective tissue.

In the midst of the granulation tissue, occasional degenerated and atrophied muscle cells may be found. When the inflammatory process subsides and the granulation tissue becomes cicatricial tissue, the heart is said to be fibrosed. The myocardial scar contains a dense development of heavy elastic fibers running parallel to one another and to the intervening collagenous fibers and adjacent muscle fibers. This scar tissue may interrupt the conduction system of the heart and cause heart-block. In suppurative myocarditis the contents of very old abcesses may become organized and even calcified.

## Changes in Size of Heart

The shape of the heart at the time of necropsy depends upon the state of rigor mortis; therefore, the relative weight should be considered with shape in determining changes in the size of this organ. The relative weight of the heart to the total body weight is approximately: horse, 0.5 to 0.6 per cent; cattle, 0.3 to 0.5 per cent; swine, 0.45 per cent; and dog, 0.8 to 2.2 per cent.

### DILATATION

This is an enlargement of the heart due to deficient emptying of the chambers during systole. It may involve the wall of a chamber or chambers completely or partially. The latter is called heart aneurysm and is due to localized injury to the heart wall. It is usually congenital however.

Dilatation may occur alone or be accompanied by hypertrophy. Occurring alone it is part of the pathologic picture of various severe infectious and intoxication diseases in which there is myocardial degeneration or myocarditis. It is seen also in fat and old animals that are overexercised (fat hogs, racing and hunting dogs, race horses). The left ventricle is most often affected. In heaves of horses and in pneumonia of all animals, however, the dilatation occurs on the right side of the heart. In dogs the right chambers may be dilated because of the presence of large numbers of heart worms (Dirofilaria immitis).

Rarely is cardiac dilatation bilateral except in animals affected with severe myocardial degeneration. Occasionally an animal is seen which presents a chronic bilateral cardiac dilatation due to valvular stenosis affecting both the tricuspid and mitral valves, and very rarely even involving the pulmonary and aortic semilunars.

Enlarged right heart with dilated pulmonary artery is designated cor pulmonale. It is a chronic condition with the sequence of cardiac changes being first, hypertrophy and later, dilatation. The cardiac and vascular changes are the result of hindrance to pulmonary circulation as occurs in chronic emphysema, pulmonary fibrosis, or any long-standing lung lesion which decreases the total pulmonary capillary bed. The presence of heart worms (Dirofilaria immitis) in the right heart accompanied by a form of arteriosclerosis (endarteritis obliterans) involving the branches of the pulmonary artery is a special type of cor pulmonale occurring in dogs.

Grossly, the lumen of the heart chamber is oval rather than conical. The wall is thin and flabby. The apex is rounded. The papillary muscles and chordae tendineae are stretched and flattened. With the stretching of the heart wall, the valve in the affected chamber is pulled outward so far that it fails to close the opening completely. This is termed valvular insufficiency or incompetence.

The effects of the valvular insufficiency arising from cardiac dilatation are observed best in aged dogs. They develop symptoms of congestive heart failure. In well advanced cases the dogs cough, are cyanotic and dyspneic, and show signs of ascites and subcutaneous edema. These effects are caused by reduced cardiac output and decreased cardiac return arising from the weakened organ and inefficient valves. The failing organ therefore allows blood to accumulate in the organs (chronic passive congestion). The tissues, consequently, suffer from hypoxia and lack of nutrients.

Occasionally the wall of the right ventricle of a chronically dilated heart may bulge at its thinnest point. This constitutes a heart aneurysm. There is always the possibility that the aneurysm may rupture. It is impossible for the animal to bleed to death into the pericardial sac, but as soon as enough blood escapes (cardiac tamponade) to prevent the heart from going into diastole, death occurs.

HYPERTROPHY

This is an enlargement of the heart due to increase in the heart musculature (an increase in size of muscle cells) as a result of increased function over a period of time, usually at least a month. It may appear alone or be accompanied by dilatation (Fig. 14.5).

A good example of cardiac hypertrophy accompanied by dilatation occurs in cattle in the Rocky Mountain states. The combined conditions are found in many of the cattle that pasture at an altitude above 8,000 feet. Because the circulatory disturbance which arises from the chronic cardiac enlargement results in edema of the brisket, the disease is called brisket disease by the cattlemen (Fig. 5.1).

At Colorado State University, where this disease has been studied most extensively, it has been noted that in clinical cases there is marked right ventricular hypertrophy and mild septal hypertrophy. The lesions are not so marked in experimental cases. One way the syndrome has been produced is by constricting the pulmonary artery about 50 per cent. This pulmonary arterial lesion results in cardiac hypertrophy, congestive hepatic fibrosis, and anasarca. It is reasoned from this research that primary pulmonary disease in mountain cattle may cause the hindrance to circulation necessary for the development of the brisket disease syndrome. Colorado clinicians have observed that brisket disease cattle generally have primary pulmonary lesions of some kind.

Hypertrophy can affect the whole heart or only a portion of it. Since increased function is usually due to a hindrance to circulation, the degree and location of hypertrophy depend upon the location and nature of the hindrance. Hindrance can be intracardial or extracardial.

**1. Intracardial hindrance** is due to valvular defects. Stenosis or insufficiency of the aortic semilunars produces hypertrophy of the left ventricle. Lesions of the mitral valve affect the left atrium. These lesions may lead to passive hyperemia of the lungs and eventually to hypertrophy of the right ventricle. Hypertrophy of the right ventricle is also produced by stenosis or insufficiency of the semilunars of the pulmonary artery.

**2. Extracardial hindrance.** Left ventricle hypertrophy may be due to chronic focal interstitial nephritis (dogs). Right ventricle hypertrophy is due to chronic pulmonary circulatory disturbances (heaves, chronic interstitial pneumonia).

Grossly, the heart is enlarged. The affected walls are thickened, firm, and rubber-like. The weight may be doubled. If accompanied by dilatation, the lumen also becomes enlarged.

The factor which may limit the progress of cardiac hypertrophy is a decrease in myocardial nutrition. As the myocardium increases in thickness, it becomes more and more difficult for coronary blood to reach every muscle fiber during the periodic rest periods (diastole). Not only do the fibers fail to get sufficient nourishment but any metabolites formed by them accumulate in and around the fibers. As a result the hypertrophy ceases, and if the heavy work which caused the hypertrophy continues, the fibers begin to degenerate and atrophy. The thickened, more powerful myocardium then can no longer compensate for the increased work it is called upon to perform. A state of decompensation has then begun which may terminate in cardiac failure.

The effects of cardiac failure are felt throughout the body. First of all, the weak right heart cannot adequately transfer blood from the venae cavae to the lungs, and the left heart cannot move it with sufficient force into the aorta. As a consequence, the arteries are underfilled and the veins overfilled. The organs suffer from hypoxia and carbon dioxide retention. The stimulation of the respiratory center is indicated by polypnea at first and dyspnea later. The renal filter is injured by passive congestion and hypoxia giving rise to albuminuria. Passive congestion of the abdominal viscera results in indigestion and

<br/>

hydroperitoneum, in congestion of the thoracic organs, and in hydropericardium and pulmonary edema (dyspnea). The congested mucous membranes become slate-colored (cyanosis).

## Parasites

Sarcosporidia are parasitic sporozoa found in the horse, ox, sheep, and pig. They become located in striated muscle fibers, both skeletal and cardiac. Geographically this parasite appears to have world-wide distribution.

The myocardial fibers and striated muscle fibers of the esophagus and diaphragm are especially favorite places of localization for this parasite. Grossly, in mild or moderate infections the cysts go unnoticed. In heavy infections, when muscle fibers are viewed longitudinally, minute, oval or eliptical grayish spots indicate the presence of cysts located in the fibers. Microscopically, the sarcocysts are well delineated in sections stained with hematoxylin and eosin. The cysts displace the contents of the muscle fibers at the place where they are located. Each sarcocyst is filled with hematoxylin-stained spores. No reaction to the parasite is displayed either by the parasitized cells or by those around it. It is conceivable, however, that in a heavily infected heart the myocardial fibers would be weakened, which might lead to some degree of myocardial failure. Furthermore, sarcosporidia contain a strong neurotoxin (sarcocystin) which, when injected into rabbits, mice, sparrows, rats, sheep, and some other animals, causes depression, paralysis, and death. This effect of sarcosporidia must be kept in mind when examining a heavily parasitized animal in which there is no other apparent cause of death.

## Tumors

**Primary tumors** of the myocardium are rare. Fibromas and myxofibromas have been reported. They are usually pedunculated, project into the heart cavity, and are covered with endocardium. The most frequent of the **secondary tumors** is lymphosarcoma in cattle (Fig. 14.6). Among 40 unselected cases of lymphosarcoma of cattle reported by Feldman, 50 per cent had cardiac involvement. The growths are circumscribed and project into the pericardial sac or into the heart cavity or are diffuse. The immature lymphocytes infiltrate the myocardium and cause atrophy of the muscle fibers (Fig. 14.7). In horses occasionally are seen melanosarcomas and fibrosarcomas; in dogs, metastatic carcinomas, hemangiosarcomas, and rhabdomyosarcomas.

A rare tumor of much interest in dogs is the heart base tumor. In most instances the tumor, which is situated subepicardially at the base of the heart, springs from

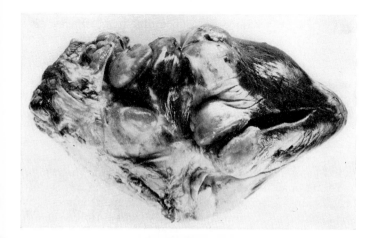

Fig. 14.6 — Lymphosarcoma of the heart of a cow. Numerous nodules involve the myocardium. Similar tumors involved the omentum, intestine, and uterus. (Feldman, Jour. A.V.M.A.)

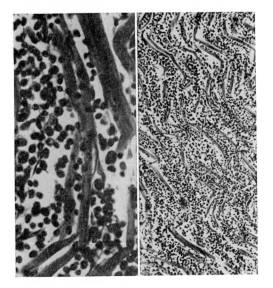

Fig. 14.7 — Lymphosarcoma of the myocardium of a horse. The lymphoblasts have pushed in between the muscle fibers and have caused them to atrophy. ×110 and ×310. (Iowa State University Veterinarian.)

the aortic body, the carotid body, or an island of thyroid tissue which may be located in the myocardium. These tumors are generally located at the root of the aorta or pulmonary artery. If they are derived from the aortic body or the carotid body, they consist of neoplastic neuroepithelium, and if they arise from an island of misplaced (ectopic) thyroid gland, they have some resemblance to thyroid tissue. They may or may not metastasize. Located, as they are, close to the large blood vessels at the base of the heart, they have a marked effect upon cardiac action and usually cause cardiac insufficiency with its chain of associated lesions.

## ENDOCARDIUM

### Local Disturbances of Metabolism

A focal **calcification** of the elastic fiber in the endocardium is occasionally encountered in horses, cattle, dogs, and foxes. It occurs most frequently in the left auricle. The endocardium presents several hard, rough, small protuberances and ridges. Calcification is also observed occasionally in the aorta in the form of plaques. The question of etiology is unsettled. It is not clear whether calcification is preceded by injury or whether it origi-

nates as a result of a local or general disturbance of calcium metabolism. **Melanosis** of the endocardium is observed mostly in sheep and calves. The pigmented cells are distributed diffusely among the elastic fibers of the endocardium.

### Disturbances of Circulation

Endocardial hemorrhages are the only circulatory disturbances which need emphasis. Practically everything which has been said about epicardial hemorrhages can be repeated here. It can be said safely that endocardial hemorrhages, however, occur more frequently than epicardial. One will notice that they occur more often in the left ventricle than in the other heart chambers. Endocardial hemorrhages may have more serious effects than those of the epicardium because they may exert pressure on the impulse-conducting system (bundle of His and the Purkinje fibers). The result may be a disturbance of the rhythmic beating of the heart.

Subendocardial ecchymotic hemorrhages of the left ventricle are seen frequently in animals that have been killed for necropsy. Often no apparent reason for their presence can be detected. They are generally referred to as **agonal** hemorrhages. It is presumed that they result from violent, terminal beating of the heart.

## Endocarditis

The causes of endocarditis are bacteria and toxins. A single inoculation is not sufficient. More or less constant infection over a considerable period is necessary. Therefore, it is not usually seen in acute septicemic diseases but in chronic ones (swine erysipelas, chronic strangles in horses, *Corynebacterium pyogenes* and streptococcic infection of cattle and hogs, white scours of calves, navel ill of foals).

In dogs experimental endocarditis can be produced by virulent strains of streptococci obtained from a variety of sources. Less virulent strains produce the condition as well as the more virulent ones, the only difference being that it requires a longer period of time and increased doses of the organisms. This emphasizes the danger to the heart of chronic streptococcic infections in other parts of the body.

At the Angell Memorial Animal Hospital, Boston, Mass., in the course of one year 6.6 per cent of 600 dogs and cats necropsied had vegetative valvular endocarditis. It was usually secondary to active or latent infections with pyogenic microorganisms. The causative organisms were hemolytic and nonhemolytic streptococci and staphylococci, *Pseudomonas aeruginosa,* and *Escherichia coli.* These organisms were isolated from the primary infected foci, valvular vegetations, heart blood, and blood stream. General signs of the endocardial infection are fever, neutrophilic leukocytosis, and a rapid sedimentation rate. Special signs are heart bruits, cardiac weakness, sudden lameness, and pain. The latter two arise from embolism to other parts of the body.

Any portion of the endocardium may be involved, but most frequently the valves (valvular endocarditis or valvulitis). Because of the presence of tiny, beadlike, warty nodules on the valves, this is also called **verrucose endocarditis,** and possibly because the lesions resemble the head of a cauliflower plant, it is often called **vegetative endocarditis.**

**Macroscopic appearance.** Macroscopically, there appear at first small, circumscribed, yellowish-white, fluffy patches upon the valves or mural endocardium. On the atrioventricular valves they appear usually on the atrial side; on the semilunars, on the ventricular side. They are nearly always near the free edge of the valves. Later these foci appear firmer, grayish white and wartlike (Fig. 14.8).

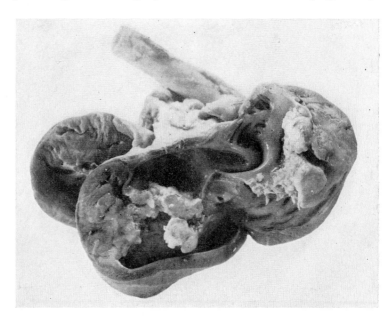

Fig. 14.8 — Chronic endocarditis of the tricuspid valve of an 8-week-old pig due to a streptococcic infection. (Bullard, Jour. A.V.M.A.)

With continued enlargement they lead to valvular stenosis or insufficiency.

**Microscopic appearance.** Microscopically, the patches referred to under Macroscopic appearance are white thrombi, which consist of platelets and leukocytes and rest upon the inner elastic membrane. The endothelium has disappeared. Hyperemia, hemorrhage, and leukocytic infiltration of the subendocardium are present. Later, organization of the thrombus by very vascular granulation tissue occurs (Figs. 14.9, 16.1, 15.14); later still, cicatrization and possibly calcification. Bacteria may be present, and their presence prevents complete organization of the thrombus. Their action also produces surface necrosis (ulcers), and continuous irritation produces excessive granulation tissue. Because of the infection, the underlying granulation tissue also contains more leukocytes. Especially noticeable is a zone of leukocytes beneath the necrotic infected areas. Plasma cells are numerous in the granulation tissue.

**Results of endocarditis.** The results of chronic valvulitis are: (1) Embolism in other parts of the body by means of sterile portions of thrombi or portions of thrombi containing pyogenic bacteria. The sterile emboli cause infarcts, especially in the kidneys. The septic emboli produce metastatic abscesses in various organs (pyemia). (2) Changes in the lumen of the heart valves; stenosis or insufficiency. Stenosis impedes blood flow, increases the work of the heart chamber affected, causes dilatation and, eventually, hypertrophy of its wall. In insufficiency the valve does not close completely and consequently results in a backflow of blood during systole. This causes over-filling and dilatation of the chamber, which should empty. This eventually leads to hypertrophy. Below are given the effects of insufficiency and stenosis of the various heart valves upon the heart and other organs:

### Tricuspid

**Insufficiency.** There is accumulation of blood in the right atrium resulting in dilatation and eventually hypertrophy of that chamber; passive hyperemia in the vena cava leading to passive hyperemia of the

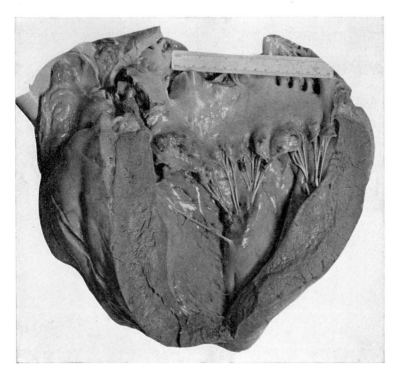

Fig. 14.9 — Mitral valve of a horse showing fibrosis following chronic valvulitis due to a streptococcus. Note the smooth surface of the thickened valve. (Department of Veterinary Pathology, Iowa State University.)

liver, hepatic cirrhosis, passive hyperemia of the kidneys, induration of the kidneys; hydroperitoneum, hydrothorax, and hydropericardium.

**Stenosis.** There is incomplete filling of the right ventricle; accumulation of blood in the right atrium with the same results as in insufficiency of this valve.

### Pulmonary Semilunars

**Insufficiency.** There is a return flow of blood from the pulmonary artery into the right ventricle, leading to dilatation and hypertrophy; accumulation of blood in the right atrium and general venous stasis.

**Stenosis.** There is accumulation of blood in the right ventricle; dilatation and hypertrophy of the right ventricle; accumulation in the right atrium and general venous stasis.

### Mitral

**Insufficiency.** There is accumulation of blood in the left atrium; dilatation and eventually hypertrophy; incomplete emptying of the pulmonary vein; passive hyperemia and induration of the lung; eventual hypertrophy of the right ventricle due to increased pressure in the pulmonary artery; later accumulation of blood in the right atrium with hypertrophy, and passive hyperemia of the large veins. From the clinical standpoint this condition is designated **congestive heart failure with pulmonary hypertension.** Clinical evidences of it are enlarged heart (cardiomegaly), right ventricular hypertrophy, dyspnea due to pulmonary congestion, cyanosis, jugular pulse, and abdominal edema (ascites) resulting from hindrance to venous return, and enlarged liver (hepatomegaly).

**Stenosis.** There is incomplete filling of the left ventricle; accumulation of blood in the left atrium with the same results as in mitral insufficiency.

### Aortic Semilunars

**Insufficiency.** During diastole there is a return flow of blood from the aorta into the left ventricle; dilatation and hypertrophy; stasis of blood in the left atrium and lungs.

**Stenosis.** There is stasis of blood in the left ventricle; dilatation and hypertrophy of the left ventricle; stasis of blood in the left atrium and lungs.

## ARTERIES

### Breaks in Continuity

Spontaneous rupture occurs mostly in the aorta of the horse just above the junction of the valve cusps. Hemorrhage occurs into the pericardial sac. Ruptures occasionally occur in the abdominal branches of the posterior aorta of the horse (parasitic aneurysms). Rupture of the aorta has been reported in dogs in which the artery has been infected with the nematode *Spirocerca lupi*. The fibrotic nodules containing the worms usually are located dorsally in the vessel wall and they rupture ventrally where the vessel wall undergoes degeneration, necrosis, and calcification. Aortic ruptures caused by dissecting aneurysms are sometimes a serious condition in large male turkeys between 10 and 24 weeks of age. Experimentally it is associated with feeding a ration high in protein and fat. Alterations, mostly degenerative and fibroblastic proliferative, involving the intima and media, pave the way for blood to escape into a space between the media and adventitia. The resulting aneurysm usually ruptures.

### Thrombosis and Embolism

Thrombi and emboli are more frequent in the arteries than in the veins. They are most important in horses. The etiological agents are:

(1) Larvae of *Strongylus vulgaris*, which locate in the anterior mesenteric artery and its branches (Fig. 17.16) (See page 472). They produce an arteritis with an accompanying thrombosis which causes stenoses of the vessels. Portions of thrombi may become emboli, pass farther down the vessels, and result in infarction in portions of the cecum and colon (thromboembolic colic) or in the muscles of the posterior limbs (intermittent lameness). Under favorable conditions the thrombi may become organized.

(2) Bacteria, as in severe mastitis where the resulting infarction may terminate in necrosis and gangrene of one or more quarters.

## Local Disturbances of Growth and Cell Metabolism

### ATROPHY

Atrophy is of importance only in involutionary processes occurring in the navel vessels after birth and in the uterine vessels after abortion or parturition. Hyaline degeneration and calcification usually accompany the atrophy. The vessel finally has the appearance of a fibrous string.

### HYALINE DEGENERATION

Nieberle states that hyaline degeneration is encountered frequently in the spleens of old dogs but appears to have no serious effects. It is also observed in chronically inflamed tissues, involuting vessels, in branches of the splenic artery in hog cholera, and in tumors.

### CALCIFICATION

**Calcification of the media** probably occurs more frequently than is supposed. It affects the larger vessels and occurs either in vessels that have been injured or in uninjured vessels as an expression of a primary disturbance of calcium metabolism. It may involve the intima or the media or both. Involvement of the media is most important. It is observed in old cattle and horses most frequently and usually occurs in the thoracic and abdominal aorta. The macroscopic appearance varies. At first the intima appears normal. Later, small, irregular, elevated patches with borders raised and centers depressed appear. Microscopically, at first, a very fine granular precipitate of calcium salt appears between the cells. Later on, the salt is adsorbed by the elastic fibers and forms a mantle around them. The fibers lose their contractility and appear stretched. Later still, the muscle fibers are affected. The calcified foci act as foreign bodies and produce an inflammatory reaction. The intima at first is not involved. Later it becomes hypertrophied (compensatory).

**Calcification of the intima** occurs in cattle and horses in the thoracic aorta (Fig. 14.10). The condition is manifestation of a disturbance of calcium metabolism or is the result of an inflammatory process of the intima. The disturbance in calcium metabolism occurs most often in young animals. At first, fine scaly foci appear in the intima. Later these become larger and the surface rougher. The microscopic appearance is similar to that of medial calcification except the changes are confined to the intima. Hyperplasia of the connective tissue is greater so that it encroaches upon the lumen.

## Arteriosclerosis

The literal meaning of the word arteriosclerosis is "hardening of the arteries." In man the most frequent type of the condition is characterized by thickening of the

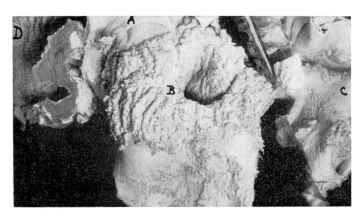

Fig. 14.10 — Calcification of the heart and contiguous vessels in a cow.

A, aortic semilunar valves (normal);

B, raised, irregular calcified areas on intima of aorta;

C, similar raised areas in pulmonary artery;

D, roughened calcified endocardium (auricle).

(Goldberg, Jour. A.V.M.A.)

intima due to proliferation of connective tissue. The connective tissue undergoes hyaline degeneration, lipoid infiltration, and calcification. These intimal changes cause a loss of elasticity and contractility of the vessel wall. A less common type of arteriosclerosis in man is one characterized by extensive destruction, atrophy, and calcification of the media of small and medium-sized vessels. In man the condition is rather common in the latter third of the normal span of life. The etiology of the condition is still being studied.

In domestic animals there is no condition which compares exactly with human arteriosclerosis. Pathologists, however, in attempting to produce in animals a condition similar to that in man, have discovered that chickens, dogs, cats, swine, rabbits, and various captive wild mammals and birds are subject to a spontaneous form of the disease. In chickens, sclerosis of the coronaries, the aorta, and its large branches is apparently quite common. In these vessels the first indication of the sclerosis is the presence of bright yellow, smooth, unelevated circular spots. These later become raised (plaques) and encroach upon the lumen of the vessels. Sometimes these elevations assume the form of white or yellow ridges which run lengthwise to the arteries.

An unsettled question relative to these lesions is whether they are primary in the intima or media. Canadian researchers have proof that they begin in the media as tiny foci of hydropic degeneration. Young foci become infiltrated with so-called foam cells — large macrophages filled with fat. Later, free fat and empty clefts (the site of cholesterol crystal deposits) appear. With these changes there is also some debris from necrosed cells and calcium deposits.

While the disturbance appears to begin in the media it soon extends to the adventitia and intima. In the adventitia there is lymphocytic infiltration, so extensive at times as to cause a nodular out-pouching of the vessel wall. In the intima in these same areas the internal elastic lamina is often partly destroyed or duplicated. At these places the endothelial cells are either swollen (hydropic) or have proliferated and become hydropic. Fibroblasts may appear in these areas of thickened intima (plaques).

The cause of arteriosclerosis in chickens has not been determined. Infection has been ruled out. Feeding a ration high in cholesterol does not increase the incidence of the disease but does hasten the development of the lesions.

Spontaneous arteriosclerosis of adult dogs probably is more common than is generally believed. It occurs in the aorta and coronaries. The cause is not known. Since it occurs at places of greatest stress in the aorta, it is conjectured that it may be traumatic, but its more frequent occurrence in old dogs leads one to believe that it is an aging process. Faulty nutrition as a causative factor cannot be ignored however.

The gross lesions are not difficult to detect when the aorta is opened and the intima inspected carefully. The lesions are slightly elevated, round to oval areas (plaques), white to yellow in color, fibrous in consistency, and 0.1 to 2 mm. up to 1 to 2 cm. in diameter. When the coronary arteries are affected, there may be signs of myocardial infarction arising from thrombosis if the lesions are young, or areas of myocardial scarring (fibrosis) if the lesions are old.

The pathogenesis of the plaques appears to be as follows: In the intima the normal pattern of the internal elastic lamina is disrupted. It becomes duplicated, split, or fragmented. This is reported to be a rather constant feature of the intimal plaques in dogs. There is fibroblastic proliferation of the inner layer (next to the lumen) of the intima together with the deposition of a mucoid ground substance in this newly formed connective tissue. At first these fibroblasts have a helter-skelter arrangement. Later, they are arranged perpendicularly, and still later, circumferentially. This final arrangement is believed to be the result of hydrostatic pressure within the vessel lumen. In time the deposition of the mucoid ground substance is followed by the formation of collagen fibers, and still later by the elaboration of elastic fibers. In old plaques the collagen may undergo hyalinization. Late in the development of intimal plaques in dogs a slight fatty infiltration may occur, but this is not important.

In the media the changes develop in much the same manner as in the intima. First, there is a deposition of a mucoid ground substance followed by a replacement of the mucoid by collagen. Accompanying this, there is a focal degeneration or loss of the elastic fibers, a focal proliferation of smooth muscle cells, and sometimes the formation of small cysts. The medial changes do not occur in younger dogs. There is lack of agreement among researchers as to which of the changes — intimal or medial — occurs first in the older dogs.

Naturally occurring arteriosclerosis in old cats, while not as common or as severe as in dogs, resembles the disease in the latter. There is absence of lipid material in the earliest arterial lesions the same as in the dog. A slight degree of lipid infiltration may occur late in the lesion but cholesterol is not present.

About one-third of the swine over 3 years of age have plaques in the aortic arch and thoracic portion of the aorta. They are small (.5 to 1.5 mm.) to large (5 to 10 mm.), pale yellow, elongated, hard, subendothelial areas of intimal thickening. The thickening is due principally to proliferation of connective tissue. In the abdominal aorta some plaques resemble those in the dog.

At the Philadelphia Zoological Garden during a 40-year period atherosclerosis in captive wild mammals and birds has been observed to be related to age and to no other factor such as sex, diet, crowding, or concurrent disease.

Spontaneous arteriosclerosis of rabbits begins in the media. The muscle cells necrose and disappear. The elastic fibers remain intact but lose their waviness, and after the muscle cells disappear, the elastic fibers bunch up in parallel rows. Calcification is common in these lesions. The degenerating muscle cells contain very little or no stainable fat. Secondarily the intima becomes involved but the changes in the endothelium are slight. The cause of the condition in rabbits has not been determined.

**Arteritis**

ACUTE ARTERITIS

The causes are bacteria, viruses, and toxins. Avenues of entrance are: (1) from outside of the vessel extending inwardly (periarteritis); (2) by way of the vasa vasorum; (3) by way of the vessel lumen (endarteritis). The latter is of most importance. Acute arteritis is usually due to pyogenic organisms metastasizing from some suppurating process such as may occur in the uterus, at the navel, or in the joints. The lungs are a favored place for these bacterial emboli to lodge and incite an inflammatory reaction in the arteries. At the place where the intima is inflamed, parietal thrombi develop. The bacteria may become phagocytized and the thrombi disappear. If the bacteria are numerous in these thrombi, the inflammatory process extends into the vessel wall (thrombo-endarteritis).

Acute arteritis is the primary lesion in at least two viral diseases — equine arteritis and sporadic bovine encephalomyelitis. It is also the primary lesion in myoclonia congenita of suckling pigs which may also be a viral disease. In these three diseases the most prominent lesions result from the primary vasculitis.

**Equine viral arteritis.** Viral arteritis is an acute disease of equines, having many of the characteristics of equine rhinopneumonitis (influenza-abortion). In the uncomplicated form there is fever, conjunctivitis, palpebral edema, nasal mucosal hyperemia and hemorrhage, stocking, respiratory difficulty, colic, diarrhea, depression, muscular weakness, and prostration. A very important manifestation of the disease in pregnant mares is abortion.

Mortality is around 33 per cent in uncomplicated cases and probably higher in those complicated by streptococcal and other secondary infections.

**Lesions.** Microscopically, the basic tissue alteration is located in the media of small muscular arteries. In them the necrotic foci involve segments of the vessels. The endothelium and intima usually remain intact except in the most severely affected arteries, which are generally those of the intestine. If the endothelium and intima are affected, thrombosis and infarction occur. The media and adventitia, however, receive the brunt of the viral attack. In the media there is necrosis of the musculature characterized by hyaline degeneration. This leads to adventitial edema and hemorrhage and usually results in hemorrhage and edema of the surrounding tissue. Both the affected media and adventitia become infiltrated with lymphocytes.

The nature of the basic lesion, which is arteritis, makes it understandable why the gross lesions should include the following: palpebral edema, hyperemia and hemorrhage of the upper respiratory tract, pulmonary edema, pleural effusion, hemorrhages of the serous membranes, hydroperitoneum, visceral edema, splenic hemorrhages of the serous membranes, infarction, and renal and hepatic degeneration. Inflammation of the respiratory and intestinal mucosa could very well be due to secondary infection.

Following the initial stage of the fever by 24 to 72 hours there is a panleukopenia with emphasis on lymphopenia. This usually lasts 4 to 10 days.

Abortion, which occurs so often in affected pregnant mares, is believed to be due to active infection of the fetus since the virus can be recovered from the spleen and blood of the fetus. There are no inclusion bodies in the cells of the fetus.

## CHRONIC ARTERITIS

Chronic arteritis is observed in the healing of the walls of injured vessels, in thrombi undergoing organization, and in vessels in chronically inflamed areas. In horses it often follows the acute verminous arteritis of the anterior mesenteric artery and its branches. Chronic arteritis in horses is due to larvae of *Strongylus vulgaris*. The anterior mesenteric artery is the most common location. At the origin of the artery and for some distance down, the inner surface of the vessel shows thick, thrombotic masses, which usually contain several strongyle larvae. The accompanying inflammatory process extends deep into the media.

An unusual lesion sometimes occurs in the branches of the pulmonary artery in dogs that have large collections of heart worms *(Dirofilaria immitis)* in the right heart. The adult worms not only fill the right heart but also extend into the trunk of the pulmonary artery and its main branches. The larger branches of the artery may show arteriosclerosis with fibrous endothelial cushions partially obstructing the lumen. The smaller branches may have medial hypertrophy and fibrous thickening of the intima. The lumen becomes extremely small. The condition has the appearance of **endarteritis obliterans** — a form of arteritis in which the production of new intimal connective tissue obliterates the lumen of the vessel.

### Aneurysm

Aneurysm is a local dilatation of an artery or vein (Fig. 14.11). It may also occur in connection with endarteritis due to uremia in the dog and chronic arteritis due to larvae of *Strongylus vulgaris* in the horse (worm-aneurysm). The latter is most important and occurs in horses of all ages. The most frequent location is the anterior mesenteric artery and its branches. The aneurysm may become as much as six inches in diameter when involving the trunk of the anterior mesenteric artery. Aneurysms may be sacculated, large ones fusiform or spherical. The wall is usually firm and thick. The normal structure of the wall disappears, being replaced by granulation tissue which may contain calcium deposits. The inner surface is

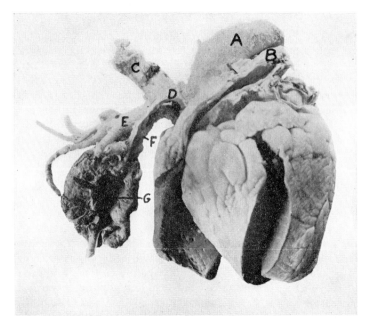

Fig. 14.11 — Heart and vessels, with brachial aneurysm, in a steer.

**A**, aorta;
**B**, pulmonary artery;
**C**, anterior vena cava;
**D**, brachiocephalic trunk;
**E**, right brachial artery with its terminal branches;
**F**, left brachial artery;
**G**, aneurysm.
(Bullard, Jour. A.V.M.A.)

rough and covered with loosely attached, or firmly adherent, laminated, thrombotic deposits. Worm larvae are in the thrombus and project from it. The results of worm aneurysm with the accompanying thrombus are thromboembolic colic, pressure atrophy upon the surrounding tissue, pyogenic infection of the thrombus with resulting pyemia, and rupture of the aneurysm with fatal hemorrhage.

**VEINS**

The pathology of veins is practically the same as that of arteries. Therefore, only certain features that pertain to veins alone will be mentioned. **Spontaneous rupture** occurs most frequently in the posterior vena cava, anterior vena cava, and portal vein. **Thrombi** in domestic animals occur in the vena cava and in the mammary, portal, and uterine veins. In the posterior vena cava and portal vein they may be associated with traumatic gastritis and hepatic abscesses. In horses they may be associated with traumatic endophlebitis of the jugular. In newborn animals, especially foals, physiologic thrombi of the umbilical veins may become infected. **Disturbances of metabolism**

are rare. Krause and Iwanoff, reporting on senile changes in the posterior vena cava of 300 cattle and 200 buffaloes, state that in animals more than 10 or 12 years old there is fibrosis of the inner portion of the wall with replacement of muscle in this part of the wall with connective tissue. They observed very little fatty change, necrosis, and calcification. No changes were noted in the anterior vena cava.

**Aneurysm** of veins is rare, but a few cases involving the subcutaneous abdominal vein (milk vein) occurring in cows are on record. The condition occurred suddenly in high-producing dairy cows (70 to 90 pounds of milk daily) and in most cases resulted in death or immediate slaughter of the animals.

**Parasitic obstruction.** It is not unusual for dogs in the South Atlantic and Gulf states to have the nematode *Dirofilaria immitis* in the right heart and pulmonary artery, but it is rare for it to be located in the hepatic veins and posterior vena cava.

**Phlebitis**

Acute endophlebitis occurs in navel infection (omphalophlebitis) of calves, lambs, and foals. Macroscopically, the wall of the umbilical vein is thickened, the

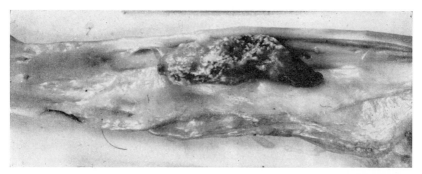

Fig. 14.12 — A 6-cm.-long thrombus of the jugular vein of a 5-month-old bull calf. (Department of Veterinary Pathology, Michigan State University.)

lumen dilated, and the vein contains thick necrotic material, after the removal of which the inner surface of the vessel appears rough and reddened. Microscopically, there is pronounced leukocytic infiltration of the vein wall. Leukocytes are most numerous in the inner layer of the wall but gradually lessen in numbers from within out. The vasa vasorum are dilated and contain numerous leukocytes. Later the inner portion of the wall becomes necrotic. Bacteria are numerous in the necrotic material. The inflammatory process extends into the adventitia. Calcium deposits in the media are physiological in these cases (involuntionary process).

Endophlebitis of the uterine veins also occurs in suppurative metritis. The changes are similar to those just described.

A periphlebitis of the jugular vein may arise as the result of improper intravenous injection or faulty technique used in taking blood samples (Fig. 14.12). In suppurative bronchopneumonia the primary inflammatory process may extend peribronchially and involve the lymph sheaths which surround the veins, and subsequently the walls of the veins themselves. This periphlebitis usually leads to inflammatory thrombosis.

## REFERENCES

Alexander, A. F., and Jensen, R.: 1959. Gross cardiac changes in cattle with high mountain (brisket) disease and in experimental cattle maintained at high altitude. Amer. Jour. Vet. Res., 20:680.

Duff, G. L.: 1935. Experimental cholesterol arteriosclerosis and its relationship to human arteriosclerosis. Arch Path., 20:81, 259.

Jones, T. C., Doll, E. R., and Bryans, J. T.: 1957. The lesions of equine viral arteritis. Cornell Vet., 47:52.

Menges, R. W., Harschfield, G. S., and Wenner, H. A.: 1953. Sporadic bovine encephalomyelitis: Studies on pathogenesis and etiology of the disease. Jour. A.V.M.A., 122:294.

Pritchard, W. R., Henderson, W., and Beall, C. W.: 1958. Experimental production of dissecting aneurysms in turkeys. Amer. Jour. Vet. Res., 19:696.

Winter, H.: 1959. The pathology of canine dirofilariasis. Amer. Jour. Vet. Res., 20:366.

# CHAPTER 15

# Hematopoietic System

The principal function of the hematopoietic system is to produce the cellular constituents of the blood. The hematopoietic system and the reticuloendothelial system are so closely associated that the activities of one cannot be listed without including those of the other. Outside of the liver, most of the reticuloendothelial cells are located in the blood-forming organs — the spleen, the lymph nodes and nodules, and the bone marrow. Since the liver in the adult animal ceases to be as important a blood-forming organ as it is in the embryo, it will not be included in the present discussion.

## LYMPH NODES

Besides producing cells of the lymphocyte series, the lymph nodes act as mechanical filters and settling chambers for the removal of bacteria, erythrocytes, and particulate substances from the lymph.

### Processes Involving Deposition of Various Substances in the Nodes

**Fat.** The deposition of fat occurs in the mesenteric nodes of fat pigs due to absorption of fat by the afferent lymphatics of these nodes. Fat appears as droplets or liquid in the lymph sinuses. Deposition also occurs in the supramammary nodes of lactating cows due to milk stasis. The fat appears microscopically in the sinus

endothelium and the reticular cells of the follicles. As a result, atrophy of the lymphoid tissue may occur. Actual infiltration with adipose tissue also may occur in fat pigs.

**Erythrocytes.** The deposition of erythrocytes in lymph nodes occurs normally to a certain extent. It practically always occurs in the renal nodes of sheep and goats. Cells appear in the lymph sinuses both free and within macrophages. In pathological conditions the number of erythrocytes may increase greatly, especially in circulatory disturbances in which there is stasis of blood such as in pulmonary hyperemia, and with the appearance of hemorrhages (hog cholera).

**Exogenous pigments. Coal dust (anthracosis)** is seen particularly in the pulmonary nodes in animals living in industrial centers or large cities or working in coal mines (mules) or around coal tipples. The pulmonary nodes of animals used in stone quarries and around gypsum and Portland cement plants may show a deposition of other mineral dusts. In the parts of the United States where severe dust storms are of frequent occurrence there is reason to believe that the frequent black and gray pigmentation of these nodes may be due to soil dust. Perhaps the deposition of hay dust may also account for the frequent occurrence of a grayish pigmentation of these nodes in ruminants and horses that have never been in the environment of other sources of lymph node pigmentation. Grossly, the medulla of the node appears black, the cortex normal gray. Microscopically, the pigment lies in the lymphoid cords of the medulla in the reticular cells.

**Endogenus pigments. Bile pigment** occurs in the portal nodes as a result of obstructive jaundice (flukes, ascarids, calculi). At first the pigment is found in the reticular cells of the lymphoid cords, later in the sinuses of the medulla. Here it is phagocytized by the sinus endothelium. **Blood pigment** is seen principally in the nodes of the limbs as a result of fracture. It collects mostly in the cortex. **Melanin** is particularly conspicuous in the lymph nodes of horses which are fading in color from dark or iron gray to gray and to white.

**Gas (emphysema).** Accumulation of gas occurs in the mesenteric nodes of swine in connection with intestinal emphysema, in the supramammary nodes of cows as a result of udder inflation, in the pulmonary nodes of horses due to pulmonary emphysema, and in the lymph nodes of the affected quarters in blackleg. Macroscopically, the nodes are enlarged, puffy, sometimes spongelike. Microscopically, gas bubbles appear in the sinuses and are surrounded by macrophages and giant cells. The lymphoid tissue may undergo atrophy.

## Lymphadenitis

### SEROUS LYMPHADENITIS

Serous lymphadenitis is found in many of the acute septicemic diseases, especially in the early stages and in the nodes draining an organ or part of the body undergoing an acute inflammation. Macroscopically, the nodes are enlarged and soft. The cut surface is moist, bulges, and is reddened. Microscopically, there are hyperemia, edema, and hemorrhage. Simultaneously with vascular changes there are alterations in the reticuloendothelium and in the lymphatic parenchyma. These changes are proliferative. In the parenchyma the resulting lymphoid hyperplasia may produce atrophy of the germinal centers. The cells of the lymphoid cords may be replaced by plasma cells.

### HEMORRHAGIC LYMPHADENITIS

Hemorrhagic lymphadenitis is frequent in the acute septicemias such as anthrax, pasteurellosis, hog cholera, and swine erysipelas. In the mesenteric nodes it is one of the lesions of enterotoxemia of suckling calves, lambs and kids, and of overfed feeder lambs. Macroscopically, the nodes are enlarged and dark red; their cut surface is moist and dark red. On the cut surface of the lymph nodes of swine this redness is confined to the outer margin and along the trabeculae. Microscopically, there is severe hyperemia and hemorrhage. In the lymph nodes of hogs the hemorrhage is in the cell-poor substance beneath the subcapsular and peritrabecular sinuses (Fig. 15.1).

### SUPPURATIVE LYMPHADENITIS

The cause of suppurative lymphadenitis is pyogenic bacteria. It occurs frequently in strangles, suppurative arthritis of hogs, and in suppurative mastitis of cows.

Macroscopically, abscesses appear in the nodes. Later these may become encapsulated. Microscopically, there is hyperemia and diffuse leukocytic infiltration, especially of the sinuses. Later, leukocytes concentrate and the tissue undergoes softening and liquefaction (abscessation). Proliferation of the sinus endothelium and of the lymphoid cells is present also.

In swine, **jowl abscesses** are caused by Lancefield's group E streptococcus, a beta hemolytic strain of the organism. The organism appears to reach the pharynx by contaminated feed and water. Afferent lymphatics convey the organism to the mandibular and postpharyngeal lymph nodes where abscesses develop. From these nodes the infection may spread down the chain of cervical nodes and into the blood stream resulting in recurrent pyrexia and leukocytosis.

**Ovine caseous lymphadenitis** is an example of suppurative lymphadenitis. This

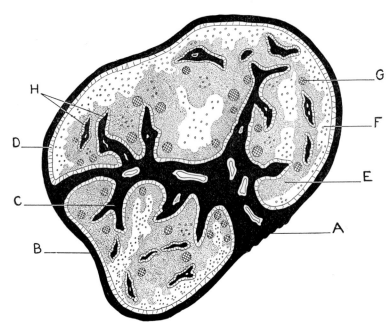

Fig. 15.1 — Schematic drawing of a lymph node of a pig:
A, hilus;
B, capsule;
C, trabecula;
D, corticular sinus;
E, lymphoid tissue of the parenchyma;
F, "cell-poor substance" of the parenchyma;
G, follicle;
H, peritrabecular sinus.

In the septicemias of swine characterized by hemorrhages, blood accumulates in the cell-poor substance. (After Seifried.)

disease, also called pseudotuberculosis, is a chronic infectious disease of adult sheep caused by *Corynebacterium pseudotuberculosis* (*Corynebacterium ovis*) and characterized by the enlargement of one or more lymph nodes which contain foci of pale greenish-yellow, caseous, or purulent material. The period of incubation and the pathogenesis are not definitely known. Since, in general, only adult sheep have the disease, it is presumed that the period of incubation is rather long. Infection may possibly occur either by way of the digestive or respiratory tracts or through wounds in the skin. Caseous lymphadenitis begins with localization of the infection but finally becomes a pyemia. There is marked general emaciation and chronic suppurative lymphadenitis of many of the nodes. The nodes may become as large as hen eggs. They present pale greenish-yellow, caseous, or purulent foci (no calcification). There is chronic bronchopneumonia in severe cases. Maddy in California reports that gross lesions of caseous lymphadenitis occur most frequently in the bronchial and mediastinal

lymph nodes and in the lungs. The lesions may resemble tuberculosis except in color and in the absence of calcification.

### CHRONIC LYMPHADENITIS

Chronic lymphadenitis is often a lesion of one of several chronic infectious diseases. Chronic lymphadenitis occurs in the mesenteric lymph nodes of cattle with paratuberculosis, in various nodes of dogs with histoplasmosis, and in the bronchial nodes of cattle with coccidioidomycosis (Fig. 15.2). The affected nodes are enlarged but usually have the normal gray appearance or may be slightly pink, and sometimes succulent.

Bovine tuberculosis is a chronic inflammation usually characterized by caseous necrosis and calcification. The enlarged, firm, gray nodes contain cheesy yellow areas which are often gritty when cut. In swine, when the lymphadenitis is due to the avian strain of the mycobacterium, there is generally no calcification and sometimes little necrosis.

In glanders, actinobacillosis, and actinomycosis a chronic suppurative lymph-

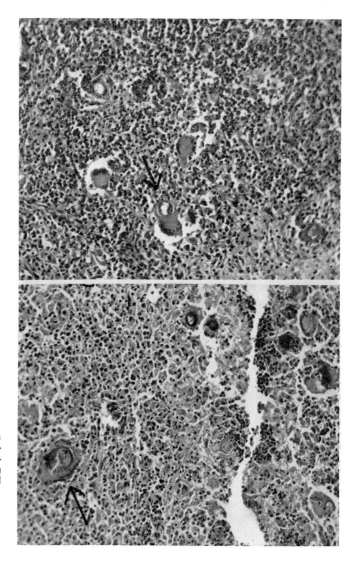

Fig. 15.2 — Chronic lymphadenitis in a cow due to **Coccidioides immitis.** Both illustrations show multinucleated giant cells containing the organisms. ×150. (Davis and Stiles, Jour. A.V.M.A.)

adenitis occurs. In any of these diseases the nodes are enlarged, usually nodular, and contain thick-walled abscess cavities. The nodes may be adherent to the surrounding tissue and therefore not moveable when palpated.

In **salmon disease** of the dog, caused by a rickettsia-like microorganism coming to the dog by ingesting fluke-infested salmon, many of the visceral and somatic lymph nodes become enlarged. In some cases they become increased in size three to sixfold. The nodes are usually yellowish, with the swollen follicles appearing as white foci. The enlargement is the result of a marked hyperplasia of the reticuloendothelial cells in both the cortex and medulla. Many of the reticuloendothelial cells contain elementary bodies. Along with the reticuloendothelial cell hyperplasia there is a depletion of lymphocytes.

## Tumors

Primary **benign** tumors of the lymph nodes are uncommon. It is difficult to find reports on lymphomas. Primary **malignant** tumors (lymphosarcomas) are common.

General lymph node enlargement is a

lesion of a lymphosarcoma which occurs most often in dogs, cattle, and swine. Because the lymphosarcoma is a chronic wasting disease the affected superficial lymph nodes may become exceptionally prominent in the living animal. A myelosarcoma may involve the lymph nodes but is an uncommon tumor.

Grossly, the lymph nodes in both myelocytic and lymphocytic sarcomas usually show some degree of enlargement. In lymphocytic sarcomas the enlargement of the nodes is generally more widely distributed throughout the body and the enlargement of individual nodes greater than in myelocytic sarcomas. In both types of sarcomas, however, all of the nodes may be involved or only certain groups. In the most severe cases, tiny, unnamed lymph nodes become sizeable nodes. The named nodes in these cases become several times larger than normal. When all of the hyperplastic lymphoid tissue of such a case is removed at necropsy and weighed, it is surprising what a large proportion of the body can become such tissue.

In the myelocytic and lymphatic sarcomas the lymph nodes usually retain their normal shape but become soft. The capsule is too small for the parenchyma so the latter bulges greatly when the node is cut in two. The bulging parenchyma is grayish, pulplike, and succulent. Small hemorrhages, foci of grayish yellow, caseous necrosis, and areas of mixed hemorrhage and necrosis may be prominent.

Histologically, in lymphocytic sarcomas one cannot recognize cortex and medulla, or subcapsular or peritrabecular sinuses of the nodes. The nodes are a solid mass of large and small lymphocytes. In chronic cases of long standing, the small cells predominate; in very acute cases, the large cells. The areas of necrosis may occur in connection with hemorrhages, or as the result of infarction arising from thrombi occurring in the nodes. In very chronic cases, attempts at organization of the old hemorrhages or necrotic areas are seen.

The changes in the nodes in myelocytic

sarcoma — the type of sarcoma less often seen — are quite similar to those in lymphocytic sarcoma, but the cells which pack the nodes are myeloblasts, myelocytes, neutrophils, and eosinophils.

**Secondary carcinoma** occurs in connection with mammary gland carcinoma of dogs and in the contiguous lymph nodes of other carcinomatous organs. **Secondary melanosarcoma** is common in old gray horses.

## LYMPH VESSELS

### Lymphangitis

**Acute serofibrinous lymphangitis** occurs in the lungs in the course of inflammatory diseases (hog cholera pneumonia, catarrhal pneumonia of dogs and horses) characterized by peribronchitis and peribronchiolitis. It occurs also in the pulmonary form of glanders. **Acute suppurative lymphangitis** arises in connection with suppurative processes in the area drained by the affected lymph vessels. **Chronic suppurative lymphangitis** is an important lesion in glanders, epizootic lymphangitis, and ulcerative lymphangitis of horses.

## SPLEEN

### Functional Disturbances

In health, the **spleen, lymph nodes,** and **bone marrow** form a cooperative team to supply and maintain an optimum number of the formed blood elements — erythrocytes, granulocytes, lymphocytes, and thrombocytes. In this function the spleen contributes many of the lymphocytes, which seem in some way to be concerned with endogenous protein metabolism and antibody-globulin production and transportation. In case of necessity, as in aplastic anemia, the spleen can assume its embryonic function of forming erythrocytes.

Besides this cytogenic function the spleen serves as a reservoir for blood, available for emergencies such as in hypoxia and severe hemorrhage. The stored blood is not whole blood but is mostly plasma containing an exceptionally high content of erythrocytes. The red cells are stored and released as needed to maintain a rather constant red cell count in the circulating blood. It is surprising that the spleen can function adequately in this respect because the organ, as it is seen in its contracted state after death, is comparatively small. However, because of its thick muscular capsule and trabeculae, it is capable of contraction after extensive dilatation. Its ability to contain large quantities of blood is facilitated by its fenestrated sinusoids and dense network of capillaries. The development of the sinusoids in the usual domestic mammals, however, is poor as compared to that in man.

With the "reservoir" function of the spleen is associated its "graveyard" function. In this latter function the organ dismantles worn out and senile erythrocytes and salvages the hemoglobin contained in them. For this purpose the organ provides large numbers of reticuloendothelial phagocytes, both fixed and wandering. These cells, together with those of the bone marrow and liver, are believed to be active in transforming hematin into hemobilirubin. The spleen retains, temporarily at least, some of the iron derived from destroyed erythrocytes, and consequently is in a continuous state of physiologic hemosiderosis. The phagocytes have the added duty of protection against infection and the formation of antibody globulins.

Even though the spleen has these important functions, its presence in the body is not indispensable for the maintenance of health or life. In its absence the bone marrow, liver, lymph nodes, and the reticuloendothelial cells in other parts of the body compensate for it.

While a normal spleen is not indispensable for health and for life, a diseased spleen can become the cause of ill health and of death. It seems strange that the organ which acts normally more or less intermittently as the reservoir for blood may at times assume the role of a continuous reservoir, and not only that, but may

permit its phagocytes to destroy the blood elements brought to it. In certain instances it destroys the erythrocytes, in some the granulocytes, and in others the platelets. Occasionally the phagocytes may destroy all three simultaneously. These conditions, referred to as forms of hypersplenism, have been studied in man and can be successfully treated by removing the abnormally functioning spleen (splenectomy).

In view of the fact that the reticuloendothelial cells of the spleen at times may develop this tendency to destroy the formed elements of the blood, it would seem that there is a possibility the reticuloendothelial cells in other parts of the body might do likewise, but this does not seem to be the case. The condition seems to be confined to the spleen and is an example of the rare phenomenon of localized hyperphagocytosis.

### Congenital and Acquired Displacements and Malformations

So-called **accessory spleens** are small spherical masses of splenic tissue attached to the visceral surface of the spleen or present in the gastrosplenic omentum. Congenital **indentations** and **grooves** are common. **Torsion** is rare but occurs more frequently in swine than in other animals due to the loose arrangement of the gastrosplenic omentum which permits considerable movement of the organ, particularly of the ventral half. The fundamental changes of torsion are present. It may result in necrosis.

### Disturbances in Continuity

**Traumatic rupture** is most frequent in the dog. It results fatally by internal hemorrhage, or healing may occur with the formation of cicatricial tissue. **Spontaneous rupture** occurs in cows in connection with lymphosarcoma, in fowls with leukosis and tuberculosis, and in horses with splenic amyloidosis. At first a subcapsular hematocyst may form. Later the capsule may rupture and permit fatal hemorrhage.

## Local Disturbances of Growth and Cell Metabolism

### ATROPHY

Senile atrophy is seen in dogs. In pigs and cattle what sometimes appears to be atrophy is really pronounced induration with subsequent contraction of the parenchyma resulting from chronic passive hyperemia.

### PROTEIN METABOLISM

**Hyaline degeneration** occurs principally in dogs during general diseases and in swine affected with cholera. Hyalin appears in the wall of the arterioles of the Malpighian corpuscles, in the corpuscles themselves, and sometimes in the reticulum and in the pulp.

**Amyloid infiltration.** Nieberle has observed amyloid infiltration frequently in dogs having tuberculosis. It has also been reported in fowls having tuberculosis. In Russia it is said to occur frequently in horses. Of late it has been reported rather frequently in horses used in serum production. Of interest in this connection are the observations made by Doerken. Material from 100 serum horses formed the basis of her study. The animals had been used for the production of serum for 2½ to 54 months. The horses had been used for the production of a variety of antiserums, but the largest number had been used in the preparation of diphtheria and tetanus antitoxins (44 and 26, respectively). Amyloidosis was observed in 60 of the 100. The percentages of its incidence distribution in the various organs of the 60 horses were as follows: spleen, 100; liver, 44; suprarenals, 34; kidneys, 21; and intestines, 12. In 8 animals amyloid infiltration led to rupture of the liver and death. Amyloidosis was relatively more frequent in horses used for scarlet fever antiserum than in those used for other antiserums. Reticuloendothelial reactions, which were present in every animal, were of three types: hypertrophy, hyperplasia, and small foci of chronic inflammation. It was not possible to determine any relation between these types of reactions and the duration of immunization or the kind of serum prepared. Reticuloendothelial reactions and amyloid infiltration appeared to have a close relationship. The cellular reaction occurred first and was necessary for the production of amyloidosis.

### PIGMENT METABOLISM (HEMOSIDEROSIS)

The amount of hemosiderin (iron-containing pigment) in the spleens of normal animals varies considerably. It is greatest in the horse, least in the dog; is greater in the old than in the young; is situated in the plasma of pulp cells, especially at the margins of Malpighian corpuscles, around arterioles, venous sinuses, and trabeculae. Therefore, it occurs most where blood is most abundant. A pathological increase occurs generally when there is increased destruction of erythrocytes. An exception to this rule is furnished by the chronic form of infectious anemia of horses.

## Disturbances of Circulation

It is difficult to differentiate between the physiologic and pathologic blood content of the spleen. Remember the normal structure of the spleen and its physiologic variation of blood content. In this connection it is necessary also to remember the action of the splanchnic, left phrenic, and vagus nerves upon the spleen. Splanchnic stimulation causes anemia of the spleen. Paralysis of this nerve, as occurs in febrile conditions, results in hyperemia of the organ. The vagus acts as an inhibitor to the splanchnic following cessation of stimulation of the latter. Stimulation of branches of the left phrenic constricts the splenic vein and causes passive hyperemia.

### PASSIVE HYPEREMIA

Passive hyperemia is the most important circulatory disturbance. Its existence may be traced to some hindrance to circulation in the splenic vein, the portal vein between its bifurcation with the splenic vein and its termination in the liver, in the liver itself, in the hepatic vein or thoracic portion of the posterior vena cava, in the right heart, and even in the lungs. Obviously, hindrances to circulation which are situated nearest the spleen will have the greatest effect. Depending upon the duration, the condition is acute or chronic. In the acute form the spleen is enlarged. Its cut surface bulges. The pulp is dark red, often cyanotic. Blood flows out readily. It occurs when death results from slow arrest of the heart's action as in myocardial degeneration and myocarditis. Under the same conditions, passive hyperemia of the liver also occurs. In abattoirs it is observed in normal animals after slaughter. The cause is not known, but it is thought to be due to splanchnic influences. The chronic form may occur in swine in the course of erysipelas with right-sided valvular endocarditis and in cattle with chronic valvular endocarditis and traumatic pericarditis. In these conditions the action of the heart is interfered with so that blood accumulates in the spleen. This is especially true if the heart involvement is located mostly on the right side. The spleen is enlarged and firm.

The cut surface is dark red. The relative proportion of interstitial tissue to that of the parenchyma is increased. The trabeculae are thickened. This increase in interstitial tissue can be determined by scraping the cut surface with a knife. In this manner the pulp is removed and the interstitial tissue remains.

## THROMBOSIS

Thrombosis of the splenic vein occasionally arises in connection with foreign-body abscess of the spleen in cattle. It is very rarely seen in horses in the splenic artery (verminous thrombosis).

## EMBOLISM

The emboli may be bland or septic. If embolism occurs in the splenic artery, total necrosis of the spleen may result. If embolism occurs in a branch of the splenic artery, an infarct occurs. This is sometimes seen in swine in erysipelas and in other species of animals that are affected with chronic valvular endocarditis.

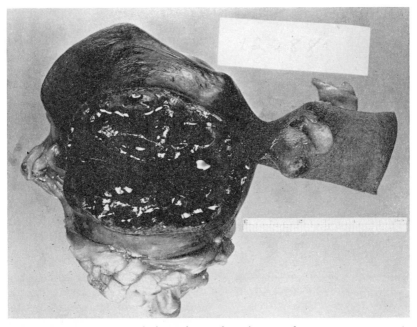

Fig. 15.3 — Hematocyst of the spleen of a dog — a frequent occurrence in dogs struck by automobiles. (Department of Veterinary Pathology, Michigan State University.)

INFARCTION

Most splenic infarcts originate as a result of embolism and thrombosis of the branches of the splenic artery. In hog cholera, however, obstructions occur in the follicular branches of the artery which also result in infarction. The obstruction is due to a combination of a hyalinization of the vessel wall and a proliferation of the endothelium. The infarcts for the most part are located at the margins of the spleen. Their bases are at the border of the organ and their apices point medially. Recent infarcts are red and bulge (Fig. 7.9). Older ones which are undergoing necrosis become white or gray and shrink.

HEMORRHAGES

Hematocysts are often seen in the spleens of dogs that have been struck by automobiles (Fig. 15.3). The hematocysts are located subcapsularly and consist of a collection of dark red, almost black blood which pushes the capsule up above the surface of the organ. They occur also in cattle with splenic lymphosarcoma. The capsule readily ruptures and results in fatal internal hemorrhage.

## Splenitis

The spleen, an organ consisting in a large degree of elements of the reticuloendothelial system, is obviously an important factor in the defensive mechanism of the body. Living and dead foreign bodies are filtered out of the blood in the spleen. The presence of such foreign substances in the spleen produces reactive processes which frequently become macroscopically apparent. Inflammatory swelling of the spleen is indicative of such processes. This is observed frequently in acute and chronic infectious diseases. Because of the structure and peculiarities of the blood flow of this organ, however, inflammatory changes in it are not always easily recognized.

ACUTE SPLENITIS

Diseases in which acute splenic swelling is especially prominent are anthrax, swine erysipelas, anaplasmosis of cattle, acute infectious anemia of horses, and *Salmonella choleraesuis* septicemia. Macroscopically, the spleen is enlarged and soft, its cut surface bulges and is dark red or black, and the parenchyma is so soft that it may flow. The trabeculae and Malpighian corpuscles cannot be detected. Microscopically, there is marked hyperemia, with collections of neutrophils, lymphocytes, and plasma cells, and swelling and finally disintegration of the reticulum.

In some viremias, such as that occurring in infectious synovitis of chickens, in which there is generalized hyperplasia of the reticuloendothelial system, the spleen is enlarged also, but the enlargement is due mostly to an increase in the number of reticulum cells and not to inflammatory cells.

CHRONIC SPLENITIS

Chronic splenitis may be characterized either by induration (increase in the reticulum) or by cellular hyperplasia (increase in the parenchyma).

The interstitial form of chronic splenitis is rarely seen. When one suspects it at necropsy, it is always advisable to examine the liver and the venous circulation as far anterior as the lungs for signs of vascular hindrance. Vascular obstruction in this area may cause lesions of chronic passive hyperemia in the spleen which resemble those of chronic inflammation. If there is one infectious disease above others in which the interstitial form of splenitis is a lesion, it is probably paratyphoid infection of calves.

Chronic splenitis in which the pulp is increased is also uncommon. Specific infectious diseases which supply good examples of it are histoplasmosis of dogs and infectious anemia of horses. In both diseases the spleen is enlarged. The splenomegaly in histoplasmosis is the result of massive macrophage proliferation. Macrophages displace most of the splenic tissue. In equine infectious anemia the splenomegaly is due to an increase in the size of the splenic nodules. The hyperplasia of

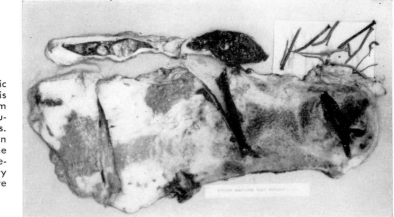

Fig. 15.4 — Acute necrotic and gangrenous splenitis in a cow resulting from penetration of the reticulum by foreign bodies. Several of the foreign bodies recovered from the reticulum are shown. (Department of Veterinary Pathology, Michigan State University.)

the nodules is interpreted to be an attempt to increase antibody production. The enlarged nodules bulge on the cut surface of the organ. There seems to be a minimum of interstitial tissue in proportion to the volume of pulp.

In some cases of porcine brucellosis the only lesion present may be a chronic nodular splenitis. There are multiple, discrete, encapsulated nodules either on the surface of the organ or deep in its parenchyma. They vary in number from few to many and are up to 4 mm. in size. Grossly, they look like tubercles of tuberculosis or parasitic nodules. They have yellow to grayish-white caseous centers, sometimes tinged with light green. Microscopically, the caseous centers are surrounded by macrophages, lymphocytes, neutrophiles, and a connective tissue capsule.

**Suppurative splenitis** may arise: (1) As a result of **septic emboli** originating from mitral endocarditis or as a result of the **metastasis of pyogenic bacteria** from more distant localized suppurative processes. In horses it occurs in connection with strangles (*Streptococcus equi*); in calves as a result of navel infection (various organisms). (2) By **penetration** of infected, sharp foreign bodies from the reticulum in cattle. The perforation canal is a firm, indurated cord running from the forestomach to the spleen. The lumen is filled with necrotic tissue. In the spleen in the vicinity of the fistulous tract are abscesses of various sizes filled with exudate (Fig. 15.4). Suppurative splenitis in cattle usually results in metastatic suppurative hepatitis and pneumonia, and terminates in death by septicemia.

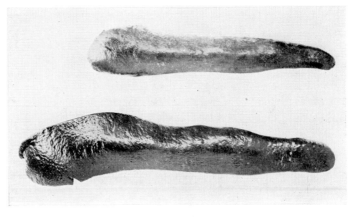

Fig. 15.5 — **Above:** Spleen of normal pig. **Below:** Enlarged spleen of pig with nutritional anemia. (Doyle, Mathews, and Whiting; Jour. A.V.M.A.)

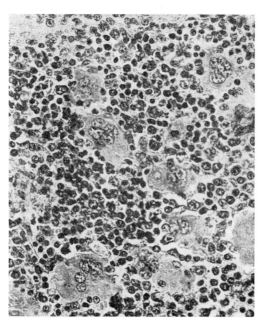

Fig. 15.6 — Splenic lesions in nutritional anemia of a pig. Note several megakaryocytes and numerous erythroblasts. (Doyle, Mathews, and Whiting; Jour. A.V.M.A.)

### The Spleen in Anemia

In nutritional anemia of young pigs the spleen is enlarged and firm (Fig. 15.5). These gross alterations are due to the presence of large numbers of erythrocytes and myelocytes. These cells occur both in dense foci — active hematopoietic centers — and diffusely distributed through-

out the spleen (Fig. 15.6). Megakaryocytes are also conspicuous. These changes are indications of bone marrow exhaustion.

### Tumors

Lymphosarcomas, myelosarcomas, and fibrosarcomas are frequently observed in the spleen. Metastatic tumors of various types are commonly observed. (See chapter on neoplasms.)

In lymphosarcoma the spleen is enlarged, usually extremely (Figs. 15.9 and 15.8). Nieberle reports cattle spleens 1 m. long by ½ m. wide by 20 cm. thick with a weight of 50 kg. or more. Frequently, there is subcapsular hemorrhage which, if the capsule ruptures, may lead to death. On the cut surface the parenchyma bulges, the gray splenic corpuscles are prominent against the dark red pulp background. In other cases the cut surface is more uniformly gray, and individual corpuscles cannot be recognized. Occasionally, there are anemic necrotic areas resembling anemic or pale infarcts. Microscopically, the changes at first consist of marked enlargement of the splenic corpuscles in which no germ center can be seen. The most prominent infiltrating cell is a medium-sized lymphocyte with a somewhat lightly stained nucleus and with indistinguishable cytoplasm. There is a diffuse infiltration of the pulp with the same type

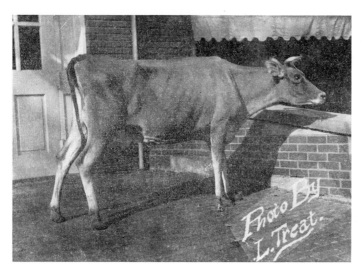

Fig. 15.7 — Lymphosarcoma in a cow. Note swelling in region of prescapular, prefemoral, and popliteal lymph nodes. (Gray, Jour. A.V.M.A.)

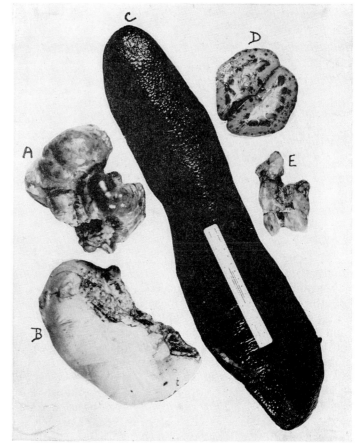

Fig. 15.8 — Organs from a pig with lymphosarcoma.

**A,** gastric and hepatic lymph nodes;

**B,** stomach;

**C,** spleen (six-inch ruler on surface);

**D,** kidney showing hemorrhages, represented by black areas;

**E,** splenic lymph nodes.

(Biester and McNutt, Jour. A.V.M.A.)

of cell (Fig. 15.9). Later, the enlarged corpuscles coalesce, and the whole parenchyma consists of a uniform infiltration of these lymphocytes. This infiltration may extend into the capsule, the trabeculae, and vessel walls; it may cause occlusion of the vessels. Descriptions of the spleen in myelosarcoma are so rare that no description will be given here.

## DISEASES OF THE BLOOD

During the early embryonic development of an animal the blood corpuscles and the endothelial cells originate in the blood islands in the splanchnopleure of the yolk sac. In later embryonic life the site of blood-cell formation shifts from this extra-embryonic location to the liver, spleen, and bone marrow. When the unborn animal ceases to be an embryo and becomes a fetus, the liver and spleen give up this cytogenic function (except for lymphocyte and macrophage formation in the spleen) but the red bone marrow continues to function throughout the remainder of fetal and on into postnatal life. When, however, in postnatal life the hematopoietic tissue of the marrow becomes incapacitated, the spleen and liver may again resume their embryonic cell-forming function. In general, diseases of the blood are actually diseases of the hematopoietic tissues.

There is much difference of opinion as to whether blood cells are formed intravascularly or extravascularly in the bone marrow. In this discussion it will be assumed that they originate extravascularly from the stem cell designated hemocytoblast. Arising from this stem cell are the following series of cells: (1) erythrocytic,

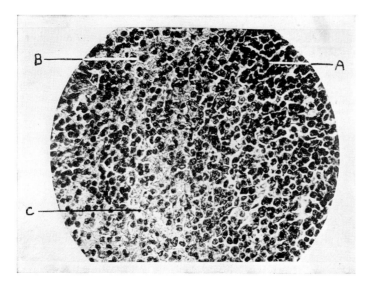

Fig. 15.9 — Spleen of a pig with lymphosarcoma. **A**, masses of lympho blasts; **B**, similar to **A** with erythrocytes interspersed (erythrocytes photographed gray); **C**, field of red cells with lymphoblasts throughout. ×300. (Biester and McNutt, Jour. A.V.M.A.)

(2) granulocytic, (3) lymphocytic, and (4) thrombocytic. Only the most important pathologic conditions which affect each series of cells will be discussed in this book. The normal blood cell and hemoglobin values for different species are given in Tables 15.1 and 15.2.

### Erythrocytic Series

The red cells pass through a series of developmental stages before they become mature. A specific maturation factor or factors are necessary for each developmental stage. These factors are chemical substances, the identity of which is known with reference to some stages and unknown in others. Those known are iron, copper, cobalt, vitamin $B_{12}$, folic acid, vita-

min C, and thyroxin. In the deficiency of any of these substances the development of the erythrocytes may be affected. For instance, in the first stage of development, i.e., from a hemocytoblast to a proerythroblast, an as yet unknown substance is necessary. This substance may be an unknown nutritional or endocrine factor. In its absence, aplastic anemia occurs. In the next stage, i.e., from a proerythroblast to a normoblast, two factors — one extrinsic and one intrinsic — are needed. The extrinsic factor is vitamin $B_{12}$, which is the actual maturation factor. The unknown intrinsic factor may promote the absorption of $B_{12}$ in the intestine. On the other hand, the vitamin folacin may be the maturation factor and vitamin $B_{12}$ may

TABLE 15.1

NORMAL BLOOD CELL VALUES FOR DIFFERENT SPECIES*

| Animal | R.B.C. | W.B.C. | Hb. % | Polys. | Lymph. | Mono. | Eos. | Bas. |
|---|---|---|---|---|---|---|---|---|
| Horse | 7,800,000 | 9,300 | 85 | 57 | 30 | 9 | 4 | 0.5 |
| Cow | 6,600,000 | 9,300 | 60 | 42 | 55 | 5 | 8 | 0.6 |
| Sheep | 10,400,000 | 7,800 | (70)† | 36 | 57 | 6 | 2.5 | 0.4 |
| Pig | 6,700,000 | 15,900 | 85 | 39 | 52 | 3 | 5 | 1.2 |
| Dog | 7,200,000 | 11,800 | 95 | 69 | 20 | 6 | 5 | 0.7 |
| Cat | 8,400,000 | 13,800 | (63)† | 57 | 33 | 6 | 5 | 0.1 |
| Chicken | 3,400,000 | 25,900 | 60 | 31 | 51 | 10 | 6 | 2.6 |
| Rabbit | 5,600,000 | 7,900 | 77 | 43 | 42 | 9 | 2 | 4.0 |
| Guinea Pig | 5,800,000 | 10,800 | 95 | 42 | 45 | 8 | 5 | 0.8 |

* Robert A. Scarborough, Yale Jour. Biol. and Med., 1930.
† Value in ( ) not accurately established.

TABLE 15.2

NORMAL BLOOD CELL AND HEMOGLOBIN VALUES FOR DIFFERENT SPECIES

| Animal | R.B.C. Millions/ cmm | W.B.C. Thousands/ cmm | Hb. gm/cc | Neutro. % | Lymph. % | Mono. % | Eos. % |
|---|---|---|---|---|---|---|---|
| Stallion[1] | 10.0 | 8.7 | 13.2 | 57.8 | 37.8 | 2.1 | 8.5 |
| Mare, pregnant[2] | 7.4 | .... | 15.0 | .... | .... | .... | .... |
| Mare, post partum 1–14 days[2] | 10.4 | .... | 14.7 | .... | .... | .... | .... |
| Mare, pregnant[1] | 9.1 | 8.1 | 12.35 | 46.0 | 47.8 | 1.2 | 4.9 |
| Mare, barren[1] | 9.6 | 9.4 | 12.98 | 55.6 | 38.5 | 2.2 | 3.5 |
| Cow[3] | 8.2 | 8.4 | ..... | 21.0 | 62.0 | 8.5 | 4.8 |
| Cow[4] | 6.3 | 8.9 | ..... | 34.7 | 41.2 | 7.9 | 14.8 |
| Sheep[5] | 11.1 | 10.4 | ..... | 28.3 | 57.3 | 10.2 | 3.7 |
| Sheep[6] | 11.5 | 9.2 | 12.4 | 21.5 | 70.5 | 2.8 | 3.7 |
| Sheep[7] | 6.0 | 10.0 | ..... | 25.5 | 61.6 | 4.3 | 8.8 |
| Dog, male[8] | 6.7 | 13.5 | 14.79 | .... | .... | .... | .... |
| Dog, female[8] | 7.4 | 12.7 | 14.55 | .... | .... | .... | .... |
| Cat[9] | 7.8 | 15.9 | ..... | 54.2 | 38.7 | 1.5 | 5.4 |
| Kitten[9] | 5.2 | 11.7 | ·.... | 52.4 | 34.0 | 1.9 | 6.6 |

[1] M. F. Hansen and A. C. Todd. Jour. A.V.M.A., 118 (1951):26–27.
[2] B. F. Trum. Amer. Jour. Vet. Res., 13 (1952):514–519.
[3] E. C. A. Samaha and C. G. Dobrovolny. Anat. Rec., 99 (1947):563.
[4] L. C. Ferguson, M. R. Irwin, and B. A. Beach. Jour. Inf. Dis., 76 (1945):24–30.
[5] J. R. Prescott, H. A. Keener, C. G. Dobrovolny, and G. P. Percival. Anat. Rec., 99 (1947):563.
[6] H. H. Holman. Jour. Comp. Path. and Therap., 54 (1944):26–40.
[7] S. A. Abramov. Veterinariya, 24 (1947):20–22.
[8] E. Marie Smith. Amer. Jour. Clin. Path., 16 (1946):457–461.
[9] W. H. Riser. No. Amer. Vet., 27 (1946):93–98.

be concerned in some way with the metabolism of folacin. In any event, when either the extrinsic or the intrinsic factor is lacking, the red cells do not develop properly. They assume a size larger than normal, which is characteristic of macrocytic anemia, and are said to undergo megaloblastic degeneration. From the normoblastic stage to the mature erythrocyte the cell passes through the reticulocyte stage. Without the required iron, copper, cobalt, vitamin C, and thyroxin the cell becomes stunted in its development, which is characteristic of microcytic anemia. When the red marrow cannot form a sufficient supply of normal erythrocytes, these underdeveloped forms are released into the general circulation.

## The Anemias

**Definition.** Anemia is a quantitative or qualitative decrease in the amount of blood in an individual. Anemia may be local or general. Local anemia is called **ischemia.** As generally used, anemia refers to a change in the erythrocytes, but it must not be forgotten that the term includes the other blood constituents, such as the leukocytes, as well.

Animals of a given size in each species and breed have a fairly well-defined volume of blood, and in that blood a rather characteristic number of erythrocytes (Table 15.3), while those erythrocytes contain a fairly constant quantity of hemoglobin (Table 15.4). Whenever a reduction occurs in the total volume (oligemia), or the quality becomes thinner (hydremia), or the number of erythrocytes is diminished (oligocythemia), or the quantity of hemoglobin decreases (oligochromemia), a state of anemia exists. In all of these states there is a reduction in the total number of erythrocytes and/or of hemoglobin. Since in anemia the erythrocytes may have the normal size, or may be enlarged or diminished in size, the qualifying adjectives *normocytic, macrocytic,* and *microcytic* are used in designating the type of condition. Furthermore, in an anemia not only may the quantity and quality of the fluid and erythrocytes be affected but also the amount of hemoglobin in each cell. This gives rise to the use of descriptive adjectives such as *normochromic* and *hypochromic* in classifying anemias. A normochrome cell contains a saturated solution of hemoglobin and, since it cannot contain a supersaturated solution of it, there is no occasion to use the word *hyperchromic*.

TABLE 15.3

NORMAL ERYTHROCYTE AND LEUKOCYTE VALUES FOR DIFFERENT SPECIES *

| Species | Erythrocytes (expressed in millions) | Leukocytes (expressed in thousands) |
|---|---|---|
| Horse.. | 7–10 | 6–12 |
| Ox.... | 5–7 | 7–10 |
| Sheep.. | 8–11 | 9–10 |
| Goat... | 13–18 | 9–12 |
| Swine.. | 5–8 | 11–16 |
| Dog ... | 5–8 | 9–10 |
| Cat.... | 9 | 11–16 |
| Fowl... | 3–6 | 30 |

\* Average number per cubic millimeter obtained by several investigators.

TABLE 15.4

HEMOGLOBIN VALUES IN HEALTH AND IN HYPOCHROMIC ANEMIA

| Species | Normal State (grams of hemoglobin per 100 cc. of blood *) | Anemic State (beginning at 70 per cent of normal) |
|---|---|---|
| Horse.. | 12.40 | 8.68 |
| Cow... | 12.03 | 8.42 |
| Sheep.. | 11.18 | 7.83 |
| Pig.... | 11.95 | 8.37 |
| Dog ... | 13.01 | 9.11 |
| Cat.... | 10.49 | 7.34 |
| Cock... | 13.50 | 9.45 |
| Hen... | 9.80 | 6.86 |

\* Values taken from Duke's *Veterinary Physiology.*

When one realizes the changes which occur in the blood in anemia, and considers them in relation to the physiology of circulation and respiration, it is easy to understand why pallor of the visible mucous membranes, palpitation, and dyspnea are signs of the blood disorder.

From the standpoint of causation there are two principal classes of anemia:

1. **Anemia due to decreased blood formation** when there is

    (a) Insufficient bone marrow (myelophthisic anemia).
    Examples: Anemia associated with leukemia (see page 292).
    Anemia associated with leukosis of fowls (see page 297).

    (b) A depression of bone marrow function (hypoplastic and aplastic anemias).
    Examples: Aplastic anemia of cattle fed trichloroethylene-extracted soybean meal (see page 372).
    Anemia of ionizing radiation (see page 86).

    (c) A deficiency of materials for the formation of erythrocytes (hypoplastic or nutritional anemia).
    Examples: Hypochromic anemia of iron and copper deficiency in suckling pigs and in Florida cattle (see pages 54 and 55).
    Hypochromic anemia of cobalt deficiency in cattle and sheep (see page 57).

2. **Anemia due to increased blood losses** which may be

    (a) Extravascular, resulting from hemorrhage (hemorrhagic anemia) (see page 375).

    (b) Intravascular, arising from hemolysis (hemolytic anemia) (see page 376).

APLASTIC ANEMIA OF CATTLE

Among the extractives which have been used in the past to remove oil from soybean meal is **trichloroethylene**. When cattle were fed sufficient amounts of this meal over rather long periods, aplasia of the bone marrow often occurred which gave rise to anemia. One to 3 pounds of the meal had to be fed daily to a cow for a period of 1 to 9 months before symptoms of a rapidly progressive and fatal aplastic anemia appeared. Most of the deaths occurred within a period of a month after the first symptoms were noticed.

The damage to the hematopoietic tissue of the marrow resulted in a reduction of erythrocytes (3 to 4½ million per cu. mm.; normal = 5 to 7 million). Since individual erythrocytes had the normal amount of hemoglobin and normal size, the anemia could be designated normocytic-normochromic as far as the individual red cells were concerned, but because of the great reduction in the total number of these cells, the quantity of hemoglobin fell to 5 to 9 gm. per 100 ml. of blood (normal = 11 to 12). Therefore, there was a state of oligochromemia. The blood changes which occurred in this condition in cattle are probably quite characteristic of aplastic anemia due to other causes.

In aplastic anemia, since the blood cannot carry the normal amount of oxygen, hypoxia of the tissues occurs. The animal tries to overcome this condition by increased respiration, but in spite of this, the tissues display oxygen hunger. This is very noticeable in the endothelium of the small blood vessels. Damage to the endothelium permits hemorrhages to occur into the subcutis, mucosa, serosa, and the parenchyma of vital organs. Due to a decrease of platelets the blood may not coagulate normally. This means that the aplastic anemia is usually complicated with hemorrhagic anemia.

Bone marrow injury is also indicated by a leukopenia. The number of leukocytes may fall to an alarmingly low number. The white cells which remain are chiefly lymphocytes. This indicates that the damage is confined mostly to the red marrow.

Poisoning of cattle by the **bracken fern,** varieties of *Pteridium aquilinum,* also has the characteristics of aplastic anemia. It is possible that the plant contains a chemical substance which destroys or depresses the bone marrow function in a manner quite similar to that of certain chemical compounds in man. There is belief also that it destroys niacin.

Among the outstanding signs of the disorder are hemorrhages of various sizes occurring throughout the body. Alterations in the blood elements link these hemorrhages with a shortage of megakaryocytes which causes a diminution in platelets. There is also a granulocytopenia followed by an erythropenia. These blood alterations point to a disturbance in the hematopoietic tissue of the bone marrow (aplastic anemia).

HYPOCHROMIC ANEMIA

Hemoglobin, as you have already learned in physiology, is a protein in which a large molecule, globin, is combined with a smaller, iron-containing molecule, hematin. Under ordinary nutritional conditions the body has available all the constituents for the formation of hemoglobin. If any element is likely to be lacking, it is iron. (See also Chapter 4). When iron is needed for hemoglobin, it must be provided either from stores of it in the body, principally in the liver, or from the outside. Even though iron is so necessary in the body, it is never present there normally in large amounts. Loss of iron from the body by excretion is negligible. If losses occur in other ways than by excretion, or if the intake of iron in the food is not adequate, an anemic state arises. The anemia occurs because the production of hemoglobin lags behind the formation of erythrocytes. As a consequence the red cells are small and pale. This type of anemia therefore is called microcytic hypochromic.

The question arises, How low must the hemoglobin content of the blood fall before a state of hypochromic anemia can be said to exist? In human medicine most authorities agree that out of a standardized 100 per cent hemoglobin, values much below 85 per cent are subnormal and that values below 70 per cent indicate an anemic condition. Based on this rule, Table 15.4 may be of value in determining the presence of a state of anemia.

The reasons for the appearance of hypochromic anemia are (1) decreased intake of iron in the body, (2) increased demand for iron in the body, and (3) increased outgo of iron from the body.

Iron intake obviously may be below the requirements of the body when it is deficient in the diet. This may be the situation in pregnant females, especially in multiparous omnivorous animals, as the sow. A supply above the normal maintenance requirements for the pregnant sow is necessary because she must confer some of her supply to her fetuses. The amount of iron in the ration may likewise be inadequate for young, rapidly growing animals. The greater demand for iron in them occurs because of the increased volume of hemoglobin in their progressively expanding mass of blood. Furthermore, an additional supply is necessary for their developing body tissues. A female that has had a hypochromic anemia during pregnancy usually gives birth to young that are not endowed with sufficient iron to prevent hypochromic anemia in themselves. This is often the case with young pigs.

Bitches, which are carnivorous multiparous animals, seldom give birth to puppies which have hypochromic anemia. The meat diet of bitches evidently supplies ample iron to be passed on to the puppies.

The intake of iron may also be low when disturbances in the gastrointestinal tract interfere with iron absorption. Such conditions as achlorhydria, a deficiency in gastric hydrochloric acid, and enteritis with diarrhea are associated with reduction in iron intake.

As stated above, iron outgo by normal excretion is not great. If the intake is adequate for normal conditions of nutrition, hypochromic anemia does not occur as the result of iron excretion. Other causes for its loss must be sought. Loss by hemorrhage is the most common. The anemia which characterizes some parasitic infections such as those caused by stomach worms in sheep and hookworms in dogs is at once both hemorrhagic and hypochromic. In hookworm anemia of dogs it has been determined that there is a marked reduction in the total number of erythrocytes, as well as a decrease in their size (microcytosis) and in their hemoglobin content (hypochromia). This type of anemia is termed microcytic hypochromic.

**Bone marrow alterations.** The changes which occur in the erythrocytes in hypochromic anemia are accompanied by changes in the bone marrow. At birth all the bones contain very vascular red marrow in which erythrocytes are formed. As the animal becomes older, areas of yellow, fatty marrow begin to form in the shafts of the bones of the limbs and extend towards the epiphyses. Finally, when the animal reaches maturity, only small areas of red marrow remain in the epiphyses. The cranial bones, ribs, sternum, pelvic bones, and vertebrae retain their red marrow throughout life in the normal animal. Normally, the red marrow of these bones supplies the necessary numbers of red cells. When the demand for oxygen increases in hypochromic anemia, the red marrow undergoes a hyperplasia in an attempt to supply more erythrocytes. This newly formed hyperplastic tissue crowds out the yellow, fatty marrow where it is present until finally the yellow marrow may be completely replaced with red marrow. In spite of the hyperplasia of red marrow, however, the production of red cells falls off because there is a deficiency of building material (iron and copper).

**Blood alterations.** As a result of the shortage of iron and copper, many of the normoblasts fail to become reticulocytes. These normoblasts that fail to mature are retained in the marrow. A few of the cells which reach the reticulocyte stage circulate in the blood with those that become erythrocytes. The latter are in diminished numbers and are small and pale (microcytic and hypochromic). The hypoxic state caused by the deficiency in the oxygen-carrying red cells acts as a stimulus to the marrow to produce more cells. This leads to the hyperplasia of red marrow.

**Other effects.** Diminished hemoglobin content and decreased red cell-numbers is reflected in the appearance of the animal. Naturally, the mucous membranes become pallid. Likewise, upon necropsy the muscles and viscera are blanched much like the tissues of an animal that has been bled. During life the anemic animal displays a general weakness (Figs. 15.10 and 15.11). Because the oxygen-carrying ability of the blood is lessened, respiration becomes more rapid (polypnea) and eventually labored (dyspnea). With in-creased respiration there is also acceler-ated heart action which, if continued long enough, results in some degree of cardiac hypertrophy and dilatation. The hypoxic state of the blood gives rise to disturbed liver-cell metabolism (cloudy swelling and fatty changes). (See Fig. 9.8. See also page 368, relative to alterations in the spleen.)

## HEMORRHAGIC ANEMIA

Anemia resulting from loss of blood is designated hemorrhagic anemia. The loss

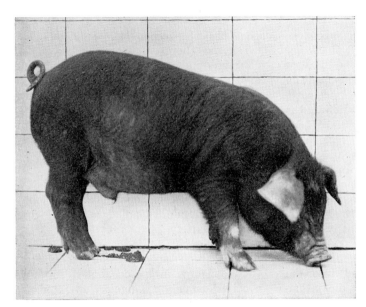

Fig. 15.10 — A non-anemic pig at 49 days of age. (Craig, Jour. A.V.M.A.)

Fig. 15.11 — A pig with nu-tritional anemia at 45 days of age. Note wrinkling of the skin which accompanies loss of weight. (Craig, Jour. A.V.M.A.)

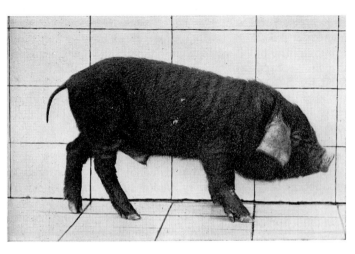

of blood may occur suddenly or gradually. Sudden losses originate when there are breaks in the continuity of blood vessels as the result of trauma, the rupture of an aneurysm, the rupture of the wall of hollow organs during overdistention and torsion of the intestine. A gradual loss of blood which may result in anemia occasionally occurs when horses are bled too often in the production of antiserums and antitoxins.

The amount of blood in the body with relation to body weight is variable in the different species of domestic animals. It is greatest in the horse, in which the amount is almost 10 per cent of the total weight, and least in rabbits, cats, and goats, in which the amount is between 6 and 7 per cent. The loss of one-third of the blood at one time usually results in fatality. Serumhorses, however, can often tolerate, without the appearance of marked anemia, the withdrawal of 25 per cent of their blood each month over a period of several years when the amounts taken at each bleeding are not excessive. On the other hand, animals with a heavy infestation of blood-sucking worms, such as sheep with stomach worms and dogs with hookworms, often show marked anemia, partly as the result of a continuous loss of blood.

Gradual loss of blood into the subcutaneous connective tissue and into the mucous membranes occurs in the intoxication which sometimes follows certain infectious diseases like strangles in horses. In this condition, which is called **purpura hemorrhagica**, there is apparently a toxic injury to the blood vessels which permits the slow escape of blood.

At the outset of the condition there are probably sufficient platelets to plug the leaks in the capillaries, but eventually the loss of platelets becomes greater than their replacement and hemorrhages become progressively more numerous and larger. There is a possibility also that the production of platelets may be inhibited.

**In sweet-clover poisoning** of cattle there is great loss of blood into the tissues and body cavities with resulting anemia. The interference with coagulation of blood in this instance is apparently a prothrombin depletion coupled possibly with an inadequate concentration of calcium in the blood. Except where the hemorrhages are present, the tissues become quite bloodless.

In 1953 in broiler chickens in the New England area a so-called **hemorrhagic disease** was first reported. Its characteristics are so variable that the disease is difficult to classify. Anemia is the only constant lesion, but many of the birds have petechial to ecchymotic hemorrhages in the subcutis and muscles of the legs and breast, and in the muscle of the gizzard. The red marrow of some bones becomes pale pink to buff yellow in color. The syndrome therefore seems to have the characteristics of both a hemolytic and aplastic anemia. The morbidity is high and the mortality low. The cause is unknown although there is a suggestion that the condition may be an allergy to chemical compounds added to the ration to control bacterial and parasitic infections.

### HEMOLYTIC ANEMIA

Anemia arising from increased erythrocyte destruction is called hemolytic anemia. A variety of hemolytic agents are responsible for this type of anemia. Among them are bacteria and viruses such as some streptococci and staphylococci, *Clostridium hemolyticum,* and the virus of equine infectious anemia. In the list also belong certain blood protozoa such as the eperythrozoa of cattle, sheep, and swine, and the anaplasma of anaplasmosis. There are also worm parasites which apparently cause anemia by elaborating hemolytic lipoid substances. Among such worms are the hookworms and ascarids. An example of a zootoxin capable of producing this condition is snake venom; of a phytotoxin, ricin; of a mineral, lead; and of organic salts, the salts of the bile acids in obstructive jaundice.

A very interesting hemolytic anemia occasionally occurs in suckling foals, pigs, and puppies. Foals that develop this *post-partum hemolytic anemia and icterus* usually appear healthy at the time of birth. Symptoms appear in the foals anywhere from 12 hours to 9 days after birth, depending upon the concentration of the hemagglutinins in the dam's colostrum and the amount of colostrum consumed by the foal. In severe cases that live a few days or recover, the erythrocyte count falls as low as 2,200,000 per cm., and icterus and hemoglobinuria appear on the second day. The spleen becomes greatly enlarged in the foals that have the greatest amount of hemolysis. Other signs of great erythrocyte destruction in these spleens are erythrophagia by the fixed and wandering phagocytes and excessive hemosiderin deposition. The Kupffer cells of the liver also become engorged with this pigment.

In cats an infectious anemia caused by *Haemobartonella felis* and characterized by the destruction of erythrocytes is probably prevalent in the United States but has attracted little attention. In a high percentage of the cases the erythrocytes decrease to less than 4 million per 100 ml. and the hemoglobin falls to less than 5 gm. per 100 ml. In blood smears, Giemsa stained, the Haemobartonellae sticking to erythrocytes assume varied forms — small and large cocci, occurring singly or in chains, and rods. They vary in size from .1 $\mu$ for the small cocci to 1.5 $\mu$ for the rods. Their presence on the red cells of the peripheral blood varies from day to day. The bone marrow attempts to compensate for the loss of red cells by releasing numerous large, immature cells (macrocytes) and also many nucleated (normoblasts) and large blue-staining cells (reticulocytes). Splenomegaly and icterus do not occur in all cases.

**Anaplasmosis** is a protozoan blood disease of cattle caused by *Anaplasma marginale*. Since the hematozoan parasite causing the disease is probably transmitted by vectors, it is not surprising that the disease has a seasonal occurrence — mostly in the summer and fall. Experimentally, ticks, horseflies, and mosquitoes have proven to be vectors. A minute quantity of infected blood, as small as .025 cc., is sufficient to transmit the infection into a healthy cow. This suggests why cases of anaplasmosis have been attributed to medical and surgical procedures which have not been carried out in an aseptic manner. Among such procedures are the bleeding of cattle for blood tests, injections with hypodermic syringes, dehorning, castration, direct transfusions, ear marking, and the use of nose tongs.

Evidence obtained by ultrafiltration of the blood of affected cattle and by electron microscopy indicates that this disease may be caused not by a hematozoan parasite but by a virus. The bodies occurring at the periphery of the erythrocytes and believed to have been the anaplasmata contain from one to seven masses of dense particulate matter, each measuring 0.2 to $0.7\mu$ in diameter, and have the characteristics of a virus. Furthermore, an ultrafiltrate of the blood is infective. If these findings are correct, it will necessitate renaming the disease.

As soon as the anaplasmata are introduced into the blood stream of a susceptible animal, they begin to reproduce in the erythrocytes. In the cells they occupy a peripheral position. In 15 to 40 days the parasites have increased in numbers to such an extent that $\frac{1}{4}$ to $\frac{1}{2}$ of the erythrocytes contain them. The animal now becomes visibly sick and has a fever. Within another week some of the erythrocytes are enlarged and have a stippled appearance. They are called "stipple" cells.

With the increase of parasites there is such a destruction of erythrocytes that the total count falls from an average of about 7 million per cubic millimeter to about 2 or 3 million. With the fall in number of erythrocytes there is also a decrease in hemoglobin — from a normal of 80 to 90 by the Talquist scale to 40 or 50. This is a hemolytic anemia characterized by oligocythemia and oligochromemia.

Macroscopically, all of the tissues and organs are icteric. The lymph nodes are edematous. This is probably due to the fact that the blood is thin, watery, and light-colored (hydremia). The heart is in a state of acute dilatation from overwork. Cardiac petechiae arise from hypoxia. The anemic and icteric lungs are emphysematous from excessive inflation consequent to the oligocythemia and oligochromemia. Bile oozes from the cut surface of the extremely icteric liver. The gall bladder is distended with flocculent, dark green, viscid bile resulting from excessive amounts of cholebilirubin. There is acute swelling of the spleen as would be expected in the presence of excessive hemolysis. The urinary bladder contains urine of a dark straw-colored hue due to the excretion of excessive amounts of cholebilirubin and urobilinogen. The urine is not bloody or tinged with hemoglobin.

If the number of erythrocytes containing anaplasmata does not exceed approximately 10 per cent, the animal may slowly recover but may remain a carrier. If the number of erythrocytes containing parasites reaches 25 to 50 per cent, about 30 to 50 per cent of the animals die.

**Eperythrozoonosis** is a disease caused by Eperythrozoa which has been found in cattle, sheep, mice, and man. The condition in pigs is caused by the protozoon, *Eperythrozoon suis*, and in acute cases is characterized by icterus and anemia. *E. parvum* may be present in the blood with *E. suis* but is apparently nonpathogenic.

The methods of transmission are unknown, but arthropod vectors, flies, and mosquitoes have been incriminated. Mechanical transmission via needles and surgery is possible. The organisms which belong to the Bartonella group are found on the erythrocytes (supracellular) and in the blood plasma (extracellular). The number of erythrocytes destroyed varies greatly and accounts for the so-called acute and mild cases of the disease. As a result of a marked destruction of red blood cells, an icterus of the hemolytic type is produced. Some animals may be found dead having shown no symptoms. The elevated temperature usually coincides with the intensity of blood infection. The period of incubation in experimental cases varies from 6 to 10 days.

Splitter is of the opinion that the lesions are quite characteristic and apparently pathognomonic if death does not take place soon after early symptoms. The blood is thin and watery (hydremia). The red blood cell count may drop as low as one to two million or lower (oligocythemia). Immature erythrocytes are produced as the anemia develops and are most numerous during the convalescent period (reticulocytosis). The hemoglobin may be as low as 2 to 4 grams (oligochromemia). The white blood cell count is usually unchanged, but in a few cases a marked leukocytosis has been noted. The spleen is enlarged and friable and in some cases three to four times normal size (splenomegaly). The body fat and other internal tissues may have a yellowish discoloration (icterus). The icterus (hemolytic type) is not constant but is usually present if the animal lives 3 to 4 days after appearance of symptoms. The stomach and intestinal contents are often discolored with orange-yellow bile. The liver may show an icteric discoloration. The gall bladder contains a thick granular or gelatinous bile. Parenchymatous degeneration is present in the kidney, heart, and skeletal musculature. A few petechiae may be present in the mucosa of the urinary bladder. Hydroperitoneum may be observed. The red bone marrow may be hyperplastic.

**Infectious viral equine anemia** is an acute or chronic viral disease of horses characterized by a gradual destruction of the erythrocytes and continuous or remittent fever. The cause is a filtrable virus, *Trifur equorum*, that is constantly present in the blood of affected horses and is capable of being transmitted by certain mosquitoes and biting flies (*Stomoxys calcitrans*). There is quite a possibility that the careless use of hypodermic needles by horsemen may be a means of transmission at race tracks. The blood of an infected horse may remain virulent for years, yet the animal may show no clinical evidence of the infection outside of occasional febrile attacks.

After entering the blood, the virus increases and exerts an injurious effect upon the erythrocytes, causing their destruction. As a consequence, the principal changes, apart from those in the blood, occur in the organs concerned with the formation and destruction of erythrocytes (bone marrow, spleen, and liver). As far as possible, the blood-forming organs attempt to replace destroyed cells with new ones. At the same time the spleen responds to an immunity reaction. Under normal conditions the destruction of erythrocytes is accomplished by the endothelial cells (macrophages) of the reticuloendothelial system. While the principal organ in the body in which this destruction appears varies considerably in the various species of animals, it is quite probable that in the horse much of it occurs in the spleen. In the early stages of infectious anemia the spleen contains an increased amount of hemosiderin due to the destruction of large numbers of erythrocytes. In chronic cases this is not usually the case. It is believed that with the advance of the disease the reticuloendothelial cells of the spleen apparently change their function from erythrocyte destruction to immunity production. The reticuloendothelial cells (Kupffer cells) of the liver assume the erythrocyte-destroying function with consequent increase of iron in the liver. The period of incubation is variable. Experimentally, it is 7 to 28 days.

Macroscopically, the lesions vary considerably according to the virulence of the infectious agent, individual resistance, stage of the disease, number of febrile attacks, the rapidity of recurrence of febrile attacks, the height and duration of fever, and the period of time elapsing between the last febrile attack and the time of death. In general, the lesions are: anemia and emaciation with serous atrophy of the fatty tissues, subserous ecchymotic hemorrhages of the peritoneum, cardiac degeneration and dilatation with epicardial hemorrhages, acute or chronic splenomegaly, splenic hemosiderosis in the early stages and hepatic hemosiderosis in the late stages, hepatic enlargement due to hyperemia and to lymphocytic infiltration of the portal sheaths, and hydroperitoneum and hydrothorax.

## Septicemic Diseases

Many diseases are characterized by septicemia and involve the entire body. They are not confined to any specific organ. Since they are distributed throughout the body by the blood stream they are discussed as diseases of the hematopoietic system.

### ANTHRAX

Anthrax is an acute, septicemic disease caused by *Bacillus anthracis*, occurring sporadically and in epizootics in herbivora and omnivora, and communicable to nearly all warm-blooded animals and to man. It is characterized by acute swelling of the spleen and by serohemorrhagic infiltrations of the subcutaneous and subserous connective tissue.

**Pathogenesis.** Experimentally, spores which enter the digestive tract do not germinate because of the unfavorable influences of the gastric juice, the presence of *Escherichia coli*, and the carbon dioxide content of the fermenting ingesta. Vegetative forms of *Bacillus anthracis* do not live long in the intestinal tract. The organisms apparently enter the body through the oral mucosa and pass to the larynx, trachea, and lungs. They can be found in all parts of the respiratory system as soon as 6 hours after ingestion but do not appear in the spleen until 24 hours or more after ingestion. From the lungs the bacilli reach the bronchial lymph nodes. It is believed that the bacilli proliferate in lymph nodes and become disseminated from them into the blood stream, resulting in bacillemia. There is concentration of the microorganisms in the spleen. In the Mississippi Delta region, horseflies transmit the disease through bites in the skin.

The dense capsule of the organism protects it against the destructive action of bacteriolytic substances in the body fluids and the phagocytes. At points where large numbers of organisms accumulate, the great amount of capsule substance swells from gradual absorption of fluid. This causes blocking of the capillaries (Fig. 7.7) and lymph vessels and results in edema. A lethal toxin also contributes to the edema. On account of the injury to the vessel walls, extensive hemorrhages develop. These occur in the center of the edematous swellings and in organs with slow circulation (spleen, liver, brain). The period of incubation is 1 to 14 days, depending upon the place and intensity of infection.

**Lesions.** There is rapid decomposition of the carcass. Rigor mortis is incomplete. Extensive serous infiltrations and extravasations of blood appear in the connective tissue in different parts of the body (subcutaneous, intermuscular, subserous in the mediastinum, mesentery, and perirenal region, submucous in the pharynx and epiglottis). With the formation of fibrin, the serous infiltration becomes fibrinous. Hemorrhages without edema may also occur. Hemorrhagic lymphadenitis and acute splenitis with extreme swelling are very prominent lesions and must always be considered in connection with a differential diagnosis. Cloudy swelling of the parenchymatous organs is present as it usually is in all acute septicemic diseases. Hemorrhagic enteritis (small intestine), and hyperemia and edema of the lungs are fairly constant. The blood becomes cyanotic and fails to coagulate, or coagulates poorly. These changes also must not be overlooked when making a differential diagnosis. A serohemorrhagic inflammation of the pharyngeal region occurs in swine.

**Termination.** Death in a few hours to several days is the usual termination.

### SWINE ERYSIPELAS

Swine erysipelas is a septicemic disease of swine of all ages but particularly of pigs weighing 50 to 150 pounds. It is caused by *Erysipelothrix rhusiopathiae* and is characterized by septicemia, unthriftiness, vegetative endocarditis, and arthritis. Swine erysipelas infection has made its appearance in turkeys in widely separated parts of the United States. It is characterized by its rapid spread in flocks, its occurrence mostly in the spring and fall, by splenic and hepatic enlargement, and hemorrhages in skeletal muscles.

**Pathogenesis.** The organisms enter the body of swine by way of the intestinal tract. Entrance through the mucous membrane is probably facilitated by injuries produced by parasites. In Germany it has been shown that the erysipelothrix can be transmitted by the ordinary stable fly (*Stomoxys calcitrans*). After the microorganism enters the blood stream, it tends to localize in certain regions (capillaries of the skin, the heart valves, and joints). In the capillaries they injure the endothelium, causing serous transudations and small hemorrhages. Occasionally, colonies of the organisms act as emboli and obstruct the capillaries, resulting in infarction and necrosis of the skin. The period of incubation is usually 3 to 5 days.

**Lesions.** In outbreaks thus far reported in the United States, the lesions observed in the field have been quite variable, depending upon the virulence of the infection and the length of time the animals have been affected. External lesions may or may not be present. If present, they vary from an erythema to a mild dermatitis to extensive sloughing of the skin (back, tail, ears). A peculiar diamond-shaped blotching of the skin is occasionally observed. The reddened areas may become more than an inch in breadth. Arthritis (carpal and tarsal joints) may be present (Figs. 15.12 and 15.13).

In the more acute cases there are only slight changes in the internal organs. Chief among them is catarrhal gastritis with numerous petechiae. The small intestine may be similarly involved. Reddening of the gastric serosa as if painted with a brush is said to be characteristic. The spleen usually presents very moderate acute swelling. Cloudy swelling of the liver can be expected. The presence of hepatic

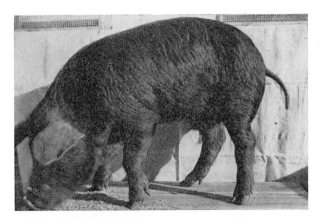

Fig. 15.12 — Arthritis in chronic swine erysipelas. (Stiles and Davis, Jour. A.V.M.A.)

degeneration may explain the occurrence of a slight icterus in some cases. Active hyperemia of the kidneys is a prominent lesion that aids in differentiating erysipelas from cholera. A characteristic cholera kidney is pale with sharply defined petechial hemorrhages, and the characteristic erysipelas kidney is swollen, uniformly dark red in color, and also contains petechiae. Pulmonary hyperemia and edema, often with petechiae, are usually conspicuous. Epiglottal petechiae are common. There is always indication of lymphadenopathy which begins as acute serous lymphadenitis but later becomes a hemorrhagic lymphadenitis. There may be a fibrinous inflammation of the serous membranes and petechiae on the serous and mucous membranes. The lesions of acute swine erysipelas, therefore, are those of an acute septicemia and are not unlike those usually produced by other infections which are capable of rapid generalization.

In the more chronic cases an important lesion is vegetative endocarditis involving especially the left atrioventricular valve but at times also the aortic and pulmonary semilunars and the tricuspid valve (Fig. 15.14). The valves display polypoid, cauliflower-like proliferations which con-

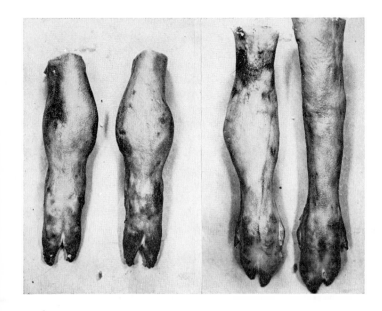

Fig. 15.13—Arthritis in chronic swine erysipelas.
**Left:** Carpal joints.
**Right:** Enlarged and normal tarsal joints.
(Stiles and Davis, Jour. A.V.M.A.)

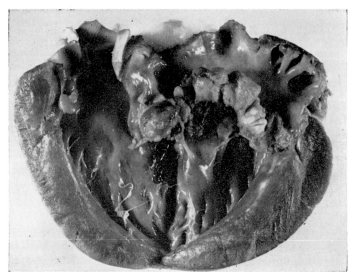

Fig. 15.14 — Vegetative valvular endocarditis of mitral valve in a pig, due to **Erysipelothrix rhusiopathiae.** (Department of Veterinary Pathology, Michigan State University.)

sist for the most part of thrombotic masses that crumble easily. These masses become organized from the underside, but bacterial growth at the surface continually irritates them. Continued irritation causes continued proliferation until finally the left auricle becomes almost filled with the thrombotic mass and dilatation of that chamber occurs. The same process occurring on the aortic and pulmonary semilunars results in severe stenosis. The changes resulting from these lesions are hydrothorax, passive hyperemia of the lungs, liver, spleen, and kidneys, and also infarcts of the latter. In the United States the heart lesions are not a constant finding, but arthritis with subsequent ankylosis seems to be a rather frequent lesion. Several joints may be involved. Necrosis and sloughing of the skin with the formation of dry, shell-like crusts over the back and side occur occasionally.

**Termination.** In untreated herds, losses from swine erysipelas on the average are about 10 to 20 per cent. About 10 to 20 per cent of a herd in which the disease exists become unprofitable because of chronic heart and joint lesions.

### AVIAN ERYSPIPELAS

The lesions of *Erysipelothrix rhusiopathiae* infection in **turkeys** are those of an acute septicemia. Beaudette and Hud-

son found hemorrhages of varying sizes in the pectoral and abdominal muscles and occasionally in the muscles of the thighs. Hemorrhages do not appear in the skin, although changes, apparently vascular in nature, leading to necrosis of the tubular leader (caruncle) of toms is reported by Madsen. Hepatic congestion and degenerative changes are rather constant. Catarrhal enteritis of the anterior two-thirds of the small intestine and hyperemia of the mucosa of the remainder of the intestine are usually present. There is acute swelling of the spleen and there are often hemorrhages in the pericardium.

### LEPTOSPIROSIS

This is an infectious disease of animals and man caused by the various species of the genus Leptospira.

Leptospirosis is characterized by extremely varied clinical manifestations. Many animals that undoubtedly are infected never show clinical signs and consequently have inconspicuous lesions. Some recover from the infection and are carriers, while others develop a rapidly fatal form of the disease. There is considerable serological evidence to show that the infection is widespread in the horse, pig, cow, and dog.

While leptospirae have been isolated from sick and normal pigs, the symptomatology of both natural and experimentally infected animals has been rather indefinite. Icterus, hemoglobinuria, and anemia have been observed in sheep affected with *L. pomona*. There are reports that *Leptospira pomona* occasionally causes abortion in cattle. The chicken is also susceptible to leptospirae.

**Pathogenesis.** Transmission occurs via food and/or water contaminated by urine or feces of infected domestic animals, rats, mice, and voles. There is a possibility of insect transmission since leptospirae can enter the ovaries of the tick and penetrate the eggs. Contact with infected animals or rodents is of considerable importance since many of these animals may act as carriers. The spirochete may pass through broken or abraded skin, or through the intact nasal or buccal mucous membranes. Hemorrhages, more common in acute cases, may be produced in tissues throughout the body and can be considered to be the result of the localized toxic effect of the leptospirae on the endothelial cells.

**Lesions.** Because there are two general types of lesions, the pathological findings vary greatly, but in the dog the cases may be classified as acute hemorrhagic and acute icteric. According to Monlux, the lesions are identical in both types except that in the icteric type there is icterus and more liver damage. Petechial and, occasionally, ecchymotic hemorrhages may be present throughout the tissues and organs, being most common in the lungs, stomach, small and large intestine, liver, kidneys, heart, gall and urinary bladders, skeletal and smooth musculature, and subserous, submucous, and subcutaneous tissues. Hemorrhages have also been observed in the brain, adrenals, parathyroids, and the uveal tract of the eyes.

Reinhard has reported that in the bovine observable lesions of focal interstitial nephritis recognized as white foci (1 to 5 mm. in diameter) are constant findings. In an occasional case, focal necrosis may be found in the liver. Hadlow and Stoenner observed proliferation of the renal tubular epithelial cells. This proliferation

of epithelial cells was accompanied by disruption or dissolution of the basement membrane. This permitted the proliferating cells to collect in masses often resembling the Langhans type of multinucleated giant cells. These, together with numerous lymphocytes, were prominent in the interstitial exudate. Hemoglobinuria, which may be very transient, is occasionally observed on necropsy. Little and Baker found bloody milk to be a more constant symptom than hemoglobinuria. Abortion may occur at any stage of the gestation period and is probably associated with the febrile period of the disease. The basic cause of abortion in cattle infected with *L. pomona* has not been determined. The reason for the abortion in sows however is obvious because the living or dead baby pigs have been infected with the organism. Icterus may be observed although it is not common. Hemorrhages in various tissues and organs may be present, particularly in the cortex of the kidney.

Microscopically, hemorrhages (petechiae, ecchymoses, and/or diffuse hemorrhage) throughout the tissues and organs are characteristic lesions of acute fatal cases. The liver, in addition to hemorrhage, may show parenchymatous degeneration (cloudy swelling and fatty change), regenerative activity (large hyperchromatic nuclei, binucleated cells, and mitotic figures), and dissociation of the normal cord arrangement. In icteric animals, bile pigment is usually present in the central canaliculi. Cholebilirubin is present in many of the hepatic cells.

The changes in the kidney may be primarily degenerative in nature, or both degenerative and inflammatory. The alterations are predominantly tubular and interstitial with only rare glomerular involvement. Regressive changes (cloudy swelling, fatty change, and necrosis) are most prominent in the proximal convoluted tubules. Detritus (desquamated and necrotic epithelial cells, and nuclear fragments) is frequently present in the tubules. Bloom reports marked vacuolar degeneration in the epithelium of the proximal convolutions. Sections, stained with Sudan III, indicated that the vacuoles (small and large) were not fat. He also found that a striking feature in all of his cases was the large number of tubules with atypical regenerated epithelium. The epithelium, depending on the degree of maturity, varied from flattened cells with large, hyperchromatic nuclei to those having a more adult appearance. In addition to petechiae in the cortex and medulla, infiltrations of macrophages, lymphocytes, plasma cells, and neutrophils were present in the interstitial tissue.

In the canine, the laboratory findings vary somewhat with the individual cases. The blood picture in many animals shows a moderate anemia and decreased hemoglobin concentration. The white blood cell count is usually high (leukocytosis) with an increase in the number of immature neutrophils (shift to the left). The blood-urea-nitrogen, and nonprotein nitrogen levels are elevated. An immediate (direct) Van den Bergh reaction is found in the blood serum of icteric cases. The bone marrow is hyperplastic, with the myeloid cells largely neutrophilic myelocytes. Urine examination reveals albumin, casts, variable specific gravity (1.010 to 1.028), acid reaction, and a moderate number of red and white blood cells in the tubules.

In a clinico-pathological study of experimental leptospirosis of calves, Reinhard reported that a transitory hemolytic anemia was always present. A neutropenia and lymphocytopenia occurred during or close to the time of fever. Albuminuria and low specific gravity were present in most cases. Albuminuria was not severe in any case. Blood chemical findings did not show the occurrence of uremia. A transitory hemoglobinuria of varying degrees was observed in some cases.

The demonstration of leptospirae by dark-field examinations of blood and urine is unsatisfactory and inconclusive. Difficulty is frequently encountered in demonstrating the organisms in tissue, although Bloom reports the observation of distinct leptospirae, particularly in the kidneys and liver of all cases when he used silver stains on formalin-preserved tissue. He found that tissue scrapings of the liver, and particularly of the kidney, when examined with the dark-field, were usually positive.

For a long time the cause of equine periodic ophthalmia has been a mystery. At times it has been attributed to various bacteria, a filtrable virus, and a deficiency of riboflavin. Now, evidence is beginning to accumulate that the cause may be leptospirae.

Recent reports tend to give causal relationship of leptospirae to periodic ophthalmia. The organism has been isolated from the aqueous humor and blood of a horse affected with the disease, and an acute iridocyclitis has been produced in foals by the injection of *Leptospira pomona*. In the latter case there was an absence of any relationship between the disease and vitamin $B_2$ (riboflavin) deficiency. Studies on equine leptospirosis at the New York State Veterinary College do not substantiate this. These studies indicate that equine leptospirosis is a very mild disease and that *Leptospira pomona* does not *per se* cause periodic ophthalmia. There was, however, a close correlation between the presence of leptospira serum agglutinins and periodic ophthalmia.

This disease is an inflammation of the eyes which recurs periodically and terminates in blindness (so-called moon-blindness). The blindness is due to a cataract or other destructive changes in the eye which are preceded by acute changes such as inflammation of the cornea with vascularization, contraction of the pupil (miosis), and the presence of exudate in the anterior chamber (hypopyon). Between the acute and chronic phases of the ophthalmia there is one of quiescence.

The extent of the changes which occur in the eye in periodic ophthalmia depends upon the number and severity of the attacks. In the acute stages of the disease there is conjunctivitis with edema of the lids, cloudiness of the cornea with marked vascularization of the cornea (keratitis), contraction of the pupil (miosis), and the presence of exudate in the anterior chamber (hypopyon). As the disease progresses, the deeper parts of the eye become involved. Along with the miosis which results from iritis and iridocyclitis, the iris may become adherent to the cornea (anterior synechia) or to the lens (posterior synechia). The lens becomes opaque (cataract), and degenerative changes develop in the retina and choroid. The resultant atrophied eye displays all of the changes of a total ophthalmitis (panophthalmia).

### HOG CHOLERA

Hog cholera is a highly contagious, pantropic viral disease of swine characterized by lesions of a septicemia and complicated often by inflammatory and necrotic processes in the lungs and intestine. While the primary infection is due to *Tortor suis*, the complications in the lungs are due to *Pasteurella multocida*, and in the intestine to *Salmonella choleraesuis* and *Spherophorus necrophorus*.

**Pathogenesis.** The virus enters the blood stream, where it is adsorbed by the erythrocytes. It produces more or less pronounced changes in the endothelium of the capillaries and other blood vessels, and also in the walls of the smaller blood vessels. The most prominent changes in the endothelium and vessel walls are degenerative in nature. In prolonged cases the most prominent change is proliferation of the endothelium. These changes are believed to provide a satisfactory explanation for the presence of small hemorrhages and foci of necrosis which characterize this disease.

In most cases, secondary inflammatory changes occur in the stomach and intestine, together with their lymph nodes, and in the lungs. *Salmonella choleraesuis* is the most frequent secondary invader in the stomach and intestine, and *Pasteurella multocida* in the lungs. The former is a frequent normal inhabitant of swine intestine, and the latter is a common saprophyte in the respiratory tract of healthy hogs. Both organisms apparently find favorable conditions for their propagation in a hog affected with cholera virus. Therefore, associated with the primary anatomical alterations of pure cholera, there may also be present alterations characteristic of **pasteurellosis** and of **infectious necrotic enteritis.**

As a consequence, the clinical and pathological pictures of cholera in the field are quite variable, depending on the secondary infection. (See also the pathogenesis of infectious necrotic enteritis and pasteurellosis, pp. 420 and 483.) The first animals to die in a herd, probably those having least resistance, show acute catarrhal inflammation of the mucous membranes and numerous hemorrhages (**viral lesions**). Other cases, animals of greater resistance and which therefore survive the effects of the virus, show the changes which constitute the secondary lesions or complications of cholera (pneumonia and enteritis). The period of incubation is at least 4 days, generally 13 to 18 days.

**Lesions.** Microscopically, there is general lymphadenitis with the earliest and most characteristic changes in the cervical and thoracic nodes. The inflammatory process is serous. Unless one keeps in mind the peculiarities in the structure of swine lymph nodes and the manner of lymph flow in them, it is not easy to understand why hemorrhage is confined principally to the periphery of the node. Neiberle believes the erythrocytes which collect in the cell-poor substance of the periphery are derived from petechiae in the region drained by the particular node. In the follicular arteries of the spleen, these vascular changes lead to cone-shaped infarcts (Fig. 7.9). In the kidneys they result in petechial hemorrhages (Fig. 7.3). In the central nervous system, encephalitis and meningitis are present in most of the cases. In the blood there is a decrease in the number of leukocytes — a leukopenia. The leukopenia is really a lymphocytopenia which is associated with marked atrophy of the lymphoid tissue in the lymph nodes and spleen. The atrophy may be the result of pressure produced by accumulations of blood in the spleen and lymph nodes, i.e., by hemorrhages. There is a possibility also that lymphopoiesis may be inhibited by the hog cholera virus.

The macroscopic changes in uncomplicated hog cholera are, first of all, small hemorrhages, the location and distribution of which vary considerably in different cases. The places where they are sought most frequently are in the kidneys, urinary bladder, epiglottis and larynx, heart, lungs, mucosa of the large intestine, mucosa of the small intestine, gastric mucosa and serosa, the serosa of the small and large intestine, and lymph nodes. Equally important gross lesions are splenic infarction and splenic passive hyperemia, pneumonia, pulmonary hyperemia, erythema and cutaneous hemorrhages of the abdomen, catarrhal cecitis and colitis, and catarrhal gastritis. The passive hyperemia is most prominent in organs having a vast capillary network such as the spleen and lungs. It also occurs in the skin. In these places it is probably the result of weakened cardiac action due to the effect of the virus on the myocardium. The inflammatory reactions, pneumonia and enteritis, which occur late in cholera are caused by *Pasteurella multocida* and *Salmonella*

*choleraesuis.* "Button ulcers" of the large intestine (Fig. 15.15) have long been recognized as a lesion of hog cholera. In some cases they arise from hyperplastic and abscessed lymph nodules of the mucosa or submucosa, and in others from infarcts of the mucosa or submucosa occurring secondary to thrombosis of small arteries. The thrombi in turn owe their origin to the proliferation of the vascular endothelium which is a histological change produced by the cholera virus.

For 286 naturally infected hogs Kernkamp recorded the frequency of occurrence of the lesions of cholera. The results are shown in Table 15.5.

### BLUE TONGUE

Blue tongue is an acute viral disease, chiefly of sheep, characterized by a swollen, blue tongue, catarrhal inflammation of the upper respiratory and the gastrointestinal tracts, and often by inflammation of the sensitive laminae of the feet and the coronet. It is prevalent in the summer, especially in wet seasons. When it was principally a disease of Africa and Near East countries it was only of academic interest in the United States, but after its appearance in the Southwestern States at the beginning of the present half-century, interest in it quickened.

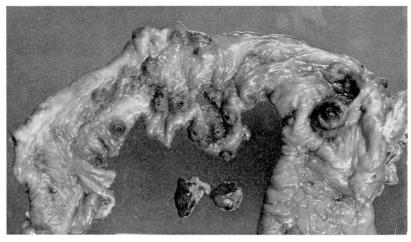

Fig. 15.15 — Button ulcers of the large intestine in chronic hog cholera. (Department of Veterinary Pathology, Michigan State University.)

TABLE 15.5

FREQUENCY OF OCCURRENCE OF LESIONS IN HOG
CHOLERA BASED ON OBSERVATION OF 286
NATURALLY INFECTED HOGS

| Lesions | Percentage Occurrence |
|---|---|
| 1. Renal hemorrhages............ | 92 |
| 2. Hemorrhagic lymphadenitis..... | 82 |
| 3. Urinary bladder hemorrhages.,.. | 78 |
| 4. Splenic infarction and hyperemia. | 59 |
| 5. Laryngeal hemorrhages........ | 58 |
| 6. Pneumonia.................. | 45 |
| 7. Pulmonary hyperemia.......... | 42 |
| 8. Cardiac hemorrhages.......... | 32 |
| 9. Pulmonary hemorrhages........ | 25 |
| 10. Intestinal (large) mucosal hemorrhages............... | 25 |
| 11. Cutaneous cyanosis and hyperemia.................. | 25 |
| 12. Enteritis (large intestine)....... | 15 |
| 13. Intestinal (small) mucosal hemorrhages............... | 10 |
| 14. Gastric mucosal hemorrhages.... | 9 |
| 15. Intestinal (small) serosal hemorrhages............... | 7 |
| 16. Intestinal (large) serosal hemorrhages............... | 6 |
| 17. Gastric serosal hemorrhages..... | 5 |
| 18. Gastritis.................... | 4 |

(H. C. H. Kernkamp)

Blue tongue virus is transmitted by a vector, which in the Southwestern States is probably a gnat (*Culicoides variipennis*). The period of incubation appears to be less than a week.

**Pathogenesis and lesions.** In the early febrile stage the disease is a viremia, but later, perhaps for a period of a month or longer, the virus is localized in the tissues.

The virus injures the smaller blood vessels in the connective tissue, causing hyperemia, edema, and hemorrhage — a serohemorrhagic infiltration. Coagulative necrosis of the skeletal muscles occurs in many animals. Anemia and leukopenia indicate that the hematopoietic tissues are affected also.

The fever has a duration of 5 to 6 days, and with it the tongue becomes blue or purple as a result of the serohemorrhagic infiltration. The buccal mucosa becomes red for the same reason. This type of oral lesion easily leads to erosions, and the erosions to ulcers and gangrene because

of the presence of saprophytes and pyogens.

From the oral lesions extension of the inflammation down the respiratory and digestive tracts becomes apparent by signs of pneumonia and enteritis. When the mouth lesions begin to heal, lameness may give indication that laminitis and coronitis are present. Wool-shedding accompanies the emaciation.

**Termination.** In the Southwestern States the mortality in affected flocks is reported to be 5 to 30 per cent. It is greater in lambs than in older sheep, and greater also in animals that have the pulmonary and enteric complications. Death may occur in 8 to 10 days in acute cases.

## FOWL PEST

Fowl pest, or fowl plague, is an acute, highly contagious pantropic viral disease of birds resembling fowl cholera and characterized by a rapid course and high mortality. It was never present in the United States until the period from August, 1924, to March, 1925. The cause of fowl pest is a filter-passing virus, *Tortor galli*. It is present in all body fluids, secretions, and excretions. It is believed to be present in the erythrocytes. It is said that the cutaneous prick of a needle that has been dipped in the blood of an affected bird is sufficient to transmit the disease. On the other hand, external parasites do not transmit the disease. The pathogenesis has not been determined. The period of incubation is usually 3 to 5 days.

**Lesions.** Highly characteristic are hemorrhages in the mucosa of the proventriculus and ventriculus. Hemorrhages frequently are present in the periventricular fat and mesentery, rarely in the epicardium, trachea, larynx, pharynx, and pleura. Enteritis occurs in about half of the cases. A serous or serofibrinous collection of fluid appears in the abdominal cavity in about 25 per cent of the cases and in the pericardial sac less frequently. Hyperemia of the vessels in the yolk capsules of the ovary and in the comb and wattles, and also edema of the comb and wattles, are of frequent occurrence.

**Differential diagnosis.** Fowl pest is differentiated from fowl cholera by the rarity of subepicardial petechiae, the absence of inflammatory processes in the intestine and lungs of many cases, by rabbit inoculation, by the absence of bacteria in the tissues, by hemorrhages of the proventriculus, and swelling of the kidneys and engorgement of the vessels of the serosa of the egg yolks.

TOXOPLASMOSIS

Toxoplasmosis is a protozoan disease caused by *Toxoplasma gondii*. Its prevalence among domestic animals is extensive. So far the disease has been reported in dogs, cats, sheep, mink, cattle, and swine. In the mink it is caused from eating infected meat.

**Pathogenesis and lesions.** While the mode of transmission is unknown, there is experimental evidence to show that infection probably takes places by ingestion. Transplacental transmisson occurs in dogs and swine. The organism is also shed in the milk of infected dogs and swine. The finding of gastric and intestinal ulcers due to the toxoplasma strengthens the belief that the parasite usually enters through the digestive tract.

The small intracytoplasmic parasites may occupy various tissue cells and cause the cells to enlarge greatly (Fig. 15.16). Such cells packed with a large number of the tiny parasites are called pseudocysts. They are difficult to recognize with the low-power objective. The parenchymatous cells of almost any organ, endothelial cells, and macrophages may become pseudocysts. They remind one of heart and skeletal muscle fibers which contain sarcosporidia. The important differences are: (1) the pseudocysts are much smaller than sarcocysts; (2) the parasites contained in the pseudocysts are not nearly so large; and (3) the pseudocysts are usually found in the presence of necrotic tissue and an inflammatory reaction, although some pseudocysts may be found in cells quite removed from the area of destruction and inflammation.

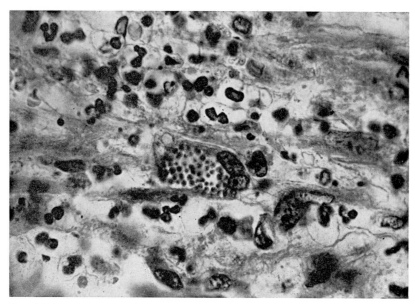

Fig. 15.16 — A giant cell containing a large number of toxoplasmata in the intestinal muscularis externa of a dog. (Department of Veterinary Pathology, Michigan State University.)

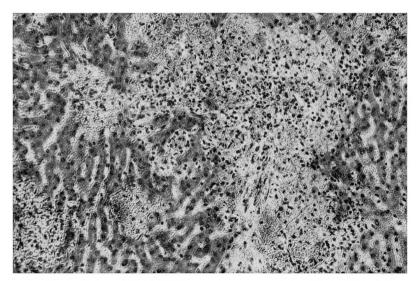

Fig. 15.17 — Focal hepatic necrosis in toxoplasmosis. Toxoplasmata are present in cells at the periphery of the necrotic foci but cannot be seen readily at this magnification. (Department of Veterinary Pathology, Michigan State University.)

The lesions consist of foci of necrosis (Fig. 15.17). While macrophages are present, they do not accumulate as they do in the fungous infections. Toxoplasmata are usually found in cells at the border of the sharply defined necrotic foci. When lesions originate in the mucosa of the stomach and intestine, ulcers usually result.

## Tumors

Tumors of the blood (leukemias) are discussed in the chapter on neoplasms.

## REFERENCES

Beasley, J. N., Davis, D. E., and Grumbles, L. C.: 1959. Preliminary studies on the histopathology of experimental ornithosis in turkeys. Amer. Jour. Vet. Res., 20:341.

Beaudette, F. R., and Hudson, C. B.: 1936. An outbreak of swine erysipelas infection in turkeys. Jour. A.V.M.A., 41:475.

Bohl, E. H., and Ferguson, L. C.: 1952. Leptospirosis in domestic animals. Jour. A.V.M.A., 121:421.

Cordy, D. R., and Gorham, J. R.: 1950. The pathology and etiology of salmon disease in the dog and fox. Amer. Jour. Path., 26:617.

Creech, G. T.: 1921. The bacillus of swine erysipelas isolated from urticarial lesions of swine in United States. Jour. A.V.M.A., 12:139.

Dalrymple, W. H.: 1917. Anthrax. Jour. A.V.M.A., 3:831.

Doll, E. R.: 1952. Observations on the clinical features and pathology of hemolytic icterus of newborn foals. Amer. Jour. Vet. Res., 13:504.

Hadlow, W. J., and Stoenner, H. G.: 1955. Histopathological findings in cows naturally infected with *Leptospira pomona*. Amer. Jour. Vet. Res., 16:45.

Hjarre, A., and Berthelsen, H.: 1938. Researches concerning the white-blood picture of infectious anemia of horses. (Translated title.) Proc. 13th Int'l Vet. Cong., 1:259.

Hubben, K.: 1959. The pathogenesis of infectious synovitis of chickens. Univ. of Penn. Vet. Ext. Quart., 154:77.

Kernkamp, H. C. H: 1939. Lesions of hog cholera: Their frequency of occurrence. Jour. A.V.M.A., 95:159.

————: 1939. The blood picture in hog cholera. Jour. A.V.M.A., 95:525.

Little, R. B., and Baker, J. A.: 1950. Leptospirosis in cattle. Jour. A.V.M.A., 116:105.

Lucker, J. T., and Neumayer, E. M.: 1944. The production of anemia in lambs by hookworms, *Bunostomum trigonocephalum*. Jour. Parasit., 30:10 Suppl.

Maddy, K. T.: 1953. Caseous lymphadenitis of sheep. Jour. A.V.M.A., 122:257.

Marsh, H.: 1931. The bacillus of swine erysipelas associated with arthritis in lambs. Jour. A.V.M.A., 31:57.

Monlux, W. S.: 1948. Leptospirosis IV. The pathology of canine leptospirosis. Cornell Vet., 38:199.

Naftalin, J. M., and Cushnie, G. H.: 1954. Pathology of bracken poisoning in cattle. Jour. Comp. Path. and Therap., 64:54.

Olafson, P., and Monlux, W. S.: 1942. Toxoplasma infection in animals. Cornell Vet., 32:176.

Osebold, J. W.: 1951. An approach to the pathogenesis of fern poisoning in the bovine species. Jour. A.V.M.A., 119:440.

Pritchard, W. R.: 1956. Studies on trichloroethylene-extracted feeds. Amer. Jour. Vet. Res., 17:425.

————, Rehfeld, C. E., and Sautter, J. H.: 1952. Aplastic anemia of cattle associated with ingestion of trichloroethylene-extracted soybean oil meal. Jour. A.V.M.A., 121:1.

Reinhard, K. R.: 1951. A clinical pathological study of experimental leptospirosis of calves. Amer. Jour. Vet. Res., 12:282.

Sanger, V. L., Yacourtz, H., and Moore, E. N.: 1956. Micropathological changes in an experimental hemorrhagic syndrome in chickens fed sulfaquinoxaline and suggested cause of the disease. Amer. Jour. Vet. Res., 17:766.

Sautter, J. H., Rehfeld, C. E., and Pritchard, W. R.: 1952. Aplastic anemia of cattle associated with ingestion of trichoroethylene-extracted soybean oil meal. II. Necropsy findings in field cases. Jour. A.V.M.A., 121:73.

Schwartzman, R. W., and Besch, E. D.: 1958. Feline infectious anemia. Vet. Med., 53:494.

Seifried, O.: 1931. Histological studies on hog cholera. I. Lesions in the central nervous system. Jour. Exper. Med., 53:277.

————, and Cain, C. B.: 1932. Histological studies on hog cholera. II. Lesions of the vascular system. Jour. Exper. Med., 56:345.

————, and Cain, C. B.: 1932. Histological studies on hog cholera. III. Lesions of the various organs. Jour. Exper. Med., 56:351.

Splitter, E. J.: 1948. Studies in anaplasmosis. Kans. Agr. Exper. Sta., Tech. Bul. 66.

————: 1950. *Eperythrozoon suis*, the etiologic agent of icteroanemia or an anaplasmosis-like disease in swine. Amer. Jour. Vet. Res., 11:324.

Stein, C. D.: 1935. Infectious anemia or swamp fever in horses: A review of the Bureau of Animal Industry's investigations. Jour. A.V.M.A., 40:312.

Stiles, G. W.: 1946. Anaplasmosis in cattle. U.S.D.A. Circ. 154.

Van Es, L.: 1937. Anthrax in swine. Jour. A.V.M.A., 43:331.

————, and McGrath, C. B.: Swine erysipelas, Nebr. Agr. Exper. Sta., Res. Bul. 84.

Vestal, C. M., and Doyle, L. P.: 1938. The effect of confinement on suckling pigs and its influence on the hemoglobin content of their blood. Ind. Agr. Exper. Sta., Bul. 426.

# CHAPTER 16

# Respiratory System

## FUNCTIONS AND DISTURBANCES

The exchange of oxygen and carbon dioxide in the lungs is, of course, the all-important function of the respiratory system. The functions of the individual parts of the system are in general related to this principal activity. For instance, the upper air passages prepare the air for entrance into the lungs by adding moisture and warmth to it. The larynx regulates the amount of air which can enter. The tracheal rings prevent collapse of the tube when it is bent or otherwise compressed. The great elasticity and vascularity of the lung parenchyma favors the exchange of gases. The gaseous exchange is further facilitated by the smoothly gliding surfaces of the visceral and parietal pleurae, by the action of the negative thoracic pressure, and by the free movements of the diaphragm and certain of the thoracic and abdominal muscles.

Besides these functions concerned primarily with external respiration, this system has other important duties. In it is lodged the termination of the olfactory nerve, the normal functioning of which determines in large part the value of hunting and watch dogs, and of bloodhounds. In male animals, of some species at least, the normal functioning of this nerve may be an important factor in breeding operations. The organs of phonation, also located in the respiratory tract, may be of no particular value to some species of domestic animals. In hunting and watch dogs, and bloodhounds, however, they are of first importance.

Furthermore, the respiratory system possesses many protective devices against the entrance of harmful agents. Hairs in and around the nostrils, ciliated epithelial cells, mucus-producing cells, the reflexes of sneezing and coughing, and the action of the epiglottis are all familiar mechanisms in this respect.

Lastly, the respiratory system functions in heat dissipation through the evaporation of water from the lungs. This is especially important in canines.

From the standpoint of health there are three chief requisites for the normal functioning of external respiration:

1. The necessity of the proper supply of air to the alveoli.

2. The unhindered passing of oxygen from the alveoli to the capillaries and of carbon dioxide from the capillaries to the alveoli.

3. The need of an adequate supply of blood containing its normal constituents and moving at a normal rate.

Changes from the normal with respect

to any of these three factors result in disturbances to inspiration, expiration, or both. In the following chapter it will become apparent that interferences to respiration can originate within the organs of this system or can be due to influences acting outside of the system. Hindrances within the system can be related to circulatory disturbances, inflammation, changes in the size or shape of the air passages, and the presence in them of inanimate foreign bodies, parasites, and tumors. Hindrances arising from influences operating outside the respiratory organs can be located in the head and neck region, in the thorax, or in the abdomen. Furthermore, the seat of the trouble may lie in the cardiovascular system or in the nervous system.

In the head and neck region, interference with respiration may result from pressure by tumors, by dilatation of the esophagus, or by enlarged lymph nodes. In the thorax painful or chronic conditions may offer the interference. Fractured ribs, pleuritis, and pleural adhesions are examples. Furthermore, disturbances in the continuity of the lung tissue, the thoracic wall, or the diaphragm may result in changes in the intrathoracic pressure. In addition, fluid such as blood, lymph, or inflammatory exudate may collect in the thoracic cavity. In the abdomen the hindrances to respiration may be associated with gaseous and alimental gastric and intestinal distension, or the accumulation of fluid in the abdominal cavity.

Disturbances in the cardiovascular system whose effects hinder respiration are those which permit blood to accumulate in the lungs, those in which there is a deficient supply of blood, and those in which changes have occurred in the constituents of the blood, particularly the erythrocytes. In the central nervous system, lesions which cause pressure, and irritants which stimulate or depress the respiratory center, do not interfere with the passage of air into or out of the lungs but do interfere with the rate of breathing.

## NOSE AND ACCESSORY UPPER RESPIRATORY PASSAGES
### Disturbances of Circulation

Active hyperemia always occurs at the beginning of inflammation. Passive hyperemia results from hindrances to circulation in the heart and lungs. Hemorrhage (epistaxis) results from trauma, chronic diseases of the heart and lungs in which there are obstructions to circulation, acute septicemic diseases, and ulcers.

### Rhinitis

Rhinitis among domestic animals is probably of as frequent occurrence as it is in man. Because of the environment and habits of many of the species of animals, it is surprising that the prevalence of rhinitis is not greater than it is. For the most part, the irritants responsible for the inflammatory reaction enter the upper air passages directly. The rhinitis, however, which is a part of some of the acute and chronic infectious diseases, may have its origin hematogenically. It is customary to refer to the rhinitis which occurs independently as a **primary rhinitis,** and that which is a partial manifestation of some of the acute and chronic infectious diseases as a **secondary rhinitis.**

Primary rhinitis may be caused by (1) physical irritants such as dust, and foreign bodies of even greater size, by (2) chemical agents such as irritating gases and smoke, by (3) animal parasites such as the larvae of the sheep botfly (*Oestrus ovis*), and by (4) bacteria such as *Spherophorus necrophorus, Pseudomonas aeruginosa, Brucella bronchiseptica*, streptococci, and staphylococci. In turkeys a virus and a pleuropneumonia-like organism may operate simultaneously to cause rhinitis.

As a part of specific infectious diseases which may involve many other parts of the body also, rhinitis may be caused by *Streptococcus equi, Malleomyces mallei,* equine influenza virus, rinderpest virus, pasteurella, swine influenza virus, *Hemophilus suis,* canine distemper virus, *Brucella bronchiseptica,* fowl-pox virus, and fowl laryngotracheitis virus. The rhinitis of A-avitaminosis of poultry needs separate mention in this connection. Obviously, it is not primarily an infection, but the epithelial proliferation and metaplasia of the nasal mucosa in this deficiency disease afford an easy entry for bacteria which complicate the primary condition.

## ACUTE CATARRHAL RHINITIS

Acute catarrhal rhinitis occurs in the early stages of several animal diseases which are often characterized by more severe respiratory involvement in the later stages. Examples of such diseases are infectious rhinitis and influenza of pigs; distemper of dogs; roup, diphtheria, and A-avitaminosis of poultry; and acute infectious rhinitis (snuffles) of rabbits.

The mucosa of the nasal passages is reddened, swollen, and covered with a seromucous exudate. In sections the usual changes which characterize a catarrhal inflammation are prominent such as hyperemia, edema, and leukocytosis of the mucosa, excessive formation of mucus by the goblet cells, and the accumulation on the epithelium of a mucous exudate containing leukocytes and desquamated epithelial cells.

Of special economic importance to turkey raisers is an **infectious sinusitis** which is caused by a virus. The mucosa of the infraorbital sinus, among other parts of the respiratory system, is the seat of lesions. The mucosa becomes thickened as a result of hyperplasia and hypertrophy of the epithelium and of the mucous glands, and also as a result of a serous and lymphocytic infiltration of the lamina propria. The goblet cells increase in numbers and become very active. The sinuses become filled to bulging with the exudate. The escape of the exudate is impeded by the closure of the opening of the sinus into the nasal cavity. As the condition progresses there is an increase in connective tissue in the upper part of the mucosa and the formation of nodules of lymphocytes in the deeper part.

**Equine Influenza (Rhinopneumonitis).** This is an acute viral disease of equines formerly believed to be two distinct diseases — influenza and viral abortion. There is strong evidence now that they are different manifestations of a single viral infection. It is an acute pantropic viral disease of horses appearing enzootically and characterized by catarrhal inflammation of the mucous membranes, especially of the respiratory tract and eyes, and often, among pregnant mares, by abortion.

The principal effect of the virus is on the lymphoid-macrophage system. Initially there is a rapid decrease of lymphocytes in all the lymphoid tissues. This results in an early lymphopenia and almost coincides with an elevation of temperature. This initial lymphoid hypoplasia is followed by a lymphoid hyperplasia. Among the cells which proliferate are the undifferentiated pericytes of Maximow which occur around small blood vessels. The perivascular proliferation of them is most prominent in organs and tissues not rich in lymphoid cells. These changes involving the lymphocytes are accompanied by an infiltration with macrophages into the walls of blood vessels. The lymphoid-macrophage infiltrations occur in various parenchymatous organs such as the liver, kidneys, adrenals, brain, and meninges, and result in vascular and degenerative changes. They also occur in cutaneous and mucous epithelium where they cause hyperemia, hemorrhage, degeneration, and erosion. Pregnant mares may abort. The uterine mucosa is not seriously involved, and aborting mares usually recover as soon as mares do after normal parturition. The fetal membranes are usually expelled with the fetus. Most abortions occur when the majority of the mares are in the ninth and tenth months of gestation, although a considerable number also occur in the eighth and eleventh months.

Lesions in aborted fetuses are foci of hepatic degeneration and necrosis. Epicardial and pulmonary hemorrhages are present. Hydrothorax as well as subpleural and interstitial edema of the lung occurs. Cells at the border of the necrotic foci in the liver contain granular or homogeneous, acidophilic, intranuclear inclusions. Similar inclusions occur in the bronchial, bronchiolar, and alveolar epithelial cells.

### ACUTE SUPPURATIVE (PURULENT) RHINITIS

Acute suppurative (purulent) rhinitis is the typical inflammatory process of the nasal mucosa in equine strangles and avian infectious coryza. Severe infestation with botfly (*Oestrus ovis*) larvae of sheep affords another excellent example.

There are collections of a creamy, yellow pus on the nasal mucosa and in the recesses of the turbinates. The mucosa is red, swollen, and in strangles in particular, studded with nodular swellings. These nodules are swollen lymph follicles which may later undergo central necrosis and suppuration. They may then rupture on the surface of the mucosa and become small ulcers.

**Strangles.** Both this disease and equine influenza are frequently spoken of as forms of shipping fever of equines. They are epizootic infectious diseases that occur in so-called green horses and mules which have undergone shipment or otherwise been exposed to the disease. Strangles is an acute infectious disease of young horses, asses, and their hybrids caused by *Streptococcus equi* and occurring sporadically or epizootically. It is rather easily transmitted and is characterized by a purulent or suppurative inflammation of the mucosa of the upper air passages associated with a suppurative inflammation of the regional lymph nodes and sometimes by metastasis to more distant lymph nodes.

Streptococci reach the surface of the nasal mucosa, colonize, and multiply there. They either penetrate the mucous glands, from which they pass into the lymph spaces of the mucosa, or are carried through the epithelium and into the lymph spaces by phagocytes. Then they are carried in the lymph vessels to the nearest lymph node and sometimes from this node to neighboring and even more distant nodes. The bacteria incite a suppurative inflammatory reaction wherever they localize. Very rarely, stallions may transmit the infection to the external genitals of mares by coition. The period of incubation is 4 to 8 days.

There is an acute purulent or suppurative rhinitis accompanied by an acute suppurative lymphadenitis. The mandibular lymph nodes are most commonly affected, but all the principal nodes of the head may show abscesses.

Strangles is rarely fatal. Occasionally, it is complicated by septicemia, pyemia, chronic valvular endocarditis (Fig. 16.1), suppurative peritonitis, catarrhal pneumonia, hemiplegia, or diplegia laryngis, retropharyngeal abscess with edema of the glottis and possibly suppurative pneumonia, and suppurative cerebrospinal meningitis by metastasis of the infection by way of the lymphatics following the olfactory nerves. An occasional complication or sequel of strangles is **purpura hemorrhagica,** also called petechial fever. Apparently, it is a bacterial intoxication because it cannot be transmitted artificially with the secretions or blood of affected animals. It is sometimes a sequel to other suppurative and necrotic processes, principally in horses. The most prominent characteristics of purpura hemorrhagica are extensive edematous infiltrations of the subcutaneous connective tissue accompanied by hemorrhages into the edematous areas. Hemorrhages also occur in the mucous membranes and in the internal organs. The hemorrhages are believed to be due to damage to the capillary endothelium and to a deficiency in blood platelets. Secondary inflammation and necrosis may occur so that death is frequently the termination.

**Canine distemper** is an acute infectious disease of young carnivora (dogs, jackals, ferrets, foxes, mink, and fitches) characterized by fever, acute catarrhal inflammation of the mucous membranes which often leads to pneumonia, and in many cases is further characterized by nervous symp-

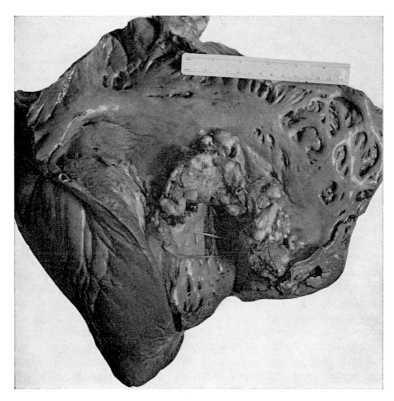

Fig. 16.1 — T r i c u s p i d valve of a horse with chronic valvulitis following strangles. Healing in this valve was retarded by the presence of streptococci. Note ulceration of surface of the much thickened valve. (Department of Veterinary Pathology, Iowa State University.)

toms. There is some question about the etiology of canine distemper, but it is quite generally conceded that it is due to a filtrable virus, *Tarpeia canis*, and that *Brucella bronchiseptica* is an almost constant secondary invader and perhaps is responsible for the major part of the gross lesions. While *Brucella bronchiseptica* is the chief secondary invader, other pathogens have been isolated from distemper-infected dogs. Conjunctivitis is often due to *Staphylococcus pyogenes* (var. *albus*) and gastroenteritis to various species of Salmonella.

The question about etiology arises chiefly for two reasons. First, canine distemper is not the only disease of dogs characterized by fever, rhinitis, pneumonia, and nervous disturbances. There are several having similar manifestations. Secondly, the causative virus appears to exist in more than one form, that is, there seem to be types or variants which cause a variety of reactions in dogs. This has given rise to the term canine distemper complex, which embraces such forms of the disease

as hard pad and paradistemper. Some prominent students of the disease do not consider these to be separate and distinct disease entities but simply varied reactions to different strains of the virus.

In Britain there are three types of distemper virus — types A, B, and C. Type A causes a disease similar to the old-fashioned febrile distemper. It is potentially neurotropic. In England, during several passages through dogs and ferrets, it acquired a new character, that of producing a nervous form of distemper in puppies. From this experiment it was concluded that the virus can be trained, so-to-speak, to produce the nervous form of distemper.

The experiments of DeMonbreun indicate that the distemper virus is cytotropic in character and attacks cells from all three germinal layers. It, however, has a special affinity for vascular endothelium, cells of the reticuloendothelial system, epithelial cells, and nerve cells. In these cells both cytoplasmic and nuclear inclusions are present. Wharton and Wharton have determined that the virus also invades the erythrocytes and produces two effects in them. One effect is upon the glycolytic enzyme and results in a hypoglycemia. The other effect is upon the factors controlling the destruction of hemoglobin and results in acute anemia. The virus is present in the blood at the onset of the disease but disappears with the decrease in sugar and hemoglobin. Incubation is 4 to 8 days.

In peracute cases, which are rare, there is considerable fluid in the pericardial sac and perhaps a few petechiae in the myocardium. In acute cases, which are common, the lesions are catarrhal rhinitis, tracheitis, bronchitis, and pneumonia, and sometimes fibrinous pleuritis. Frequently, catarrhal gastroenteritis, serous lymphadenitis of the thoracic and abdominal nodes, considerable serous fluid in the pericardial sac, petechiation and fatty degeneration of the myocardium, and cloudy swelling and fatty degeneration of the renal coretx and liver are present. Slight acute swelling of the spleen is occasionally present. Usually, there is catarrhal conjunctivitis and sometimes ulcerative keratitis. Pustular exanthema of the abdomen and inner surface of the thighs and external otitis are said by some to occur in half of the cases.

In the experimental form of distemper, fever appears early, followed by paralysis in 1 to 2 weeks. Paralysis begins in the hind limbs first, extends anteriorly, and is due to inflammation in the gray matter of the cord and brain (poliomyelitis and polioencephalitis). It is accompanied by hyperkeratosis of the pads (hard pad) in some cases.

The presence of specific inclusion bodies in canine distemper is becoming more significant from the standpoint of diagnosis. This becomes apparent when it is realized that dogs and foxes have two diseases in common, canine distemper and fox encephalitis, which sometimes have similar symptoms but have inclusion bodies in different locations. In canine distemper they are primarily in the epithelium and in fox encephalitis in the endothelium. This fact is now taken advantage of in differentiating the two diseases histopathologically. Further, the presence of the inclusions in canine distemper is receiving greater attention as a means of making an accurate diagnosis of this disease.

Both cytoplasmic and nuclear inclusions occur in canine distemper. The cytoplasmic type is more common. The two types often appear simultaneously. In foxes, both kinds are present.

The cell inclusions in canine distemper are found principally in the epithelium which lines the passageways of the body such as the urinary, respiratory, and gastrointestinal tracts, and in the ducts of some of the glands, particularly the liver, pancreas, and salivary glands. The bodies also occur in the neurons and neuroglia of the brain, in the reticuloendothelial cells of the lymph nodes and spleen, and most often in the epithelium of the adrenal medulla. In dogs the presence of intracytoplasmic inclusions has been demonstrated in circulating neutrophils, and in fluorescent antibody studies it has been shown that these inclusions contain the specific viral antigen of canine distemper. Inclusion bodies are present in the transitional epithelium of the urinary tract in 90 per cent of the fatal cases of distemper among mink and foxes. As in rabies the bodies do not appear until late in the disease. They can be demonstrated in properly stained smears of bladder and bronchial epithelium of animals that die of distemper or that are destroyed late in the disease. From living animals, nasal epithelial cells containing inclusion bodies can be obtained by the use of nasal swabs.

The number of cytoplasmic inclusions in a cell may vary from 1 to 10, rarely 20. They are irregular in shape, but the majority are round or elliptical. The inclusions usually adapt themselves to the shape of the cell. Their size varies from beginning visibility to that of the nucleus or larger. Nuclear inclusions are usually single, round, or elliptical. Some nearly fill the nucleus but others are much smaller.

## ACUTE FIBRINOUS AND NECROTIC RHINITIS

Acute fibrinous and necrotic rhinitis are often associated with one another. The best examples of these forms of rhinitis occur in the later stages of malignant catarrhal fever of cattle, in rinderpest which occurs on the Philippine Islands but not in continental United States, in calf diphtheria, necrotic rhinitis (bull nose) of pigs, and in fowl diphtheria.

The fibrinous form is superficial in extent; the necrotic form deep. The rather tough, tenacious exudate in the fibrinous form is easily removed and leaves no defect in the epithelium. In the fibrinonecrotic form, the removal of the exudate leaves a defect in the mucosa. If necrosis predominates in the process, the dead mucosa has a rough, dull, yellowish-gray appearance.

**Bovine malignant catarrhal fever** is an acute, noncontagious disease of cattle characterized by a severe inflammation of the mucous membranes of the upper respiratory passages, the upper digestive tract, the conjunctiva, and frequently of the meninges and brain.

There is belief that the cause of malignant catarrhal fever is a virus. In the early stages the disease possesses the characteristics of a viscerotropic viral disease, especially of the influenza type, but later the characteristics of a neurotropic disease appear also. The belief that the cause is a virus is based partly upon the presence of cytoplasmic inclusion bodies in the nasal epithelium and in certain nerve cells. The belief is strengthened by the fact that in some instances the disease can be transmitted from animal to animal, but this succeeds only when blood or lymph node suspensions of an affected animal are injected into a healthy animal. This leads one to suspect that the virus sticks to body cells. In artificial transmission experiments the period of incubation is 14 to 37 days when lymph node suspensions are used. Transmission does not seem to take place by direct contact.

Although bovine malignant catarrhal fever is frequently diagnosed in the United States, proof is lacking that the disease actually exists. The authors are not aware of a single case in which the viral agent has been isolated and identified.

Subcutaneous and intramuscular edema of the head and throat region are the usual lesions. In the beginning, acute catarrhal stomatitis, pharyngitis, rhinitis (often accompanied by sinusitis), tonsillitis, laryngitis, and tracheitis are prominent lesions. Along with these changes there is acute catarrhal conjunctivitis. Soon, this catarrhal inflammation may give way to a severe fibrinous inflammation with which there may be foci of necrosis (ulceration), especially in the mouth, nose, and larynx. There is general lymphadenitis, which is hemorrhagic in type in the nodes of the head and upper cervical regions, and serous in character in other parts of the body. The myocardium, liver, and kidneys show marked degenerative changes and often a distinct inflammatory reaction. The epicardium may be studded with petechiae, particularly along the coronary grooves. Pulmonary edema, with areas of atelectasis and foci of bronchopneumonia, is relatively common. The pneumonia usually involves the anterior lobes of the lungs. Acute splenomegaly is a fairly constant lesion. In the later stages of the disease a serohemorrhagic meningitis and encephalitis often can be found. Death usually occurs within 10 days.

Cytoplasmic inclusion bodies occur in the nasal epithelium, Purkinje cells of the cerebellum, and in the cytons of the nerve cells forming the nuclei of the glossopharyngeal and vagus nerves. The inclusion bodies are not uniform in type or staining characteristics. There are both granular and homogeneous types. They are polychromatic in their staining.

In transmission experiments the presence of a nonsuppurative encephalitis accompanied by degenerative changes and the presence of inclusion bodies in the cytons of the glossopharyngeal and vagus nuclei suggest why the disease at times has some of the characteristics of neuro-tropic viral disease.

### CHRONIC RHINITIS

Chronic rhinitis sometimes develops from the acute form. In this manner acute purulent rhinitis of strangles may give rise to the chronic form. Often in horses chronic rhinitis accompanies chronic alveolar periostitis and chronic sinusitis. In cattle it may develop as an extension of a sinusitis frontalis following dehorning. In sheep it is of frequent occurrence as a result of *Oestrus ovis* larvae infestation. In pigs spirochetes may be a secondary cause of chronic rhinitis (rhinohyperplasia). Specific forms of chronic rhinitis are those produced by *Malleomyces mallei, Actinobacillus lignieresi, Actinomyces bovis, Spherophorus necrophorus, Mycobacterium tuberculosis,* and *Pseudomonas aeruginosa.*

In swine there are two important forms of chronic rhinitis. They are infectious atrophic rhinitis and rhinohyperplasia (bull nose).

**Glanders.** A rather out-of-date synonym for glanders is farcy. It is an infectious, usually chronic disease of horses, asses, and mules, involving the lymphatic system of the upper air passages, lungs, and skin. It is caused by *Malleomyces mallei* and characterized by the formation of small nodules which have a tendency to degenerate, form ulcers and abscesses, and later heal, leaving characteristic cicatrices. Occasionally, carnivora become infected. Man is susceptible.

The organisms enter the body generally by way of the digestive system. They enter the lymph vessels of the intestinal wall, pass to the mesenteric lymph vessels, thence by way of the thoracic duct to the blood stream. By means of the blood the organisms are distributed to all parts of the body, but apparently colonize only in organs or tissues pre-eminently susceptible (lymphatics of the respiratory tract and skin). After colonizing, they stimulate a proliferation of macrophages and fibroblasts, which results in the formation of **nodules.** Subsequently, lymphocytes pass from the periphery and lodge between the cells of the nodule. The center becomes soft, and necrosis occurs. If the nodule is located near the surface, it ruptures in the direction of least resistance. Otherwise, caseation and calcification of the central necrotic mass occur. An outer connective tissue capsule infiltrated with numerous eosinophils develops. If the nodule ruptures on a mucous surface, an **ulcer** results, leaving behind, upon healing, a **star-shaped scar.** Ulcers may coalesce, forming large, irregularly shaped **ulcerated patches.** The inflammatory process may ex-

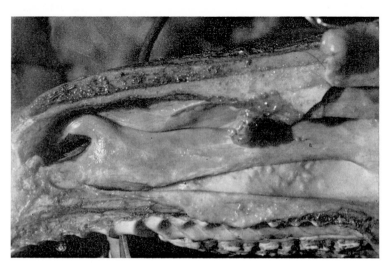

Fig. 16.2 — Nodules and scars of glanders on the nasal septum and turbinates of a horse. (E. E. Thompson.)

tend along lymphatics, forming knotty strands, especially in the subcutis. A conglomeration of nodules in the lymph nodes results in enlarged, knotty nodes. The period of incubation is variable but usually of rather long duration, perhaps several weeks, sometimes months.

Lesions in the upper air passages consist of gray or yellowish, prominent nodules the size of millet seeds, surrounded by a tumefied, brightly reddened area (Fig. 16.2). These break down and form ulcers which at first are round and smooth bordered; later, as a result of progressive tissue destruction, they become irregular in outline with rough raised borders. Small primary ulcers coalesce to form larger ones. The ulcers heal and leave behind irregular star-shaped, reddish or white scars. In the skin and subcutaneous tissues, nodules may develop which rupture at the surface and form ulcers with ragged borders and which discharge a yellowish-gray or reddish viscid pus. The lymphatics between the nodules and ulcers are enlarged and filled with coagulated lymph, yellowish white in color. The regional lymph nodes are enlarged and firm, due to proliferation of connective tissue, and contain small pus foci. In the lungs there may be small tubercle-like nodules which by

extension may result in large pneumonic areas. In the early stages the lung may feel as though it contained shotgun pellets; in more advanced cases conglomerate masses of nodules may be mistaken for tumors. At times the nodules may be found in the liver, spleen, bone marrow, kidneys, adrenals, testicles, brain, myocardium, and skeletal muscles. In Figure 16.3 the lesions are in an unusual place, the colic lymph nodes.

**Infectious atrophic rhinitis** of swine begins as a catarrhal inflammation. The irritant, which may be a virus accompanied by trichomonads and various bacteria, appears to enter the mucosa of the turbinates in scattered foci and to cause a catarrhal inflammatory reaction characterized by desquamation of the surface epithelium and a lymphocytic infiltration of the lamina propria. As the inflammation progresses the desquamation becomes more conspicuous and the reaction extends to the outer layer of the periosteum of the turbinate. The serous and mucous glands of the mucosa become distended with secretion, and since their mouths are closed by inflammatory swelling, the glands become tiny cysts. As the reaction becomes more chronic there are proliferation of the connective tissue in the

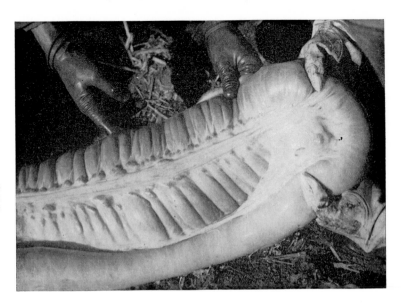

Fig. 16.3 — Glanderous colic lymph nodes in a horse. (E. E. Thompson.)

lamina propria and a low grade arteritis with constriction of the vessel lumina. Eventually, the process extends through the external layer where the osteoblasts are located. The osteoblasts proliferate, but in spite of their large numbers they are unable to form bone. As a result, bone formation in the turbinates ceases, and the bone already present becomes rarefied by decalcification. Finally a turbinate will completely atrophy (Fig. 16.4) and only a dense irregular fibrous band will remain to indicate its place of attachment to the nasal bone.

The growth and development of the dorsal turbinate is closely related to the growth of the nasal bone to which it is attached. When growth of the turbinate is interfered with, the growth of the nasal bone is likewise disturbed. As a consequence, atrophy of the turbinate on one side results in decreased growth of the associated nasal bone and causes the snout to be deflected laterally. Bilateral atrophy of the turbinates leads to bilateral arrested development of both nasal bones, and the face becomes "dished" and the skin over the snout wrinkled.

In Maryland an inclusion body rhinitis has been described which may be an early stage of atrophic rhinitis. Round and stellate nuclear inclusions occur in ballooned cells of the mucosal glands of the turbinates. Accompanying inflammatory changes result in shrinkage of the turbinates.

Inclusion bodies in rhinitis are reported not to occur in pigs over 4 weeks of age. Usually the pigs are 2 to 4 weeks of age. In both Canada and Scotland, where this form of rhinitis is more prevalent, researchers are not certain whether the condition is or is not a stage in the pathogenesis of atrophic rhinitis. In Canada, in

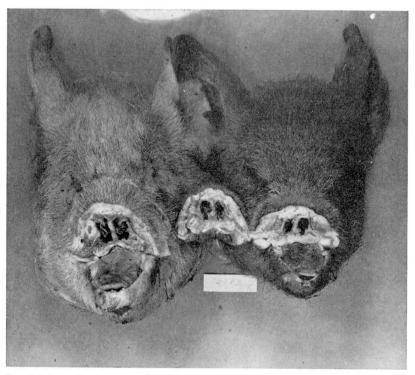

Fig. 16.4 — Infectious atrophic rhinitis. The turbinates in the specimen at the left were in an early stage of atrophy; those in the specimen at the right had completely atrophied. (Department of Veterinary Pathology, Michigan State University.)

a study of the pathogenesis of artificially induced atrophic rhinitis, inclusion bodies were not found.

In **rhinohyperplasia (bull nose)** of swine the face also becomes distorted, and there is bulging of the facial bones. The inflammatory reaction is apparently due to a mixed infection of *Staphylococcus pyogenes* in association with *Bacillus subtilis* (a saprophyte), *Spherophorus necrophorus, Pseudomonas aeruginosa,* and spirochetes.

The inflammatory process extends from the nasal mucosa into the paranasal sinuses, the facial bones, and subcutis of the face and snout where it is characterized by necrosis, suppuration, and massive connective tissue proliferation. The collections of pus and necrotic tissue in the bones and sinuses which cause the face to bulge suggested to swine raisers the name bull nose for the condition (Fig. 16.5). Pressure exerted by the collections of pus, necrotic tissue, and accompanying fibrosis closes the nasal passages and causes difficult breathing.

While the infection is supposed to enter through the nasal mucosa, there is relatively little damage done to it compared to the alterations which occur in the sinuses, the facial bones, and the subcutaneous tissues over the face and snout. In many cases Howarth found only localized edematous areas in the mucosa. When the changes in the mucosa are compared to those occurring in the sinuses, facial bones, and subcutis of the face, one wonders whether the infection actually enters by way of the nasal mucosa.

The tissue changes which occur where the lesions are most conspicuous have a great similarity in appearance. Whether the changes be in the sinuses, the bones, or in the subcutis, there is always a central area of necrosis and suppuration and sometimes even gangrene. This central area is enclosed in a thick capsule of proliferating fibrous connective tissue. Between the central necrotic and suppurative core and the outer thick capsule of connective tissue there is a zone containing numerous spirochetes (Fig. 16.6).

### Catarrh of the Guttural Pouches

Catarrh of the guttural pouches is usually secondary and occurs rarely. The pouches may contain concretions and are probably most often involved if they are congenitally enlarged. Sisson reports the case of a yearling colt with a pouch which had the capacity of 6 quarts.

### Tumors

The occurrence of carcinomas in the nasal passages of animals is not uncommon. For the most part they are carcinomas which are located in the nasal

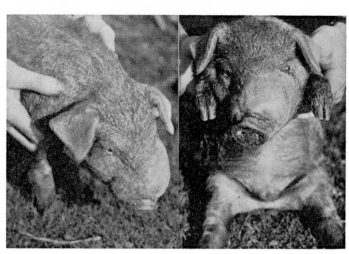

Fig. 16.5 — Chronic necrotic rhinitis (bull nose) in pigs. (Howarth, Jour. A.V.M.A.)

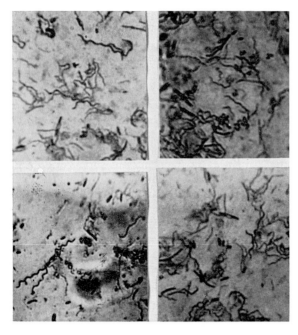

Fig. 16.6 — Spirochetes in smears prepared from rhinohyperplasia in pigs and also from scirrhous cord in pigs, foot-rot in sheep, and thrush in horses. ×1,500. (Howarth, Jour. A.V.M.A.)

passages proper or in the paranasal sinuses. In sheep and cattle, in some European countries in particular, they seem to involve the mucosa of the ethmoid bone. In horses and sheep soft, edematous fibromas (nasal polyps) are frequently observed.

### LARYNX

#### Disturbance of Growth

Atrophy of the laryngeal muscles occurs in horses as a result of the paralysis of the left recurrent laryngeal nerve (hemiplegia laryngis). Causes of the paralysis may be pressure by tumors, enlarged lymph nodes, enlarged thyroids, aneurysms, esophageal diverticula, or abscesses along the course of the nerve. Mechanical irritation of the recurrent laryngeal nerve and perhaps congenital defects involving it are also to be considered as etiological factors. This nerve supplies motor fibers to all the laryngeal muscles except the cricothyroideus. The paralysis is usually left-sided only.

Macroscopically, the laryngeal muscles appear like fish flesh and are atrophied. Only the fascia of the cricoarytenoideus may remain. The arytenoid cartilage sinks into the laryngeal lumen. The vocal cords approach the median line. The entrance to the lateral ventricle dilates so that inspired air is caught and the rima glottis is closed.

Microscopically, the muscle cells show various degenerative changes, atrophy, and myolysis (Fig. 16.7). As a result of the myolysis and fatty degeneration, some of the sarcolemmas may be empty. The muscle cells which remain are separated by considerable connective tissue. The connective tissue may show myxomatous or mucoid degeneration. There are also degenerative changes in the recurrent laryngeal nerve.

#### Disturbances in Circulation

Hemorrhages in the larynx are fairly frequent in some acute septicemic diseases. They appear as petechiae and ecchymoses on the epiglottis and are quite constant in hog cholera. Edema of the glottis is mostly inflammatory in nature. Other causes are foreign bodies (bones in dogs), dust on army marches (horses), and abscess of the postpharyngeal lymph nodes (strangles in horses). Marked edema can

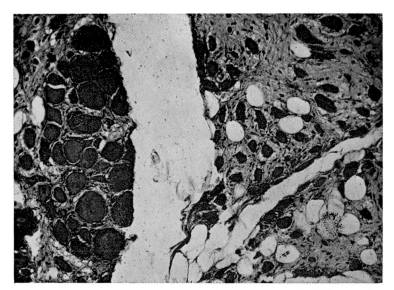

Fig. 16.7 — Atrophy and coagulative necrosis in the left cricoarytenoideus muscle of a horse due to degeneration of the left recurrent laryngeal nerve. (Department of Veterinary Pathology, Iowa State University.)

occur only where there is loose connective tissue, i.e., where the submucosa is well developed such as on the lingual surface, base of the epiglottis, and false vocal cords.

### Laryngitis

The occurrence, etiology, and tissue changes in laryngitis are the same as for rhinitis. Emphasis should be placed upon the fibrinonecrotic laryngitis seen in calf and pig diphtheria (*Spherophorus necrophorus* infection), in the diphtheritic form of fowl pox, and in the ulcerative form in glanders.

A chronic suppurative laryngitis is especially troublesome in sheep. It occurs wherever sheep are raised but is reported to be especially prevalent in the western United States. Chronic abscesses develop in the region of the arytenoid cartilages and often involve the cartilages themselves. The inflammatory process sometimes extends to the softer tissues of the larynx and causes edema of the mucosa with closure of the glottis and death from suffocation. In other cases the abscesses rupture into the larynx, allowing the pus to flow down the trachea and bronchi into the lungs. These sheep die of aspiration pneumonia.

Awns of barley and oats are believed to be the most common cause of this form of laryngitis in sheep, but the awns and barbs of such plants as foxtail, pigeon grass, wild oats, and star thistles are also probable causes.

### TRACHEA

#### Changes in Form

**Congenital.** The free ends of the tracheal rings may bend into the lumen of the trachea, or the rings may be flattened dorsoventrally. This occurs sometimes in horses. **Acquired** changes of form may result from compression by thyroid tumors (in dogs) and by tuberculous bronchial lymph nodes (in cattle).

#### Disturbances of Circulation

**Hemorrhages** are observed mostly in acute septicemic diseases and in bacterial intoxications. Examples are anthrax, pasteurellosis, hog cholera, and purpura hemorrhagica.

#### Tracheitis

The occurrence of tracheitis is the same as for rhinitis and laryngitis. Pathologically, the forms are identical. A contagious **acute catarrhal tracheobronchitis** (kennel cough) occurs in dogs. It is a self-limiting disease with a period of incubation of 5 to 10 days and a course of 2 to 3 weeks.

The cause is unknown. The **suppurative** form of tracheitis sometimes occurs as a result of retrotracheal strangles abscesses rupturing into the trachea. A **hemorrhagic** form is common in pasteurellosis of cattle and sheep. The **necrotic** and **gangrenous** form is occasionally due to improper medication (kerosene and other irritants introduced into the trachea). A **chronic** form, as a result of tracheotomy, presents some special characteristics. It has a polypoid nature which changes somewhat upon cicatrization. In dogs a chronic diffuse polypoid type is reported to have been encountered occasionally; the cause is unknown. Specific forms are seen in tuberculosis, glanders, actinomycosis, swine influenza, and laryngotracheitis, infectious bronchitis, and pneumoencephalitis (Newcastle disease) of fowls, and infectious sinusitis of turkeys.

### INFECTIOUS LARYNGOTRACHEITIS

This disease first appeared in the United States in 1922. It is an acute viral disease of chickens characterized by a sudden onset and acute respiratory symptoms arising from an inflammation of the larynx and trachea. The cause is a filtrable virus, *Tarpeia avium*, which apparently possesses a selectivity for the mucous membrane of the respiratory tract. The virus will pass through coarse but not through fine filters. In winter the virus lives 6 to 9 days in the litter. At other times it dies quickly.

Among chickens of all ages there are also two other filtrable viral diseases quite similar to infectious laryngotracheitis. They are infectious bronchitis and pneumoencephalitis (Newcastle disease).

**Pathogenesis and lesions.** The course of the disease is so rapid that this has not yet been determined fully. Seifried's investigations seem to justify the conclusion that the virus attacks the epithelial cells first, penetrating the submucosa afterwards. It gives rise to edema, cellular infiltration, and hemorrhage. Secondary invaders may aggravate the condition. Inclusion bodies are found in the nuclei of the epithelial cells of the trachea in the early stages of the disease. In all of the affected birds the virus can be found in the tracheal exudate; in 60 per cent, in the spleen; and in 30 per cent, in the liver. It is probably carried to the latter two organs by the blood. It has no apparent affinity for them. In acute cases the virus is eliminated for as many as 10 to 15 days. Some birds become carriers. Acute catarrhal or hemorrhagic inflammation of the upper larynx and trachea are the principal lesions. Death may result from asphyxiation due to occlusion of the trachea and larynx (Fig. 16.8).

### INFECTIOUS BOVINE RHINOTRACHEITIS

A new disease of cattle made its appearance in feed lots in Colorado in 1951 and in dairy herds in California in 1953. It is characterized by sudden onset, fever, diminished milk secretion, drooling, nasal discharge, dyspnea, and severe inflammation of the upper respiratory passages and trachea.

The cause is a virus which Madin, York, and McKercher discovered. It will pass through a fine glass sintered filter and will survive storage at $-70°$ C. for at least 7 months, and at $37°$ C. for at least 96 hours. The period of incubation is unknown. Jensen and his colleagues observed that the disease made its appearance anywhere from 10 to 150 days after cattle entered the feed lot and that it occurred in any season of the year. The course generally is short, 3 to 7 days. In the Colorado outbreaks the morbidity rate was approximately 10 per cent and the mortality rate about 6 per cent.

**Lesions.** The principal organs affected are the nasal passages, including the paranasal sinuses, larynx, trachea, and sometimes the bronchi and bronchioles. The mucosa and submucosa of these parts are in a state of acute suppurative and necrotic inflammation. On the mucosa, which at first displays a suppurative inflammatory reaction, foci of necrosis appear. The latter enlarge and coalesce, causing areas of the mucosa to slough. This gives the mucosa of the larynx a

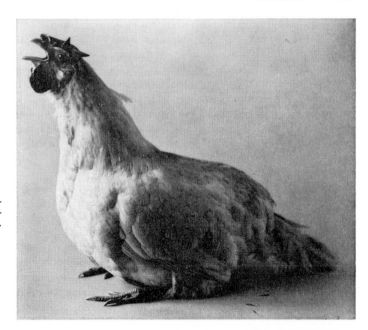

Fig. 16.8 — Infectious laryngo-tracheitis. Note attitude during inspiration. (J. R. Beach, Jour. A.V.M.A.)

diphtheria-like appearance. The submucosa in general is thickened by inflammatory edema containing fibrin and a variety of leukocytes — predominantly neutrophils, lymphocytes, and large macrophages. In the most severe cases the inflammatory process extends to the bronchi and bronchioles. The supramammary lymph nodes share in the reaction and become enlarged as a result of acute serous and hemorrhagic inflammation. In very severe cases the rhinotracheitis may terminate in bronchopneumonia.

In experimentally infected animals intranuclear inclusion bodies have been observed in the epithelial cells of the upper respiratory tract as soon as 36 hours after infection and have remained through 60 hours.

## BRONCHI

### Changes in the Bronchial Lumen

#### BRONCHOSTENOSIS

Bronchostenosis, a narrowing of the bronchial lumen, may be due to changes in the bronchial wall and is frequent in bronchitis, especially with involvement of the small bronchioles. The mucosa swells,

thick folds develop, and the lumen becomes narrow. Stenosis may also be due to pressure from the outside. Pressure may be exerted by enlarged tuberculous lymph nodes or tumors involving lymph nodes (lymphosarcoma). The results of stenosis depend upon the degree of closure. Complete closure produces collapse of the lungs (atelectasis); partial closure causes dilatation or ballooning of the lungs (emphysema).

#### BRONCHIECTASIS

Bronchiectasis is a dilatation of a bronchus. There are two ways in which this condition arises: (1) With the increase in thickness of the bronchial wall in chronic bronchitis, the elastic and muscular fibers disappear and are replaced by connective tissue. The consequent loss of elasticity in the bronchial wall allows the exudate to accumulate in the lumen and results in stretching or expansion of the bronchi. (2) In chronic peribronchitis, upon the contraction of the newly formed connective tissue around the bronchus, an outward tension is exerted upon the bronchial wall with a consequent dilatation resulting.

The dilatations in the bronchi may assume the cylindrical or the saccular form (Fig. 16.9). The cylindrical dilatations are most frequent in the apical lobe of cattle. Macroscopically, the main bronchus and later several of its branches are dilated cylindrically and tightly filled with viscid mucus. The mucosa is gray and very thin. Microscopically, there is a cellular infiltration of the propria and a disappearance of the elastic and muscle fibers, and glands. The bronchial wall may eventually consist only of a narrow band of connective tissue together with an unaltered epithelium stretched over the infiltrated propria.

The saccular form is frequent in sheep and swine in the course of pulmonary strongylosis (lungworm disease). Masses of parasites inhabit the saccular dilatations which arise as a result of a chronic bronchitis and peribronchitis with thickening of the bronchial wall and the surrounding tissue. The volume of the affected lobe or portion of the lung is diminished and the consistency leathery. The surface is nodular much like that of a liver affected with nodular cirrhosis. The color is gray or grayish red, and mottled. When the lung is cut, the elevations on the surface correspond to the sac-like dilatations of the bronchi which are extremely thick walled. The lung parenchyma has been replaced by connective tissue. The organ has the appearance of consisting almost entirely of the dilated, thick-walled bronchi.

The saccular form of bronchiectasis has been encountered in dogs and cats in Ontario. Roentgenograms have been of aid in diagnosing the condition.

### Bronchitis

In the majority of cases the inflammation does not remain confined to the large bronchi but extends to the smaller ones and to the lung parenchyma. The result then is bronchopneumonia. This is especially true in young calves. The forms of bronchitis correspond to similar inflammatory processes of the upper air passages. In adult cattle acute bronchitis resulting from massive invasions of the bronchi by immature forms of *Dictyocaulus viviparus* occurs occasionally and resembles so-called acute pulmonary emphysema clinically. Chronic bronchitis arising from feeding dusty hay, and perhaps from other causes, may lead to chronic diffuse alveolar emphysema (heaves) of horses. In calves and yearlings lungworms may incite a chronic catarrhal bronchitis.

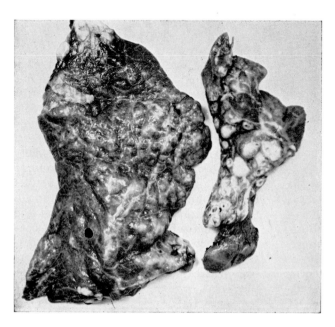

Fig. 16.9 — Saccular form of bronchiectasis associated with chronic pneumonia in the lung (apical lobe) of a cow. At **left**, a surface view; at **right**, a cross section. (Department of Veterinary Pathology, Michigan State University.)

## NEWCASTLE DISEASE

Pneumoencephalitis, more commonly called Newcastle disease, is a viral disease of chickens, pheasants, and turkeys caused by *Tortor furens*.

**Pathogenesis and lesions.** The disease appears about 3 days after exposure. It begins as a mild respiratory disease which lasts 3 to 5 days but often terminates in a nervous disturbance which may be characterized by tremor, circling, twisting of the neck, or paralysis.

The lesions in the respiratory tract are quite similar to those of infectious bronchitis. In addition to these changes the birds have encephalitis and petechiae in the heart, gizzard, and proventriculus. No cell-inclusion bodies are present.

The central nervous system lesions occur chiefly in the cerebellum and medulla. They consist of hyperemia, endothelial proliferation, and degeneration of neurons of the vestibular, medial reticular, and cerebellar nuclei and of the Purkinje cells.

In very young birds the mortality rate approaches 100 per cent. Even in old birds it is about 15 per cent. Regardless of the age, the losses are great.

## AVIAN CHRONIC RESPIRATORY DISEASE

Chronic respiratory disease of chickens and turkeys is a viral infection involving, for the most part, the upper and lower parts of the respiratory system. In chickens a prominent characteristic of the disease is air sac infection, and in turkeys sinusitis.

The disease occurs most frequently in the growing birds, particularly those in broiler plants, but it is also a disease appearing in laying houses. The primary cause is a pleuropneumonia-like organism classed with the viruses. *E. coli*, which is a common secondary invader in field cases, increases the severity of the infection. Stress factors associated with the primary cause of the disease are vaccination for Newcastle disease and infectious bronchitis. Concomitant infection with the viruses of those diseases is possible. Some recovered birds probably become carriers of the virus.

**Pathogenesis and lesions.** The infection probably is most often aerogenic. The virus localizes chiefly in the paranasal sinuses, the trachea, the bronchi and lungs, and the air sacs. Usually all of these parts are not involved simultaneously. Furthermore, when more than one is involved they are not affected to the same degree. Some of these organs may not be involved at all.

In the four sites mentioned, paranasal sinuses, trachea, lungs and bronchi, and the air sacs, the initial reaction is a mucous inflammation. The usual changes of congestion, edema, leukocytic infiltration and minute hemorrhages are present. Where the surfaces are covered with a mucous membrane there is a mucocellular (catarrhal) exudate in the lumen of the organ. In addition to this there is usually a hyperplasia of the epithelium and a loss of the cilia (deciliation).

Superimposed on this mucous inflammation, other changes occur which follow one or the other of two patterns, or a combination of both. They are:

Minute foci of lymphocytic infiltration having the appearance of lymphoid nodules but containing no germinal centers. These occur in the lamina propria of the involved mucous membranes, in the interbronchial septa of the lungs, and on the visceral surface of the air sacs. There is reason to believe that these are produced by the virus.

Chronic inflammatory foci in the lungs and on the surface of the air sacs. There is circumstantial evidence that this reaction is the result of secondary *E. coli* infection. Severe field cases display this type of lesion. In the lungs there are grayish consolidated foci with necrotic cores replacing the catarrhal exudate in the bronchial lumina. These cores are sheathed by a layer of macrophages and giant cells. Beyond and around this sheath is a peribronchial pneumonitis. A similar change involves the surface of the air sacs. In either the lung or air sacs, invasion of the inflammatory process by fibroblasts and angioblasts indicates the chronicity of the disease.

## INFECTIOUS BRONCHITIS

Infectious bronchitis is a disease of chickens caused by the virus, *Tarpeia pulli*, which belongs to the influenza group. The disease is not a viremia.

**Pathogenesis and lesions.** The virus enters the body by the respiratory tract and after a short period of incubation causes a catarrhal tracheitis and bronchitis. The tracheal mucosa and submucosa in particular become thickened due to edema and diffuse leukocytic infiltration. The epithelium of the trachea remains intact. Serous and mucous exudate collects in the lumen. The inflammatory swelling, together with the accumulated exudate, gives rise to difficult respiration. The inflammatory reaction may extend to the bronchi and to the air sacs, causing the thin, transparent lining of the sacs to become opaque. Exudate sometimes collects in the sacs. There are no lesions in the nervous system and no cell-inclusion bodies.

Unless the affected birds die, the disease runs a self-limiting course in 3 to 5 days. Very young chicks may die because the trachea and bronchi become occluded with caseous plugs. Among chicks beyond 3 weeks of age, few die of the disease.

## LUNGS

### Changes of Air Content: Atelectasis and Emphysema

#### CONGENITAL ATELECTASIS

Congenital atelectasis, an intrapulmonary decrease in the air content of very young animals, appears as sharply circumscribed collapsed areas in the lungs. The finding of complete atelectasis in a dead, newborn foal is of significance when one is called upon to determine whether or not the foal met the requirements for stallion service-fee exemption.

In many sections of the country the mare owner is liable for the service fee if the colt stands and nurses.

Obviously, complete atelectasis in a newborn foal would be evidence that the animal did not even breathe, to say nothing of standing to nurse.

#### ACQUIRED ATELECTASIS

Acquired atelectasis is caused by pressure exerted upon the lungs which reduces the intrapulmonary air content. This pressure may have its origin (1) within the lungs, e.g., tumor, (2) within the thoracic cavity but outside the lungs, e.g., hydrothorax and hydropericardium, and (3) within the abdominal cavity, e.g., tympanites. Atelectasis also results from bronchostenosis due to collections of inflammatory exudate and parasites. This is common in lungworm infestation of calves, sheep, and pigs. In the acute and chronic catarrhal bronchiolitis which is a part of the lesions in catarrhal pneumonia, the inflammatory swelling of the bronchiolar mucosa and the accumulation of exudate in the bronchioles furnish the requirements for the occurrence of atelectasis. This can be demonstrated to good advantage in calf pneumonia.

Atelectasis due to hydrothorax disappears at the upper limits of the fluid in the thoracic cavity. In atelectasis due to bronchostenosis, there is a sharp lobular demarcation between the atelectatic and air-containing portions of the lungs. Air which is retained in these atelectatic lobules at the beginning is gradually absorbed.

If the atelectasis is of short duration, the collapsed lung gradually returns to normal. If the airless condition is of long duration, chronic edema will occur because of blood stasis in the area of low intrapulmonary pressure. The chronic edema in turn gives rise to an interstitial fibrosis. The lung then resembles the spleen and is said to have undergone splenization.

#### ACUTE ALVEOLAR EMPHYSEMA

Acute alveolar emphysema is a compensatory increase in air content of the alveoli in a functioning portion of a lung and occurs when other portions are incapacitated because of pneumonia, atelectasis, or other processes. The lung returns to normal after the escape of the increased amount of air.

In Canada an acute alveolar emphysema has been reported in cattle that feed on rape, kale, and turnip tops. The alveoli become greatly distended and frequently rupture so that what begins as an alveolar emphysema becomes an interstitial form of the condition. The emphysema is accompanied by congestion and edema (Fig. 16.10).

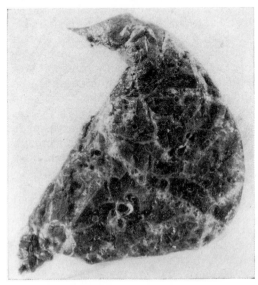

Fig. 16.10 — Acute alveolar and interstitial pulmonary emphysema in a cow. (F. W. Schofield.)

Grossly, in the Canadian cattle, all the lobes show emphysema accompanied by congestion and edema. Were the condition a pure emphysema, the voluminous lobes would be light in weight, but the accompanying congestion and edema cause them to be heavy. Large ballooned areas occur where the air has caused extensive alveolar destruction. Where air escapes into the interlobular septa, beading occurs. Bloody froth fills the bronchi and trachea. Unlike the appearance in pneumonia the lungs present the same appearance throughout.

Histologically, there is rupture and collapse of alveoli. Capillaries are empty where pressure due to the air is greatest and gorged where the pressure is less. The enlarged alveoli may contain lymph and a few neutrophils. Interlobular septa are thickened by edema, and fissures are filled with air.

## CHRONIC FOCAL ALVEOLAR EMPHYSEMA

Chronic focal alveolar emphysema occurs in lungworm infestation of calves, sheep, and swine. Strong inspiratory effort permits air to pass places in the bronchi which are constricted by an inflammatory process or occluded by worms, but expiratory effort is too weak to force the air out again. Air, therefore, accumulates in the lungs behind the constricted or occluded portions of the bronchi. There is, therefore, an increase in the intrapulmonary air content. Macroscopically, there are sharply defined foci involving one or more lobules. These areas are prominent because of their pallor and large volume. In pigs they occur along the basal border of the diaphragmatic lobes. The emphysematous areas are cone-shaped, with the base of the cone at the pleura, and the apex pointing in. When the cone-shaped area is opened from its apex to its base, parasites and exudate are found in the bronchus at the apex. In calves and sheep the emphysematous areas have no favored location but may involve a few lobules or several lobules at widely scattered places or may even cause the distension of a whole lobe. Microscopically, the alveoli are dilated and the interalveolar septa are thinned. Many alveoli coalesce to form larger ones. A mild chronic inflammatory reaction in the bronchi infested with the parasites results in a narrowing of the bronchial lumen. To compensate for this there is a hypertrophy of the bronchial musculature. The mild chronic inflammation of the bronchi also results in a hyperplasia of the peribronchial lymphoid tissue.

## CHRONIC DIFFUSE ALEVOLAR EMPHYSEMA

Chronic diffuse alveolar emphysema occurs particularly in the horse (heaves). The condition is preceded by a bronchitis which increases respiratory effort. This causes weakening of the elastic fibers and ballooning of the alveoli, which in turn impairs the capillary circulation producing stasis of blood in the right side of the heart, leading to chronic right cardiac dilatation and hypertrophy, tricuspid insufficiency, hydropericardium and general venous hyperemia, and also edema. Congenital weakness of the fibers and strong respiratory efforts in hard work are sometimes mentioned also as possible etiological factors. Macroscopically, there is pallor and increased volume. The lung is puffy, crepitates when cut, and shows a smooth, dry cut surface. Numerous lymph follicles are conspicuous as translucent miliary foci. Microscopically, the alveoli are ballooned; their walls in part are atrophied; the bronchial mucosa is diffusely thickened; lymphadenoid tissue in the whole lung is increased.

### INTERSTITIAL EMPHYSEMA

Interstitial emphysema is frequent in kosher-killed animals. Bellowing during estrum or after separation from a newborn calf may cause it in cows. It may occur in old hunting dogs. It is extensive in pulmonary strongylosis, gangrenous pneumonia, and also in trauma of the lungs due to penetrating objects. Macroscopically, large and small vesicles arranged like a string of beads under the pleura and in the interlobular connective tissue are prominent. Large vesicles lead to compression atelectasis of neighboring lobules. Forced respiratory efforts may cause these large vesicles to rupture. This permits air to escape into the interstitial tissue and into the thoracic cavity. From there it may escape through the thoracic inlet into the subcutis of the cervical region. From there it ascends to the top line of the animal where it may be found located subcutaneously from the poll to the base of the tail.

## Local Disturbance of Pigment Metabolism

Melanosis is commonly observed in the lungs. It occurs mostly in calves and is usually a partial manifestation of a more or less general congenital melanosis. It disappears with age. Macroscopically, there are sharply defined areas of pigmentation having a lobular arrangement; black lobules border on pigment-free lobules. Those involved are partially or completely pigmented. Microscopically, the pigment is present in the interlobular and interalveolar connective tissue, adventitia of vessels, and peribronchial tissue. The nuclei are obscured by pigment in the cytoplasm of the cells.

## Disturbances in Continuity

Perforations and rupture are due to foreign bodies in the bronchi, rumen, and reticulum, penetrating objects from without, fractured ribs, necrotic areas in pneumonia, or squeezing during transport. The seriousness of the condition depends upon the extent of the damage done to the lung and the entrance of bacteria. In the case of penetration of foreign bodies from the reticulum of cows, the danger from bacterial infection is especially serious.

## Disturbances in Circulation

### PASSIVE HYPEREMIA

Passive hyperemia is due to (1) cardiac disease (myocardial weakness or lesions of the valves of the left heart), and (2) increased intra-abdominal pressure (bloat). Macroscopically, the color of the lung is dark red, the consistency is firmer than normal, and there is increase in size. The lung crepitates only a little when cut; the cut surface is dark red, smooth, and moist. The bronchial lymph nodes of swine have dark red margins underneath the capsule and along the trabeculae extending into the medulla. Microscopically, the capillaries, extremely dilated, are tortuous so that they project into the alveolar lumen. The alveolar epithelium is swollen and desquamated at times. There may be slight proliferation of the interalveolar tissue.

In mitral stenosis the two rather consistent changes that occur in the small pulmonary vessels are medial hypertrophy in the muscular pulmonary arteries and a development of a distinct media in the arterioles.

### HYPOSTATIC CONGESTION

Hypostatic congestion occurs in moribund animals due to heart weakness. Blood collects in the most ventral portions of the lungs because the force of the heart is not sufficient to return all the blood to this organ. Hypostasis is most frequent in the ventral and anterior portions of the diaphragmatic lobe on the side on which the animal lies at the time of death. The congestion may lead to hemorrhage and edema if the animal lives long enough, and occasionally hypostatic pneumonia may result.

## EDEMA

Edema is an accumulation of lymph in the alveoli, bronchi, and interlobular connective tissue of the lung. The fluid in the alveoli prevents the entrance of air. In the bronchi the fluid and air become mixed, forming froth.

Edema of the lungs may result from cardiac weakness, cardiac anomalies (Fig. 16.11), obstruction to circulation in the heart or liver, and incoordination of the ventricles. It usually accompanies pulmonary passive hyperemia. In sheep it is a frequent lesion in severe stomach worm infestation.

Edema occurs in the course of pulmonary inflammation. In cattle, horses, and swine the edema frequently appears in the peribronchial and interlobular tissue. Here it usually occurs in connection with a peribronchial extension of a primary bronchitis; this is especially true in swine influenza, in hog cholera, and in contagious pneumonia of horses. A peribronchial gelatinous infiltration extends in radiating fashion into the surrounding tissue.

Macroscopically, an edematous lung is distended and firm. Its color varies from deep pink to red, depending upon the etiology. The tissue pits on pressure, and on incision crepitates very little. From the cut surface of the lung there flows a watery, foamy exudate, pale yellow to pale pink in

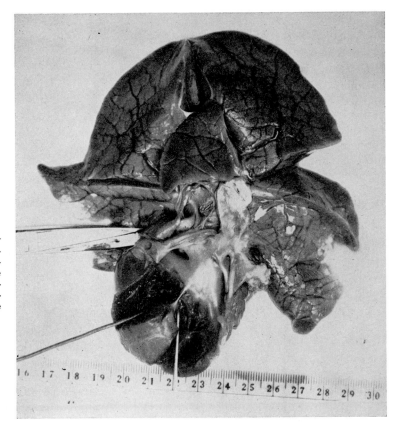

Fig. 16.11 — Interlobular edema of the lung associated with absence of interatrial septum in the heart of a pig. (Department of Veterinary Pathology, Michigan State University.)

color. The flow of lymph becomes greater with pressure. The larger bronchi are filled with froth. Microscopically, the alveoli are filled with a finely granular, coagulated fluid, and a small number of isolated erythrocytes, leukocytes, and detached epithelial cells.

### HEMORRHAGE

The causes of pulmonary hemorrhage are: trauma; erosion of vessels due to degenerative, necrotic, or suppurative processes in the lungs (glanders, tuberculosis, and pulmonary gangrene); passive hyperemia in heart diseases; and severe bacterial and viral intoxications such as occur in purpura hemorrhagica, pasteurellosis, hog cholera, and anthrax. The hemorrhages vary in size and distribution.

Blood that has been aspirated by slaughtered animals, especially by those that have been kosher-killed, collects in foci that have a distinct lobular arrangement. Clots are found in the bronchi and bronchioles, but no changes occur in the walls of these air passages. The capillaries and larger vessels in these slaughtered animals are empty.

### EMBOLISM

Emboli usually lodge in the first and second lateral branches of the pulmonary artery. Their size and appearance vary. Organization of them is frequent; only connective tissue strands across the lumen may remain. In cows the emboli may be portions of thrombi of the uterine veins in cases of severe suppurative endometritis. In pigs a common type of pulmonary emboli is ascarid larvae. Vegetative endocarditis of the tricuspid valve is occasionally the source of pulmonary emboli. Massive pulmonary embolism causes death by mechanical obstruction. The cause of death from showers of small emboli has not been satisfactorily explained. It may be by mechanical means or by a reflex mechanism.

### THROMBOSIS

Thrombi may occur in branches of the pulmonary artery in severe acute septicemic diseases (hog cholera, pasteurellosis). They may also appear in pneumonia when a peribronchial extension of bronchitis involves the peribronchial blood vessels.

### INFARCTION

Hemorrhagic infarction of the lung is common. If an embolus occludes a branch of the pulmonary artery when the heart is normal, the lateral branches of the artery supply the anemic area, and normal circulation is restored within a short time. With heart defects, the force is weak, blood accumulates in the area ahead of the occlusion, and an infarct results. The infarcts may be single or multiple. They appear as prominent, dark red areas which are firm and bulge on the cut surface. They are cone-shaped, with the base of the cone at the visceral pleura and the apex pointing into the organ. The thrombus or embolus is at the apex. Microscopically, there is stasis of blood in the vessels. The alveoli and bronchioles are filled with blood, and the normal architecture is nearly absent. Later there is an inflammatory border.

## Pneumonia

Pneumonia (inflammation of the lungs) is of common occurrence among all species of domestic animals. Since most cases of pneumonia are caused by bacteria and viruses, one can readily understand why the inflammatory exudate of one sick animal can easily contaminate the feed and water of all the healthy animals in the herd or flock. This accounts for the presence of several cases of pneumonia among a group of animals in a short period of time.

**Etiology of pneumonia.** Much of what has been said about the etiology of rhinitis can be repeated with reference to the cause of pneumonia. Thus, as with rhinitis, pneumonia can be primary or secondary. The causes of **primary pneumonia** are irritants that enter the lungs mostly by way of the upper air passages. Among such irritants are physical influences, e.g., dust and other foreign bodies, hot and cold air; chemical agents, e.g., smoke and war gases, anesthetics, and medicinal agents improperly given; bacteria and molds, e.g., staphylococci, streptococci, *Corynebacterium pyo-*

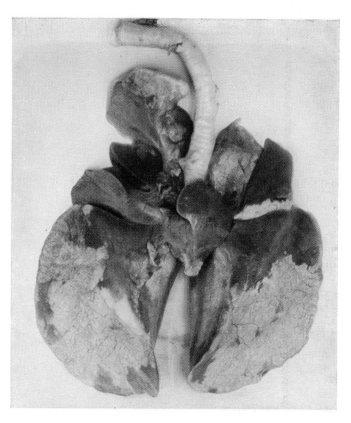

Fig. 16.12 — Pneumonia in an aged ewe. The reddened areas are either consolidated or atelactatic. The lighter areas are either normal or emphysematous. (Department of Veterinary Pathology, Michigan State University.)

genes, *Pseudomonas aeruginosa*, *Escherichia coli*, *Salmonella choleraesuis*, and *Aspergillus fumigatus*. *Brucella abortus* has been shown to be a cause of fetal pneumonia in calves. The viruses of laryngotracheitis and infectious bronchitis of chickens, of sinusitis of turkeys, and of feline distemper also belong in this category.

In certain instances a single kind of microorganism which has been recovered from a pneumonic lung cannot by itself cause pulmonary inflammation. This organism, however, in combination with another kind of organism isolated from the same case, can produce pneumonia. This has been proven experimentally in lambs. In them a virus, a pleuropneumonia-like organism, and a Pasteurella obtained from pneumonic lesions of lambs did not cause pneumonia singly, but a combination of any two of them did cause illness. When the lambs were stressed by alternately subjecting them to heat and cold or by administering large doses of cortisone, pneumonia did not develop, but when stress was applied in combination with 2 or 3 of the infectious agents, all the lambs became sick.

Often the irritant produces an inflammation of the upper respiratory tract which extends down the trachea, bronchi, and bronchioles into the alveoli. Sometimes the primary cause is believed to be a microorganism which may inhabit the respiratory tract as a saprophyte, but which, under conditions that are detrimental to the health of the animal, becomes pathogenic and capable of producing pneumonia. There is some evidence that the Pasteurellae act in this manner in cattle and swine. Certain parasites furnish an exception to the rule that the irritants causing most primary pneumonia enter the lungs by way of the upper respiratory tract. Among these parasites are the larvae of the lungworms of cattle, sheep, swine, and foxes and the larvae of swine ascarids which are brought to the lungs from the intestine by the blood stream.

**Secondary pneumonia** is the result of a hematogenic infection which arises during a specific infectious disease that is also characterized by other pathologic disturbances. Examples of the etiological agents of such pneumonias are the viruses of equine contagious pneumonia, bovine contagious pleuropneumonia (eradicated from the United States in 1892), and members of the Pasteurella group. Many of the pneumonias which occur in the acute, more or less general infectious diseases owe their origin to an organism which invades the lungs after the primary causative agent has already initiated a rather mild inflammatory process. Such organisms are *Pasteurella equiseptica* in equine contagious pneumonia and equine influenza, *Hemophilus suis* in swine influenza, *Pasteurella suiseptica* in hog cholera, and *Brucella bronchiseptica* in canine distemper.

**Predisposing causes.** When considering the causes of pneumonia, one should not lose sight of the importance of predisposing or accessory factors which make animals more susceptible to respiratory infection. Such factors would embrace exposure to sudden changes in weather, especially when rain is accompanied by a marked fall in temperature; confinement to damp, drafty stables or houses; fatigue from work and from shipping or trucking; the detrimental effects of dipping for external parasites in the winter; and the debilitating effects of nutritional deficiencies.

**Pathogenesis.** The pathogenesis of pneumonia depends upon the avenue of entrance of the irritant. When the irritant enters the lungs by way of the upper air passages, a rhinitis, laryngitis, tracheitis, and bronchitis may precede the inflammation of the bronchioles and the lung parenchyma. Often, however, the inflammation begins first of all in the bronchi and bronchioles and extends into the alveoli by way of the lumen of these tubes or through their walls into the surrounding lung parenchyma. When the infection extends through the walls of the bronchi and bronchioles, a peribronchitis and peribronchiolitis arise first, and later a pneumonia. Regardless of whether the inflammatory process travels down the tubes or through their walls into the lung parenchyma, the end result is that a combination of bronchitis and pneumonitis occurs which is called **bronchopneumonia.** This type of pneumonia, in its beginning, usually has a lobular distribution, but by the time it has caused the death of the animal the lobular pattern of the affected areas has disappeared, and large portions of lobes or even entire lobes may be involved (Fig. 16.22). A suggestion of the earlier lobular arrangement, however, often can be seen in the mostly normal lung at the edge of a pneumonic area. These newly inflamed lobules denote a recent extension of the process into healthy portions of the lung.

The lobes most often affected are those in which the bronchi tend towards the vertical direction rather than the horizontal when an animal is standing or is lying on the sternum. It is reasonable to believe that in bronchi directed horizontally, infectious agents are more likely to be, trapped by mucus and engulfed by phagocytes than in those directed vertically. In the latter, infectious agents may be carried quickly direct to the ventralmost portions of the lobes where the conditions are more favorable for them to increase and produce lesions. However, when pigs are in the usual recumbent position (on the side, not on the sternum), the direction of the bronchi is not favorable for the entrance of infectious agents.

The irritant causing pneumonia may reach the lungs not only by way of the upper air passages but also by way of the blood stream. Such a hematogenic type of pneumonia accompanies some of the acute specific infectious diseases, especially those which are septicemias. The same infectious agent which attacks the other organs may localize in the lungs.

Another type of hematogenic pneumonia arises from pyogenic infections localized in other parts of the body (Fig. 11.6). Septic emboli bring the bacteria from the primary focus of infection. A frequent site of such infection is the uterus of the cow following the retention of fetal membranes. Since the septic emboli in the blood stream may reach any part of the lung, the resultant foci of suppurative inflammation (abscesses) have a rather widespread distribution. The inflammation may extend radially from the abscesses so that large pneumonic areas result. This type of inflammation is designated **metastatic suppurative pneumonia.**

In the pathogenesis of pneumonia a third avenue of entrance of the infection is believed to be important. The organisms may reach the lungs by the lymphatics and therefore can be said to be lymphogenous in origin. By this route the infection passes through the epithelium of the oral and nasal cavities, is conveyed by the lymphatics to the lymph nodes of the head and cervical region, and enters the venous circulation just anterior to the heart.

There are favored areas in the lungs in which the lesions become located. Those areas are the lowermost portions of the apical and cardiac lobes, the anteroventral portion of the diaphragmatic lobes, and most of the intermediate lobe. These locations obviously apply only to the lungs of species which have these lobes. These are the portions of the lungs that are situated most anteriorly and ventrally in the thoracic cavity. Their location may account for their frequency of involvement. Large secondary bronchi extend into these portions of the lung from the primary bronchi near the origin of the latter. This permits infected secretion or exudate from the upper air passages to gravitate directly into the lower portions of all of the lobes. Furthermore, it may be that infection has a better opportunity to establish itself in these areas of the lungs because they are the parts having the most restricted movement during respiration. This is partly due to the fact that in respiration the movement of the anterior series of ribs is limited. They are short and rather straight ribs and, as a consequence, rotate less than the posterior ones that are longer and greatly curved. It is possible that other portions of the lungs benefit by the massaging action of the greater rib movement and also by the rhythmic changes of position of the diaphragm.

In the pathogenesis of the pneumonia which accompanies some of the acute specific infectious diseases, the condition of the heart may be an important factor. The blame for conditions favorable to the development of inflammation of the lungs may be placed on the myocardial weakness which occurs in these infections. With the myocardial weakness comes some degree of pulmonary hyperemia and edema, especially in the dependent parts of the lungs — the ventral portions of the lobes. This stagnation of blood in the lung capillaries probably injures the capillary endothelial cells and makes it easier for infectious agents to invade the tissues and incite an inflammatory reaction. This also may explain why in debilitated animals penumonia is so frequently the final pathologic process responsible for death. This terminal pneumonia develops in the areas of hypostatic congestion — the ventral portions of the lobes.

Since pneumonia usually begins in the lowermost portions of the lobes, any extension of the process must be in a dorsal direction. This is the case. The extension is brought about by means of the inflammatory exudate. It flows up the bronchi and bronchioles from the affected areas when an animal is in the recumbent position. After flowing up these passages it enters others that are not involved and carries the infection into new areas. The infection can pass from one alveolus to another through the pores in the alveolar walls. Raising the infected exudate by coughing and aspirating it upon inspiration results in further spread of the disease process.

**Macroscopic appearance.** Inflammation of the lungs begins with a patchy distribution of areas of consolidation in the lower portions of the apical lobes of both lungs. These are reddened areas that are slightly swollen and liver-like in consistency. As the disease progresses, similar changes occur in the lower portions of the other lobes. In animals that die of pneumonia, the early, more or less isolated consolidated areas have enlarged and coalesced.

Furthermore, the lesions have extended in an upward direction until a large portion and in some cases nearly entire lobes have become involved (Fig. 16.12). By this time the color of the lung first affected has changed from red to a yellowish or grayish red. Small excised pieces of this lung sink completely in water.

At the edge of the large consolidated areas there are often sharply outlined patches of more recently consolidated lung. In addition there are multiple, anemic, puffy distensions of the functioning lung parenchyma next to the consolidated areas or a rather general increase in the volume of all the remaining more or less healthy lung. This is compensatory alveolar emphysema. Air may also accumulate in portions of the lung as a result of being trapped by plugs of exudate in the bronchi. If many alveoli rupture, air escapes into the interlobular septa as well. This constitutes interstitial emphysema. Often at other places along the border of the pneumonic lung next to the functioning lung, depressed, dull red areas appear. They are collapsed lobules caused by the occlusion of their bronchi with plugs of exudate and with subsequent absorption of the trapped air. These lobules are in a state of atelectasis.

The pleura of the consolidated lung often is covered with a rough, dry, grayish or yellowish fibrinous exudate. The inflammation has extended from the lungs to the pleura by way of the superficial or pleural set of lymphatics which drain from the lung towards the pleura. If the cause of the pneumonia is a pyogen, the exudate is purulent and empyema may be the result.

The interlobular septa in the inflamed areas are also affected and become thickened. The bronchial and mediastinal lymph nodes are practically always enlarged. Their subcapsular sinus may be reddened (hemorrhagic lymphadenitis) or the whole node may be edematous (serous lymphadenitis).

The cut surface of the consolidated lung bulges above that of the normal lung. Its color in the early stages is rather uniformly red, but when it is squeezed, bubbles of mucopurulent or purulent exudate rise up out of the bronchi and bronchioles. Later the reddened cut surface is mottled with gray or yellow.

In man there is a lobar pneumonia, a specific type of pulmonary inflammation caused by a pneumococcus. Unlike the usual pneumonia of domestic mammals, it is characterized by the formation of large amounts of fibrinous exudate like that shown in Figure 16.13. With modern therapeutics it is rapidly becoming rare. In animals there is nothing that quite compares with it. The cut surface of such a lung in man is dry and granular due to the abundance of fibrin in the exudate.

With rapid recovery the affected portions of the lung of animals become less voluminous. The color returns from a grayish red to normal. The parenchyma ceases to be solidified and becomes soft and pliable. The lung regains its normal crepitancy. Excised portions float in water, although at times much like a heavily laden ship. The process by which the exudate is liquefied and removed is called resolution.

If recovery is not rapid, that is, if resolution is delayed, organization of the ex-

udate may result (Fig. 16.14). Fibroblasts invade the exudate in individual alveoli. When the exudate in many adjacent alveoli in one portion of the lung becomes replaced by fibroblasts, a large area of organization is the result (Fig. 16.15). In these areas there are a few alveoli devoid of exudate scattered throughout the newly formed connective tissue. These alveoli have cuboidal epithelium instead of simple squamous. Occasionally in these organized areas the epithelium of the bronchi undergoes a metaplasia, becoming stratified squamous instead of pseudostratified in type.

The description just given is for bronchopneumonia in cattle, sheep, and swine. In so-called progressive pneumonia of sheep in western United States, *Corynebacterium pyogenes* associated with *Pasteurella oviseptica* are organisms which have been isolated but not proved to be the cause of the disease. Similar alterations in the inflamed lungs occur in ovine caseous lymphadenitis caused by *Corynebacterium pseudotuberculosis* and in calf pneumonia in which various pyogens play a part in the etiology. Abscesses, miliary to hazelnut in size, often contain pale greenish pus. Subpleural abscesses project above the

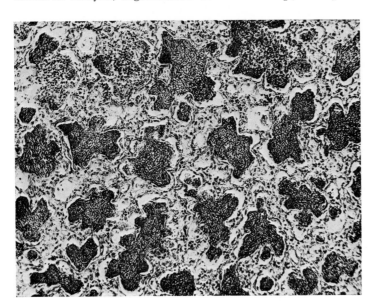

Fig. 16.13 — An area showing a distinct fibrinous exudate in in a 7-month-old calf with pneumonia of 3 days' duration. (Department of Veterinary Pathology, M i c h i g a n State University.)

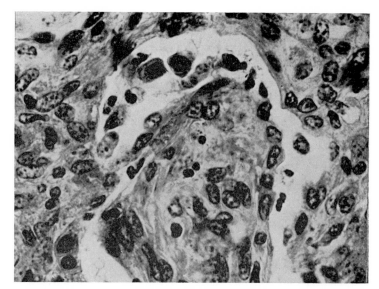

Fig. 16.14 — Organized exudate in an alveolus. ×650. (Department of Veterinary Pathology, Michigan State University.)

surface. The overlying pleura is thick and rough. The presence or absence of a capsule around the abscesses gives an indication as to their age.

**Microscopic appearance.** In the early stages the bronchi and bronchioles show catarrhal inflammation. In their lumina is a mucous exudate containing desquamated epithelial cells. Later the exudate is invaded by leukocytes, among which the neutrophils are so numerous that the exudate is purulent. In the mucosa of the bronchi and bronchioles the capillaries are congested. If the duration of the inflammation is prolonged, there is proliferation of connective tissue around the small bronchioles. The inflammation radiates from the walls of the bronchi and bronchioles into the adjacent alveoli, and through them to others beyond (Figs. 16.16, 16.17, 16.18). In this area the interalveolar capillaries become distended. Macrophages and

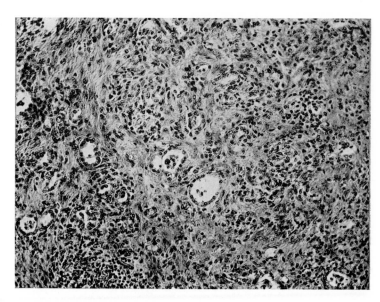

Fig. 16.15 — Lung of a 4-month-old calf with pneumonia of 18 days' duration. Note effects of organization of exudate and interalveolar fibrosis. ×140. (Department of Veterinary Pathology, Michigan State University.)

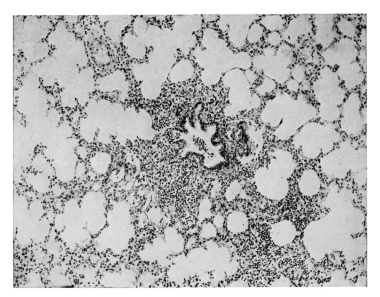

Fig. 16.16 — Peribronchial pneumonia in a 1-month-old calf. ×100. (Department of Veterinary Pathology, Michigan State University.)

lymphocytes invade the alveoli. The macrophages persist in the exudate and may become exceedingly large and conspicuous. Sometimes they form giant cells. An occasional megakaryocyte must not be mistaken for multinucleated giant cells. Megakaryocytes are seen at times both in health and disease in the lungs of mammals of all ages. They are increased in numbers, however, in infections and also in postoperative states, thromboembolic

diseases, and in anemias. They break up into thrombocytes.

Fibrin in the cellular exudate is not readily seen, and when it does occur in abundance, it may fill the alveoli in a rather circumscribed area (Fig. 16.13). It may be seen to extend from one alveolus to another through pores in the alveolar wall (Fig. 16.19). Along with the accumulation of exudate in the alveoli there often is considerable destruction of the

Fig. 16.17 — Peribronchiolitis in the lung of a 14-week-old calf with pneumonia of 1 week duration. ×130. (Department of Veterinary Pathology, Michigan State University.)

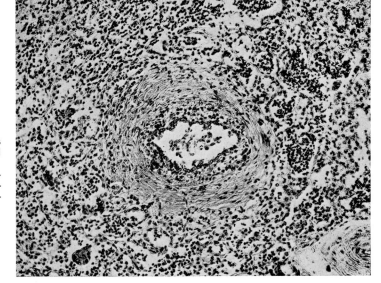

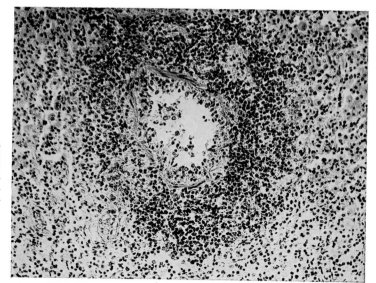

Fig. 16.18 — Peribronchiolitis in the lung of an 8-week-old calf with pneumonia of 12 days' duration. ×150. (Department of Veterinary Pathology, Michigan State University.)

walls of the alveoli. At other times there is a mild proliferation of connective tissue between the alveoli (Fig. 16.20). In the most severely affected areas the inflammation may extend into the branches of the pulmonary veins and result in thrombosis. The thrombosis in turn causes areas of necrosis. This is referred to as **necrotizing pneumonia.**

Sections made at the periphery of the pneumonic areas are almost sure to show either areas of over-distended alveoli (emphysema) or of collapsed alveoli (atelectasis).

The interlobular septa become thickened as the result of a serous, fibrinous, or hemorrhagic exudate which also contains neutrophils, lymphocytes, and macrophages. The interlobular lymph vessels are distended with erythrocytes and leukocytes.

With recovery the lung undergoes reso-

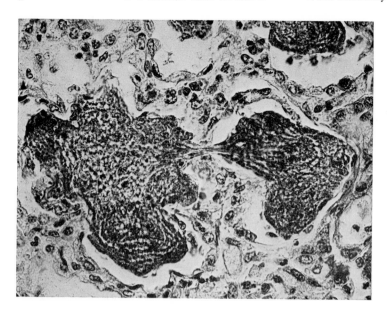

Fig. 16.19 — Two adjacent alveoli filled with fibrinous exudate and with fibrin extending through pore in alveolar wall. ×650. (Department of Veterinary Pathology, Michigan State University.)

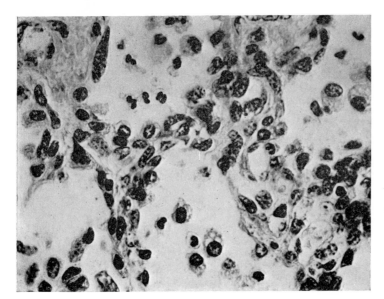

Fig. 16.20 — Early interalveolar fibrosis in the lung of a 4-month-old calf with pneumonia of 18 days' duration. ×550. (Department of Veterinary Pathology, Michigan State University.)

lution. The amount of the exudate commences to diminish, and the alveoli again begin to admit air. In the alveolar exudate there are degenerating and disintegrating leukocytes. The exudate is undergoing autolysis, leukocytic-enzyme digestion, and absorption. Regeneration of the epithelium soon follows unless there is delayed resolution, necrosis, or suppuration.

The sinuses of the bronchial and mediastinal lymph nodes are engorged with erythrocytes or distended with lymph containing neutrophils. The pleura is thickened because of the presence of hyperemia and serofibrinous exudate containing neutrophils and leukocytes.

**Disturbed function.** The exudate in the air passages and alveoli displaces air and interferes with its free passage causing labored respiration. The exudate also stimulates coughing. Exudate in the air passages alters the quality of respiratory sounds as detected by the stethoscope, while consolidation of the lungs changes the normal resonance as determined by percussion. Failure of the blood to get sufficient oxygen and to rid itself readily of carbon dioxide causes speeding up of respiration. The heart compensates by accelerating its rate. Interference with circulation in the consolidated portions of the

lung increases the labor of the right side of the heart. At the same time toxic substances originating in the inflamed area or as a result of the general infection which may have brought on the pneumonia may weaken the myocardium through degenerative changes. These disturbances in the cardiovascular system are reflected in the pulse. The heat-regulating center is upset by the bacterial toxins and by the products of tissue destruction. A rise in body temperature occurs. The products of tissue destruction stimulate the formation of leukocytes in the general circulation.

### THE PASTEURELLOSES

**Pasteurellosis of cattle.** Shipping fever of cattle is a common feed-lot disease in the United States and Canada. Cattle shipped from the ranges in western United States to the feed lots in the Midwest or from western Canada to Ontario and Quebec are frequent victims of this respiratory disease. While *Pasteurella multocida* and *Pasteurella hemolytica* can often be isolated from the lungs of affected cattle, these same organisms will not usually reproduce a similar severe disease in calves. It appears that stress influences, such as those to which animals are subjected while in transit, and possibly exposure to infection by a virus, or pleuropneumonia-like organisms are necessary to cause the disease.

In very acute cases, only lesions of a septicemia are present. Hyperemia of the internal organs, hemorrhages on the mucous and serous membranes, and cloudy swelling of the parenchymatous organs can be found. In subacute cases, edema, gelatinous infiltration, and hemorrhages in the subcutis of the head, throat, and neck are present. The mucous membranes of the head and neck region are in a state of catarrhal, fibrinous, or hemorrhagic inflammation. There is acute hemorrhagic lymphadenitis of the regional nodes. Either with or without the subcutaneous edema, there may be involvement of the organs of the thoracic cavity (**pectoral form**) or of the organs of the abdominal cavity (**intestinal form**). In either case, lesions of a septicemia are present.

In the pectoral form, which is the more common, there is usually bilateral consolidation of the lower one-third to two-thirds of all the lobes of the lungs. The inflammatory exudate is rich in fibrin, and hemorrhage occurs into the bronchi and bronchioles. Interlobular edema is usually present (Fig. 16.21). Lymph vessels draining the lungs, and blood vessels in the consolidated areas are often thrombosed. The thrombosed blood vessels are accompanied by infarcts. Areas of the lung bordering the pneumonic portions may display atelectasis, and functioning lung is almost always emphysematous. Complications may be gangrene, abscessation, and fibrosis.

In the intestinal form hemorrhagic enteritis is an important lesion.

**Pasteurellosis of sheep** is an infectious disease, especially of feeder lambs, characterized in acute cases by manifestations of septicemia, and in subacute and chronic cases by inflammatory disturbances of the respiratory system. In Montana pasteurellosis occurs principally as a pneumonia of lambs less than a month old. Two species of the organism cause the disease — *P. multocida* and *P. hemolytica*. Both organisms may be found in the upper respiratory tract of healthy lambs. *P. hemolytica* is the cause of an acute septicemia of lambs.

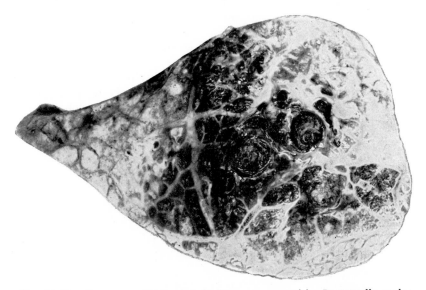

Fig. 16.21 — Severe acute pneumonia in a cow caused by **Pasteurella multocida.** The marked interstitial edema gives the lung a marbled appearance. In the specimen the light areas are infiltrated with leukocytes and the dark areas are congested and hemorrhagic. (Department of Veterinary Pathology, Michigan State University.)

In severe infection the organisms multiply rapidly in the body and produce death quickly by septicemia. If the infection is less severe or if the resistance of the animal is high, a chronic infection results, manifested by progressive emaciation and anemia. Secondary infection is then likely to occur in the internal organs, and *Pasteurella multocida* may disappear from the blood stream. Secondary lesions resulting are bronchopneumonia (common), and arthritis and tendinitis (less frequent). An important secondary invader is *Corynebacterium pyogenes*. It acts in this role in the so-called lunger disease of sheep on ranges in the western United States. The primary pleuropneumonia in this disease has quite generally been thought to be due to *Pasteurella multocida*, although recent experimental work has not confirmed this belief.

In very acute cases subcutaneous edema of the anterior half of the body, inflammation of the air passages (frequently a hemorrhagic inflammation), abomasitis and enteritis, hemorrhagic lymphadenitis, petechiae in the serous membranes and kidneys, and sometimes early bronchopneumonia and interlobular edema are present. Occasionally an atypical form of pasteurellosis occurs in lambs. It is characterized by an acute diffuse nonsuppurative meningoencephalitis in which foci of leukocytic infiltration and perivascular cuffing, as are found in listerellosis, are

lacking. In subacute cases there are pneumonia (Fig. 16.22), fibrinous pleuritis and pericarditis associated frequently with the pneumonia, fibrinous or fibrinohemorrhagic tracheitis and bronchitis, and sometimes catarrhal or fibrinous rhinitis. In chronic cases, late fibrinous pneumonia with encapsulated necrotic foci (secondary abscess formation due possibly to streptococci, *Escherichia coli*, *Corynebacterium pyogenes*) and occasionally serofibrinous arthritis are found.

**Pasteurellosis of swine,** also called swine plague, is usually a sporadic, occasionally a herd, disease of hogs caused by *Pasteurella multocida* and characterized sometimes by a septicemia but usually by a pleuropneumonia with focal necrosis. It is doubtful that the disease ever exists as a primary infection. It is generally believed, however, to be a serious secondary affection in debilitating diseases such as hog cholera, swine influenza, and infectious necrotic enteritis. In Canada, where hog cholera is uncommon, swine plague is reported to be common.

In peracute cases (rare), hemorrhagic lymphadenitis, pulmonary edema, usually a few petechiae in the mucous surfaces, and reddening of the skin of the abdomen are the lesions. In acute cases (more frequent), thoracic lesions are more or less constantly present and consist of a fibrinous pneumonia with or without multiple necrotic foci, interlobular edema, bron-

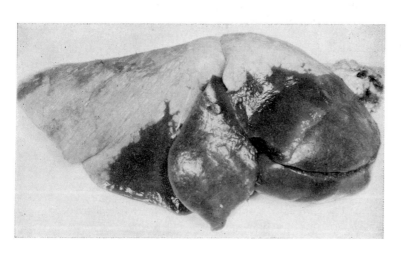

Fig. 16.22 — Pneumonic lung in hemorrhagic septicemia in a sheep. A similar lesion characterizes the pectoral form of the disease in cattle. (Colo. Agr. Exper. Sta.)

chial edema, fibrinous pleuritis, fibrinous pericarditis, and hemorrhagic lymphadenitis of the peribronchial nodes. In the abdominal cavity catarrhal gastroenteritis and petechiae frequently can be found. There may be early focal fibrinonecrotic cecitis and colitis. This, however, is secondary to the Pasteurella infection and is probably caused by *Salmonella choleraesuis* which enters the mucosal hemorrhages of the intestine. The kidneys show hyperemia and sometimes anemic infarcts. In chronic cases emaciation, suppurative pneumonia (secondary infection), suppurative lymphadenitis (peribronchial and mesenteric nodes), and serofibrinous or suppurative arthritis are the lesions.

**Pasteurellosis of rabbits** (acute snuffles, infectious nasal catarrh) is an acute infectious disease caused by *Pasteurella multocida* and characterized by a catarrhal inflammation of the respiratory organs, frequently terminating in pneumonia and resulting in death. This disease must not be confused with chronic rhinitis and sinusitis (also called snuffles) due to *Brucella bronchiseptica* (primary invader) and *Staphylococcus aureus* (secondary invader). In chronic snuffles the secondary invader is believed to be responsible for the chronicity of the disease. Acute snuffles (Pasteurella infection) is often fatal, but chronic snuffles is usually not fatal except in very young rabbits.

**Fowl cholera,** an acute septicemic disease of domesticated birds, characterized by fever, and manifested by weakness, prostration, and a profuse diarrhea, is the avian form of pasteurellosis. The disease apparently is more acute in geese than in the domestic fowl. In geese it has the special designation of goose septicemia. Death usually occurs within a few hours in both chickens and geese.

The organism enters by way of the digestive tract, passes through the intestinal epithelium into the lymph spaces, eventually enters the blood stream, multiplies rapidly, and causes death probably by means of toxic substances which exert a negative chemotactic action upon the phagocytes. The period of incubation is variable — 24 hours to a week.

In acute cases (most common) there will be found cutaneous hyperemia (pectoral and abdominal regions), passive hyperemia of the comb and wattles (only occasionally anemic), general hyperemia of the internal organs, petechiae on the heart (frequently), a fibrinous or gelatinous exudate in the pericardial sac (less frequently), hemorrhagic enteritis (quite constant), focal hepatic necrosis (frequently), pulmonary hyperemia, or catarrhal or hemorrhagic pneumonia. In chronic cases there are multiple caseous foci in the lungs, liver, and intestinal mucosa, suppurative arthritis, and fibrinous pleuritis and pericarditis.

**Tularemia** is an acute septicemic disease of several species of mammals and birds, chiefly wild animals. It is caused by *Pasteurella tularense*, which, among wild animals at least, is transmitted by the bite of insects, principally ticks. Among domestic mammals reports indicate that natural transmission has occurred in sheep, and that ticks have been the mechanical vector. It is also a disease of man contracted by handling infected animals (Fig. 16.23). Since the cottontail rabbit (*Sylvilagus floridanus*) is the animal in which tularemia is encountered most often, the lesions described below will be for that animal.

**Pathogenesis.** After the organism enters the blood through the bite of a vector, it multiplies and invades the vascular endothelium, the pulmonary alveolar epithelium, hepatic cells, and the reticuloendothelial cells of the liver, spleen, and lymph nodes. The presence of the bacteria together with the damage to the endothelium of the capillaries and venules furnish the proper setting for the development of thrombi. The infected thrombi give rise to small foci of necrosis, especially in the spleen, liver, and their lymph nodes.

**Lesions.** The spleen is enlarged and dotted with numerous minute white spots which are foci of necrosis. The splenic

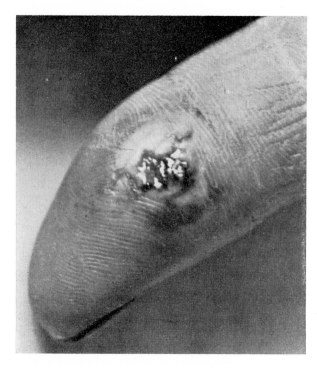

Fig. 16.23 — Tularemic ulcer on thumb following handling of infected rabbit. (Graham and Thorp, Jour. A.V.M.A.)

enlargement is due to hyperemia. The foci of necrosis occur both in the follicles and in the pulp. The liver is likewise enlarged because of congestion, and is similarly studded with tiny white foci of necrosis. These are foci of coagulative necrosis at points where bacterial emboli are present. Degeneration of the hepatic epithelium occurs around the emboli, but there is no infiltration of neutrophils nor proliferation of fibroblasts. Hepatic cells and Kupffer cells at the margin of the foci of necrosis contain the pasteurellae. In the hepatic and splenic lymph nodes, small foci of caseous necrosis are present. In sections the reticuloendothelial cells appear swollen and contain nuclear fragments and bacteria.

### VIRAL PNEUMONIAS

**Swine influenza** is an acute viral disease of swine of seasonal occurrence (late fall, early winter) and characterized by a sudden onset (the whole herd may become affected within 24 to 48 hours), inflammation of the upper respiratory tract with rapid recovery in uncomplicated cases, and bronchopneumonia and death in complicated ones. This disease was first recognized in 1918 at the same time that the great wartime human influenza epidemic occurred. The most recent researches indicate that the etiological agents are related. The virus of swine influenza, *Tarpeia alpha*, together with *Hemophilus suis* or *Pasteurella multocida* introduced into the nasal mucosa, produce the disease. The virus alone produces only a very mild, scarcely recognizable illness with a progressive atelectasis and with little or no pulmonary congestion. The virus with *Hemophilus suis* produces slight congestion, atelectasis of the ventral portions of all or almost all of the lobes of the lungs, and a catarrhal bronchitis with peribronchial pneumonia. The virus with *Pasteurella multocida* produces atelectasis, catarrhal pneumonia, fibrinous pleuritis, fibrinous pericarditis, and in some cases a fibrinous peritonitis. The virus has a specificity for the respiratory epithelium. It is regularly present in the turbinates, tracheal exudate, and lungs of infected swine but not in the spleen, liver, kidneys, mesenteric lymph nodes, colon mucosa, brain, or blood.

In nonfatal cases mild catarrhal rhinitis, pharyngitis, laryngitis, and tracheitis are the lesions. There is serous lymphadenitis of the cervical, mediastinal, and mesenteric nodes. Frequently, there is hydroperitoneum and usually acute swelling of the spleen. In convalescent animals there may be lung abscesses, bronchiectasis, chronic adhesive pleuritis, and connective tissue increase of the alveolar walls. In fatal cases, which are often those that have been exposed to adverse weather or shipping conditions, atelectasis of most or all of the lobes of the lungs, catarrhal bronchitis with peribronchial catarrhal pneumonia, fibrinous pleuritis, and pericarditis are the lesions. Alveolar and interstitial edema are often present also. Rapid recovery occurs within 2 to 6 days in uncomplicated cases with at least some degree of immunity. One to 4 per cent of the cases die of complications. In pigs that contract swine influenza during shipping, at garbage-feeding plants, or at the time of vaccination for hog cholera, the losses may be much greater. *Pasteurella suiseptica* has been found to be associated with the virus of swine influenza in such outbreaks.

**Viral porcine pneumonia** is a chronic diffuse pneumonia which is not acute and short-lasting like the pneumonia of swine influenza. The primary cause is a virus which produces mild lesions that become transformed into more severe lesions by a pleuropneumonia-like organism and Pasteurellae. The mild viral lesions consist of peribronchial lymphoid hyperplasia. The pleuropneumonia-like organism alone causes a serositis, an alveolarcell proliferation, and a lymphocytic infiltration of the pleura. Together these mildly pathogenic microorganisms cause a chronic pneumonia. A similar pneumonia occurs in calves, sheep, and laboratory rats.

It is much easier for the virus of porcine pneumonia to establish itself in the lungs and cause lesions if it enters the body at the time ascarid larvae are migrating. Experimentally, pneumonia is ten times more common in pigs having ascarid larvae migrating at the time of infection than in those which do not. The combination of viral infection simultaneously with larval migration produces a pneumonia similar to severe field cases.

**Feline pneumonitis** is a highly contagious respiratory disease of cats caused by the virus *Miyagawanella felis* (a member of the psittacosis-lymphogranuloma-pneumonitis group) and is characterized by pyrexia, debilitation, sneezing, coughing, a mucopurulent discharge from the eyes and nose, and low mortality. Synonyms include feline influenza, infectious coryza, cat cold, and feline distemper.

It has been shown by experimentation that the virus can be transmitted via the intranasal but not the parenteral route of inoculation. The incubation period after exposure by inoculation or direct contact varies from 6 to 10 days.

The lesions, consisting of inflammation (serous to mucopurulent), are principally in the conjunctival membranes and the respiratory tract. Even though many affected cats do not show symptoms of pneumonia, it is known that during the acute stage they have pneumonic lesions, patchy in distribution and suppurative in nature. Some necrosis may be present. The affected alveoli are filled with macrophages and neutrophils. Cytoplasmic elementary bodies may be found in the macrophages.

**Psittacosis,** also known as parrot fever, is an acute septicemic disease of parrots and parakeets (psittacine birds) caused by the Rickettsia *Miyagawanella psittacii* and characterized by fever and diarrhea. The infection is transmissible to man, in whom it is usually characterized by pneumonia. The lesions are those of a septicemia. General hyperemia of the viscera, ecchymoses on the serous surfaces, focal necrosis of the liver, spleen, and kidneys, pneumonia, and air sacs filled with a serous or sero-fibrinous fluid are present. Inclusion bodies are present in the epithelial cells of the small intestine, ureter, renal secreting tubules, and bile ducts, in reticuloendothelial cells and mesothelial cells of parrots, in the epithelium of the renal collecting tubules in parakeets, and in macrophages and alveolar epithelial cells in the lung and hepatic cells in man.

**Ornithosis** is the disease in non-psittacine birds caused by the psittacosis-ornithosis virus. The disease in man contracted from diseased birds is also termed ornithosis. The disease has most often occurred in turkeys and in individuals working in turkey processing plants and in poultry diagnostic laboratories. The disease affects turkeys of all ages. Mortality is greatest in young turkeys. The period of incubation in the field is about 21 days.

Gross lesions in turkeys are chiefly subacute and chronic inflammation of the air sacs and serous membranes of the thoracic and abdominal cavities, involving both the parietal and visceral layers. The type of inflammation is variable — purulent, fibrinous, or fibrinopurulent. In addition, the spleen, liver, and kidneys are swollen. The spleen is dark purple in color, the kidneys gray, and the liver irregularly gray and green. Invariably there is severe pneumonia. The disease resembles the air-sac syndrome of chickens and turkeys.

## VERMINOUS PNEUMONIAS

Verminous pneumonia is a chronic bronchopneumonia occurring most often in swine, young cattle, sheep, and goats. Since the cause and pathogenesis vary somewhat from the pneumonia already described, this kind of pneumonia needs special consideration. The worms which invade the lungs are the larvae of strongyles. They become sexually mature and reproduce in the lungs. Because they inhabit the lungs for a considerable period of time during their development, they produce a pneumonia which has a protracted course.

**Pathogenesis.** The larvae enter the body in the feed and water. In the intestine they penetrate the mucosa and invade the small blood and lymph vessels of the villi. The larvae which enter the blood vessels are carried directly to the lungs by way of the portal vein and the intervening parts of the circulatory system. Those which penetrate the lymphatics transfer to blood vessels in the mesenteric lymph nodes and arrive at the same destination by the same route as the others. In the lungs the immature worms leave the capillaries and enter the alveoli, where they continue their development. As they reach maturity they migrate to the bronchioles and bronchi. Their movements and their waste products here act as irritants which stimulate a low-grade inflammatory reaction that is usually aggravated by bronchogenic infection. Early stages of the invasion of the larvae may not give rise to marked symptoms but can be detected by histological examination. As the worms approach maturity they cause increasing irritation, and as a result more extensive tissue changes develop and symptoms appear.

**Macroscopic appearance.** Consolidated areas are either quite widely scattered or have become so numerous and extensive that they have coalesced to form large solidified areas (Fig. 16.24). These areas are somewhat increased in volume, are firm in consistency, and vary in color from red to grayish red to grayish yellow, depending upon their age. The oldest lesions are grayest and also the firmest because they contain much newly formed connective tissue. The pleura over these areas may be inflamed. Mucopurulent exudate can easily be expressed from the bronchi and bronchioles which contain mature worms, eggs, and embryos.

The walls of bronchi which enclose masses of worms and exudate become distended (bronchiectasis) and thickened. The chronic inflammatory reaction radiates from these bronchi into the surrounding lung parenchyma. This means that there is not only a bronchitis and peribronchitis but also a peribronchial pneumonia.

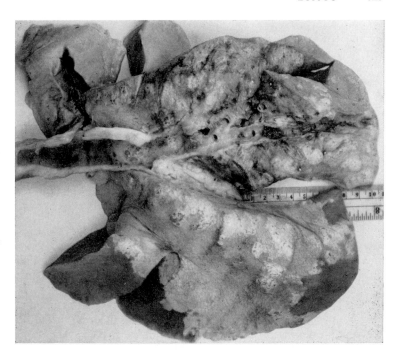

Fig. 16.24 — Verminous (lungworm) pneumonia in a ewe. Foamy edema is present in the trachea, and there are lungworms in the bronchi. The dark areas are pneumonic and the pale, puffy area is emphysematous. (Department of Veterinary Pathology, Michigan State University.)

Masses of the exudate containing worms occlude the passage of air back and forth in the bronchi and bronchioles and result in areas of atelectasis and emphysema. The chronic cough incited by the constant irritation in the air passages further aggravates the emphysema by causing such extensive rupture of alveolar walls that air escapes into the interlobular septa (interstitial emphysema).

**Microscopic appearance.** The histological changes occurring in verminous pneumonia are progressive. Generally their course of development is 60 to 80 days or more.

The youngest lesions consist of tiny areas of inflammation scattered throughout the lungs. Centrally in each focus are larvae surrounded by a cellular exudate containing many eosinophils. Bordering the focus is a zone of hyperemia. Other nodules which are older may contain dead larvae imbedded in cell debris and exudate containing many lymphocytes a n d eosinophils. Large macrophages and even giant cells are often prominent in these foci. The border of these small lesions consists of granulation tissue.

The largest inflamed areas involve bronchi and the surrounding tissue. The bronchi are filled with purulent exudate containing active adult worms. The bronchial mucosa has been completely destroyed. Often the leukocytic infiltration and connective tissue proliferation in the bronchial walls have been so extensive that only the presence of cartilaginous plates identifies the nature of the original structures. In some of the alveoli in the neighborhood of these bronchi are ova and embryos. In these same areas the interalveolar septa are thickened. Lymph nodules along the bronchi increase in size.

In well-advanced cases of verminous pneumonia there is a confluence of lesions like the one just described. The condition then becomes a diffuse chronic bronchopneumonia. In swine lungs the terminal stages of verminous pneumonia are marked by the presence of peribronchial lymphoid hyperplasia, stenosis of bronchi, and chronic emphysema.

### INTERSTITIAL PNEUMONIA

For the most part interstitial pneumonia is caused by viruses that have an affinity for pulmonary tissues. The alveolar walls become thickened because of an infiltration of leukocytes and a proliferation of fibroblasts. The leukocytes are chiefly lymphocytes, plasma cells, and macrophages. At times there are neutrophils. Thick bands of reticulum fibers are present on both sides of the exudate next to the alveolar lining. From these bands delicate fibrils of reticulum extend into the exudate. Focal emphysema, microatelectasis, and hemorrhages usually accompany these alveolar-wall changes. Metaplasia and desquamation of the alveolar epithelium can also be expected as well as occasional giant cells. In animals there is usually peribronchial lymphoid hyperplasia also. Viral pneumonia in calves, pigs, and lambs is of this type.

## MYCOTIC PNEUMONIA

Mycotic pneumonia is an inflammation of the lower respiratory organs, including the air sacs of birds, caused principally by the mold *Aspergillus fumigatus* (Fig. 16.25) and characterized by an inflammatory exudate in which the mold grows luxuriantly. *Aspergillus fumigatus* is widespread in nature in moldy materials which may be used for poultry-house litter, and also on moldy grain. It is therefore relatively easy for the mold spores to enter the respiratory tract, either from breathing dust-laden air containing the spores or by aspirating the spores which are on moldy grain. Because of its prevalence in brooder houses, it is often called **brooder pneumonia.** The inflammatory exudate in the trachea, bronchi, lungs, and air sacs, particularly the abdominal sacs, is of the suppurative type. When only the vegetative form of the mold is in evidence, the exudate has a gray, stringy appearance. This is due principally to the mycelia of the mold which permeate the trachea, bronchi, and air sacs. When the mold spores appear, the exudate has a distinct greenish color and reminds one of the green scum which grows on the tops of jars of preserved fruit which have not been hermetically sealed. The lesions in the lungs usually have a focal distribution. The termination of mycotic pneumonia is frequently death.

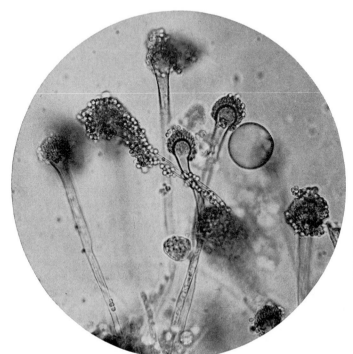

Fig. 16.25 — Part of a colony of **Aspergillus fumigatus** from the lung of a chicken. ×400. (Department of Veterinary Pathology, Iowa State University.)

## METASTATIC SUPPURATIVE PNEUMONIA

This disease is most frequent in cattle, swine, and horses. Rather common etiological agents in swine are *Corynebacterium pyogenes, Pseudomonas aeruginosa, Salmonella choleraesuis, Spherophorus necrophorus,* and possibly *Pasteurella multocida;* in cattle, *Corynebacterium pyogenes* and streptococci from suppurative endometritis and suppurative mastitis; in horses, *Streptococcus equi* in strangles and *Shigella equirulis* in navel ill. Macroscopically, miliary or larger abscesses are rather widely and quite uniformly scattered throughout the lungs. The abscess borders are hyperemic and edematous, and surrounding the abscesses is a zone of pneumonia. The abscesses may become encapsulated, undergo organization, and finally terminate in a scar in the lung parenchyma.

Abscesses which are disseminated are characteristic of metastatic pyogenic infections. Large, single abscesses like the one shown in Figure 16.26 are more likely to originate from bronchogenic infection.

## GANGRENOUS PNEUMONIA

This is a putrefactive decomposition of necrotic pulmonary tissue. It is caused by microorganisms capable of producing putrefaction of dead tissue. These bacteria may be of bronchogenic or hematogenic origin; the former is most frequent. The primary necrosis in the lungs is due to the aspiration of foreign material such as medicine (medication pneumonia), anesthetics (narcosis pneumonia), food (foreign-body pneumonia), or pus. It may also be due to the penetration of foreign bodies from the forestomachs.

The macroscopic appearance of gangrenous pneumonia is quite varied. The basic alterations are those of fibrinous or suppurative pneumonia. The putrefactive changes occur in the hepatized areas. There may be dirty gray miliary nodules which coalesce, or miliary to pea-sized putrefying foci with greenish, pasty contents. These are areas of liquefaction. They may become large enough to involve lobules or groups of lobules. These areas of putrefaction are irregular in outline.

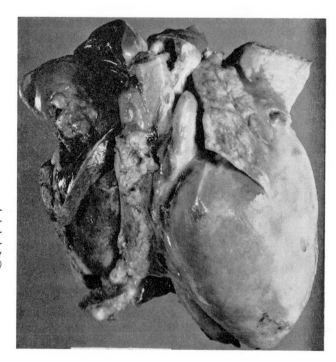

Fig. 16.26 — A single, massive abscess in a dog, the type of lesion usually resulting from bronchogenic infection rather than hematogenic infection. (Department of Veterinary Pathology, Michigan State University.)

They have a putrid odor. Air escapes from areas of decomposing lung tissue and from large areas of emphysema. At first it causes only pneumothorax, but later the air escapes through the thoracic entrance into the subcutis of the neck. Eventually the subcutaneous emphysema of the neck and shoulder may extend dorsally and be located along the topline of the animal from the poll to the base of the tail. If the animal does not die, healing occurs by organization beginning in the interlobular tissue and around the larger bronchi.

Microscopically, at first, a suppurative-necrotic bronchitis and bronchiolitis is most prominent. This process extends in a radiating manner around the bronchi and bronchioles into the lung parenchyma, producing multiple foci of the same type of inflammation. These necrotic foci coalesce and may undergo liquefaction. In cattle extensive interlobular edema and emphysema are present.

### PULMONARY ADENOMATOSIS

Pulmonary adenomatosis is a disease of domestic animals that is characterized by hyperplasia and hypertrophy of the septal cells of the lung. Pulmonary adenomatosis and pulmonary emphysema are the terms usually used to describe the disease in cattle. The disease in sheep is more commonly known as Montana progressive pneumonia, jagzeikte, maedi, or epizootic adenomatosis. Silo-fillers disease is the current popular term used to describe the disease in the human being.

The prevalence of pulmonary adenomatosis in cattle is not known. However, descriptions of the disease have been so numerous and from so many widely scattered areas in the United States that it is suspected the disease is quite common. Calves, yearlings, and adults of all ages are affected. The majority of the animals are feeder cattle that are 1 to 2 years of age. No breed predisposition has been observed. One animal, several animals, or the entire herd may be involved. Most cases of the disease have occurred during the summer and fall months, and it is particularly prevalent in areas where drouth has been present. Apparently the retardation of growth associated with drouth alters the chemical constituents of the feed, resulting in a greater incidence of the disease.

The respiratory symptoms are usually somewhat different from those observed in the more common diseases of the lung. The respirations are extremely deep and much more frequent than in cattle affected with pneumonia. Usually the animals do not appear to be particularly ill except for the rapid respiratory rate. Rhinitis and conjunctivitis, usually observed in infectious respiratory diseases (pneumonia), are not present. The temperature of the individual depends upon the external temperature of the surroundings. In warm weather there is quite a noticeable temperature elevation, rising to as much as 105° F. In cooler weather the temperature rise is only slightly above normal.

The course of the disease in the herd is usually slow, extending over a period of several weeks from the time the first animal is observed to be ill. In a few herds the disease is very acute and many animals are involved at the same time. Frequently the disease terminates in death; the more severe cases die within 24 hours after they are first observed to be ill. Less severely affected animals will live a week or more.

The condition is due to some form of food allergy or intoxication, and it will become progressively worse unless the animals are given a different type of feed. In some cases a definite amount of feed will produce the disease and bring about the death of the individual. As little as 150 pounds of feed will produce symptoms and even death of feeder cattle. The disease can apparently occur with all types of feed. In most cases the animals have been on a finishing ration for several weeks. The disease is observed in cattle that have consumed moldy sweet potatoes.

Jagzeikte, or Montana progressive pneumonia, has been recognized in sheep for many years. The disease occurs in sheep that are over 2 years of age and usually appears in flocks at the time they are driven or moved from one area to another. Although it is generally believed a viral agent is present in the lungs of affected sheep, there is still considerable question if the viral agent is actually the cause of the lung alterations.

Maedi, epizootic adenomatosis, and jag-zeikte are described in Iceland. There is some question as to whether these are the same disease or represent three distinct entities. The etiology has not been adequately demonstrated, although there is some evidence to indicate it is infectious.

Lungworms in sheep, particularly the *Muellerius* species, cause a chronic irritation of the lung resulting in proliferation of the septal cells. The lung of the ovine is very sensitive to mild chronic irritation and responds with hyperplasia and hypertrophy. It would appear that mild environmental stimulants found in dust or feed may be responsible for the pulmonary reaction in jagzeikte, Montana progressive pneumonia, maedi, and other adenomatous reactions of the sheep lung. The isolation of viral agents of questionable pathogenicity from the lung is to be expected since it has been well demonstrated that numerous viral agents and pleuropneumonia-like organisms can be found in most organs and especially in those tissues of the digestive and respiratory tracts. No one has satisfactorily demonstrated and described a viral agent from the lungs of sheep that reproduces the clinical disease consistently. The infectious agents isolated may be a contributing stimulant but it is doubtful if they are the basic etiologic agents. The complicated methods used in attempting to obtain infection in an environment not distantly removed from the normal location of the disease may be sufficient to produce a lung reaction and do not represent the passage of an infectious etiologic agent. The disease is not transmitted to susceptible animals when infected sheep are introduced into flocks in areas where the disease does not naturally

occur. This is additional evidence to indicate that the disease is probably not infectious, or if it is infectious, factors other than just a viral agent must be present if the disease is to be reproduced.

Pulmonary adenomatosis is observed in horses that have consumed *Crotalaria dura*. It has not been determined if other species of *Crotalaria* will produce similar lesions.

Swine affected with pleuropneumonia-like organisms and viral porcine pneumonia show a pulmonary adenomatous type of reaction. The lesion is observed primarily in the cardiac lobe, posterior portion of the apical lobe, and anterior portion of the diaphragmatci lobe. Apparently the mild stimulation produced by these organisms causes a proliferation of the septal cells.

During the past few years a serious respiratory disease known as silo-fillers disease has been observed in man. It occurs in those individuals working in the vicinity of silos from which a brown gas, primarily nitrogen dioxide, is escaping. The gas is evolved in the process of fermentation of corn silage shortly after it has been placed in the silo. After the fermentation process is complete, the silo is no longer dangerous. A similar respiratory disease is observed in men employed in feed mills and elevators where considerable feed dust is present. Similar lesions can be produced in the lungs of cattle and guinea pigs following the inhalation of nitrogen dioxide.

**Macroscopic appearance.** The principal lesions found at necropsy are quite constant whether the disease involves cattle, horses, sheep, guinea pigs, or humans. The entire lung is involved either as a diffuse alteration or as multiple focal areas of consolidation. The lungs are voluminous and do not collapse when the thoracic cavity is opened. Often the imprint of the ribs can be seen upon the lungs. The lesions are not limited to the anterior ventral portion of the lungs as is usually seen in bronchopneumonia. The involved lung tissue has a reddish-pink, slightly cyanotic appearance resembling the thymus gland in color and consistency. The degree of consolidation depends upon the length of time the animal has been ill. If the disease has been present for a considerable period of time, a complicating bronchopneumonia is sometimes observed in the anterior ventral portion of the lung. Upon incision of the lung an abundance of pink foamy fluid flows from the cut surface, indicating extensive pulmonary edema. Considerable white foam is found in the bronchi and trachea.

Portions of the lung that are not hepatized show a marked alveolar pulmonary emphysema. Interstitial pulmonary emphysema is prominent due to the over-distention of the alveoli and rupture of the alveolar walls which allows air to escape into the interstitial tissue of the lung. When the air enters the interstitial tissue it migrates to the hilus of the lung and then escapes into the mediastinum. From there, at times, it passes through the anterior thoracic inlet and appears under the skin of the neck and shoulders. Occasionally the gas follows the large vessels posteriorly and accumulates in the perirenal region.

There is an acute general passive hyperemia. The heart is slightly or moderately dilated. Both the heart and visceral alterations are due to the reduction in the area of the capillary bed in the lung and the interference with the exchange of gases.

**Microscopic appearance.** Histological examination of the lung does not reveal the acute inflammatory reaction associated with viral or bacterial diseases. Phagocytic cells are few in number unless a secondary complicating pneumonia or bronchitis is present. The outstanding lung lesion is the marked hyperplasia and hypertrophy of the septal cells. In the more advanced cases the alveolar walls are completely covered with one or more layers of septal cells, and at times the entire alveolus is filled with these cells. Many desquamated septal cells are present in the lumen of the alveoli. Alveolar and interstitial pulmonary emphysema are prominent lesions. Hyperplasia and hypertrophy of the bronchial

epithelium are usually observed. The lumen of the bronchi contains many septal cells and desquamated bronchial epithelial cells.

It is obvious that the cause of the dyspnea is due to the interference with the exchange of gases between the lumen of the alveoli and the blood vascular system. The layer or layers of septal cells lining the alveoli prevent the free exchange of gases between the lumen of the alveoli and the blood. The air is not able to enter some alveoli because they are completely filled with septal cells. The bronchial involvement interferes with the tidal air flow.

In sheep considerable fibrosis of the lung may occur since the disease usually persists over a long period of time. Fibrosis is also a prominent pulmonary reaction in the human.

Bacteriological examination of the lung does not result in the isolation of microorganisms unless a complicating bacterial infection is present.

PNEUMOCONIOSIS

**Anthracosis** occurs in city dogs and mining mules. **Chalicosis** occurs in mules and horses used in stone and lime quarries and around cement plants. Pneumoconiosis is not a serious condition. Macroscopically, there are numerous, uniformly distributed, pigmented foci. There may also be pigmented lines in the interlobular connective tissue. Microscopically, the exogenous pigment may be free in the alveoli, in macrophages, in the alveolar epithelium, in the walls of the interlobular lymph vessels, and in the peribronchial lymph nodes. In the lymph nodes it is located in the lymph cords of the medulla. There may be moderate connective tissue proliferation in the region of the peribronchial deposits.

It has been demonstrated experimentally that it is not necessary for dust particles to be phagocytized at all in order to become located within the lung tissue. Direct penetration of the alveolar lining by fine particles is possible. Physical influences which make this possible are the fluctuating pressures that occur during respiration and the constant movement of the lung tissue.

PULMONARY OSTEOARTHROPATHY

In man there is a rare disease called generalized hypertrophic osteoarthropathy which has also been reported occasionally in domestic animals, particularly in dogs. It is associated with an intrathoracic disease. In dogs the associated disease has been either pulmonary tuberculosis or primary or secondary pulmonary tumors. Skeletal changes occur which are related to the shafts of the leg bones. There is periosteal proliferation with the formation of several layers of new cortical bone. Surrounding the bony proliferations there is an accompanying fibrosis. Roentgenograms of the swollen legs and feet reveal the arthropathy. (See the chapter on the skeletal system.)

**Tumors**

Primary and secondary tumors of the lung are common. (See the chapter on neoplasms.)

**Classification of Lung Lesions According to Location**

The classification of lung lesions according to location makes it possible for lung diseases to be diagnosed on gross examination. In most instances it also indicates the probable etiology. The schematic sketches (Figs. 16.27, 16.28, and 16.29) show the basic alterations that occur in the lung.

Illustrations of hyperemia and edema are not included in the drawings. These two changes are, however, quite easily recognized. The lungs are larger than normal and are not hepatized. The pulmonary vessels are engorged with blood and the lung has a cyanotic color. When the lung is incised, blood flows from the cut surface. White foam is present in the trachea and bronchi. Samples of tissue removed from the lung will float when placed in water.

Hyperemia and edema of the lung may be unilateral or bilateral. Unilateral lesions are usually the result of the influence of gravity on the circulatory system in animals that are recumbent and remain on one side for a long period of time, or in those individuals whose cardiac output is not sufficient to maintain a blood pressure that will overcome the influence of gravity. As a result, blood accumulates in the ventral lung. The condition is usually termed hypostatic congestion.

Hypostatic congestion must be differentiated from post-mortem congestion. Post-mortem congestion occurs when the blood, under the influence of gravity, accumulates in the lung that is ventral in the dead animal. Post-mortem congestion is distinguished from hypostatic congestion by the absence of foam in the trachea and bronchi. Air must be passing through the pulmonary passages and be mixing with the edematous fluid if foam is to be produced. Since respiratory excursions are not occurring in the dead individual, no foam will be present in post-mortem congestion.

Bilateral edema and congestion of the lung occur when the influence of gravity is equal in both lungs. They are associated with cardiac failure, hypoproteinemia, exhaustion, the vascular alterations associated with shock, and the first stage of bronchopneumonia.

Drawing A (Fig. 16.27) shows the distribution of the lesion in bronchopneumonia. It is located in the anteroventral portion or the dependent portion of the lung when the animal stands and moves in a normal position. Because of the influence of gravity on the blood vascular system, passive hyperemia occurs in this portion of the lung if any impairment of circulation is present. Since there is difficulty in maintaining normal blood circulation in the ventral portion of the lung in pulmonary and cardiac diseases, it is in this portion of the lung that pneumonia is most likely to occur because the body defense mechanism is impaired by the passive hyperemia that is present. Lesions in the anteroventral portion of the lung will be found in the pneumonia associated with shipping fever, canine distemper, viral pneumoenteritis of calves, chronic heart disease, and debilitating diseases in which passive hyperemia and edema are present.

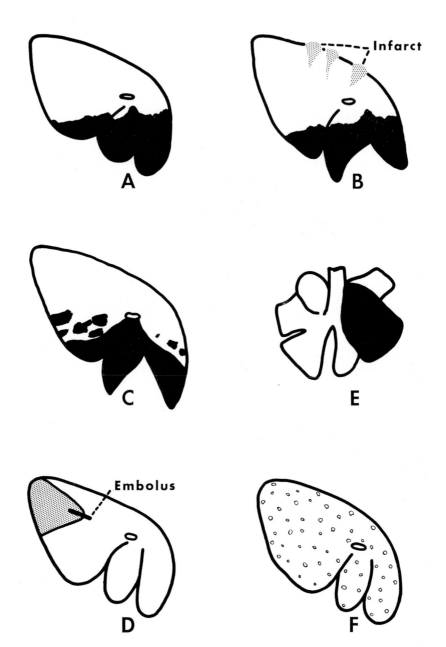

Fig. 16.27 — Classification of lung lesions.

Drawing B (Fig. 16.27) reveals the typical lung lesions of hog cholera. A bronchopneumonia is seen in the anteroventral portion of the lung. In addition, one or more red infarcts may be found in the dorsal portion of the diaphragmatic lobe of the lung. The base of the infarct will protrude above the dorsal border of the lung.

Drawing C (Fig. 16.27) depicts the type of lung lesion seen in the pneumonia associated with pleuropneumonia-like organisms in swine. The lesion suggests that an inhalation type of bronchial pneumonia is present. The infectious material coming down the trachea passes into the bronchi and then, under the influence of gravity, settles into the ventral portions of the lung immediately under the tracheal bifurcation. As a result, the pneumonia involves the entire cardiac lobe, the anteroventral portion of the diaphragmatic lobe, and the posteroventral portion of the apical lobe. Patchy areas of pneumonia may be found in the ventral portion of the lung anterior and posterior to the location described in the preceding sentence if considerable bronchitis is present. The disease spreads through the lung by bronchial extension.

Drawing D (Fig. 16.27) represents the lung alteration occurring as the result of pulmonary embolism when the embolus is large. The centripetal force of the blood carries the large embolus into the diaphragmatic lobe of the lung because the blood flow into this lobe is greatest. The embolus will be found in the pulmonary artery approximately at the junction of the posterior and middle thirds of the diaphragmatic lobe. The portion of the lung supplied by the artery is slightly reduced in volume, and the surface shows a slight depression as compared to the surrounding tissue. Infarction of the area does not occur unless the embolus is septic or pneumonia is present.

Drawing E (Fig. 16.27) shows a torsion of the right cardiac lobe of the lung of a dog. This lesion is often diagnosed as pneumonia instead of a torsion because the rotation of the lobe is overlooked.

Drawing F (Fig. 16.27) reveals the location of the lesions when the pulmonary emboli, such as bacteria or tumor cells, are small. Because of their small size, the centripetal force of the blood is not exerted and the emboli are distributed throughout the lung.

Drawing G (Fig. 16.28) shows the location of the lesions in gangrenous pneumonia as the result of inhalation or medication. The material that pours into the lung enters the ventral portions of the lung below the entrance of the bronchi into the lung. As a result, the necrotic areas will be found in the entire cardiac lobe, the anteroventral portion of the diaphragmatic lobe, and the posteroventral portion of the apical lobe.

Drawing H (Fig. 16.28) indicates the location of the suppurative or gangrenous pneumonia resulting when foreign bodies originating in the reticulum pass through the diaphragm and penetrate the lung.

Drawing I (Fig. 16.28) locates the site of the suppurative or gangrenous pneumonia when large septic emboli are carried into the lung by the blood stream.

Drawing J (Fig. 16.28) indicates the complication that may result when large septic emboli as shown in drawing I are present in the lung. The exudate from the suppurative or gangrenous lesions in the diaphragmatic lobe enters the bronchi, and under the influence of gravity it settles into the ventral portions of the lung, producing secondary suppurative or gangrenous lesions.

Drawing K (Fig. 16.28) illustrates the type of lesion seen in typical Pasteurella pneumonia or in contagious pleuropneumonia in horses and cattle. The basic lesion is a bronchopneumonia as is shown in drawing A (Fig. 16.27). In addition, throughout the area there are multiple foci of necrosis as the result of vascular damage and infarction in the area. If saprophytic organisms are present, gangrene may be the result in these necrotic areas.

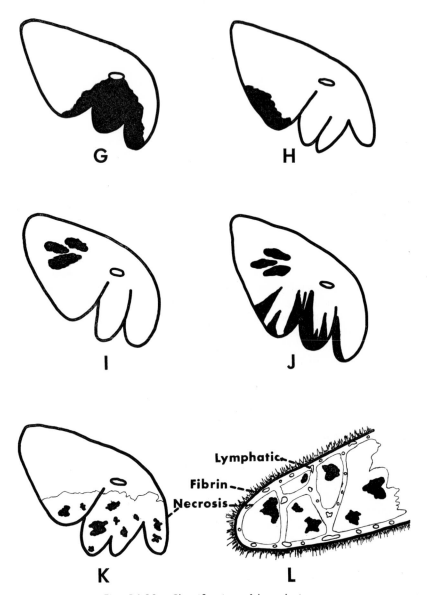

Fig. 16.28 — Classification of lung lesions.

Drawing L (Fig. 16.28) is an enlargement of a portion of a lung showing the alterations that occur in Pasteurella pneumonia or contagious pleuropneumonia of cattle and horses. Note the wide interlobular septa and pleura as the result of the exudate that has accumulated in these structures. Distended lymphatics can be seen in both the pleura and the septa. The surface of the lung is covered with a layer of fibrin.

Drawing M (Fig. 16.29) shows the type of alterations observed in the lungs infected with lungworms of the *Dictyocaulus* and *Metastrongylus* species. The parasites are located in the bronchi of the dorsoposterior portion of the diaphragmatic lobe. Because of bronchial obstruction, bronchitis, and pneumonia, V-shaped areas of alveolar emphysema intermixed with areas of atelectasis and inflammation are present.

Drawing N (Fig. 16.29) is a sketch of the posterior border of the diaphragmatic lobe showing the enlargement of the edge of the lung as the result of the alveolar pulmonary emphysema that occurs when lungworms are present as indicated in drawing M.

Drawing O (Fig. 16.29) illustrates the location of the lesions in the lungs of animals infected with *Muellerius* and *Aelurostrongylus* species of lungworms. These parasites are found in the pulmonary alveoli and the blood vessels of the lung. They are present throughout the lung but are most numerous in the diaphragmatic lobe.

Drawing P (Fig. 16.29) locates the site of the primary lesion of tuberculosis in the lung of the bovine, canine, and feline. It is found in the mid-dorsal portion of the diaphragmatic lobe.

Drawing Q (Fig. 16.29) shows the alterations that occur in pulmonary adenomatosis in cattle, sheep, and horses. The lung is larger than normal, meaty in consistency, and shows extensive areas of both alveolar and pulmonary emphysema. Multiple areas resembling foci of hepatization are scattered throughout the lung.

Frequently, a complicating bronchopneumonia is present in the anteroventral portion of the lung.

Drawing R (Fig. 16.29) represents the pulmonary atelectasis that occurs in the ventral portion of the lung when hydrothorax is present. The line between the atelectic and the normal lung is straight and horizontal in the apical lobe but is curved in the diaphragmatic lobe. This curve in the diaphragmatic lobe occurs when considerable fluid is present in the pleural cavity, and because of the buoyancy of the lung the pulmonary tissue is compressed in a dorsal direction. When the pleural fluid escapes at the time the thoracic cavity is opened at necropsy examination, the pressure on the lung is removed and the lung returns to its normal position. When the lung is observed at this time, the line between the atelectic and normal lung tissue will curve in a ventral direction.

Drawing S (Fig. 16.29) shows a cross section of the atelectic lung described in drawing R.

Drawing T (Fig. 16.29) illustrates another alteration of the lung seen in hydrothorax. As the lung floats on the pleural fluid the dorsal compression of the lung is so great that a crimping of the ventral border of the diaphragmatic lobe occurs. When the fluid pressure is released at necropsy examination, the lung returns to its normal position and the site of the crimp is indicated by a narrow area of atelectasis that extends into the diaphragmatic lobe in a dorsoanterior direction.

## PLEURA

### Abnormal Contents of the Pleural Cavity

**Abdominal viscera** may enter the cavity as a result of congenital and acquired openings in the diaphragm (diaphragmatic hernia) (Fig. 16.30). **Foreign bodies,** such as nails, pieces of bailing wire, and various other sharp metallic objects, may penetrate from the forestomachs of cattle. Penetration is usually slow; therefore, a local fibrinous pleuritis develops.

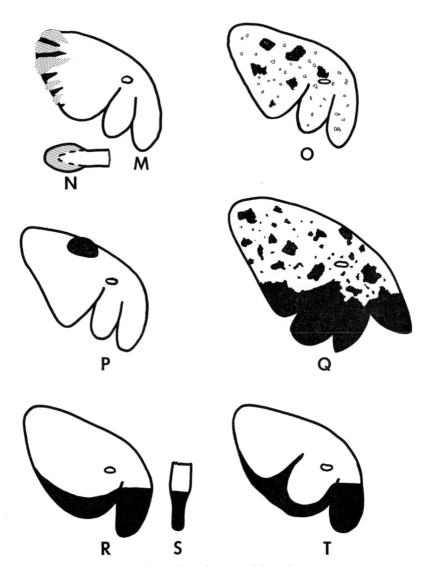

Fig. 16.29 — Classification of lung lesions.

Later the body may become encapsulated. **Air (pneumothorax)** may result from trauma of the thorax (fractured ribs), trauma of the lungs (foreign bodies penetrating from the forestomachs), spontaneous perforation of the lung (rupture of an abscess in the lungs). **Fluid (hydrothorax):** see circulatory disturbances. **Blood (hemothorax)** usually results from trauma. **Pus (pyothorax):** see suppurative pleuritis.

## Circulatory Disturbances

**Hemorrhages.** Petechiae of the pleura appear in some acute septicemic diseases (hog cholera, anthrax, pasteurellosis) and in purpura hemorrhagica. Their location is in the subserous tissue. Large collections of blood (hemothorax) are usually due to trauma. **Hydrothorax** is a collection of clear, pale yellow fluid in the pleural cavity in the absence of inflammatory

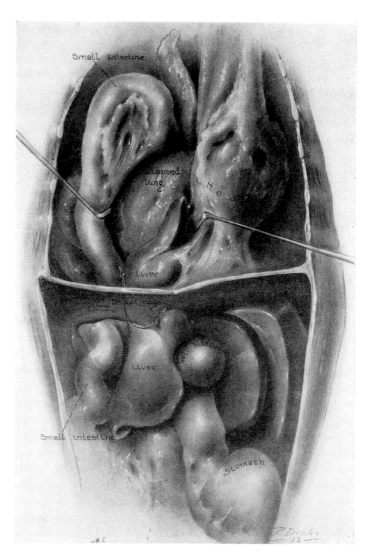

Fig. 16.30 — Abdominal viscera of a 1-year-old fox terrier in thoracic cavity (diaphragmatic hernia). (J. G. Hardenbergh, Jour. A.V.M.A.)

changes. The fluid is a transudate from the vessels. It is seen in connection with chronic passive hyperemia due to chronic heart, lung, and kidney diseases or general hydremia as occurs in liverfluke and stomachworm infestations of sheep.

### Pleuritis

Pleuritis in general is caused by the same traumatic and infectious agents as pneumonia. The infections reach the pleura by the extension of pneumonia to the pleura or by hematogenic introduction as in some of the acute septicemic diseases. The course may be acute or chronic.

#### SEROUS, SEROFIBRINOUS, AND FIBRINOUS PLEURITIS

These forms of pleuritis occur in equine contagious pneumonia, calf pneumonia, hog cholera, swine influenza, canine distemper, fowl cholera, and pasteurellosis. Macroscopically, there are varying quantities of serous fluid containing fibrin flocculi. The fluid may cause compression atelectasis. The pleura is rough, lusterless, and dry. It seems paradoxical to say that the pleura is dry when it has already been stated that in the pleural cavity there is a variable amount of serous fluid. The condition of dryness is more apparent than real. The appearance of dryness is due to the presence of fibrin upon the parietal and visceral pleura. The maximum amounts of fluid reported are: horse, 15 to 20 liters; dog, $\frac{1}{2}$ to 5; swine, 2 to 10. Microscopically, the serous membrane in serous pleuritis remains intact. In the fibrinous form it disappears. In all forms the propria is edematous and the subpleural vessels are dilated. In the fibrinous form, the fibrinous exudate is rich in leukocytes. The termination of the serous and fibrinous forms is either by absorption of the serous exudate and of the fibrin which is digested by the leukocytic enzymes followed by regeneration of the serous membrane, or by organization of the exudate with the formation of adhesions between the visceral and parietal pleurae if the exudate is so extensive that it cannot be liquefied and absorbed.

#### SUPPURATIVE PLEURITIS

A diffuse form results from an extension of suppurative pneumonia to the pleura. A focal form is seen mostly in pigs in the region of pulmonary abscesses caused by *Corynebacterium pyogenes*. Small encapsulated abscesses containing pale green pus appear on the pleura.

## REFERENCES

Baker, J. A.: 1942. A filtrable virus from pneumonia and diarrhea of calves. Cornell Vet., 32:202.

——: 1944. A virus causing pneumonia in cats and producing elementary bodies. Jour. Exper. Med., 79:159.

Biberstein, E. L., and Kennedy, P. C.: 1959. Septicemic pasteurellosis in lambs. Amer. Jour. Vet. Res., 20:94.

Boidin, A. G., Cordy, D. R., and Adler, H. E.: 1958. A pleuropneumonia-like organism and a virus in ovine pneumonia in California. Cornell Vet., 48:410.

Carter, G. R., and Schroder, J. D.: 1956. Virus pneumonia of pigs with special reference to the role of pleuropneumonia-like organisms Cornell Vet., 46:344.

Cole, C. R.: 1946. Changes in the equine larynx associated with laryngeal hemiplegia. Amer. Jour. Vet. Res., 7: Part I, 69.

DeMonbreun, W. A.: 1937. The histopathology of natural and experimental canine distemper. Amer. Jour. Path., 13:187.

Doll, E. R., Bryans, J. T., McCollum, W. H., and Crowe, M. E. W.: 1957. Isolation of a filtrable agent causing arteritis of horses and abortion by mares. Its differentiation from equine abortion (influenza) virus. Cornell Vet., 47:3.

Dunkin, G. W., and Laidlaw, P. P.: 1926. Studies in dog distemper. II. Experimental distemper in the dog. Jour. Comp. Path. and Therap., 39:213.

Findlay, G. M., MacKenzie, R. D., and Stern, R. O.: 1937. The histopathology of fowl pest. Jour. Path. and Bact., 45:589.

Gillespie, J. H., McEntee, K., Kendrick, J. W., and Wagner, W. C.: 1959. Comparison of infectious pustular vulvovaginitis with infectious bovine rhinotracheitis virus. Cornell Vet., 49:287.

Graham, W. R.: 1953. The pathology of shipping fever in feedlot cattle. Jour. A.V.M.A., 123:198.

Hagen, K. W.: 1958. Enzootic pasteurellosis in domestic rabbits. I. Pathology and bacteriology. Jour. A.V.M.A., 133:77.

Hennigar, G. R., and Ferguson, R. W.: 1957. Pulmonary vascular sclerosis as a result of *Dirofilaria immitis* infection in dogs. Jour. A.V.M.A., 131:336.

Hofstad, M. S.: 1945. A study of infectious bronchitis in chickens. I-III. Cornell Vet., 35:22.

Jensen, R., Griner, L. A., Chow, T. L., and Brown, W. W.: 1955. Infectious rhinotracheitis in feedlot cattle. I. Pathology and symptoms. Proc. 55th Meet. U.S. Livestock Sanit. Assn., 189.

——, Griner, L. A., Chow, T. L., and Brown, W. W.: 1955. The pathology of rhinotracheitis of cattle. Proc. 55th Meet. U.S. Livestock Sanit. Assn., 189 and 199.

Jungherr, E., and Minard, E. L.: 1944. The pathology of experimental avian pneumoencephalitis. Amer. Jour. Vet. Res., 5:125.

——: 1949. The pathology of experimental sinusitis of turkeys. Amer. Jour. Vet. Res., 10:372.

Langham, R. F., Thorp, F., Ingle, R. T., and Scholl, L. B.: 1942. Some observations on the pathology of pneumonia in the food-producing animals. Amer. Jour. Vet. Res., 3:139.

Larin, N. M.: 1959. "Nervous distemper" in dogs. I. Its features and experimental transmission. Vet. Rec., 71:447.

Lillie, R. D., Francis, E., and Parker, R. R.: 1936. The pathology of tularemia. Nat. Inst. Health, Bul. 167.

MacKenzie, A.: 1959. Studies on lungworm infection of pigs. III. The progressive pathology of experimental infections. Vet. Rec., 71:209.

Madin, S. H., York, C. J., and McKercher, D. G.: 1956. Isolation of the infectious bovine rhinotracheitis virus. Science, 124:721.

Maurer, F. D., Jones, T. C., Easterday, B., and DeTray, D.: 1955. The pathology of rinderpest. Proc. Book, A.V.M.A., 201.

Orcutt, M. L., and Shope, R. E.: 1935. The distribution of swine influenza virus in swine. Jour. Exper. Med., 62:623.

Pattison, I. H.: 1956. A histological study of a transmissable pneumonia of pigs characterized by extensive lymphoid hyperplasia. Vet. Rec., 68:490.

Schwartz, B., and Alicata, J. E.: 1932. Ascaris larvae as a cause of liver and lung lesions in swine. Jour. Parasit., 19:17.

Seifried, O.: 1931. Histopathology of infectious laryngotracheitis in chickens. Jour. Exper. Med., 54:817.

Shope, R. E.: 1931. Swine influenza. I. Experimental transmission and pathology. Jour. Exper. Med., 54:349.

Simpson, C. F., Wade, A. E., Dennis, W. R., and Swanson, L. E.: 1957. Pathological changes associated with *Dictyocaulus viviparus* infections in calves. Amer. Jour. Vet. Res., 18:747.

Stamp, J. T., Watt, J. A. A., and Thomlinson, J. R.: 1955. *Pasteurella haemolytica* septicaemia of lambs. Jour. Comp. Path. and Therap., 65:183.

Stenius, P. I.: 1952. Bovine malignant catarrh. A statistical histopathological and experimental study. Inst. Path., Vet. Coll., Helsinki, Finland, and State Vet. Med. Inst., Stockholm, Sweden.

Thompson, W. W., and Fabian, F. W.: 1932. Molds in the respiratory tract of chickens. Jour. A.V.M.A., 33:921.

Underdahl, N. R., and Kelley, G. W.: 1957. The enhancement of virus pneumonia of pigs by the migration of *Ascaris suum* larvae. Jour. A.V.M.A., 130:173.

Van Roekel, H., Gray, J. E., Shipkowitz, N. L., Clarke, M. K., and Luchini, R. M.: 1957. Chronic respiratory disease complex: Etiology and pathology. Mass. Agr. Exper. Sta. Bul., 486:61.

Wharton, D. R. A., and Wharton, M. W.: 1934. Canine distemper: The disease and nature of the virus. Amer. Jour. Hyg., 19:189.

# CHAPTER 17

# Digestive System

## FUNCTIONAL DISTURBANCES

Diseases of the various parts of the oral cavity interfere with prehension, mastication, and insalivation of food. Undernourishment of the animal is associated with these conditions if they persist long enough. Since mastication stimulates the flow of gastric secretion, a hindrance to the proper chewing of food leads to diminished stomach secretions. Poorly masticated food contains an insufficient quantity of secretion and must remain longer in the stomach to become saturated with fluid. This favors fermentation and putrefaction. Masticatory movements mechanically cleanse the oral cavity of mucus and bacteria. Inhibition of these movements permits a profuse growth of organisms capable of producing acid fermentation in the oral cavity. Dental tartar, dental caries, stomatitis, and pharyngitis occur more often in connection with this type of bacterial flora. Salivation or ptyalism is a functional disturbance occurring in some forms of stomatitis such as appear in foot-and-mouth disease and in poisonings such as mercurialism, iodism, plumbism in cattle, and fagopyrism. In these cases the disturbed function is a result of direct or indirect nerve irritation. Salivation also occurs in paralysis or partial paralysis of the lips and of the pharynx as is seen in encephalitis and in rabies. In these diseases the condition is due to inability to retain saliva in the mouth or to swallow.

Diseases of the pharynx, like diseases of the mouth, interfere with food consumption and lead to undernourishment. Because the paths of food and air conduction cross in the pharynx, this organ is often the seat of origin of serious pathologic conditions in the lower respiratory organs. These processes owe their development to disturbed function of the epiglottis which may arise from alterations in its structure. Failure to function permits food and drink to be aspirated into the lower air passages and lungs, resulting in tracheitis or gangrenous pneumonia.

Diseases of the esophagus of rather long standing disturb nutrition because of their effect on deglutition. Often, though, pathological processes involving the esophagus have more alarming effects. Large collections of food in the esophagus causing choke, or food accumulating as a result of paralysis of this organ, may press upon and cause paralysis of the vagus nerve. Furthermore, the accumulated food, by exerting pressure, acts as a physical irritant, and by its fermentation acts as a chemical irritant, causing inflammation. There is then the possibility of rupture of the esophagus. Rupture of the organ allows the escape of food and drink into the surrounding tissues or even directly into the thoracic cavity. Suppuration and putrefaction then lead to the death of the animal.

In ruminants, partial or complete obstruction of the esophagus, either by processes inside or outside the organ, interfere with regurgitation of the food boluses and eructation of gas. The result is a gaseous or tympanitic distension of the forestomachs, particularly of the rumen.

In ruminants, especially in cattle, functional disturbances of the reticulum and rumen are of frequent occurrence and of prime importance. The reasons for this are that these two organs serve as very necessary maceration and fermentation tanks in the digestion of cellulose. The reticulum has been designated the "starter" tank because it is filled with a fluid medium containing beneficial bacteria and protozoa — a fluid which flushes each bolus before it enters the cardia at the beginning of the regurgitation process. Upon the return of the bolus to the rumen this organ functions as the fermentation tank. The bacteria and protozoa in it digest about 60 to 90 per cent of the roughage consumed by an animal.

Cellulose digestion is only a part of the contribution made by these microorganisms in the digestive process. They themselves constitute about 10 per cent of the dry matter in the rumen. For their own use they synthesize most of the essential amino acids and many of the vitamins. When these microorganisms pass from the rumen to the intestine, the animal appropriates these necessary nutrients for its own use.

Another contribution to the nutrition of the animal is made by the by-products of ruminal fermentation — three short-chain, volatile fatty acids: acetic, propionic, and butyric. A large part of these is absorbed by the rumen mucosa and then utilized as nutrients by the animal. The proper removal of these acids by absorption reduces the acidity of the rumen contents, this reduction being necessary for the optimum growth of the desirable bacteria and pro-

tozoa. The acidity is further reduced by the neutralizing action of the large amounts of the alkaline saliva which reach the rumen. The pH of the rumen contents is kept at approximately 7. If, for any reason, bacterial and protozoan digestion ceases and saliva continues to flow, the rumen contents become alkaline. As soon as the alkalinity reaches pH 7.5, contractions of the rumen cease. From a review of the foregoing functional activities of the rumen, one realizes that in health there must be a balance among the several factors involved, i.e., (1) the quantity and quality of the bacterial and protozoan populations must be optimum; (2) suitable and adequate nutrients (carbohydrates, nitrogen, minerals, and water) to support these microorganisms must be supplied in the ration of the animal; (3) the bacteria, protozoa, and medium for their growth must be thoroughly mixed by efficient ruminal muscular contractions; (4) there must be no hindrance to prehension, mastication, insalivation, deglutition, or regurgitation; (5) gases formed by fermentation must be eructated; and (6) volatile fatty acids must be absorbed. Functional disturbances arise whenever the balance is upset by (1) disease of any of the organs or parts which participate in the total process, (2) inadequate intake of food and water, (3) innutritious food, (4) excessive consumption of food, (5) sudden change of food, and (6) intake of drugs or chemicals which kill or inhibit the growth of the desirable bacteria and protozoa.

Overdistention with food (impaction) and dilatation with gas (tympanites or bloat) are two common disturbances of the rumen. When they occur, the functions of other organs are simultaneously affected. Pressure upon the other abdominal viscera, the diaphragm, and the thoracic organs interferes with both circulation and respiration, and may terminate in death by asphyxia. There is a possibility also that prior to death the rumen or the diaphragm may rupture.

In the simple stomach, pathologic processes do two things, principally, to the normal activities of the organ. They (1) hinder its movements, and (2) affect the quantity and quality of its secretions. Some of the disease conditions which involve the stomach act over a period of time long enough to cause an atony of the gastric musculature. When this happens, the stomach movements become weak, and food is not mixed thoroughly with fluid. In the horse, dog, and pig, where the food is said to accumulate in layers one above the other, this movement, of course, may not be so important in this respect. In animals such as the ruminants, where kneading movements are important, atony results in insufficient mixing and maceration. These ingesta become a suitable medium for the growth of fermentative and putrefactive bacteria. The excessive amount of gas formed distends the stomachs and must be expelled by eructation or by passage posteriorly.

Accumulation of food in the stomach hinders its movements and has a similar effect on respiration and circulation as does alimental dilatation of the forestomachs in ruminants. It has the added effect that in the dilated simple stomach the secretions are inhibited. The reason is that the stretching and compression of the blood vessels and glands disturb their functions.

The movements of the stomach are increased in force when there are hindrances to the passage of food through the pylorus. Increased movements also occur when chemical substances stimulate the nerves of the gastric mucosa or its musculature either directly or indirectly. The powerful contractions force the contents into the intestine, or the diaphragm and abdominal muscles are brought into play and vomition occurs.

It was stated above that diseases of the stomach not only interfere with its movements but also with the character of its secretions. A change in the chemical reaction of the gastric contents to neutrality or alkalinity due to a reduction in hydrochloric acid favors the growth of fermentative and putrefactive bacteria. The prod-

ucts of the action of these microorganisms are irritating to the gastric mucosa and cause gastritis. An excess of hydrochloric acid produces a hyperacidity which is characterized by gastric pain and vomiting.

In the intestine various saprophytic and commensal bacteria, yeasts, molds, fungi, and protozoa are always present. Many of them are helpful in the digestion of food. Under normal conditions they are not injurious because the healthy epithelium is a barrier to them. In addition, the acid reaction in the first part of the intestine keeps their number to a minimum. In the posterior parts of the intestine the action of bile makes conditions unfavorable for their growth in numbers sufficient to harm the animal. Furthermore, the normal rate of passage of ingesta and feces through the intestinal canal does not permit long contact between the organisms and the epithelium. Besides these factors there may be other means of defense against the entrance of these microorganisms into the mucosa.

When conditions prevent the normal passage of the contents along the intestine or when the mucosa is injured, these saprophytes and commensal microorganisms may invade the tissues. It is possible that these organisms prepare the way for their own entrance. It may be that when conditions are suitable for their superabundant growth, their products of fermentation, such as lactic, butyric, and acetic acid, and such gases as hydrogen sulfide and methane, may injure the epithelium, especially in very young animals. Through these injuries the organisms may be able to pass.

Absorption of the digested food is hindered by alterations in the intestinal mucosa, especially if the changes are diffuse. When the tissue changes are localized and not too numerous, sufficient absorption can take place in the normal areas between the lesions. Absorption is also restricted when peristalsis is increased because the digested food is not in contact with the mucosa sufficiently long. If the increased peristalsis takes place along the whole course of the intestines or only in the colon, the fecal material becomes thin and watery due to deficient absorption. Such accelerated peristalsis is incited by a stimulation of the sensory nerves of the intestinal mucosa and transfer of the stimulus to the motor nerves of the intestinal musculature. With the increased movements of the intestine there is practically always a hypersecretion of the intestinal glands and a transudation from the capillaries of the mucosa. Local irritants of various kinds which will be mentioned later may do this. Continued hindrance to absorption from the large intestine results in emaciation and general tissue dehydration.

It has already been stated that absorption from the intestine is interfered with when there are lesions in the intestinal wall that restrict absorption and when increased peristalsis hurries the ingesta along so rapidly that absorption is incomplete. Incomplete as the absorption of nutrient material is, enough toxic substances which are produced within the diseased intestine may be absorbed so that the animal will suffer from an intoxication. Furthermore, there may be a loss of blood from the intestinal lesions great enough to give rise to a general anemia. All of these factors may combine to cause the death of the animal.

The passage of ingesta and feces through the intestine may be retarded or completely prevented by several factors which may operate in the lumen of an intestine, in its wall, or even outside of the tube. Insufficiently masticated and insalivated food, food of poor quality or unsuitable for the species or age of the animal, food not moistened with sufficient fluid, general fatigue, chilling, excitement, and other factors are important in this connection. The retardation of the passage of intestinal contents may be due to a narrowing or complete closure of the intestinal lumen by foreign bodies, tumors, enlarged mesenteric lymph nodes, scars, adhesions, and various types of intestinal displacements. When the closure occurs suddenly, the functions of the intestine are disturbed similarly as they are in gaseous and alimental distention of the simple stomach and the intestine. In addition to these changes, others of a more profound nature occur in the intestinal displacements. They owe their character to serious circulatory disturbances which arise in the displaced portion of the intestine. Regardless of the type of intestinal malposition, the underlying tissue changes are similar because the vascular changes which initiate them are of the same nature. These vascular changes consist of either a twisting or a pinching of the vessels in the displaced intestine. Since the effect of this torsion or pressure closes the lumen of the thin-walled veins more than that of the thicker-walled arteries, blood is forced into the displaced portion faster than it can be removed. The chain of results which then occurs in the displaced intestine is: hyperemia with edema and hemorrhage, malnutrition of the tissues, and retention of metabolites leading to degeneration and death of the cells, and possibly to putrefaction of them by saprophytes in the ingesta in the lumen. Death occurs from loss of blood in the area, absorption of toxic material from the abdominal cavity, inflammation of the peritoneum, and shock.

When the closure of the intestinal lumen occurs gradually, chronic alimental dilatation takes place anteriorly to the stenosis. Accompanying the dilatation there is a compensatory hypertrophy of the muscle coats of the distended portion of the intestine.

Pressure upon the nerves of the intestinal mucosa and wall either from within or without stimulates powerful muscular contractions in the intestine. When the pressure is continued, the smooth muscle tires and paresis occurs. Some chemical substances in the intestinal contents have a similar action. The resultant spasmodic movements may be reversed so that ingesta and even feces may be forced forward into the stomach. When this occurs in swine or dogs, the animals may vomit intestinal contents. In the horse this anti-peristalsis may result in gastric rupture.

Strong muscular spasms of the intestine are associated with excruciating pain, the so-called colicky pain. The pain is believed to be due to stretching of the sensory nerves of the intestine. Much of the pain may originate in the nerves of the mesentery which are pulled upon when long sections of the intestine contract. Pain is also prominent when the nerves of dilated portions of the intestine are stretched.

## MOUTH AND PHARYNX

### Stomatitis and Pharyngitis

The prevalence of inflammation of the oral cavity and pharynx among domestic animals is fairly common, yet of remarkably less frequency than would be surmised when considering the nature of much of the food and the eating habits of some of the species. As with rhinitis and pneumonia, stomatitis and pharyngitis may be of primary or secondary occurrence. In the first case, the irritant enters the mouth directly from the outside world and injures the oral mucosa. In the second case, the inflammation in the mouth is a partial manifestation of a more general disease.

Physical influences which cause stomatitis and pharyngitis are most commonly traumatic in character. Depending upon the species of animal affected, the objects producing the trauma may be awns, spines, barbs, and thorns of plants, slivers of wood, broken glass, discarded razor blades, pieces of corn cobs wedged into the roof of the mouth, accumulations of dental tartar, rubber bands around the tongue, pieces of wire caught in the teeth, harsh bits and war bridles, and sharp teeth and instruments. A physical influence less commonly the cause of stomatitis and pharyngitis is heat. Occasionally, animals are drenched with liquid food or stimulants sufficiently hot to produce some degree of burn in the mouth.

Chemical substances that produce inflammation in the anterior part of the digestive tract are some of the caustic alkalis, and corrosive acids and their salts which animals may get accidentally or which may be used as medicinal agents in a too concentrated form. Among these chemical irritants belong certain acrid substances of some plants which may be eaten at times when forage is scarce. Not only do stomatitis and pharyngitis originate from the direct action of chemical substances on the oral mucosa, but also from the withholding from the diet of other chemical agents which are necessary for the maintenance of a healthy oral epithelium. These two substances are vitamin A and nicotinic acid (niacin).

A third group of irritants which cause stomatitis and pharyngitis are the microorganisms. The list includes bacteria, viruses, yeasts, and molds. Many of the bacteria are filth-borne, that is, they are ones that are omnipresent in the insanitary surroundings of animals. Some of these are *Spherophorus necrophorus, Pseudomonas aeruginosa, Escherichia coli, Corynebacterium pyogenes*, staphylococci, and streptococci. Others, such as *Actinomyces bovis* and *Actinobacillus lignieresi*, are linked up principally with the eating of straw of rye and barley. Viruses which fall into this group are those of foot-and-mouth disease, vesicular stomatitis, rinderpest, and fowl diphtheria. Two yeasts in particular have been reported principally in stomatitis of chickens, i.e., *Monilia albicans* and *Oidium pullorum*. Molds, rusts, and mildew in damaged forage have also been incriminated as causal agents.

### CATARRHAL STOMATITIS

The primary form is due to traumatic, thermic, chemic, and infectious agents. The secondary form occurs in other diseases such as catarrhal gastritis and specific infectious diseases. Macroscopically, the mucous membrane, chiefly in the region of the soft palate and pharynx, is reddened and swollen diffusely or in irregular streaks or patches. The tongue papillae are enlarged. The tonsils and lymph follicles of the mucosa are swollen. Due to the occlusion of the mouths of mucous glands, small glassy retention cysts rise above the surface. Grayish-white or brownish-gray adhesive exudate appears on the tongue and in the recesses of the mouth and pharynx. It is sometimes mixed with food. A fetid odor is due to bacterial decomposition. Microscopically, there are hyperemia, edema, and leukocytosis of the mucosa. There is also desquamation of the epithelium. An exudate of mucus, leukocytes, desquamated epithelial cells, bacteria, together with food particles, lies upon the mucosa. Crypts of the tonsils are filled with plugs of exudate consisting of desquamated epithelial cells, leukocytes, and bacteria.

## VESICULAR STOMATITIS

Vesicular stomatitis occurs mostly in horses and cattle. Etiologically, thermic, chemic, and infectious agents are important. This form of stomatitis is seen in foot-and-mouth disease, infectious vesicular stomatitis, and in infectious vesicular exanthema. These specific forms are differentiated from the others epidemiologically. Macroscopically, vesicles appear in the mucosa of the lips, tongue, gums, dental pad, and hard palate. Their size varies from 1 to 2 millimeters to $2\frac{1}{2}$ centimeters and larger. They are filled with clear, serous exudate which is the result of hydropic degeneration. The overlying covering of epithelium breaks and leaves a hyperemic eroded surface over which the epithelium regenerates rapidly (Fig. 17.1).

**Foot-and-mouth disease,** or aphthous fever, is an acute, highly contagious viral disease of cloven-footed animals, characterized by the formation of vesicles and erosions on the mucous membranes and skin (mouth, interdigital spaces, udder). The disease is caused by *Hostis pecoris*, which can produce the experimental disease in dilutions of one to ten million. In the initial stages of the disease the virus is present in the blood. It is always present in the lymph of the vesicles. Three types of the virus have been found in Europe.

The virus may reach the epithelium in the region in which it localizes either by direct contact or by way of the blood stream. In either case, the manner in which the changes are produced is the same. Two to 7 days after the virus enters the epithelium, **vesicles** (Fig. 17.2) and **erosions** develop in this manner: The epithelial cells in foci begin to enlarge and undergo hydropic degeneration. The intercellular bridges disappear, and the cells consequently become loosened from one another. Their nuclei become pyknotic. Separation of the epithelium is aided by edematous fluid arising from the hyperemic vessels of the papillae of the skin.

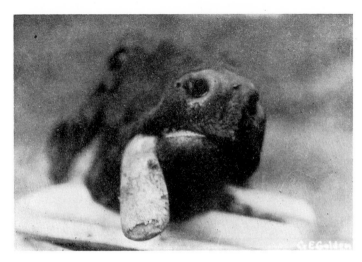

Fig. 17.1 — Foot-and-mouth disease. Erosion at tip of tongue. (Golden, Jour. A.V.M.A.)

Adjacent foci, thus filled with edema and with fluid arising from cells undergoing hydropic degeneration, fuse to form small vesicles. Small vesicles coalesce to form larger ones. Internal pressure of the vesicles becomes great and the superficial

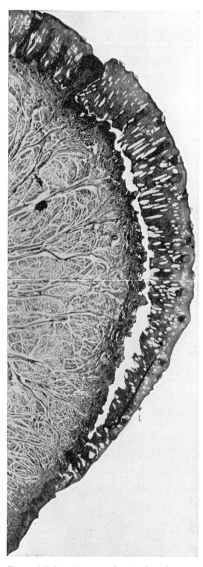

Fig. 17.2 — Foot-and-mouth disease vesicle in glossal epithelium of a cow. Papilla acts as an anchor for the epithelium at one end of vesicle. ×7.5. (Tissue, Rosenbusch; photo, Benbrook and Sloss.)

covering becomes increasingly thinner and also soft due to excessive amounts of saliva. These factors, coupled with attempts at mastication or with the characteristic smacking movements of the mouth which occur during this disease, result in rupture of the vesicles and the formation of erosions (Fig. 17.1) which heal in 5 to 8 days.

Besides the vesicles and erosions in the mouth, on the teats, and in the interdigital spaces (Fig. 17.3), there may be acute catarrhal inflammation of the respiratory and digestive systems. The vesicles develop almost simultaneously and rupture within 24 hours. Secondary pyogenic infection usually complicates the foot lesions. As a result, ulcers are frequent.

**Vesicular stomatitis** is a rather benign, acute viral disease of horses, cattle, and swine, characterized by the formation in the buccal mucosa of vesicles which rupture in a short time leaving in their places reddened erosions. It is caused by a filter-passing virus, *Hostis equinus,* which occurs in the blood during the whole course of the disease. Two types of the virus have been found in the United States.

The pathogenesis is probably not materially different from that of foot-and-mouth disease, except that the virus of vesicular stomatitis has a selectivity only for the buccal mucosa (occasionally for the skin on the teats and around the feet of cows). The virus produces small, reddened patches on the buccal mucosa at first, especially on the tongue. These are quickly followed by grayish-red vesicles, varying in size from a dime to a dollar. They are filled with a clear or yellowish hydropic fluid. Several may coalesce to form a large vesicle. They rupture in a very short time, leaving reddened erosions. Several of these may become confluent and result in large, irregular-shaped, eroded patches. Healing with regeneration of the epithelium occurs rather quickly (8 to 15 days). The period of incubation is usually 2 to 5 days.

**Vesicular exanthema of swine,** caused by *Hostis exanthematis,* is an acute, self-limiting, viral disease characterized by the formation of vesicles on the snout, in the nostrils, on the lips and oral mucosa, or between the digits of the feet, around the coronary band, on the footpads, and on the skin of the dewclaws. In sows nursing pigs, the vesicles occur on the teats. These lesions are preceded and accompanied by fever. The vesicles soon rupture to form erosions which usually heal rapidly.

The disease made its appearance in the United States in California in 1932 but has occurred in several other states. Practically every outbreak has begun in garbage-fed pigs.

The disease is communicable as a result of direct infection; only slightly by indirect infection. Cattle, sheep, goats, and guinea pigs are not susceptible to the virus, and horses only slightly, even by artificial inoculation. The period of incubation by artificial infection is on the average about 48 hours.

The lesions of vesicular exanthema of swine are confined to three parts of the body: (1) oral mucosa, including the snouts and nostrils, (2) feet, including the dewclaws, (3) teats of sows nursing pigs.

The lesions begin as vesicles varying in size from 2 to 3 mm. in diameter up to those large enough to cover the top of the snout or a whole footpad. A succession of vesicles may occur so that the last ones appear as late as 96 hours after the first. The vesicles develop in the stratum malpighii. At an early stage the lesion has a center of cellular debris floating in serous fluid. Around this center the epithelial cells are necrotic but maintain their normal position, but outside this zone the cells are ballooned (hydropic degeneration), the intercellular bridges are stretched, and fluid is present between the cells. Neighboring vesicles coalesce. There are no inclusion bodies. The vesicles soon rupture and form erosions which heal rapidly unless they become infected with pyogenic bacteria. The lesions may occur in only one place or in all the places where they usually develop.

Swine on concrete feeding floors frequently have excessive wear of the hoof and, as a result, they become extremely sore-footed, are lame, and show locomotor disturbances somewhat similar to those observed in vesicular exanthema.

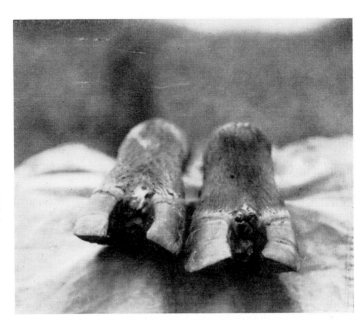

Fig. 17.3 — Foot-and-mouth disease. Slough of skin on coronary band, the result of ruptured vesicles. (Golden, Jour. A.V.M.A.)

## ULCERATIVE STOMATITIS

Ulcerative stomatitis results from trauma (foreign bodies, sharp teeth, dental tartar, sharp instruments) and chemicals (acids, alkalis, corrosive salts). In cattle and sheep in California the awns of yellow bristle grass (*Setaria lutescens*) cause serious ulcerative stomatitis. Penetration of the barbs into the dorsal surface of the tongue and into the dental pad and lower gums results in deep ulcers in the mucosa and underlying tissues. The craters of the ulcers contain cell debris surrounded by young granulation tissue which is infiltrated by leukocytes. Plant barbs may penetrate deeply into the floor of the ulcers. Ulcerative stomatitis may complicate catarrhal stomatitis or appear in connection with diseases of the digestive organs or with specific infectious diseases (foot-and-mouth, vesicular stomatitis, fowl pox, canine distemper). In cattle there are three diseases which clinically have oral erosions and ulcers that appear identical. They are viral diarrhea, mucosal disease, and infectious ulcerative stomatitis.

Ulcerative stomatitis appears also as a lesion of nicotinic acid deficiency (black tongue) in dogs, and A-avitaminosis (nutritional roup) in chickens and poults.

The lesions consist of erosions and ulcers. The erosions consist of a circumscribed loss of epithelium. Therefore, they are superficial. The ulcers involve the propria and submucosa and are therefore deep. Macroscopically, the ulcers are round, oval, or irregular, ragged areas varying in size from a pinhead to a 5-cent piece, at times larger. Their base is reddened or covered with white epithelial shreds. Microscopically, the base and margin of the ulcer are hyperemic and infiltrated with leukocytes. Erosions heal by regeneration of the epithelium, but ulcers heal by the formation of scar tissue.

## FIBRINOUS AND NECROTIC STOMATITIS AND PHARYNGITIS

In veterinary literature these forms are frequently considered under the heading diphtheritic inflammation. The reason is that the two forms are often combined and have the appearance of a false membrane. This form consists of a superficial or deep inflammation, rarely diffuse, usually circumscribed, characterized by a dirty grayish-yellow, grayish-white, or gray, dry membranous deposit upon the mucous membrane, the nature and cause of which are varied. At times it is characterized principally by epithelial necrosis and fibrin formation on the mucous membrane (fibrinous or croupous stomatitis); at other times by more or less deep coagulative necrosis of the mucous membrane with more marked fibrin formation (fibrinonecrotic or diphtheritic or diphtheroid stomatitis); at still other times by pure necrosis without fibrin formation (necrotic stomatitis).

Fibrinous and fibrinonecrotic stomatitis occur alone or in combination. The fibrinonecrotic form frequently follows the fibrinous. In calves, lambs, foals, and pigs the cause is often *Corynebacterium pyogenes* and *Spherophorus necrophorus;* in chickens two yeastlike fungi, *Monilia albicans* and *Oidium pullorum*. In rinderpest and in fowl diphtheria it is a filtrable virus; in black tongue of dogs, a deficiency of niacin. In malignant catarrhal fever the cause is now believed to be a filtrable virus. Microscopically, the exudate consists of a fibrinous network in the meshes of which are leukocytes and necrotic epithelium. The exudate is often in layers. The propria of the mucosa is infiltrated with inflammatory exudate. If the inflammation is more severe, the mucosa becomes necrotic and infiltrated with fibrin.

Necrotic stomatitis is caused by thermic, chemic, and bacterial agents. Macroscopically, alkalis and acids produce necrotic areas that vary somewhat in color, depending upon the agent. These irritants penetrate more deeply in the mucosa of the pharynx. Sloughing of the necrotic tissue leaves erosions and ulcers which heal, leaving a scar. Similar changes may occur in the esophagus and stomach. *Spherophorus necrophorus* is the most frequent bacterial cause in calves (so-called diphtheria), pigs (necrotic stomatitis), and sheep (lip and leg ulcerations) (Figs. 17.4, 17.5, 22.4). A necrotic tonsilitis is of rather common occurrence among pigs. It is usually associated with the penetration of oat hulls and grain beards into the crypts of the tonsils and an infection with streptococci.

On the edges of the tongue, inner surface of the cheeks, on the gums, sometimes on the palate, pharynx, and tonsils are single or multiple, sharply circumscribed, dirty, grayish-red or grayish-yellow, firm, dry, cheesy foci which are very variable in size. They extend deeply into the underlying tissue, have a reddish border, and later a granulating base. If the necrosed tissue sloughs off, a deep ulcer with a granulating base results. This may heal, leaving a scar. Necrotic stomatitis and pharyngitis may give rise to lesions in other parts of the body. Microscopically, the necrophorus infection shows coagulative necrosis of the cells. The necrotic area either contains no fibrin at all or only a little. At the margin of the necrotic area is a zone of inflam-matory reaction (leukocytic infiltration and fibroblastic proliferation). Numerous necrophorus organisms are present at the margin of the living tissue.

**Calf diphtheria.** This form of necroba-cillosis is an ulcerative inflammation of the oral and pharyngeal mucosa of nursing calves, which often occurs as a stable infection and is usually fatal.

On the borders of the tongue, inner surfaces of the cheeks, on the gums, sometimes on the soft palate, and especially on the pharynx, larynx, and tonsils, there are single or multiple, sharply circumscribed, round or linear, dirty grayish-red or grayish-yellow, firm, dry, cheesy foci of coagulative necrosis. See Figure 17.5 for illustration of a similar condition in a lamb. The necrotic areas project prominently above the surrounding more or less normal mucosa and extend into the submucosa, even to the musculature and underlying bone. At first, they are not so sharply defined but later become marked off by a red zone, and finally by a white connective tissue capsule. If the necrotic mass is pulled off, a

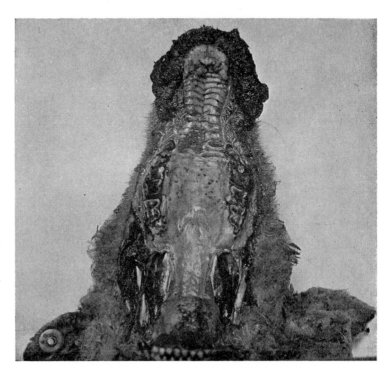

Fig. 17.4 — Contagious ec-thyma lesions in the mouth of a ewe. Note ulcers on lips, dental pad, hard pal-ate, and tongue.

deep bleeding ulcer remains. This may heal by means of the processes of granulation and cicatrization. However, death usually occurs in 4 to 5 days. The histological appearance is that of a coagulative necrosis.

## SUPPURATIVE AND GANGRENOUS STOMATITIS

If, as a result of trauma of the mouth, pyogenic bacteria gain entrance to the loose submucous and intermuscular connective tissue, a deep-seated inflammation (phlegmon) results. In the connective tissue there are hyperemia, edema, a yellowish gelatinous infiltration, and small hemorrhages. Later these areas may undergo definite suppuration. Swelling may extend to the larynx and result in dyspnea and asphyxia. If putrefactive, instead of pyogenic, bacteria enter, the tissues become soft, grayish-green or grayish-brown in color, and the offensive odor of gangrene becomes strong. Gas vesicles may also appear in the necrotic tissue. If the tongue is involved, the gangrenous portion may slough.

## ACTINOBACILLOSIS AND ACTINOMYCOSIS

**Actinobacillary and actinomycotic glossitis** may develop when grain awns and

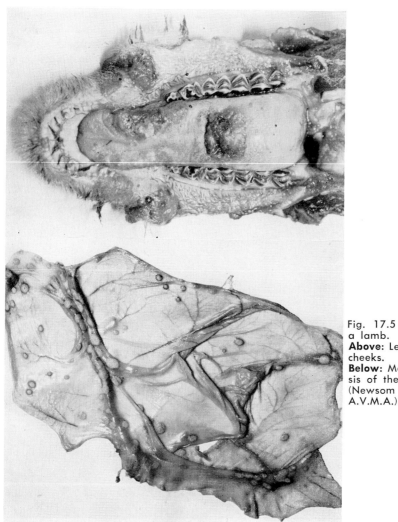

Fig. 17.5 — Necrobacillosis in a lamb.
**Above:** Lesions on tongue and cheeks.
**Below:** Metastatic focal necrosis of the rumen.
(Newsom and Cross, Jour. A.V.M.A.)

other similar hard plant fibers penetrate the tongue, and the alveolar cavity between the molars and the gum in cattle, and carry in with them *Actinobacillus lignieresi* and *Actinomyces bovis*. In the tongue these foreign bodies often penetrate the groove or depression (so-called food cavity) anterior to the eminence of dorsum. When the tongue is extended for food, the cavity opens; when the tongue is retracted, the cavity closes. Beards which are caught in it may penetrate the mucous membrane and give rise to ulcers. These are usually small, funnel-shaped depressions with a round or oval opening into which have entered the grain beards, plant barbs, or hairs. Microscopically, the ulcers are lined with connective tissue heavily infiltrated with leukocytes. Colonies of *Actinomyces bovis* or *Actinobacillus lignieresi* are found in foci of neutrophilic infiltration (Fig. 17.6). In close proximity to the colonies are macrophages. Some of these form large multinuclear giant cells which have phagocytized colonies of the organisms.

In swine, abscesses of the pharyngeal region are of great economic importance. The abscesses usually involve the lymph nodes of the area and are referred to by swine raisers and packing house workers as feeder boils, **jowl abscesses,** or cervical abscesses. It has been reported that in some abattoirs these abscesses are responsible for condemnation of heads up to as high as 7 per cent. In one study over 85 per cent of these abscesses were caused by a *beta* hemolytic streptococcus.

### Tumors

The most frequent tumors in the oral cavities of dogs are viral papillomas. They usually occur in large numbers and have the usual gross and microscopic appearance of papillomas. They disappear spontaneously in 1 to 3 months if not removed. Squamous-cell carcinoma of the tonsils is reported to be an important tumor of dogs in London, England. In dogs in the United States squamous-cell carcinomas of the tongue (Fig. 17.7) and other parts of the oral cavity are reported occasionally. Adamantinoma (ameloblastoma), a tumor derived from the epithelium associated with the enamel organ, has been reported most often in cattle. Benign and malignant melanomas, while generally occurring in the skin, are occasionally seen in the oral cavities of dogs.

### SALIVARY GLANDS

**Foreign bodies.** Kernels of grain, beards, plant fibers, and splinters of wood may be found in the ducts of the parotid and submaxillary glands. They produce inflammation and occlusion of the duct and may form the nucleus for salivary concretions.

**Concretions.** Sialoliths are most frequently encountered in the horse. They are usually located in the ducts of the parotid

Fig. 17.6 — Lesion, typical of actinomycosis and actinobacillosis, occurring in the tongue of a cow. The four bodies in the dense collection of neutrophils are awns or barbs of plants. Colonies of the disease-producing organisms can be seen at their periphery. ×150. (Department of Veterinary Pathology, Iowa State University.)

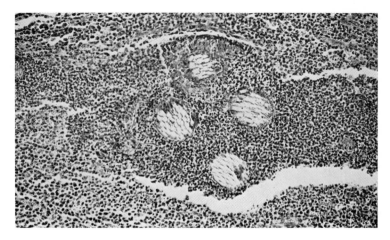

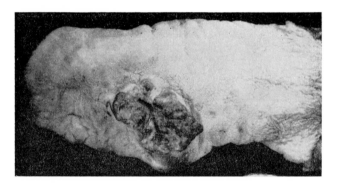

Fig. 17.7 — Squamous-cell carcinoma of the dorsal surface of the tongue of a 7-year-old dog. The tumor cells infiltrated to the ventral surface and metastasized to the mandibular lymph node. (Department of Veterinary Pathology, Michigan State University.)

and submaxillary glands a short distance from the external opening. They usually occur singly, vary in size from 1 to 10 cm., are ovoid in shape, and weigh up to 600 gm. The largest one in the Iowa State University collection weighs 368 gm. Long ones may be broken, and the broken surfaces may become faceted. Their color is white or yellowish. Their cut surface displays concentric rings. Often, there is a foreign body in the center.

In the Iowa State University collection a pin forms the nucleus of one. Sialoliths consist of calcium carbonate, other salts, and organic material. They produce stasis of salivary juice, dilatation of the duct, distension, and finally, atrophy of the gland.

**Dilatation of the ducts** results from stasis of secretion due to occlusion by foreign bodies, concretions, injury, and stricture. The wall of the duct is thinned by stretching, or thickened by chronic inflammation. The secretion is thicker and more viscid than normal.

**Atrophy** of a salivary gland is due to occlusion of the duct and stasis of secretion (pressure atrophy). The lobules decrease in size, disappear, or remnants of them become cystic. There is an increase in connective tissue to replace the atrophic glandular tissue.

**Fistula** of a salivary gland results from an injury to the gland or duct which permits saliva to flow out of an unnatural opening. Fistulas are also caused by abscesses. The flow of saliva through the fistula prevents healing, and the epithelium of the duct at the place of injury may join the epithelium of the skin.

**Inflammation.** The catarrhal form of sialadenitis may be primary or secondary. The primary inflammation of the parotid gland is most frequent. Secondary inflammation of the submaxillary gland occurs in rabies. The suppurative form of inflammation in any of the glands is due to pyogenic bacteria entering by way of the duct along with foreign bodies, or entering from the immediate neighborhood by way of the lymph, or entering from other suppurative centers by way of the blood (strangles). It results in either a diffuse polymorphonuclear infiltration (phlegmon) or in a circumscribed suppurating focus (abscess). The latter may rupture in the mouth or on the outer surface and produce a fistula. Repair occurs through the formation of granulation and cicatricial tissue. The chronic form of sialadenitis is due to trauma, chronic inflammation of the duct, or *Actinomyces bovis* or *Actinobacillus lignieresi* infection. It leads to connective tissue proliferation and atrophy of the parenchyma.

**Cysts.** Cyst formation in the sublingual gland is called ranula. The cyst lies under the tongue between the frenum linguae, may measure as much as 8 cm. in diameter, is fluctuating, and contains a viscid, grayish-yellow or brownish, clear or turbid, odorless fluid. The cyst is lined with cylindrical epithelium. It occurs most frequently in the dog and cow. It is a retention cyst arising from occlusion of the duct of the sublingual gland.

## ESOPHAGUS

Changes in the size of the lumen. Narrowing (stenosis) may be congenital or acquired. There are two kinds of the latter: (1) **Compression stenosis,** which is due to pressure from the outside of the esophagus by tumors, goiter, tuberculous lymph nodes, abscesses, actinomycotic new growths, aneurysms, and diverticula. (2) **Obturation stenosis (choke),** which is due to occlusion of the lumen from within by foreign bodies, food boluses, chronic inflammatory processes, parasitic nodules, tumors (Figs. 13.28, 13.29, 17.8), submucous abscesses and phlegmon, and strictures. Either form of stenosis results in difficulty or prevention of swallowing, which may lead to undernourishment. Regurgitation of food and eructation of gas are prevented; therefore, tympanites occurs in ruminants. Stasis of food in front of the stenosis leads to dilatation and diverticulum formation. Slight stenosis may result in compensatory hypertrophy of the musculature anterior to the stenosis.

**Widening of the lumen (dilatation)** may be congenital (rare) or acquired (horses and cattle). (1) **Ectasia** is a uniform, spindle- or cylindrical-shaped dilatation. It may be due to stenosis (accumulation of food anterior to a stenosis, also posterior in ruminants), injuries which encircle the esophagus (rare), or relaxation of the esophageal musculature due to disturb-ances of innervation (vagus). (2) **Diverticulum** is a one-sided sacculated dilatation. It may be due to traction by cicatricial tissue on the outside of the esophagus or to rupture of the muscle coats due to accumulation of food in the esophagus. In the diverticulum, decomposition of accumulated food, epithelial maceration, inflammation, ulcers, and gangrene may result. Difficulties in deglutition, rumination, and eructation of gas (chronic bloat) also occur in ruminants.

**Foreign bodies** consist principally of improper food (insufficiently masticated or insalivated, or very large, angular, or sharp pieces) or substances not food (sticks, wire, stones, fetal membranes, milk teeth, hair balls). They may cause complete or partial stenosis, pressure necrosis, inflammation, perforation, phlegmonous and gangrenous processes, pressure on the trachea, blood vessels, and nerves, or, occasionally tympanites in ruminants, leading to asphyxia.

**Disturbances in continuity.** Perforations and ruptures may be caused by many of the foreign bodies mentioned above, also by trauma from the outside, and abscesses. They may lead to phlegmon and gangrene of the surrounding tissues, pleuritis and pericarditis, stricture, or esophageal fistula.

**Esophagitis.** Superficial inflammation is rare because the thick, superficial cornified

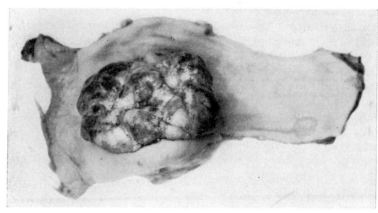

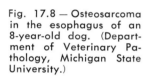
Fig. 17.8 — Osteosarcoma in the esophagus of an 8-year-old dog. (Department of Veterinary Pathology, Michigan State University.)

epithelium protects against agents producing inflammation. Furthermore, the irritant is in contact with the mucosa only a very short time. Forms of the inflammation are the same as for stomatitis. In the catarrhal form in dogs and swine, there is more mucus than in other animals. A special type of ulcerative esophagitis occurs in A-avitaminosis or nutritional roup of chickens and poults. A focal, and at times a diffuse, necrotic esophagitis in turkeys may possibly be due to *Trichomonas gallinae*. **Viral diarrhea** of cattle is characterized by the presence of linear and irregularly shaped erosions of the esophageal mucosa. As a result of this, 80 to 90 per cent of the mucosa may be lost.

**Hyperkeratosis.** In cattle with hyperkeratosis caused by highly chlorinated naphthalenes, rounded, papillary proliferations of the mucous membranes and underlying connective tissue form in the esophagus as well as in the mouth, and occasionally in the omasum.

### Tumors

Reports of tumors of the esophagus in domestic animals are quite rare. Most of the available reports are concerned with carcinomas in cats, papillomas in cattle, and fibrosarcomas and osteosarcomas in dogs. In old cats carcinomas are reported to occur at the thoracic inlet and almost encircle the lumen of the esophagus. They usually metastasize. Papillomas of the esophagus of cattle appear not to be related to the contagious warts so common to this species. In dogs malignant connective tissue tumors have been observed. Seibold and his colleagues have reported an interassociation of malignant connective tissue tumors and the lesions produced by the roundworm *Spirocerca lupi*. The tumors are usually fibrosarcomas and osteosarcomas. They usually develop in the caudal portion of the esophagus in the area commonly the site of Spirocerca infection. They are polypoid in shape and cause death by esophageal occlusion or by metastasis to other organs.

Seibold and co-workers have made another interesting observation in their study of the association of *Spirocerca lupi* infection and esophageal tumors in dogs. The bodies of the thoracic vertebrae adjacent to the involved Spirocerca lesions display exostoses, a lesion which they designate as deformative ossifying spondylitis. The thoracic vertebrae most often affected are the sixth, seventh, and eighth. These lesions are presumed to be the result of Spirocerca migration. In some cases the aorta in the affected region showed aneurysmal scarring which also seemed to be caused by migration of the worm.

### INGLUVIES (CROP) OF BIRDS

**Impaction** is the result of retention of normal or pathological crop contents such as grass and feathers, leading to dilatation and to occlusion of that portion of the esophagus anterior to the proventriculus. The following may occur: acute catarrhal ingluvitis, perforation or rupture of the crop, asphyxia due to pressure upon the trachea, or death by starvation.

**Necrosis** is caused mostly by caustics and corrosives which the birds get accidentally or which are used in too great concentrations as medicinal agents in the drinking water.

**Ingluvitis** appearing in the acute catarrhal form is most frequent. It is caused by mechanical irritation (foreign bodies, caterpillar hair); chemical irritation (phosphorus, oxalic acid); alimentary intoxication (spoiled feed, fermentation, and putrefaction occurring during impaction); infection; and parasites (capillarids). Two yeastlike fungi, *Monilia albicans* and *Oidium pullorum*, produce an ulcerative ingluvitis. The ulcerative form also occurs in fowl A-avitaminosis. It may also be due to *Trichomonas gallinae* in turkeys. Ground seeds of corn cockle produce a hemorrhagic type which may become necrotic.

**Pendulous crop** in turkeys is either a temporary or permanent distention of the organ with liquid or semiliquid contents. The crop may become so greatly distended that almost one-third of the weight of the bird may be crop contents. The cause has not been determined. In some flocks it has been associated with the ration and in others it has appeared to be heritable.

## FORESTOMACH OF RUMINANTS

### Displacements

**Diaphragmatic hernia** of the reticulum has been reported. In the few cases on record it has occurred in the lower diaphragm in the xyphoid region either to the left or right of the mid-line. The reticulum projects through a circular ring to which it is adherent by fibrous bands. The heart and lungs become displaced and compressed.

### Foreign Bodies

Because of the manner of prehension and mastication of cattle, many metallic objects, such as pieces of baling wire, nails, small bolts, and metal tag fasteners from feed bags, are ingested. The heavier objects lodge in the reticulum. Their lodgement is facilitated by the nature of the mucosa of this organ. Blunt foreign bodies (concretions) may remain for years without causing apparent injury. Sharp foreign bodies assisted by the ruminatory movements may penetrate the wall of the reticulum (traumatic gastritis, traumatic pericarditis). Larger and more rounded bodies may occlude the openings of the forestomachs, preventing rumination and eructation by way of the esophagus or preventing passage of ingesta to the abomasum. This may result in impaction and tympany.

Sharp metallic foreign bodies gravitate to the anteroventral wall of the reticulum. Here they may become fastened in the mucosal folds which form the honeycomb-like cells of the reticulum.

### Disturbances in Continuity

#### PERFORATIONS

Perforations occur chiefly in cattle, usually in the reticulum, but in the rumen occasionally, and in the other stomachs rarely. They may be due to agents operating from the outside or inside.

**External perforations** of the rumen such as trocharization also open the peritoneal cavity, but general peritonitis rarely develops. Fibrinous adhesions, which give way to connective tissue adhesions, form and unite the parietal peritoneum to the visceral peritoneum. If the opening fails to close, a ruminal fistula results. Abscess formation may occur.

**Internal perforations** are usually produced by sharp metallic objects lying in the reticulum. As stated above, these objects, for the most part, are pieces of baling wire, nails, and metal tag fasteners from feed bags. Where extensive surveys have been made relative to the cause of traumatic gastritis, pieces of baling wire have been incriminated most often and miscellaneous sharp metallic objects least. Traumatic gastritis occurs most often during the period from October to May, the period during which cattle are usually stable-fed and also when cows are most often in advanced pregnancy. In California traumatic reticulitis occurs in about 20 per cent of the beef cows and 80 per cent of the dairy cows and bulls.

Penetration by sharp objects is assisted by the reticular movements, abdominal pressure, pressure of the gravid uterus, fetal movements, parturition, diaphragmatic movements, and any other pressure upon the forestomachs (casting). Penetration is usually slow and may be complete or incomplete. At the point of penetration, at first there is hemorrhage. Then begins the development of a chronic inflammatory process with the formation of connective tissue which becomes cicatricial tissue. Besides the foreign body, the fistulous tract contains a purulent, putrefactive exudate. When the foreign body reaches the serosa, a local fibrinous peritonitis is produced. Fibrinous adhesions form first; later they become organized and unite the peritoneum of the reticulum to the peritoneum of the adjacent organs. Bacteria (*Corynebacterium pyogenes, Spherophorus necrophorus, Actinomyces bovis, Escherichia coli,* cocci, and putrefactive microorganisms) may accompany the foreign body and produce suppurative and gangrenous processes.

The foreign body may penetrate the diaphragm, pericardial sac, heart, lung, liver, or spleen. Traumatic pericarditis and myocarditis (Fig. 14.3), and traumatic pleuritis are the most common complications. Splenitis, hepatitis, pneumonia, bronchitis, and subcutaneous and subserous emphysema are less common.

Fatal hemorrhage resulting from the penetration is very rare because there are no large vessels in the area ordinarily penetrated. There is always the possibility, however, that after reaching the heart the sudden penetration of the right coronary artery may lead to death by cardiac tamponade.

Serious nerve involvement leading to atony of the rumen or reticulum may result if an important nerve becomes pierced or if an abscess caused by the foreign body encroaches upon a nerve.

Important changes relative to the number and kinds of leukocytes in the blood occur as a result of traumatic reticulitis and pericarditis. There is an increase in the total number of leukocytes. Among the neutrophils there is a very noticeable increase in the immature forms (unsegmented cells) and a moderate increase in the mature forms (segmented cells), while at the same time there is a relative decrease in the lymphocytes. While a total leukocyte count and a differential count are both important in the diagnosis of chronic traumatic reticulitis, the differential count usually shows the greater deviation from normal. The more complicated the cases are, the more likely is the total number of leukocytes to be increased, and the normal ratio of lymphocytes to neutrophils is more likely to be markedly changed.

**Rupture** of the rumen occasionally occurs and may be due to trauma from without or overdistension from within. One must always differentiate between ante-mortem and post-mortem ruptures.

## Dilatation of the Forestomachs

The rumen and reticulum are usually affected. According to the etiology, they are classified as: tympanitic and alimental dilatation.

### TYMPANITIC DILATATION

Tympanitic dilatation of the rumen and reticulum is commonly called bloat, or more technically designated meteorism or tympanites. The dilatation may be the result of gas accumulation during excessive fermentation of ingesta or the result of the inability of the animal to expel the gas by eructating. Distention from excessive fermentation probably is unusual because a ruminant normally can eructate free gas as rapidly as it is formed. Inability to eruct gas is believed to be the more common reason why bloat occurs.

According to its duration, which is usually dependent upon the cause, bloat is acute or chronic. Generally it is easier to explain why bloat can be chronic than why it can be acute. It is obvious that any continued hindrance to eructation in the esophagus or in the wall of the rumen will be associated with chronic bloat. Such hindrance, either within or without the esophagus, can be traced to tumors (Fig. 17.9), abscesses, foreign bodies, enlarged lymph nodes, constrictions, and diverticula. In the rumen such hindrance can come from conditions which lessen contractions of the ruminal wall. Examples of such conditions are: atony, paresis, serosal adhesions, and diffuse tumor formations (lymphosarcomas).

There is uncertainty about the actual cause of many cases of acute bloat. Except in cases of esophageal choke, its sudden onset, alarming symptoms, and often fatal termination are usually associated with sudden changes of feed, particularly when stable-fed cattle are turned to legume pasture. The probability of the occurrence of bloat at that time is increased if the plants are wet with dew or rain.

Among the theories advanced for the explanation of bloat are the following: (1) Some legumes contain hydrocyanic acid, which causes paralysis of the ruminal and reticular musculature. (2) Some legumes contain an excessive amount of the enzyme phosphatase, which in association with arsenates accelerates fermentation with the production of large amounts of carbon dioxide. (3) Unusual quantities of hydrogen sulfide derived from the fermenting ingesta act as a paralyzant to the ruminal muscularis. (4) Green plants lack the stiff fibers necessary to scratch the ruminal mucosa as a stimulus for the reflex which results in contraction of the ruminal musculature. Much credence has been given to this theory because the customary practice of cattlemen to prevent bloat is to give the animals a big feeding of hay immediately before turning them out to pasture. The presence of the fibers of the dry roughage mixed with the green forage is believed to be sufficient to stimulate the contraction of the rumen.

Veterinarians and cattlemen have always recognized two types of bloat — dry and frothy. The latter is the more serious because animals are able to eruct free (dry) gas but not frothy gas. The ruminal contents in frothy bloat are permeated with myriads of gas bubbles, and the distended upper part of the rumen is filled with foam. Someone has said that the condition in the rumen is like the suds produced in a laundry washer after the detergent is added. The animal cannot eruct the froth.

The underlying cause of froth formation in the rumen has not been determined. Saponin, a glucoside found in plants and used in the manufacture of liquid soaps, has been incriminated, but attempts to cause frothy bloat by introducing it into the rumen have not been successful. A water-soluble protein which is found in fresh legumes has been shown to be capable of forming a stable foam like that present in cases of bloat. In the very complex physiochemical processes which characterize ruminal digestion, changes in surface tension and viscosity of the fluid apparently are related to the formation of froth. Both the apparent surface tension and relative viscosity vary considerably in relation to feeding times, kinds of feed, and amounts of water consumed. Experimentally it has been determined that a sudden change from feeding alfalfa hay to fresh ladino clover is associated with a period of high surface tension, increased viscosity, deep ruminal fermentation, and froth formation. Defoaming agents such as turpentine and methyl silicone reduce surface tension of rumen fluid.

In acute bloat due to legumes, rather large amounts of toxic gases are formed from the proteins in the feed. The gases which are particularly toxic are carbon dioxide, carbon monoxide, and hydrogen sulfide. When the intraruminal pressure is increased, as in bloat, these gases are more readily absorbed and are thought by some to cause a paralysis of the motor nerves in the muscularis externa of the rumen. These gases, absorbed into the blood, contribute to the cause of death in bloat.

In either acute or chronic tympanitic dilatation, gas accumulates in the upper part of the rumen. The gas is a mixture of carbon dioxide, carbon monoxide, methane, nitrogen, oxygen, and hydrogen sulfide. Distension of the rumen and reticulum stimulates the sensory nerves in these organs and results in muscular contractions. After long-continued distension, however, partial sensory and motor paralysis occurs. Finally the organ may rupture.

Death usually comes before this occurs because the bloat initiates a chain of other pathologic processes which give rise to alarming symptoms. The distended rumen compresses the other abdominal organs and especially interferes with the venous circulation of the abdominal cavity, because veins are more easily compressed than arteries. The diaphragm is pushed forward, resulting in partial pulmonary atelectasis which leads to diminished gas exchange in the lungs. Signs of air hunger ensue — respirations increase and the mucous membranes become cyanotic. The animal may die of asphyxiation.

## ALIMENTAL DILATATION

Acute alimental dilatation (impaction) is the result of overfeeding or of atony of the musculature of the forestomachs. A common cause is the overfeeding of concentrates or chopped feed which swell readily in the rumen. When the alimental dilatation is the result of atony of the forestomachs, the condition usually makes its appearance late in the winter in cattle that have been wintered on coarse fibrous forage. An insufficient supply of water may be a contributing factor. The results of alimental dilatation are abnormal distension of the wall of the rumen, difficult contraction of the musculature, acute motor insufficiency, and fermentation. The condition either subsides or death occurs due to the absorption of the toxic products of food decomposition, to inanition, or for the same reasons as in acute tympany. In experimentally overfed sheep, histamine and tyramine have been identified as toxic constituents in the rumen contents.

### Atony of the Rumen

Loss of tone (atony) of the musculature of the rumen probably occurs most often when this part of the ruminant stomach is overworked from attempting to digest large quantities of innutritious roughage over extended periods. It occurs frequently in late winter under the same conditions that give rise to chronic alimental dilatation (chronic impaction). The conditions may be different manifestations of the same underlying ruminal disturbance.

In some cases at least, the underlying cause of rumen atony is to be found in the quality of the hay fed. Hay produced on some soils is deficient in phosphates and sugar. Hay of this composition will not support an adequate microflora and microfauna in the rumen. Without the necessary microorganisms, ruminal fermentation and digestion diminish. The contents of the rumen then change in character. They become heavy, pasty, and doughy. Rumination decreases. The volatile fatty acids derived from normal cellulose digestion in the rumen are lacking. They are needed as a source of energy for the animal. Without them, and without the movement of sufficient nutrients from the rumen into the intestine, the animal shows signs of inanition or wasting. The entire musculature, including that of the rumen, is affected; that is, it shows some degree of atony.

A condition similar to that just described occurs after ruminants have had various disturbances in the rumen — disturbances which destroy the necessary bacteria and protozoa, such as bloat, engorgement, infections, and medication with agents such as antiferments and antiseptics.

### Disturbances in Growth

#### HYPERPLASIA

In the western United States there is an unusually high incidence of **ruminal parakeratosis** in lambs fattened on pelleted feed. The cause has not been determined. The parakeratosis involves only the papillae. Those of the anteroventral sac are most often affected. Affected papillae are enlarged, discolored, and leathery. Histologically, the epithelium of an individual papilla is thickened because of hyperplasia of the malpighian layer and accumulation of excessive layers of keratinized, nucleated cells on the surface. Ingesta and bacteria cling to the roughened surface.

### Rumenitis

Rumenitis in cattle is traumatic or nontraumatic in origin. The traumatic form is caused by various types of foreign bodies which are ingested by cattle. While such cases are numerous, those that are nontraumatic far outnumber them. In both traumatic and nontraumatic cases *Spherophorus necrophorus* is usually present. Because of this, there is quite a possibility that the microorganisms can be transported from the site of the ruminal inflammatory reaction to the liver by the portal system. There is strong circumstantial evidence that hepatic abscesses are related to the rumenitis.

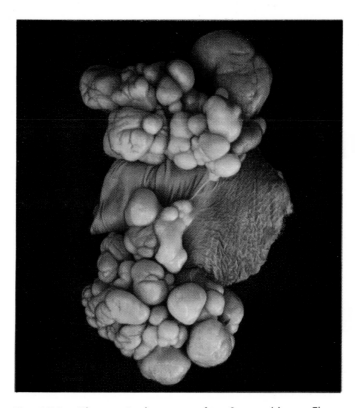

Fig. 17.9 — Fibromas in the rumen of an 8-year-old cow. There were about 120 in a rather circumscribed area. Tumors like these sometimes occur in the atrium ventriculi of the rumen and encroach upon the cardia. When they do, they may result in chronic alimentary and tympanitic dilatation of the rumen. (Department of Veterinary Pathology, Michigan State University.)

Areas of rumenitis are frequently found in the anterodorsal and anteroventral sacs of the organ. Indications of the inflammation are quite varied. About two thirds of the cases are characterized by an acute reaction in the mucosa and submucosa. As a part of the acute reaction, foci of necrosis up to 5 cm. in size may be present. In the remaining, chronic cases, villi may be lost in areas up to 20 cm. in size and pigment in areas up to 15 cm. in size. In cases that have gone on to the repair stage, as many as 75 scars have been observed. Other evidences of a long course are foci of thickened mucosa and submucosa due to fibroplasia, pits due to great loss of epithelium, and nodules resulting from proliferation of epithelium or connective tissue.

Viral diarrhea of cattle is a condition in which erosions may occur in the ruminal mucosa. They are usually shallow and are located in the pillars. Similar erosions may involve the epithelium of the omasal laminae.

## STOMACH

### Displacements

**Diaphragmatic hernia** of the stomach is seen occasionally. **Invagination** of the stomach into the duodenum is rare. **Torsion** of the stomach occurs in old dogs of the heavier breeds. The reason is that the pylorus is moveable so that when the stomach is full this portion can swing quite readily. Body movements which exaggerate this swinging (rolling, running up or down stairs, spinning) may produce torsion.

The esophagus, together with the stomach attachments at the lesser curvature, acts as a fixed point for the rotation, which is clockwise. The torsion is generally more than 180° (one-half turn) but less than 270° (three-quarter turn). This closes both openings of the stomach, twists the vessels supplying it, and leaves the organ wrapped in the lesser omentum. Gastric tympany arises, causing pressure on the lung, and resulting in polypnea. Blood flow into the gastric arteries is impeded less than the outflow by the veins so that passive congestion occurs. The stomach contents become blood-tinged, and the gastric hydrochloric acid changes the color of the accumulated fluid to brown. The venous outflow from the spleen is involved in the torsion, and results in extreme passive congestion of that organ. Coma, with anemia of the visible mucous membranes, is an indication of shock.

**Displacement of the abomasum** of dairy cows occurs rather frequently. The body and the pyloric part are subject to displacement. The fundus has attachment to the reticulum so that its movement out of position by itself is difficult. Displacement of the pyloric part is also restricted because it is attached to the liver by the lesser omentum. The body, however, especially its greater curvature, apparently is easily displaced if the proper conditions arise. Late pregnancy and parturition in dairy cows that are fed large amounts of concentrates and fine hay seem to provide these conditions. It is believed that the gravid uterus in such animals displaces the rumen enough to permit the greater curvature of the body of the abomasum to slip under the ventral sac of the rumen. Gas then accumulates in the displaced portion and causes it gradually to encroach upon the space between the visceral (left) surface of the rumen and the left parietal peritoneum. In extreme cases the distended abomasum may push up as far as the paralumbar fossa. For this to occur it seems reasonable to assume that the rumen and liver must rotate slightly clockwise.

When a cow with this condition is necropsied in the usual position (left side down), no evidence of the displacement can be seen except the enlarged, tympanitic abomasum when the right body wall is removed. Removal of the side permits the distended organ to slip out of its misplaced position.

Such abomasal displacement results in signs of chronic indigestion, continuous ketonuria which does not yield to treatment, and high-pitched tympanitic sounds heard on auscultation along the rib-line on the left side. The blood cell count is not affected. A trocharized sample of the contents of the displaced abomasum contains gastric juice (Liptak test).

**Torsion** of the abomasum is rare because of its attachments to the reticulum, rumen, omasum, and liver.

### Acute Gastric Dilatation

Acute gastric dilatation is caused by ingestion of an excessive amount of food (alimental dilatation) or by excessive gas formation (tympanitic dilatation), or by a combination of both. Accessory causes are reflexive closing of the pylorus, atony of the gastric musculature, diseases of the stomach wall, hard work immediately after feeding, or poor teeth. In horses it may be due to sudden closure of the intestinal lumen; in dogs, to torsion of the stomach; and in foxes, to heavy feeding after a period of insufficient feeding and to excessive feeding of cereals. In acute dilatation the stomach may be enlarged three or four times. There is spasmodic pain followed by relaxation and possible paralysis of the musculature. Stretched muscle fibers may rupture. There is compression upon the neighboring organs, particularly the diaphragm and lungs. Pressure upon the thoracic organs results in hindrance to respiration and circulation. The diaphragm may rupture. Atony of the stomach may persist if the termination is not fatal.

### Chronic Gastric Dilatation

Chronic gastric dilatation is rare. It may follow the acute form or appear in chronic catarrhal gastritis. Sometimes it is the result of the continuous feeding of easily fermentable food. In northwest Nebraska, on the bottom-lands of South Dakota, and in the Pacific Northwest, it occurs in horses that have been poisoned by plants belonging to the genus *Senecio*. It may also be due to stenosis of the pylorus or of the small intestine. In chronic gastric dilata-

tion there may be compensatory muscle hypertrophy or chronic induration of the gastric wall, chronic catarrhal gastritis, and digestive and nutritional disturbances.

### Disturbances in Continuity

**Perforations** are caused by trauma from the outside or from the inside (foreign bodies, corrosives, peptic ulcers in calves, *Gasterophilus* larvae in horses). Peritonitis results more frequently than in perforation of the forestomachs, otherwise the results are the same. **Rupture** occurs most frequently in the horse and fox. The causes are trauma, powerful gastric constrictors (physostigmine), and tympanitic and alimental dilatation (most common). The rupture usually occurs on or near the greater curvature if due to dilatation. The tear is always greater in the muscularis and serosa than in the mucosa. Death usually takes place in 1 to 8 hours. If postponed longer, a fibrinopurulent peritonitis develops.

### Abnormal Content

**Foreign bodies** of various kinds are observed frequently in the stomachs of dogs. In cattle their occurrence is rare as compared with foreign bodies in the forestomachs. Sand may appear in the stomachs of horses shipped in cars bedded with sand, also in horses fed on picket lines; in cattle and sheep pastured on sandy land or pastures recently flooded; in pigs rooting in sand; or in baby chicks kept in brooders with sand used as litter. Coal is a frequently found foreign body in the stomachs of pigs in sections of the country where it is customary to feed slack. When ground corn-cobs are used as litter in brooder houses, they often furnish a source of foreign bodies for baby chicks. The effects of foreign bodies depend upon their character. Small, blunt ones are harmless; larger, blunt ones may obstruct the pyloric orifice; rough, angular ones may produce erosions, hemorrhages, and inflammation; sharp ones may perforate the stomach mucosa and wall. **Concretions.** Gastroliths are rare; hair balls and food balls are seen mostly in cattle and swine. Any of these may occlude the pylorus and duodenum.

### Circulatory Disturbances

Pathological **active hyperemia** of the stomach occurs as a part of the inflammatory processes, while **passive hyperemia** occurs as a result of obstruction in the portal circulation and chronic heart diseases. **Edema** is seen in connection with passive hyperemia.

Pigs, mostly between 10 and 14 weeks of age, sometimes become affected with an edema of the stomach, which is one manifestation of an edema which may become so extensive as to constitute a state of anasarca. Signs of the **edema disease** are edema of the eyelids, face, ears, and body cavities. There may be incoordination or even paralysis of the fore and hind extremities. A period of coma precedes death. One of the most constant lesions is edema of the stomach wall. Edema is present chiefly in the submucosa, which may become 2 to 3 cc. thick. The edema is the result of an enterotoxemia arising from a toxin produced by a hemolytic strain of *Escherichia coli* of a particular serotype. The toxin is formed in the intestine and, after absorption into the blood, apparently increases the permeability of the capillary endothelium for fluid.

**Hemorrhages** occur in septicemic diseases (anthrax, hog cholera, pasteurellosis) and as a result of passive hyperemia. Hemorrhages may also be produced by foreign bodies and parasites, and by the erosion of blood vessels by ulcers and tumors. Blood free in the stomach lumen soon turns brownish black in color due to the action of the hydrochloric acid.

### Necrosis

Necrosis of the gastric mucosa may be diffuse or focal. Diffuse can be expected in an area of infarction arising from thrombosis of a branch of one of the gastric arteries, but this is rare because of the abundant anastomoses of these vessels. In animals it is much more often the result of caustic or corrosive chemicals; hence the condition occurs rather frequently in garbage-fed swine.

Focal necrosis in the form of erosions and ulcers is not so common in domestic mammals as in man, where gastroduodenal ulcers attract so much attention. It is seldom that a duodenal ulcer is seen in a domestic animal in conjunction with gastric ulcers. Gastric ulcers in animals are frequently associated with gastritis or gastroenteritis. Coarse feed and various kinds of foreign bodies can be the irritants. In swine, ulcers sometimes occur as one of the lesions in chronic cholera, chronic plague, chronic erysipelas, and chronic infectious necrotic enteritis. In some of these diseases a petechial hemorrhage in the mucosa may give a starting point for an ulcer. Ulcers also have been reported in glanders of horses and in foot-and-mouth disease of cattle. In horses, they may appear in the esophageal region of the stomach, where large numbers of the larvae of some of the gasterophili are attached.

In pigs under a year of age there may be a causal relationship to the occurrence of nutritional anemia (Kernkamp, 1945). In dogs, gastric ulcers are occasionally associated with the uremic state which arises from acute nephritis in an animal that already has chronic nephritis.

Why gastric (abomasal) ulcers are so common in calves is a matter of conjecture. They may arise from traumatic injury produced by plant fibers which have been eaten before the calf has developed its forestomachs. They may, however, result from injury due to the pressure exerted by the other compartments of the stomach upon the abomasum, especially the rather heavy omasum. One theory used to explain the frequent occurrence of gastric ulcers in man in that the stomach is injured by being pinched between the vertebrae and liver. In domestic mammals this is not the case. In ruminants, however, the position of the abomasum does permit it to be squeezed more than the stomachs of other animals. In support of this theory it is reported that pregnant cows, animals in which a still greater pressure is exerted upon the abomasum, have gastric ulcers more often than nonpregnant cows.

Ulcers then may arise from (1) local circulatory disturbances or from (2) traumatic injury. Factors contributing to the pathological process are (*a*) local injury of the stomach mucosa, and (*b*) the digestive action of the gastric juice upon the injured tissue. The local circulatory disturbances are hemorrhages. They are important because they may occur in various infectious and toxic diseases. The traumatic injuries arise from coarse feed and foreign bodies.

Macroscopically, the ulcers are variable in size, round or irregular, and are variable in depth from slight erosions to complete perforation (Figs. 11.7 and 11.25). The centers of the ulcers are depressed because the necrotic tissue is digested. Their color is dirty brown. Microscopically, the ulcers at first are structureless. The necrotic mucosa shows evidences of digestion. The base and rim show hyperemia and hemorrhage, but in the early stage there may be no marked inflammatory reaction. Ulcers may extend to the muscular coats and serosa. They usually develop rapidly (3 to 4 days). Perforation may occur in 6 to 7 days. Most ulcers heal slowly by the formation of granulation tissue which becomes scar tissue. The scar becomes covered with regenerated epithelium. At times the ulcer may progress to perforation resulting in peritonitis and death. Incomplete perforation leads to local fibrinous peritonitis, organization of the exudate, and adhesions to the neighboring organs.

In viral diarrhea of cattle ulcers occur in the abomasal mucosa. The lesions are sharply circumscribed, depressed areas with raised borders. Their size is 1 to 15 mm. Beneath these areas the lamina propria is edematous and moderately infiltrated with leukocytes.

## Gastritis

Gastritis frequently occurs in most species of domestic animals. This is not to be wondered at, considering the fact that the feed of such animals is frequently not of their own choice. Often the feed contains an excess of easily decomposed or fermentable ingredients, sometimes too much coarse fibrous material, and at other times irritating substances. Frequently, sudden and radical changes are made in the character of the food. Work and racing animals are often fed too heavily when they are fatigued, and food and milk-producing animals are overfed when they are closely confined. Then, too, the feeding and drinking utensils and appliances, and also the places where the animals feed and drink, are frequently insanitary, with the result that bacteria and bacterial decomposition products may be ingested and cause gastric irritation. In addition to the factors just mentioned, and also in addition to many of those which have already been mentioned as causes of stomatitis, gastritis may be caused by some parasitic roundworms such as the stomach worms of horses, cattle, sheep, and swine, and by the larval forms of some insects such as the bots or larvae of the gasterophili in horses.

Gastritis, like so many other pathological processes in the body, may be primary or secondary. Many of the causes of primary gastritis have just been listed or suggested. Excellent examples of infectious diseases of animals in which gastritis occurs secondarily are canine distemper, hog cholera, swine erysipelas, and bovine and ovine pasteurellosis.

### ACUTE GASTRITIS

The etiology of **catarrhal gastritis** is thermic, chemic, bacterial, or traumatic injury. Secondarily, it accompanies some specific infectious diseases (canine distemper and hog cholera). Macroscopically, there are redness and swelling of the mucosa, an increased amount of mucus, and often small hemorrhages and erosions. Microscopically, there are hyperemia, abnormal mucus formation, desquamation of epithelium, and leukocytic infiltration. **Hemorrhagic gastritis** is similar in appearance to catarrhal except there is marked reddening due to hemorrhage. It is observed in some infectious intoxication diseases (pasteurellosis, uremia of dogs) and in poisonings caused by caustic and corrosive chemical agents. **Fibrinous gastritis** is produced by more intense irritants. **Necrotic gastritis** occasionally occurs in hog cholera. In baby pigs a necrotic gastritis is characteristic of transmissible gastroenteritis. The necrotic form also occurs in blacktongue of dogs. **Suppurative** or **purulent gastritis** is rare. The cause may be streptococci and *Corynebacterium pyogenes* through trauma, and streptococci by hematogenous metastasis (strangles).

**Parasitic gastritis** is usually characterized by a combination of the changes which occur in the basic types of inflammation. Special mention should be made of the gastritis in horses and calves whose stomachs are heavily parasitized with *Trichostrongylus axei*. In both horses and calves, raised circular lesions about 1 to 2 cm. in diameter are irregularly distributed over the stomach mucosa, which is rather uniformly and severely inflamed. The highly reddened surface is covered with mucus. Microscopically, the inflammation is most severe in the areas which have the raised appearance. In these areas desquamation of the mucosa and marked edema of the tunica propria occur.

Gastritis in cattle caused by *Ostertagia ostertagi* also presents special features. The abomasal mucosa is inflamed and thickened by the presence of the adult and immature forms of the worm, both in the superficial and deep aspects of the lining membrane. Macroscopically, the fundic and pyloric mucosa is involved in a patchy or diffuse granularity having a surface appearance of minute cobblestones. Many of the small granular lesions contain a small dark red spot. The tops of the abomasal folds are inflamed and sometimes ulcerated, the ulcers seldom being more than 4 to 6 mm. in diameter. The submucosa of the folds is edematous. Microscopically, the tiny nodules contain developing worms, singly or in groups. The worms lie in the gland crypts. The presence of several worms in one crypt gives rise to a cyst. The epithelium of such glands becomes atrophied and may disappear. The surrounding lamina propria may or may not show an inflammatory reaction. In the fundus the parietal cells are present, but the chief cells may be replaced by mucous cells. The mucosa may undergo a superficial necrosis with parasites, neutrophils, and eosinophils present in the necrotic tissue.

CHRONIC GASTRITIS

The etiology is the same as for the acute gastritis but must operate for a longer period of time. Secondarily, it occurs in chronic gastric dilatation and in hepatic cirrhosis. In either case it is an accompaniment of circulatory disturbances. In chronic gastric dilatation there is a partial state of anemia, and in hepatic cirrhosis a passive hyperemia. In both conditions there is lessened local resistance to infection. Macroscopically, the wall of the stomach is thickened and the mucosa covered with thick, viscid, glassy mucus. Sometimes in the mucosa small cysts appear which are retention cysts due to occlusion of the mouths of glands. If the lymph follicles show hyperplasia, nodules appear on the surface. Microscopically, there are hyperplasia of the glands, epithelial desquamation, increase in interstitial connective tissue, hypertrophy of the muscle fibers, and inflammatory cell infiltration.

**Tumors**

Tumors of the stomach are rare and are usually primary. Only one deserves attention, and that is the lymphosarcoma of the abomasum of cattle (Fig. 13.18).

**INTESTINE**

**Changes of Position**

HERNIA

Hernia is a condition in which viscera pass from body cavities without a break in the continuity of the skin, serosa, or mucous membranes. Applied to the intestine it infers that a portion of the organ protrudes through a congenital or acquired opening in the abdominal wall. An external hernia usually consists of a sac, a **ring,** and the **contents of the sac** (Fig. 17.10). The sac consists of the protruded peritoneum. The ring may be a congenital fissure, a weak place in the abdominal wall due to trauma, or a place at which nerves and blood and lymph vessels or ducts leave the abdominal cavity (inguinal canal, femoral ring, navel ring). The contents of the hernial sac may be portions of any of the abdominal viscera and also peritoneal fluid. Hernias are designated ventral (Fig. 17.10), umbilical, inguinal, scrotal, femoral, perineal, or diaphragmatic (Fig. 16.30), according to their location.

Including diaphragmatic hernia in this list raises the question about a fine distinction made in classifying hernias as **true** or **false.** In a true hernia of the diaphragm the protruding portion of the ab-

dominal organ is covered by the stretched peritoneum and pleura of the diaphragm. In false hernia the peritoneum and pleura are torn so that the protruding viscus is not covered by them.

Hernias are either reducible or irreducible. They become irreducible due (1) to incarceration or strangulation of the hernial contents, (2) to the contents becoming too firm, or (3) to adhesions forming between the contents and wall. The first factor, incarceration, is most dangerous. It may occur as a result of straining. When it occurs, arterial blood can enter, but venous blood cannot readily leave the incarcerated loop of intestine. Therefore, passive hyperemia, hemorrhage, and edema result. The loop of intestine becomes cyanotic and edematously swollen, and contains a hemorrhagic exudate. Bacteria and toxic products in the decomposing ingesta in the loop of intestine lead to

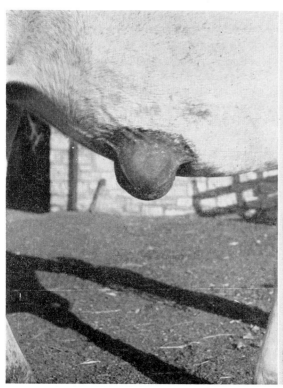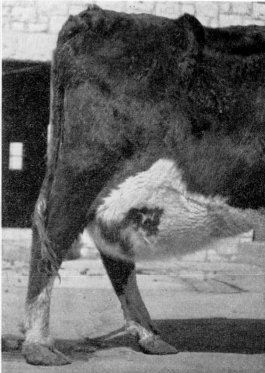

Fig. 17.10 — **Left:** ventral hernia in a horse. **Right:** ventral hernia in a cow. (Frank, Jour. A.V.M.A.)

peritonitis, necrosis, and gangrene, and, if the animal lives long enough, rupture of the intestinal wall occurs. The second cause of irreducible hernias is related to the contents of the hernia. They become too firm as a result of. the accumulation of gas, ingesta, or secretions in the loop of intestine. These substances may accumulate because of paralysis of the musculature of the incarcerated portion. Adhesions between the sac and the loop of intestine, the third factor responsible for irreducible hernia, may result from a chronic inflammatory process in the hernial sac which may arise from traumatic influences.

### INTERNAL STRANGULATION

Internal strangulation of loops of intestine may result when these portions pass through congenital or acquired openings in the omentum, mesentery, or ligamentous attachments of abdominal viscera. The pathological processes accompanying such strangulation of the intestine are essentially the same as those described for strangulated hernia. Peritonitis, shock, and death within 24 to 36 hours are the usual outcome.

### VOLVULUS

Volvulus of the jejunum and ileum occurs most frequently in the horse and consists of a 180°, or more, rotation of the intestine on the long axis of the mesentery. Volvulus sometimes occurs physiologically, but becomes pathologic only when disturbances result. Overfilling of a portion of the intestine with gas or ingesta, or the hindrance of peristalsis by other organs may be factors in the pathological production of volvulus. When it occurs, the mesentery becomes twisted around its dorsal attachment.) Peristaltic movement continues for a time in the loop causing it to continue to rotate and assume a snail-shell formation. The continued twisting increases the strangulation of the mesentery and intestine. The twisted portion of intestine becomes occluded, gas forms in it, arterial blood flows into the area, but venous blood flowing out is impeded. Therefore, passive hyperemia, edema, and hemorrhage arise in the involved portion.

There is an exudate both inside and outside of the loop. As much as 15 liters of the hemorrhagic exudate have been reported in the abdominal cavity. Gangrene and rupture of the affected portion of the intestine may occur. Death results within 12 to 24 hours due to intestinal occlusion, putrefactive intoxication, shock, and acute anemia resulting from loss of blood in the twisted portion.

### TORSION OR ROTATION OF THE LARGE COLON OF THE HORSE

The left dorsal and ventral parts of the colon, and the diaphragmatic and sternal flexures are movable; the right dorsal and ventral parts are relatively fixed. In torsion the left dorsal part may turn laterally or medially (usually the latter) around the left ventral part (Fig. 17.11). Usually it is a 360° twist. The place at which the torsion is exerted is at the two anterior flexures. Occasionally, torsion occurs along the course of the right dorsal and ventral parts almost as far posteriorly as their middle. Two occlusions result. Ingesta collects in the lumen in front of the first one; gas and hemorrhagic exudate collect between the two. The cause is often a mechanical influence such as violent rolling. Predisposing factors are the length of the free parts of the colon, width of the peritoneal band between the left dorsal and ventral parts, peritoneal adhesions between the parietal peritoneum and the peritoneum of the left ventral portion, and temporary fluctuations in the fullness of the portions of the freely moving parts of the colon. The results of torsion of the colon are similar in many respects to those of volvulus of the small intestine and to tympanitic dilatation. Death usually occurs within 6 to 10 hours.

### TORSIONS AND VOLVULUSES OF MINOR IMPORTANCE

Torsion or rotation of the cecum occasionally occurs in the horse, cow, and pig. The place of torsion is in the body of the cecum near the two orifices. Another displacement, caused by violent body movements, is a kinking of the colon at the pelvic flexure in the horse. Another is the

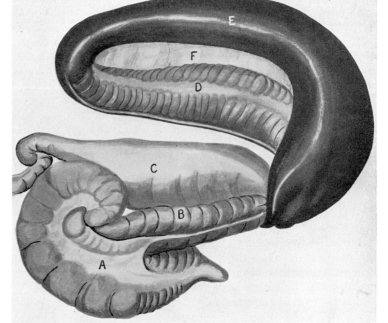

Fig. 17.11 — Drawing of a torsion of the great colon of a horse.
**A,** cecum;
**B,** right ventral colon;
**C,** right dorsal colon;
**D,** left ventral colon;
**E,** left dorsal colon;
**F,** peritoneal band between left dorsal and ventral parts.
(After Nieberle and Cohrs.)

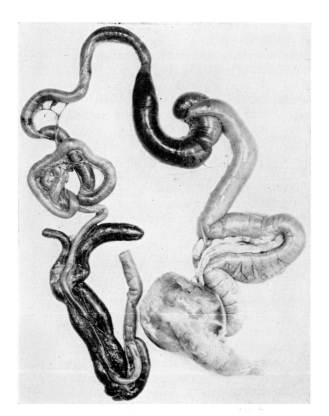

kinking of the small colon and small intestine of the horse as a result of peritoneal adhesions between the intestine and abdominal wall.

INVAGINATION

Invagination, or intussusception, is a telescoping of a section of the intestine into the portion following (Fig. 17.12). It is believed that it frequently occurs physiologically and becomes pathologic only

Fig. 17.12 — Invagination of small intestine in a turkey. The intestine, mostly duodenum, cephalic to the invagination is distended with ingesta and gas. Ceca show lesions of histomoniasis. (Department of Veterinary Pathology, Michigan State University.)

when circulatory disturbances result. Invagination occurs more frequently, perhaps, when peristalsis is increased. It may take place as a result of constriction of the circular muscle at a given point with increased peristalsis of the longitudinal musculature. The constricted portion under these conditions may be forced into a following relaxed portion (Fig. 17.13). The constricted portion carries with it, of course, a portion of the intestine anterior to it, together with the mesentery of the invaginated portion. Therefore, two sections of intestine, one within the other, become ensheathed by a third portion. In small animals the invagination may reach a length of 5 to 10 cm., in larger animals 20 to 30 cm. It can extend in as far as the length of the mesentery or farther if the mesentery tears. The condition occurs in all species of animals but most often in dogs and cattle. It usually appears in the small intestine (jejunum).

Macroscopically, due to venous compression, there are passive hyperemia, edema, hemorrhage, and necrosis. The affected portion of the intestine is swollen, firm, red or bluish red, and slightly curved (Fig. 17.14). The mesentery is pulled into the neck of the intussusception. Fibrinous adhesions form between the two contacting serous surfaces. The condition results in occlusion of the intestine, stasis of ingesta, gas formation, acute dilatation of the stomach, and vomiting of intestinal contents in dogs and swine. There is the possibility that sloughing of the invaginated portion may occur and that, subsequently, healing at the neck of the intussusception may occur by the formation of granulation tissue and regeneration of the epithelium. The resulting scar tissue produces a girdle-shaped stenosis. Ordinarily, death results, however, as the result of acute intoxication, shock, peritonitis, tympany, or gastric rupture.

### EVERSION OF RECTUM

Eversion of the rectum is an extrusion of the rectum through the anus. Rectal prolapse is caused by pressure from increased peristalsis, constipation, and weakness of the perirectal tissues of the sphincter ani. Macroscopically, a portion of the intestine projects from the anus and curves downward. It becomes hyperemic and gelatinously infiltrated, at times hemorrhagic and torn. It usually becomes traumatized and dessicated. Sometimes it is covered with ulcers or necrotic areas. The prolapsed intestine easily becomes gangrenous.

Fig. 17.13 — Schematic drawing of an intestinal intussusception.

A, entering segment;
B, returning segment;
C, portion of mesentery whose vessels are being compressed;
D, portion of intestine containing the invagination.

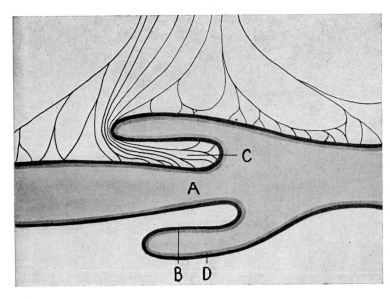

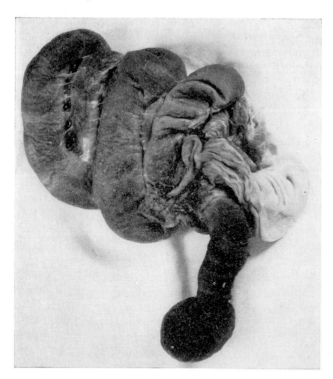

Fig. 17.14 — Intussusception of the ileum into the cecum of a pig. The cecum has been opened to expose the invaginated portion of the ileum. (F. W. Schofield.)

## Changes in the Size of the Lumen

### STENOSIS AND OBTURATION

Narrowing (stenosis) and closure (obturation) of the intestinal lumen owe their origin (1) to factors on the outside of the intestine or in its wall which may compress the lumen, such as enlarged lymph nodes and organs, tumors, adhesions, parasitic nodules, and abscesses; (2) to factors located within the lumen which cause obstruction, such as foreign bodies, concretions, masses of parasites, tumors, hematocysts, abscesses, chronic inflammatory proliferations, invagination, and impaction with ingesta or feces; and (3) to strangulation resulting from incarceration, torsion, and volvulus.

The results of stenosis are stasis of ingesta anterior to the narrowing, and in chronic cases compensatory muscle hypertrophy in this region. Dilatation of the intestine usually accompanies the hypertrophy. Bacterial decomposition of the ingesta often results in acute or chronic ca-

tarrhal enteritis, necrosis, and ulceration. The results of obturation are impaction anterior to the obstruction and increased peristalsis giving way later to paralysis of the musculature. Bacterial decomposition and fermentation of the ingesta result in an intestinal intoxication and tympanites. Later, gastric dilatation may occur. Carnivora and swine may vomit intestinal contents. In dogs a definite indicanuria develops which is attributed to intestinal putrefaction resulting from the stasis of ingesta and feces. After manifestations of collapse, death occurs within 24 hours by putrefactive intoxication, shock, gastric rupture, or tympanites.

### DILATATION

**Acute tympanitic dilatation** is caused by abnormal fermentation of ingesta, the swallowing of large quantities of air (wind-sucking horses), and hindrance to the expulsion of gas. It is frequent in the horse (flatulent colic). The results are distension of the abdomen, pressure upon the diaphragm, and gastric dilatation.

Acute and chronic alimental dilatation (impaction) occurs chiefly in the horse and dog. In dogs it is caused by voluntary suppressed defecation because of an enlarged prostate, painful conditions of the anal region (inflammation of the anal glands, anal sacs, circumanal glands) or of the abdominal wall. In horses it is caused by atony or paralysis of the intestinal musculature, by dry, coarse, or insufficiently masticated food, by diminished secretion, intestinal adhesions, stenoses, obstructions, cecal and colic artery occlusion, and atresia of the anus or rectum. The results are similar to those of intestinal obstruction.

### Alterations in the Intestinal Contents

**Abnormal coloring.** Retardation of passage of ingesta results in feces becoming darker than normal. A decrease of bile results in feces becoming lighter than normal. Blood originating in or entering the anterior alimentary tract becomes chocolate colored in the posterior part and sometimes black and tarry due to the action of hydrogen sulfide. Medicinal agents may alter the color. **Alterations in consistency.** Thin, fluid consistency points to increased secretions, decreased absorption, increased peristalsis, and passive hyperemia; also to lack of absorption due to enteritis. Thickened consistency points to retention in the intestine. The contents become greasy if undigested fat is present. **Putrefactive decomposition** takes place in stenosis and obstruction. Gas is produced as the result of fermentation, and a putrefactive odor as the result of protein decomposition. **Pathologic secretions** and **exudations** may be mucus, fibrin, blood, and pus, depending upon the type of inflammation. **Foreign bodies** of various kinds may be found such as sand in herbivora, coal and sand in pigs, grass and bones in carnivora, blood vessels of fetal membranes in cows, intestinal parasites in all animals. The results vary with their character, size, shape, and number. **Concretions,** such as enteroliths, food, and hair balls occur but often

cause no damage. Occasionally, they form an obstruction.

### Disturbances in Continuity

#### PERFORATIONS

Perforations may originate from the exterior (punctures and gunshot wounds); or from the interior (foreign bodies, parasites, ulcers, abscesses). Rapid penetration produces a wound with a hemorrhagic, smooth, or ragged border, swollen and soiled with ingesta. There are blood clots in the ingesta in the neighborhood of the perforation. Slow penetration produces a wound with a thickened margin (chronic inflammatory reaction). The serosa is covered with fibrin. Ulcers produce cone-shaped perforations with the apex at the serosa. Abscesses may rupture in adhesions between the intestine and the abdominal wall and show a ragged, thin border covered with pus. The results of perforation vary according to their size, location, and nature. Rapid perforations lead to acute peritonitis; slow ones to adhesions and localized peritonitis, abscess, or fistula formation.

#### RUPTURE

Rupture may be due to trauma (violent thrusts) or to distension. Accessory causes are any factors that lower the resistance of the intestinal wall. In horses rupture may occur at the stomach-like dilatation of the large colon, at the greater curvature of the base of the cecum, and at the beginning of the small colon. Macroscopically, the border of the tear is typical of ante-mortem rupture. The tear begins in the serosa and muscular coats, and if not complete the mucosa may protrude. The amount of ingesta in the abdominal cavity depends upon the size of the opening. The ingesta is distributed throughout the cavity by peristaltic movements and becomes entangled in fibrinous deposits on the serosa. Fluid in the abdominal cavity is derived from the ingesta, from the hemorrhage, and from the inflammatory process. Gas and sometimes concretions appear in the cavity. In the horse, death occurs within 1 to 6 hours by putrefactive intoxication or shock. If the animal lives longer, fibrino-purulent peritonitis may develop. Occasionally, there is fatal hemorrhage. In small ruptures the termination may not be fatal because the opening may become encapsulated as a result of the localized inflammatory process.

In sheep, perforations made by the larvae of the nodule-producing roundworm (*Oesophagostomum columbianum*) are scarcely recognized because they consist only of minute hemorrhages in the mucosa of the small and large intestine. In the wall of the intestine, however, the larvae cause a severe focal chronic inflammatory reaction in the form of a connective tissue nodule, in the center of which pale greenish caseous exudate accumulates. These nodules, which may be very numerous, occasionally rupture. Those opening into the intestine result in small ulcers. Those breaking through the peritoneum may give rise to local peritonitis with adhesions.

## Intestinal Emphysema

Intestinal emphysema is a rather frequent condition among swine, even in normal pigs that have reached the abattoir. Gas-filled vesicles varying in size up to about 2 cm. in diameter occur in the lymphatics of the mesentery near the place of attachment to the intestine and in the lymphatics of the wall of the intestine, principally in the jejunum and ileum. The etiology of the condition is not known. Biester and associates have produced it experimentally in pigs fed a deficient diet. Macroscopically, there are solitary, multiple, or conglomerate masses of gas-filled vesicles, which are sometimes pedunculated. At first the wall of each vesicle is clear or translucent. Later the wall may become red because of inflammation. Vesicles in the mucosa and submucosa occasionally project into the lumen of the intestine. Microscopically, there is gas in the lymph vessels and lymph nodes. The wall of the vesicles is lined with macrophages, many of which have grouped themselves to form foreign-body giant cells which enclose bubbles of gas. The surrounding connective tissue is infiltrated with lymphocytes and numerous eosinophils.

## Circulatory Disturbances

### PASSIVE HYPEREMIA

The acute form of intestinal passive hyperemia is due to sudden impediment to the venous outflow which usually owes its origin to some intestinal displacement such as a hernia, torsion, intussusception, or prolapse. The color of the intestinal wall is dark bluish- or brownish-red. The venous network is injected. There is edema with transudation into the abdominal cavity and intestinal lumen. Hemorrhages occur. The serosa becomes covered with fibrin. Later, gangrene and rupture may result. Chronic passive hyperemia of the intestine is due to hindrance to the blood flow in the portal system for a longer period of time. The subserous and mesenteric veins are injected. The mucosa is bluish-red and thickened. There is edema and later proliferation of connective tissue. The end result may be chronic catarrhal enteritis.

In edema disease of pigs edema of the mesentery of the coiled colon (mesocolon) is a characteristic lesion.

### THROMBOSIS AND EMBOLISM

Portal thrombosis is rare. Thrombosis of the intestinal arteries is very common in the horse and is due to larvae of *Strongylus vulgaris*. The most frequent location of the thrombosis is in the right branch of the anterior mesenteric artery, the branch which supplies the cecum and the ventral colon (Fig. 17.15). The series of changes which involves this artery is as follows: (1) Larvae of the very common intestinal roundworm, *Strongylus vulgaris*, irritate the wall of the artery and produce an acute arteritis. (2) A thrombus containing the larvae forms at the site of irritation (Fig. 17.16). (3) The thrombus partially or completely blocks the lumen of the artery so that an aneurysm forms at this

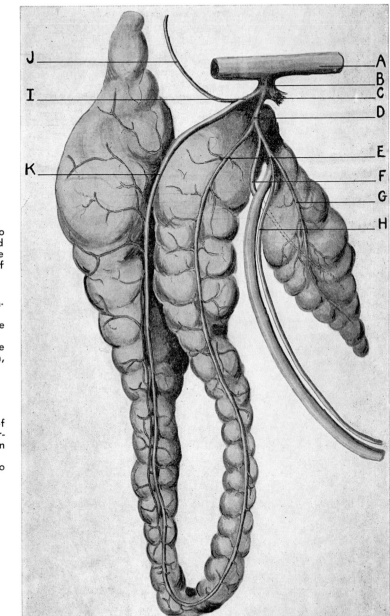

Fig. 17.15 — Drawing to show the principal blood vascular supply of the great colon and cecum of the horse.

A, posterior aorta;
B, root of anterior mesenteric artery;
C, left branch to the small intestine;
D, right branch to the great colon, cecum, and ileum;
E, ventral colic artery;
F, lateral cecal artery;
G, medial cecal artery;
H, ileal artery;
I, anterior branch of anterior mesenteric artery to dorsal colon and small colon;
J, middle colic artery to the small colon;
K, dorsal colic artery.

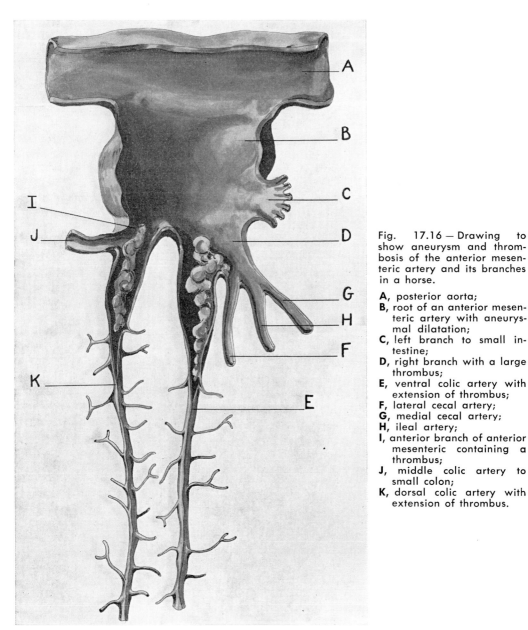

Fig. 17.16 — Drawing to show aneurysm and thrombosis of the anterior mesenteric artery and its branches in a horse.

A, posterior aorta;
B, root of an anterior mesenteric artery with aneurysmal dilatation;
C, left branch to small intestine;
D, right branch with a large thrombus;
E, ventral colic artery with extension of thrombus;
F, lateral cecal artery;
G, medial cecal artery;
H, ileal artery;
I, anterior branch of anterior mesenteric containing a thrombus;
J, middle colic artery to small colon;
K, dorsal colic artery with extension of thrombus.

point and also dorsally to it. (4) The larvae continue to irritate the vessel wall, and as a consequence, the arteritis becomes chronic and a fibrosis of the wall develops. The fibrotic arterial wall is less elastic than the normal vessel wall and therefore becomes stretched, but cannot contract. Because of this the aneurysm at this point becomes progressively larger and its wall thinner until occasionally under extraordinary strain it may rupture. Calcification of the wall may accompany the fibrosis, but this only makes the wall still less elastic. (5) The thrombus begins to undergo liquefaction and organization. As long as worm larvae are present, complete organization cannot occur because the larvae constitute a constant irritant. If the aneurysm is not large and the thrombus becomes organized completely, the arterial wall at this point becomes greatly thickened and the vessel lumen quite small. The aneurysm above this constriction then generally becomes enlarged.

The thrombosis of the right branch of the anterior mesenteric artery may have the following effects on the ventral colon and the cecum: (1) Blocking of the artery by the thrombus causes anemia in the portions of the intestine just mentioned. This is usually more serious in the cecum than in the ventral colon because the latter may still get an adequate blood supply from the dorsal colic artery. (2) The anemia is associated with poor nutrition of the musculature of the ventral colon and the cecum. This leads to atony of the musculature of these organs. (3) The atony is accompanied by diminished peristalsis. (4) Diminished peristalsis at a time when the ration consists of coarse, fibrous, relatively innutritious food leads to alimental dilatation (impaction colic). This is further provoked by an inadequate supply of water. On the other hand, decreased peristalsis along with succulent, fermentable food results in gaseous dilatation (gas colic).

What has been said so far about thrombosis of the anterior mesenteric artery has

been with reference to the right branch. The left branch, the one which supplies the small intestine, is seldom involved. The anterior branch sends the relatively unimportant middle colic artery to the small colon, and the very important dorsal colic artery to the dorsal colon. The origin of this latter branch is the seat of verminous or worm thrombi rather frequently but not so often as is the ventral colic artery. If the dorsal colic artery alone is involved, the consequences are not so serious, but when it, along with the ventral colic artery, is the site of thrombi, then the chain of events just described for the cecum can occur in the great colon.

The presence of a thrombus in the right branch of the anterior mesenteric artery of a horse always constitutes a threat to the origin of an even more serious pathologic process, which is embolism of the branches of the artery ventral to the thrombus. The embolus is a detached portion of the thrombus. The embolus usually lodges in the ventral colic or in the cecal arteries. The results vary depending on whether closure is partial or complete, sudden or gradual. In gradual closing, anastomosing vessels may dilate, take care of the extra load of blood, and no symptoms may appear. In the sudden closure of a single small branch of the anterior mesenteric artery, no clinical evidences are seen. If a large branch is occluded near its origin, the blood pressure falls in the affected area (temporary anemic infarct). Ischemia lasts for 1 to 2 hours, disturbing the nutrition of the capillary endothelium and injuring it so that it becomes pervious to the blood elements. Finally, blood enters these capillaries through anastomoses. Because of the occlusion of the artery which normally supplies this area, blood pressure in the part becomes diminished. As a result, the blood which flows in through the anastomosing vessels cannot be completely forced out again. It accumulates in the capillaries which have already been injured by faulty nutrition of the part, and as a consequence edema and hemorrhage occur. The whole affected area now constitutes a hemorrhagic infarct. Deficient oxidation and the accumulation of metabolites in the infarcted area result in necrosis and often gangrene. The affected portion of the intestine is dark red in color, edematously swollen; its lumen contains bloody fluid, and the serosa is covered with fibrin. Decomposition of ingesta produces tympanites and further dilates an already relaxed intestinal wall. Death results from putrefactive intoxication, peritonitis, shock, and possibly from hemorrhage.

Occasionally, in severe enteritis the irritant may pass from the lumen of the intestine into the veins and lacteals in great enough concentration to damage the endothelium of those vessels sufficiently so that clotting will occur in them. When this happens, thrombosis like that shown in Figure 17.17 results.

HEMORRHAGE

Hemorrhage of the intestine occurs in acute inflammations, septicemic diseases, various poisonings (Fig. 7.1), infarction, and passive hyperemia. In the septicemic diseases hemorrhage appears as multiple petechiae or ecchymoses. Their color is dark red, reddish brown, or almost black. They are seen in the mucosa or serosa.

On the mucosa they may appear as streaks involving the crests of the folds. In the propria mucosae are focal infiltrations of blood. The connective tissue is displaced by them. The glands of the mucosa are pushed aside and compressed. In connection with the hemorrhages which result from passive hyperemia, marked edema forces the tissues apart. In hemorrhagic infarcts the hemorrhagic infiltration is diffuse. Hemorrhage is also produced by trauma (foreign bodies, parasites), caustic substances, ulcers, and ulcerating tumors. The escape of blood may give rise to the formation of hematocysts in the submucosa and subserosa.

**Enteritis**

Most of what has been said about the occurrence and etiology of gastritis can be applied to enteritis. Often the two conditions appear simultaneously and together are called gastroenteritis. Like gastritis, enteritis can be primary or secondary. Examples which would apply to gastritis are almost equally suitable for enteritis. There are, however, a few special characteristics of enteritis which will be dealt with in the appropriate places. The general effects of enteritis — diarrhea, emaciation, and tissue dehydration — have already been mentioned under functional disturbances.

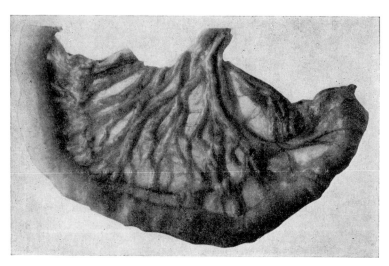

Fig. 17.17 — Thrombosis of the veins and lymphatics of the mesentery of a foal. (F. W. Schofield.)

## ACUTE CATARRHAL ENTERITIS

Acute catarrhal enteritis is the most common form but is difficult to differentiate from physiological changes occurring during digestion and also post-mortem changes. History and symptoms aid in differentiation. The tissues vary depending upon the nature of the secretion and the epithelial changes (serous, mucous, purulent, or desquamative catarrh). Macroscopically, the mucosa is reddened and swollen. The reddening is diffuse, spotted, or streaked (on the crests of folds). At necropsy, hyperemia may not be prominent although diarrhea was a symptom. Hyperemia, edema, and cellular infiltration of the propria are prominent. The villi are swollen. In severe cases the inflammatory reaction extends to the submucosa. Swelling of the solitary lymph follicles and Peyer's patches is marked. In young animals which normally have large lymph follicles, one must use caution in speaking of a pathological increase in the size of the follicles. There is a perifollicular hyperemic zone, at times hemorrhagic. If the latter is marked and if the post-mortem examination is not performed immediately after death, the color may be black due to the presence of hydrogen sulfide. Superficial epithelial defects (desquamation, erosions, ulcers) are common. The consistency of the contents of the lumen varies with the nature and amount of secretion and exudate. The mucosa is covered with an abundant, slimy, cloudy exudate. Portions of the exudate are mixed with the ingesta. In sections an increase in the neutrophils is significant in differentiating pathological from physiological conditions. Eosinophils occurring in a moderate amount when intestinal parasites are present are not significant. There is an increase in goblet cells. Among the infectious diseases in which acute catarrhal enteritis is present are diarrhea of sucklings, pullorum disease of baby chicks, hexamitiasis of turkeys, paratyphoid infection of poults, viral enteritis of mink, hog cholera, canine distemper, equine influenza, and vibrionic enteritis (winter scours) of cattle.

**Parasites** such as the *Cooperia* in calves produce a marked catarrhal enteritis in the first thirty feet of the small intestine. Adult worms and larvae are present in the gland crypts and in the mucosa and serosa. In severe cases the catarrhal inflammation is mixed with foci of a fibrinonecrotic reaction with hemorrhages.

**Enteritis or diarrhea of sucklings.** This is an acute infectious disease affecting very young animals, principally calves, but sometimes foals, lambs, and pigs, characterized by profuse diarrhea and rapid emaciation. The cause is not always a single infective agent. *Escherichia coli* is the microorganism most commonly encountered in all the animals, but in foals and lambs *Salmonella typhimurium* and in calves *Salmonella enteritidis* have also been the cause. In cattle the presence of *Brucella abortus* infection in the mother is responsible for the birth of premature and weakened calves, which are more susceptible to factors which bring on this disease. Discharges from genital infections of cows may be the source of the causative microorganisms. Prenatal infection may also occur. Since bacteria often cannot be isolated from the blood and organs before the affected calves reach the moribund condition in this disease, researchers are more and more inclined to believe that some other agent is the primary cause, possibly a virus.

The bacteria enter the gastrointestinal tract by way of the mouth. They next enter the tissues of the intestinal mucosa, then the lymphatics, and finally the lymph follicles. Penetration is said to be facilitated by the absence of the mucous layer in very young calves. From the lymph follicles the organisms pass to the mesenteric lymph nodes and finally to the blood stream (septicemia). In calves when *E. coli*, fecal type I, is the cause of the enteritis called white scours, it has been observed that a septicemia usually results in calves deprived of colostrum but that when calves receive colostrum the infection remains localized in the intestine. So-called immune proteins have been shown to be present in the colostrum for 24 hours after parturition. They disappear from the milk at about the same time the calf loses ability to absorb them from the intestinal tract. The period of incubation is 1 to 3 days in animals born healthy.

The principal lesions are emaciation, acute catarrhal enteritis, serous lymphadenitis (mesenterics), fibrinous polyarthritis occasionally, cloudy swelling of the parenchymatous organs, hemorrhages of the serous membranes (heart particularly), and acute swelling of the spleen. The termination is often fatal. Calf pneumonia is often an accompaniment of or a sequel to calf diarrhea.

### PURULENT ENTERITIS

Purulent or suppurative enteritis is encountered particularly in young animals. It is caused by pyogenic organisms gaining entrance to the mucosa through injuries or ulcers. In strangles, metastatic hematogenic abscesses may occur in the intestinal wall. Involvement of the lymph follicles may result in follicular abscesses and ulcers. In the rectum, abscesses may break into the surrounding tissues (periproctal abscess).

In chickens and turkeys small abscesses caused by a mucoid encapsulated strain of *Escherichia coli* may arise anywhere in the wall of the intestine but more especially in the wall of the ceca. Grossly and microscopically they appear like the lesions caused by *Mycobacterium avium*. The necrotic centers are contained within a connective tissue capsule having multinucleated giant cells. Since Hjarre of Sweden was the first to describe the condition, it is called **Hjarre's disease.**

**Pullorum disease,** also called bacillary white diarrhea of chicks, is an extremely septicemic disease of baby chicks, occasionally, also, of poults, guineas, and ducklings. It is caused by *Salmonella pullorum* and occurs during the first three weeks of life, attended with heavy mor-

tality, the greatest loss occurring between the fifth and twelfth days after hatching. It is characterized by great prostration and a white diarrhea. It is also a chronic infectious disease of mature hens, and occasionally of roosters, which is not so readily transmitted as among chicks. It is characterized by a chronic degenerative inflammation of the ovary in hens and sometimes by serous pericarditis in roosters. It occasionally becomes septicemic in hens and then terminates fatally.

Microorganisms in the infected ovary localize in the vitelline substance which constitutes the yolk of the egg. If the bacteria are in large numbers within the yolk, the latter undergoes degenerative changes, and ovulation fails. The retained yolk undergoes further degeneration. From it, *Salmonella pullorum* may enter the blood stream and result in septicemia and death. If the microorganisms are present in small numbers, ovulation occurs. From the infected yolk, the infection may be transferred to the oviduct and result in salpingitis. If the egg containing the infected yolk is incubated, the number of microorganisms may increase, causing death of the chick before it hatches, or the chick may have sufficient strength to hatch but succumb to the disease within a few days after hatching. Normal chicks from uninfected eggs associating with this chick either inhale infected down or consume infected feces and contract the disease. The organism may produce pneumonia, an enteritis, and a septicemia. Either death occurs or the chick recovers and may carry the infection to maturity. In pullets it localizes in the ovary, and in cockerels in the testicles and pericardial sac. Adult birds may also contract the disease by association with infected ones, most frequently, perhaps, from eating infected eggs. Attempts at experimental transmission of the infection via the oviduct have failed.

In **hens,** the vitelline sacs change from a rich or pale yellow color to gray, red, or brown, sometimes greenish. The gray yolks are cheesy in consistency. The red and brown ones are semi-fluid (blood-tinged). Frequently some become bright yellow and contain a thin, oily fluid. The size of the yolks varies. Caseous ones are likely to become nearly as large as a normal yolk. Bright yellow, oil-containing ones are usually pea size and firm. Red and brown ones are intermediate in size. The shape is usually irregular, at times even angular (Fig. 17.18). Many yolk sacs are pedunculated. The pedicles may separate and leave the yolks free in the abdominal cavity, or they may become attached to the visceral or parietal peritoneum by fibrous adhesions. One must not confuse the appearance of an ovary and yolks of a hen that has suddenly ceased laying with that of pullorum disease. In **pullets** salpingitis is observed. In **roosters,** there may be suppurative pericarditis. The organism has been recovered from the testicles, but no lesions are described. In **baby chicks,** acute catarrhal enteritis, focal necrosis of the musculature of the ventriculus, myocardium, and liver, and focal suppurative pneumonia are usual. Formerly, an unab-

sorbed yolk was considered an important lesion. It is now known to be of very little or no significance, as it may be found in most normal chicks under 3 weeks of age.

Other members of the paratyphoid group of organisms, notably *Salmonella typhimurium*, produce similar lesions in young birds of various species. This organism, like *Salmonella pullorum*, can be transmitted through the egg. In turkey poults it often causes an enteritis so severe that it has the appearance of *Salmonella choleraesuis* infection in swine.

**Fowl typhoid** is an acute septicemic disease of fowls caused by *Salmonella gallinarum* and characterized by drowsiness, prostration, anemia of the mucosa and skin of the head (usually), and by a decrease in erythrocytes and an increase in leukocytes. The period of incubation is 4 to 6 days.

Anemia of the mucous and serous membranes is prominent. The most marked changes are in the liver, kidneys, spleen, and blood. The liver is enlarged and dotted with grayish necrotic foci (focal necrosis).

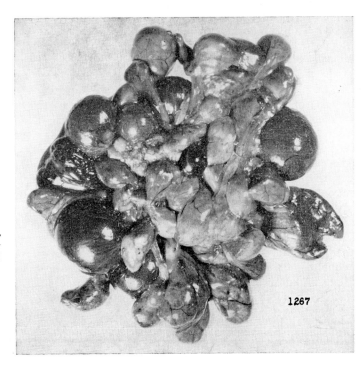

Fig. 17.18 — **Salmonella pullorum** infection of the ovary of a hen. (Hinshaw, Scott, and Payne; Jour. A.V.M.A.)

1267

Sometimes there is acute swelling of the spleen. It may show necrotic foci. The kidneys are enlarged and pale (cloudy swelling), yet slightly injected with blood. Occasionally, there is focal necrosis of the myocardium (grayish spots). The blood is pale, coagulates poorly, and shows a decrease in erythrocytes and an increase in leukocytes (particularly in neutrophils).

### FIBRINOUS ENTERITIS

Fibrinous enteritis is most frequent in cattle, swine, and cats, but it occasionally occurs in the horse and fowl. The causes are toxic agents (various medicinal substances) and bacteria (*Salmonella choleraesuis, Escherichia coli, Salmonella enteritidis*). In turkeys a fluke, *Echinostomum revolutum,* is the cause of a fibrinous inflammation of the large intestine.

Macroscopically, at times a fine fibrin network appears on the mucosa, at other times a heavy shredded membrane, at still others a diffuse, thick layer which may take the form of a tube (fibrinous cast). The color of the pseudomembrane is yellowish, yellowish gray, or grayish brown. The mucosa is hyperemic, edematous, and frequently sprinkled with capillary hemorrhages. The inflammatory reaction may extend to the submucosa. The intestinal contents are fluid and mixed with fibrin shreds and flocculi. The small intestine is affected more often than the large. From the exterior the affected portion can often be detected by its redness and the vessel injection of the subserosa. Microscopically, the membranous exudate consists of a fibrin network in the meshes of which are varying quantities of mucus, neutrophils, and desquamated epithelial cells. There is hyperemia, edema, and neutrophilic infiltration of the propria mucosae and villi. The tips of the villi may show necrosis and other parts may be devoid of epithelium. Frequently, the condition is fatal. A favorable termination occurs with loosening and evacuation of the fibrinous membrane (proteolytic action of the neutrophils next to the mucosa), and regeneration of the epithelium.

### HEMORRHAGIC ENTERITIS

This form of enteritis is caused by intense irritants of a toxic and infectious nature which injure the capillary walls. It appears in some acute septicemic diseases such as anthrax, bovine pasteurellosis, fowl cholera, and canine leptospirosis.

**Vibrio enteritis** in the swine-raising sections of the United States, particularly in the Corn Belt, hemorrhagic enteritis is a lesion of *Vibrio coli* infection. It is sometimes referred to as black scours because the blood-containing feces are black and tarry. A more correct name for the condition is swine dysentery. Grossly and microscopically, the mucosa of the small and large intestine is severely congested or hemorrhagic and is dotted with areas of focal necrosis. The ingesta and feces are mixed with blood. The stomach is usually simultaneously involved, especially the fundic portion.

The highly contagious **winter diarrhea** of stabled dairy cattle which is caused by *Vibrio jejuni* is characterized by enteritis varying from catarrhal to hemorrhagic. The hemorrhagic form deserves the name **vibrionic dysentery.** The onset of the enteritis is sudden — 3 to 7 days after exposure — and 10 to 100 per cent of a herd becomes affected. It is most severe in adult milking cows and seldom occurs in calves. A day or two before the diarrhea begins there is fever and the symptoms usually associated with elevation of temperature. During the scouring period the temperature is normal. In severe cases the feces are blood tinged because of the hemorrhagic inflammation involving the jejunum and ileum. The disease passes through a large herd in 1 to 3 weeks and through a small herd in 5 to 8 days. (In Canada a virus is reported more often to be the cause of winter scours than is *Vibrio jejuni.*)

In **histomoniasis** (blackhead) of turkeys, hemorrhagic cecitis is the primary lesion. *Histomonas meleagridis* invades the cecal epithelium, and causes hyperemia and leukocytic infiltration of the mucosa and submucosa with erosion of the epithelium.

With this there is a hyperplasia of the lymph nodules of the ceca. Within three days the inflammation has become very severe and the protozoan parasite has reached the liver by way of the portal vein. Because of the liver involvement simultaneous with that of the intestine, the disease is also called infectious enterohepatitis. In the later stages of the disease the inflammation extends through the muscularis externa and serosa so that histomonads may be present in the peritoneal cavity.

In **coccidiosis of chickens** there is a similar hemorrhagic cecitis. The ceca become dark red in color, swollen, and filled with a plug of hemorrhagic debris.

Hemorrhagic inflammation of the cecum, colon, and rectum is the principal lesion of **bovine coccidiosis**. In areas most severely affected, the surface epithelium is denuded and as a consequence there is bleeding. Where the surface is not denuded, there may be hemorrhage in the mucosa which varies from petechial to diffuse. Exudation into the mucosa often causes it to be raised into irregular ridges. The tops of the ridges may also be hemorrhagic. All stages in the development of coccidia are present in the epithelial cells of the intestinal glands, especially at the base of the latter. As the parasites mature, the cells containing them burst and release the parasites. Along with this, capillaries immediately underneath the epithelium also rupture, resulting in bleeding. These structural changes in the mucosa account for the diarrheal discharges of blood, mucus, and fibrin, and also the anemia and emaciation which are characteristic of coccidiosis.

**Enterotoxemia** of nursing calves, lambs,

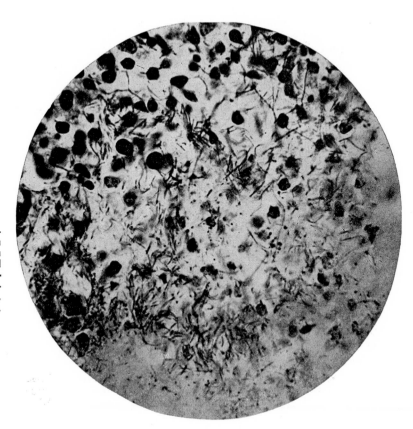

Fig. 17.19 — Fibrinonecrotic colitis in a pig due to **Salmonella choleraesuis** a n d **Spherophorus necrophorus.** ×880. (Murray, Biester, Purwin, and McNutt; Jour. A.V.M.A.)

and kids, and of overfed feeder lambs is characterized by a severe hemorrhagic enteritis which usually becomes a necro-hemorrhagic type of inflammation. The mucosa and submucosa of the jejunum, ileum, and colon are most seriously affected by the toxin of *Clostridium perfringens*, which is the cause of the condition. As a result of the hemorrhage and necrosis, many of the villi slough. The lumen of the intestine contains blood, necrotic tissue, inflammatory exudate, and the clostridial organisms. The severe inflammation may extend to the muscularis externa and serosa. A serohemorrhagic inflammation involves the adjacent lymph nodes.

FIBRINONECROTIC ENTERITIS

Fibrinonecrotic enteritis is a combination of coagulative necrosis of the mucosa and fibrin exudation in and on the mucosa. It occurs in all animals, but in the Middle West particularly in hogs. The etiology is similar to that of fibrinous enteritis, but in pigs it is most frequently caused by a deficiency of B-complex vitamins and *Salmonella choleraesuis* and *Spherophorus necrophorus* (Fig. 17.19). The former may initiate the condition and pave the way for infection by the latter.

Macroscopically, the affected areas may be superficial or deep, focal or diffuse, or confined to lymph follicles (Figs. 17.20 and 17.21). Therefore, the surface may be

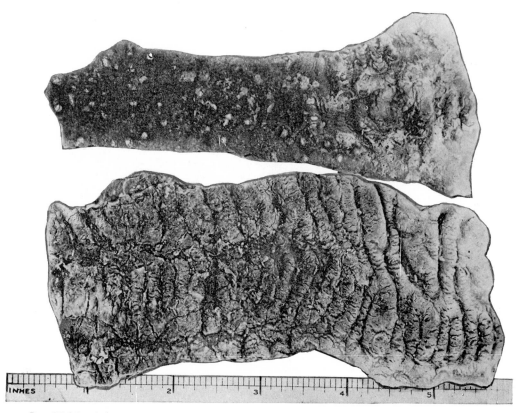

Fig. 17.20 — Infectious necrotic enteritis in a pig. **Above:** focal necrosis of the mucosa of the small colon. **Below:** diffuse necrosis of the mucosa of the large colon. (Murray, Biester, Purwin, and McNutt; Jour. A.V.M.A.)

strongly hyperemic with small, adhesive claylike deposits if the process is superficial; if deep, it may appear dry, firm, and fissured, having a color of grayish yellow, grayish brown, or grayish green. The submucosa is edematous. The intestinal contents are similar to those in the fibrinous form. The large intestine is more frequently involved than the small. The affected portion is often distinguishable externally by a hyperemic redness.

Microscopically, the normal structures of the fibrinonecrotic area are lost or nearly lost (Fig. 11.10). Bacteria are present in this area. The affected zone is variable in depth; even the submucosa may be included. A zone of inflammatory reaction separates the dead from the living tissue. Hemorrhages and edema are seen beneath this. If the process is extensive, death results; otherwise recovery occurs by digestion and sloughing of the fibrinonecrotic areas, filling of the gap with granulation tissue, and covering of the scar with regenerated epithelium. Specific infectious diseases in which fibrinonecrotic enteritis is present are hog cholera, infectious necrotic enteritis (so-called necro) of swine, rinderpest, and sometimes paratyphoid enteritis of poults (of the ceca in particular).

## NECROTIC ENTERITIS

Necrotic enteritis is quite similar to the fibrinonecrotic form except it contains less

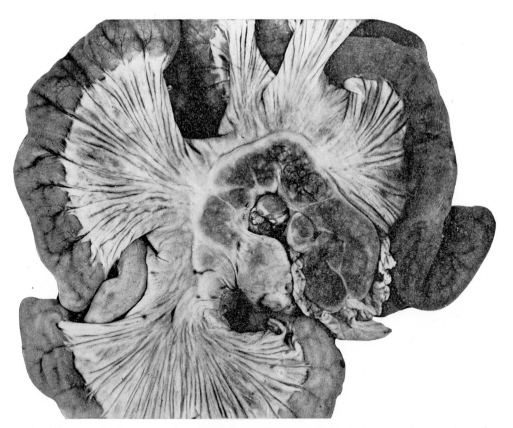

Fig. 17.21 — Infectious necrotic enteritis in a pig. Note distended mesenteric vessels and swollen lymph nodes with mottled appearance (serous lymphadenitis with focal necrosis). (Murray, Biester, Purwin, and McNutt; Jour. A.V.M.A.)

fibrin (Fig. 17.22). It is difficult to differentiate from the fibrinonecrotic form grossly. In the case of young chickens, coccidia are the cause of a very severe necrotic cecitis characterized also by much hemorrhage. In turkeys a severe necrotic cecitis (Fig. 17.12) with much exudate occurs in infectious enterohepatitis (blackhead) and sometimes in paratyphoid enteritis due to *Salmonella typhimurium.*

In young pigs (weanlings to 60 pounds) a necrotic enteritis is associated with the feeding of a ration low in protein (15 per cent or less) and deficient in some of the B vitamins (niacin, pantothenic acid, and possibly riboflavin). A ration of corn without adequate pasture is the kind which produces this nutritional type of necrotic enteritis.

The lesions are most prominent in the cecum and colon. In the early stages the lesions consist of multiple foci of mucous degeneration of the epithelium (Fig. 9.4). In these foci goblet cells increase in numbers, become excessively filled, and their nuclei become pyknotic. The crypts of Lieberkühn become gorged with mucus which is pushed up in plugs into the lumen where it becomes mixed with ingesta and feces. Because of this mixture of mucus and feces the plugs often remain adherent to the mucosa when the intestine is opened. The mucosa of the affected foci is dull and opaque. Later it becomes gray, or yellowish and cheesy. This occurs when necrosis follows the mucous degeneration. It starts at the base of areas in the mucosa which are in the state of mucous degeneration. As a consequence, the upper part of the mucosa is characterized by necrosis with a zone of inflammation located deeper.

The inflammation extends through the intestinal wall. The wall becomes thick, edematous, and the serosa covered with fibrin so that it ceases to be smooth and shiny, and becomes dull and rough. In later stages it becomes covered with fibrous tags. The colic lymph nodes display a serous inflammation.

It is reasonable to expect pigs with such lesions of the colon and cecum to develop

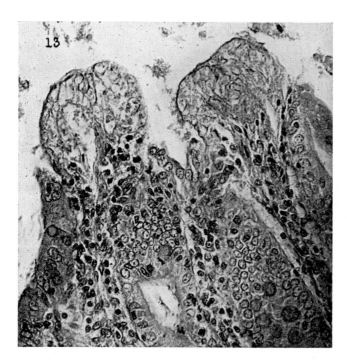

Fig. 17.22 — Necrotic enteritis due to **Isospora suis.** Loss of surface epithelium and necrosis of substantia propria of the terminal portion of villi. ×550. (Biester and Murray, Jour. A.V.M.A.)

a diarrhea, become dehydrated, cease to grow, and become runts.

**Salmonellosis of pigs and dogs.** Infectious enteritis of swine is also called necro, infectious colitis, infectious diarrhea, and pig typhoid. It is an acute or chronic infectious disease of pigs characterized by a diarrhea, emaciation, and a focal or diffuse necrotic or fibrinonecrotic enteritis. The primary cause is *Salmonella choleraesuis*. After this organism has produced the primary injury to the intestinal mucosa, *Spherophorus necrophorus* invades the necrotic tissue and multiplies deeply where anaerobic conditions prevail. Accessory factors in the cause of infectious necrotic enteritis are insanitary hog lots, whipworm infestation, coccidiosis, and the feeding of coal slack. The petechial hemorrhages of hog cholera which may occur in the intestinal mucosa also furnish an avenue of entrance for the two causative organisms.

Many cases of necrotic enteritis in pigs may owe their origin to niacin deficiency rather than *Salmonella choleraesuis* infection. In niacin deficiency the late lesions have the appearance of those of intestinal salmonellosis. Their origin is different, however, because they begin as foci of mucous degeneration of the epithelium of the large intestine. Necrosis supervenes so that the terminal lesions are almost identical even though *Salmonella choleraesuis* may not be present in the niacin-deficiency lesions.

*Salmonella choleraesuis* enters the intestinal tract and produces a primary inflammatory reaction with extensive necrosis, principally in the mucosa of the cecum and colon, occasionally in the ileum. Secondarily, *Spherophorus necrophorus* invades the necrotic tissue and causes further tissue destruction, chiefly at the base of the primary necrosis (Fig. 11.10). At first, the necrosis of the mucosa has only a focal distribution, but as the process becomes more and more extensive, the necrotic foci coalesce and the condition becomes diffuse (Fig. 17.20). Very rarely, when the bacteria are carried to the solitary lymph follicles in the submucosa, they cause abscessation. The abscessed follicles rupture into the intestine and give rise to peculiar button-shaped ulcers which occasionally characterize chronic hog cholera.

The most usual lesions are a focal or diffuse fibrinonecrotic cecitis and colitis, and occasionally ileitis (Fig. 17.20). The mesenteric lymph nodes display a serous lymphadenitis with foci of early caseous necrosis (Fig. 17.21). The parenchymatous organs undergo cloudy swelling. In severe cases the liver may show acute hepatitis with centrolobular necrosis. At times a septicemia develops in which the lesions resemble those of acute hog cholera and acute swine erysipelas. Acute swelling of the spleen is of rather frequent occurrence in this form of *Salmonella choleraesuis* infection.

The acute form of salmonellosis in swine may simulate hog cholera so closely, both from the standpoint of symptoms and lesions, that the diseases are difficult to differentiate. The reason is that the disease, which begins as a severe enteritis, soon becomes a septicemia. Besides the severe enteritis, acute swelling of the spleen is of rather frequent occurrence in this form of salmonellosis. The blood picture is that of a bacterial infection rather than a viral infection with an increase in neutrophils and a decrease in lymphocytes. Hyaline degeneration of blood vessel walls, proliferation of vascular endothelium, and resulting thrombosis are not present.

The death rate from infectious necrotic enteritis is not high. The effects on the pigs which survive, however, are alarming to the swine-raiser. Because of the extensive and often permanent injury to the mucosa of the cecum and colon, the affected animals are not capable of absorbing either nutrient materials or water. As a consequence, they become emaciated and dehydrated. They eat but do not grow.

Acute enteritis of dogs in kennels, veterinary hospitals, and dog racing tracks in Florida and other parts of the country is referred to as salmonellosis in the literature. Many mature healthy dogs harbor various species of Salmonella in the intestinal tract but do not become sick. In fact, such dogs do not develop enteritis when fed cultures of Salmonella. Debilitated dogs, puppies, and distemper-infected dogs become victims of the infections and develop a severe acute catarrhal or hemorrhagic enteritis.

**Transmissible gastroenteritis of swine.** Transmissible gastroenteritis is an acute viral disease of swine of all ages and is characterized chiefly by a severe inflammation of the gastrointestinal tract, which is responsible for the prominent signs of the disease: anorexia, diarrhea, vomiting, and dehydration with rapid loss of weight.

The virus most probably reaches the gastrointestinal tract in the food and water. The first indication of its invasion is a mild hyperemia of the gastric and intestinal mucosa which progresses down through the mucosa and submucosa to the muscularis externa. At first there is desquamation of the surface epithelium, but later there is necrosis even into the crypts of the glands. Baby pigs usually die at this point, but in older pigs the next step in the pathogenesis is an infiltration of the lamina propria with leukocytes (lymphocytes, macrophages, and neutrophils). From 1 to 7 days after exposure the pigs are definitely sick.

The most constant lesion is gastroenteritis varying from catarrhal to necrotic. There is atony of the intestinal wall and the presence of whitish, yellowish, or greenish fluid in the lumen. In baby pigs there is curdled milk in the stomach.

Changes in the kidneys begin with cloudy swelling of the tubular epithelium accompanied by congestion. This progresses to tubular necrosis.

The renal cortex appears anemic, and the medullary rays and collecting ducts are streaked with urates. The lesions are more prominent in baby pigs than in older hogs. Histologically, the gastrointestinal lesions are those described under pathogenesis. The renal lesions are those of degeneration, not nephritis. Hematologically, there is, on the average, a 49 per cent increase in leukocytes on the fourth day after exposure. The relative number of neutrophils increases while the number of lymphocytes decreases.

Among pigs less than 1 week old, 90 to 100 per cent die within 2 to 7 days after exposure. At 3 weeks of age, 30 to 60 per cent recover. Older hogs recover in 7 to 10 days.

**Viral diarrhea of cattle.** An acute infectious viral disease, characterized by multiple ulcers in the mucous membranes throughout the animal, has been described in cattle. Similar, if not identical, diseases (Indiana viral diarrhea, mucosal disease, mycotic stomatitis, malignant head catarrh) have been described in various parts of the United States. There is considerable evidence to indicate that infectious rhinotracheitis, in many instances, is probably nothing more than viral diarrhea. There is reason to believe that outbreaks of calf diphtheria may be preceded by a mild infection of this viral agent.

The disease is extremely prevalent throughout the United States, and probably the majority of animals are so slightly affected that clinical recognition of the disease is not accomplished. This probably explains why so many animals cannot be infected when inoculated with supposedly infectious material.

The viral agent is extremely infectious for susceptible cattle and spreads rapidly through the herd. The animals show anorexia, depression, and a very severe diarrhea. Animals that are still apparently normal in an affected herd may have temperatures of 105 to 108 ° F. Usually, when the diarrhea appears the temperature drops to normal or near normal. Shortly after the very severe diarrhea appears, multiple ulcers will be observed in the mouth, along the gum line, on the muzzle, and in the region of the external nares. A mucous or mucopurulent rhinitis is present, and an abundance of exudate may cover the muzzle (Fig. 17.23). In some animals there is rather profuse salivation. A serous, mucous, or mucopurulent conjunctivitis is present, and considerable ex-

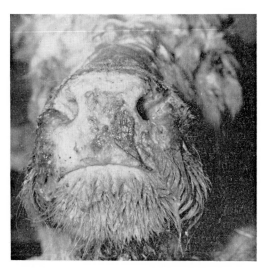

Fig. 17.23 — Viral diarrhea of cattle. Necrotic inflammation of the skin of the muzzle.

udate is encrusted on the hair below the eyes.

Abortion may follow the acute attack. When the relatively mild outbreaks of the disease in a herd occur, the association of the viral diarrhea with the wave of abortions is often overlooked, and considerable effort is made to demonstrate vibriosis, brucellosis, or leptospirosis when actually the basic disease is viral diarrhea.

Usually the cadaver is dehydrated and emaciated. An acute catarrhal inflammation is present throughout the gastrointestinal tract. Multiple ulcers with sharp borders (punched-out appearance) are found in the muzzle, the mucous membrane surrounding the external nares, tongue, dental pad, palate, gum line, esophagus (especially in the posterior 12 inches), forestomachs (particularly in the pillars of the rumen), multiple and rather shallow ulcers in the abomasum, and ulceration of the Peyer's patches and lymph follicles throughout the large and small intestine. The inflammation is most severe in the posterior 6 feet of the small intestine, where diffuse necrosis of the entire mucous membrane may be present. In some animals the necrosis also involves

the cecum and colon. One characteristic of the disease is the abundance of mucous in the intestinal tract that is especially noticeable in the region of the Peyer's patches.

The basic alteration is a catarrhal, suppurative or ulcerative inflammation of all mucous membranes. The viral agent appears to be particularly injurious to lymphoid tissue. Necrosis of lymphocytes within the Peyer's patches, lymph follicles, and lymph nodes throughout the animal is quite prominent. As a result, there is a noticeable suppression of lymphocyte regeneration. One of the characteristics of the disease is a leukopenia in which the leukocytes range from 450 to 3,100 cells per cubic millimeter.

The morbidity is usually from 33 to 88 per cent, and the mortality is usually low, ranging from 4 to 8 per cent. In a few herds a larger death loss may occur.

**Rinderpest** is an acute viral disease of cattle, occasionally of sheep, occurring chiefly in the orient. It is characterized by a typical course, destruction of lymphocytes, and necrosis of the epithelium of portions of the digestive tract.

The virus has an affinity for lymphocytes which it destroys in the various parts of the body where this tissue is prominent such as the spleen, lymph nodes, and Peyer's patches. The first indication of the attack upon the lymphocytes is karyorrhexis in the cells of the germinal centers. The destroyed cells are replaced by a cellless, fibrillar, eosinophilic matrix around which plasma cells, macrophages, and neutrophils accumulate. The lymphocytic destruction results in a leukopenia. Grossly, the spleen shows no indication of the severe histological changes which occur in it. The lymph nodes are enlarged because of edema. Peyer's patches often slough.

The virus also has an affinity for the epithelium of parts of the digestive tract. In the oral cavity, pharynx, and first portion of the esophagus the virus destroys the cells in foci in the stratum germinativum. This results in erosions which may coalesce to form irregularly shaped raw patches. These become covered with a caseous exudate consisting of ingestum, necrotic tissue, and bacteria.

The columnar epithelium of the abomasum and intestine is also attacked, and this results in denudation of the mucosal folds and villi. This results in hyperemia and hemorrhage of the lamina propria. The epithelium of the respiratory tract may be attacked also, but to a lesser degree. Other lesions occurring in affected animals are generally secondary.

**Infectious feline enteritis** is a highly contagious, rapidly spreading disease of cats, particularly kittens, which is caused by *Tortor felis*. Cats over 2 years of age appear to be quite resistant to the disease. Dogs and the usual laboratory mammals are not susceptible. The period of incubation is 4 to 7 days, usually 5 to 6. Affected cats sit in a prone position, refuse food, and display extreme lassitude.

Experimentally, the virus can be introduced into the body through any of the usual avenues of entrance for infections. Some investigators believe the virus enters the intestinal mucosa through punctures made by hookworms. Regardless of the place of entrance, the virus soon spreads throughout the body. At the height of the disease it appears in the blood, the viscera, and the excretions and secretions. In the blood the virus reduces the number of leukocytes. There is a controversy regarding which leukocytes are diminished in number. Some investigators maintain that the decrease is confined to the granulocytes, and therefore designate the disease a granulocytopenia. They also state that there is a decrease in the granulocytes, and call the disease an agranulocytosis. The decrease in granulocytes is attributable to the destruction of the bone marrow cells and an absence of differentiation of the myeloid cells. Other researchers have found a decrease in all leukocytes and prefer the designation panleukopenia. In the lymph nodes and spleen there is a proliferation of the reticuloendothelial cells. Nuclear inclusions appear in the gastrointestinal epithelium, in the epithelium of the bronchial mucous glands, in the reticular cells of the lymphoid tissue, and in the liver very early in the course of the disease and are not found in the later stages.

The principal gross lesions of infectious enteritis of cats occur in the middle third or the posterior half of the small intestine. Externally the affected portion of the intestine may be somewhat dilated and conspicuously reddened. This is because the subserous vessels are distinctly injected. Sometimes the serosa is covered with a delicate fibrin network indicating peritonitis — an extension of the inflammation from the mucosa to the serosa.

The changes within the intestine are those of an enteritis (Fig. 11.5) which may vary in intensity from a mild catarrhal form to a severe fibrinous or fibrinonecrotic form. The intestine contains a small amount of grayish-yellow or grayish-red, thin, foul-smelling fluid. The mucosa may be covered with an excessive amount of mucus, but more often there is a delicate fibrin network ½ to 1 mm. thick. The color of the mucosa is bright red, or brownish red. The mucosa is swollen and sometimes dotted with punctate hemorrhages. A very characteristic change is edema of the intestinal wall. The wall is thickened, and the cut edge has a glassy appearance due to a serofibrinous infiltration of the mucosa, submucosa, and muscularis.

Practically always there is serohemorrhagic inflammation of the mesenteric nodes. There may be a slight catarrhal gastritis. The heart, liver, and kidneys usually show the common degenerative changes which occur in severe bacterial and viral intoxications.

Due to the severe diarrhea and anorexia, affected cats become rapidly emaciated and dehydrated. Spontaneous recovery is reported to occur in only about 8.5 per cent of the cases. In some outbreaks practically all untreated cats succumb.

### CHRONIC CATARRHAL ENTERITIS

Chronic catarrhal enteritis arises from an acute catarrh or independently as a gradual slowly progressive process result-

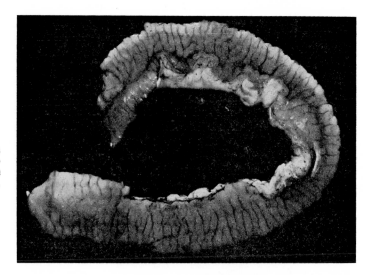

Fig. 17.24 — Chronic enteritis in a cow due to **Mycobacterium paratuberculosis.** Note thickened, corrugated mucosa. (Howarth, Jour. A.V.M.A.)

ing from parasitic infestation. It is seen also as a complication of chronic interstitial hepatitis and chronic heart disease, both of which result in chronic passive hyperemia of the intestine. The mucosa is gray in color, except in chronic hepatic and cardiac diseases, where it is bluish or brownish red. There is a hyperemic zone around the lymph follicles, and at times hyperplasia of the latter. The mucosa is covered with viscid, glassy, cloudy mucus. There is proliferation of the connective tissue and lymphocytic infiltration of the mucosa and submucosa (chronic hypertrophic enteritis). The mucosa may be smooth or granular, or pushed up into

rigid folds. Degeneration and atrophy (pressure) of the glands are prominent. Closure of the mouths of glands leads to retention-cyst formation. The newly formed connective tissue may contract (chronic atrophic enteritis) (Figs. 17.24, 17.25, and 17.26).

**Paratuberculosis (Johne's Disease).** This is a chronic infectious disease of cattle, occasionally of sheep, caused by *Mycobacterium paratuberculosis* and characterized by a chronic catarrhal enteritis which results in a profuse diarrhea leading to extreme emaciation (Fig. 17.27).

The organism reaches the intestine (jejunum, ileum, cecum, and colon), where

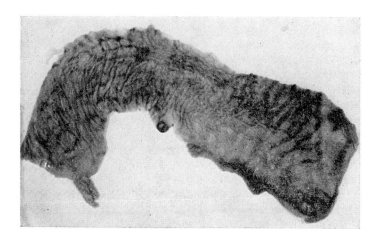

Fig. 17.25 — Chronic cecitis in paratuberculosis. Note irregular folds of the mucosa with hyperemic crests. (Howarth, Jour. A.V.M.A.)

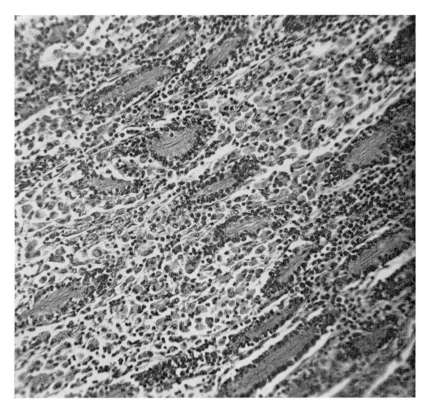

Fig. 17.26 — Lesion of paratuberculosis in the intestinal mucosa of a cow showing accumulation of macrophages between the glands, absence of necrosis, and scarcely any proliferation of connective tissue. (Department of Veterinary Pathology, Michigan State University.)

it either passes through the epithelium of the glands or is engulfed by macrophages and carried through the epithelium. In the mucosa the organism acts as an irritant and produces an inflammatory reaction. (See Figures 11.2, 11.3, and 11.4.)

From this area the organisms are carried by way of the lymph spaces to the submucosa and may there produce changes in the lymph vessels. The bacteria are next carried to the mesenteric lymph nodes, where a chronic inflammatory reaction results. The infection is apparently arrested here as lesions rarely appear elsewhere. Hagan has shown that natural infection establishes itself in very young calves and develops slowly so that lesions of sufficient extensiveness to cause symptoms do not occur until after a heifer calves for the first time — between 2 and 3 years of age.

Animals over 4 months of age are quite resistant to the infection. The period of incubation therefore is expressed in months — even years.

The lesions usually occur somewhere between the jejunum and the first part of the rectum. Macroscopically, the intestine may show no changes externally. Frequently, however, it may show variable thickening of the wall and cordlike enlargement of the subserous and mesenteric lymph vessels, distinct edema of the serosa and of the mesentery, especially at the attachment of the latter and along its vessels (Figs. 17.24 and 17.25). Alterations of the mucous membrane are especially characteristic. Increased thickness (3 to 20 times) takes place, and the formation of rigid, tortuous folds. The mucosa is pale yellowish white or grayish yel-

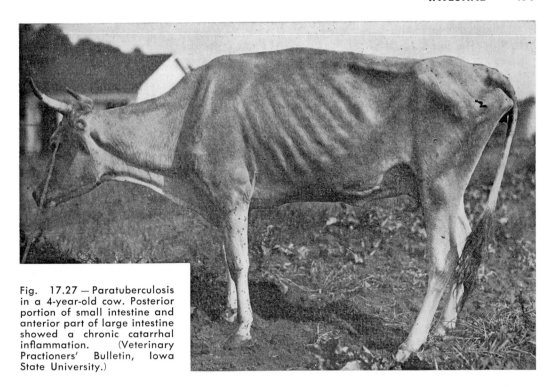

Fig. 17.27 — Paratuberculosis in a 4-year-old cow. Posterior portion of small intestine and anterior part of large intestine showed a chronic catarrhal inflammation. (Veterinary Practioners' Bulletin, Iowa State University.)

low. Here and there on the crests of the folds there is hyperemia. The mucosa is covered with adhesive, viscid, cloudy, grayish-yellow mucus. There are no nodules, necrosis, or ulcers. Only a small amount of ingesta is present.

Microscopically, the picture is also typical. The mucosa and villi are thickened (Fig. 17.26). The latter are club-shaped or wartlike. The thickening is due to the presence of macrophages which, when stained for acid-fast organisms, appear to be filled with them (Fig. 11.4). Many of these cells, filled with bacteria, can also be seen upon the epithelial surface. Often, the macrophages group themselves into multinucleated giant cells. Lymphocytes and eosinophils collect around the foci of macrophages. This paratuberculous tissue pushes the intestinal glands apart, compresses them, and results in their disappearance. The macrophages containing the microorganisms follow lymph spaces and vessels to the submucosa, the serosa, and

the mesentery. The microorganisms produce a chronic lymphangitis.

The **mesenteric lymph nodes** are enlarged and soft. They show a moist cut surface and yellowish-white foci. There is no necrosis. Microscopically, these foci consist of macrophages. The bacteria apparently exert little or no toxic action. They seem to cause irritation like foreign bodies. The changes in the lymph nodes are those of a chronic inflammatory reaction.

### Inflammation of Anal Glands

Inflammation of the anal glands of the dog is caused by trauma due to hard fecal balls and by pyogenic bacteria. It is characterized by abscess formation and may then result in the development of a fistula.

### Inflammation of Bursa Fabricii

Inflammation of the bursa fabricii in the fowl is caused by parasites, bacteria, hard feces, and foreign bodies. A chronic form may be due to the occlusion of the bursal duct. Inflammation of the bursa occurs in poults affected with A-avitaminosis. In this disease the bursae become distended with a flaky, white, urate-like substance.

### Tumors

Tumors of the intestine are not as common among domestic mammals as in man. If there is any particular tumor whose occurrence is more frequent than that of others it is the lymphosarcoma. Its occurrence is greatest in the cow, dog, and cat. A variety of other tumors have been reported, such as sarcomas, carcinomas, lipomas of the mesentery, leiomyomas, lymphangiomas, adenomatous polyps in the large intestine in cattle and hogs, and leukotic tumors in chickens. There is little difference in the incidence of tumors in the small and large intestine.

An adenoma at the anal end of the digestive tube of the dog deserves special mention. Lateral to the anus near the mucocutaneous junction are the perianal or circumanal glands — specialized sebaceous glands. Adenoma of these glands is the most common tumor of this region. It occurs most often in male dogs about 9 years of age.

The perianal glands are liver-like in structure, composed of elongated collections of large, polyhedral cells having abundant cytoplasm. Secretion canals lie between the cells similarly as bile capillaries in the liver but there are no sinusoids. An occasional bundle of skeletal muscle is interspersed among the collections of gland cells, especially at the periphery of the gland.

Microscopically, the tumor in general has the appearance of the normal gland except in volume. There is simply a hyperplasia of the gland cells, and occasionally of the ducts also. The surrounding and intervening tissue is encroached upon, and because some bundles of skeletal muscle are intimately associated with the gland, one may mistakenly get the impression that there is malignant invasion by the tumor. The gland cells, however, seldom show any anaplasia and do not metastasize. The tumor may become acutely inflamed and even ulcerate. Such tumors are painful and interfere with defecation.

## LIVER

### Functional Disturbances

The liver is the largest organ in the body and probably possesses the greatest number and variety of functions. The hepatic epithelial cells, highly specialized in their functions, are normally in direct contact with about 25 per cent of the blood of the body if the intravital distribution of blood in the liver is analogous to that occurring after death. Because of the highly specialized functions of the hepatic parenchymal cells and the vast blood supply of the organ, it is quite obvious that injuries to these cells or interference with the hepatic vascular system may have serious and far-reaching effects not only on the liver itself but also on other organs and systems.

Functional disturbances of the liver are more easily understood when one considers the changes which may affect a single unit of structure — the lobule. In doing this, one must keep in mind the principal anatomic structures which comprise the lobule — the liver cells, the blood vessels, and the bile passages. He must also keep in mind the anatomic and functional relationship of these structures to each other. At the outset of a liver disturbance any one of these structures may be the seat of the trouble, but sooner or later, because of their intimate anatomic association, the lesions affecting them spread so that eventually all parts of the lobule are involved. Since, in most cases, all of the lobules, or at least those of a particular lobe, are simultaneously exposed to the causative factor, the entire organ or large parts of it are affected in the same manner at the same time. Because of the varied and important functions of the organ and also because of its location with reference to other organs, it is not surprising that liver lesions may lead to serious and widespread disturbances in other parts of the body. Stated briefly the functions are:

**1. Secretion of bile.** Bile pigments serve no purpose, but their retention in the body results in hyperbilirubinemia and a generalized yellowish pigmentation with symptoms of an intoxication (obstructive and toxic jaundice).

Bile acids (cholic and desoxycholic) are formed in the liver from cholesterol, conjugated with tourine or glycine, and excreted in the bile as sodium salts. These bile salts activate pancreatic lipase, probably accelerate the activity of pancreatic amylase, aid in the emulsion of fat in the intestine, facilitate the absorption of fat and fat-soluble vitamins (the most important one being vitamin K) from the intestine, and act as cholagogues. When bile is not excreted, vitamin K is not absorbed, and soon prothrombin ceases to be formed. Bile is alkaline and thus aids in maintaining the most suitable reaction in the intestinal tract. Mucin or a mucin-like substance in the bile helps as a stabilizer of the fat emulsion in the intestine. While bile is not an antiseptic in the strict sense of the word, it does make the intestinal contents an unfavorable medium for the growth of bacteria which cause putrefaction.

**2. Protein metabolism.** Amino acids are deaminized, urea is formed from ammonium salts which are said to be 40 times more toxic than urea, and uric acid is converted into allantoin. The non-nitrogenous residue from the deaminization of amino acids is converted into glucose, ketone bodies, and other materials used as fuel for metabolism. In the metabolism of proteins the liver uses the amino acids to form (1) the plasma proteins — albumin, globulins, fibrinogen, prothrombin, and cholinesterases, (2) tissue proteins, and (3) protein reserves that are stored in the liver. When the structure of the liver is disturbed, the amounts of the nitrogenous constituents of the plasma are changed. Determining the amounts of the various nitrogenous constituents of the plasma then gives indica- tions of disturbed liver function and is a useful means of detecting liver disease. A test for only one such nitrogenous substance is not sufficient. Several tests may be necessary because the amounts of the various nitrogenous constituents are not altered to the same degree. The reason for this is that liver function relative to the production of some constituents is easily upset, whereas with others extensive parenchymal changes are required.

**3. Carbohydrate metabolism.** Glycogen is formed and stored in the liver. When excessive amounts of carbohydrates are absorbed from the intestine, the liver converts the excess to lipids which are stored in the regular fat depots.

**4. Fat metabolism.** In the intestine, bile salts aid in the emulsification of neutral fats in the food. After the fats are emulsified, they are hydrolyzed to produce fatty acids and glycerol which are absorbed by the intestine. In the intestinal mucosa the fatty acids and glycerol are resynthesized to fats which are characteristic for the particular species. These fats consist of a mixture of neutral fats such as comprise lard, beef tallow, mutton tallow, and chicken fat. In the mucosa these fats pass mostly into the lacteals of the villi and eventually reach the blood. Deficiency of bile, either in quantity or quality, in the intestine allows fat to pass through the intestine in an unemulsified and consequently in an unabsorbable state. This results in an excess of fat in the feces (steatorrhea).

The liver constantly removes neutral fat from the blood. This fat consists not only of that absorbed from the intestine but also some that is released by the fat depots. The liver transforms this fat into tissue fat, mostly phospholipid, which the organ gives back to the blood for use by the tissues. For this transformation of fat, choline is necessary. If choline is not present, the neutral fat accumulates in the hepatic cells (fatty infiltration).

**5. Iron metabolism.** In some species of animals, at least, the reticuloendothelial cells of the liver, along with these cells in certain other parts of the body, destroy erythrocytes. Much of the iron derived from these cells is stored in the liver.

**6. Detoxication.** Some toxic substances, particularly putrefactive products of the intestinal tract, which are brought to the liver through the portal system are made harmless by conjugation. Other endogenous substances inactivated by the liver are bacterial toxins and hormones produced in excess by the endocrine glands. Some exogenous chemical substances used in veterinary medicine are also inactivated by the liver; among these are camphor, phenol, benzoic acid, morphine, and the barbiturates. Evidences of intoxication are characteristic of some liver disturbances.

**7. Erythropoiesis.** Under certain circumstances the liver may stimulate and even participate in the formation of red blood cells and hemoglobin in mammals. In birds it is a normal site of erythrocyte production.

**8. Vitamin metabolism and storage.** Disturbed liver function interferes with the absorption of the fat-soluble vitamins A, D, K, and E in the intestine. This occurs when there is a deficiency of bile. The storage of vitamin A in the liver, the utilization of vitamin K in the formation of prothrombin by the liver, and the metabolism of some of the water-soluble vitamins, notably of thiamin, riboflavin, and niacin, are interfered with in some hepatic diseases. Not only does the liver act in the metabolism of these three members of the B vitamin complex, but the organ itself is dependent upon them for its well-being.

**9. The liver and portal vein bed,** with the spleen, act together to provide a huge blood reservoir. They control the outflow of blood into the posterior vena cava and thereby act as a major factor in the control of cardiac output. Experimentally, adrenalin causes the outflow mechanisms of these organs, especially of the liver, to relax and release blood. Just how this mechanism behaves in disease is not known, but it can be assumed that it is affected.

A review of this long list of liver functions leads one to conclude that if the structure of this organ is altered by irritants of various kinds, then the functions of the organ itself and that of other organs may also be affected. A partial list of the effects would include hyperbilirubinemia with icterus and bilirubinuria, emaciation from disturbances in the various stages of fat metabolism, excessive intestinal putrefaction and intoxication arising from it, hypoglycemia, delayed coagulation of the blood, anemia, and portal hyperemia with hydroperitoneum. Fortunately the liver, like the heart and kidneys, has a remarkable reserve power.

Functional disturbances of the liver can be detected by a variety of tests. There are one or more tests available for each function. Unfortunately the severity or extent of hepatic damage cannot be adequately measured by the tests that are available, but the presence of damage can often be ascertained by repeated testing and by using combinations of tests. The use of a combination of tests is advantageous because all functions of the liver are seldom disturbed simultaneously or to the same degree. Sometimes it is necessary to supplement the function tests with liver biopsy.

**Disturbances in Continuity**

**Rupture** of the liver is usually due to forceful blows or to squeezing. Conditions favorable to rupture are increased friability of the hepatic parenchyma and stretching of the capsule. Pathological conditions in which rupture may occur are fatty infiltration, amyloid infiltration, tumors, tuberculosis, and leukemia (leukosis). The latter two occur in chickens, particularly. The liver capsule may or may not be ruptured. If the capsule ruptures, fatal hemorrhage may occur. In the horse when rupture occurs there may be 5 to 25 liters of blood in the abdominal cavity. **Perforations** are caused mostly by foreign bodies from the forestomachs and by parasitic larvae. The former penetrate slowly and become encapsulated; the latter more rapidly and produce some hemorrhage and tissue destruction.

## Disturbances of Circulation

**Passive hyperemia** of the liver is of frequent occurrence. It is caused by any hindrance to the flow of blood in the hepatic vein, or posterior vena cava, or through the right heart or lungs. Baby pigs reared in a cold, damp environment often develop congestion and hemorrhage of the central part of the liver lobules. The condition does not make its appearance until the pigs are about 3 weeks of age. It is believed that prolonged chilling drives the blood from the skin into the viscera. The liver is the organ most affected.

The macroscopic and microscopic appearances depend upon the severity and duration of the stasis. At first, the central vein and that portion of each sinusoid where it empties into the central vein is dilated. The liver is consequently enlarged, firm, brownish red, or dark bluish red, its capsule stretched. Blood flows from the cut surface. With continued stasis, the liver cells atrophy due to pressure and disturbed nutrition. The peripheral cells undergo fatty infiltration. Therefore, the periphery of the lobule is yellowish brown or bright yellow in color, and the center is dark red. The liver has a nutmeg appearance. Later, a proliferation of the connective tissue may occur in the wall of the central vein and extend outwardly into the lobule. The liver becomes firmer due both to increased venous blood and to an increase in connective tissue. The accumulation of blood in the liver interferes with the flow of blood from the portal vein into the liver. The resultant portal hyperemia leads to splenic passive hyperemia, gastrointestinal hyperemia, and to chronic gastroenteritis if the hepatic passive hyperemia is of long duration. In the latter case, hydroperitoneum also occurs.

## HEPATIC LESIONS PECULIAR TO CATTLE

In the packing houses of the Middle West, condemnation of large numbers of bovine livers for **telangiectasis,** "sawdust," and abscesses makes it necessary to give special attention to these lesions. Because of the frequency of occurrence of these conditions, either singly or in combination in the liver of an individual animal, or because several animals from the same herd have shown the lesions, there is reason to believe that the conditions may be related. These lesions — telangiectasis, "sawdust," and abscesses — which are peculiar to cattle livers occur chiefly in feed-lot animals generally between the 40th and 80th days under full feed. From the time the animals enter the lot until they are on full feed, they are fed gradually increasing amounts of a highly nutritious ration. This is the period during which glycogen accumulates rapidly in the liver cells. The accumulation becomes so great that a state of pathologic glycogen infiltration can be said to exist. In California it has been shown that not only do the hepatic cells become heavily infiltrated with glycogen but also granules of glycogen accumulate between the liver cells and the endothelium lining the sinusoids. These two histological changes pave the way for the formation of blood cavities (telangiectasis) in the lobules. These in turn may result in so-called sawdust and abscesses. The pathogenesis of a single lesion appears to be as follows:

In foci in which hepatic-cell glycogen infiltration with its accompanying accumulation of glycogen between these cells has occurred to an extreme degree, breaks develop in the endothelial lining of the sinusoids. This permits blood to push between the hepatic cells and the endothelial lining, wash out the accumulated glycogen, and erode the liver cells. Some liver cells atrophy, others become eroded and disintegrate. In this manner a cystlike cavity arises which constitutes the primary telangiectasis. Grossly, it is a pin-point, purplish-black spot.

From a tiny telangiectasis, perhaps a lobule in size, the lesion may become larger by the coalescence of several other similar lesions.

The degenerated and necrotic hepatic cells, together with the erythrocytes mixed with them, give the whole area a homogeneous, structureless, hyalinized appearance. This phase of the lesion is termed "sawdust" because grossly it has the appearance of a gray particle of sawdust. If this necrotic focus does not become infected with *Spherophorus necrophorus* or other pyogenic bacteria which finds such areas suitable for growth, resolution and repair by regeneration occur. The necrotic tissue is digested by enzymes or removed by phagocytes. Newly formed cords of hepatic cells push into the area from the surrounding normal tissue. Because of the ability of hepatic tissue to regenerate, repair by substitution with connective tissue does not occur, or if it does occur, it is at a minimum. Even after the regeneration has taken place, the sinusoids may be ex-

tremely wide, giving rise to the large cavernous blood spaces observed in older cattle. This lesion can properly be called secondary telangiectasis.

If, simultaneously with the telangiectasis and "sawdust," the animal has a localized pyogenic infection elsewhere in the body, metastasizing bacteria may find the lesions suitable for enlodgement, with the subsequent development of abscesses. Ulcers in the rumen due to *Spherophorus necrophorus* are examples of lesions found in association with abscess development in telangiectasis and "sawdust."

In this description of the pathogenesis of the hepatic lesions only a single focus has been described. Such lesions can be single or multiple and can have local or disseminated distribution. As yet the cause of the condition is unknown. Apparently some agent capable of causing a primary focal necrosis initiates the process. Vinylite-corrosion models of the hepatic vascular system show that the telangiectases occur principally in connection with the terminal interlobular branches of the portal vein.

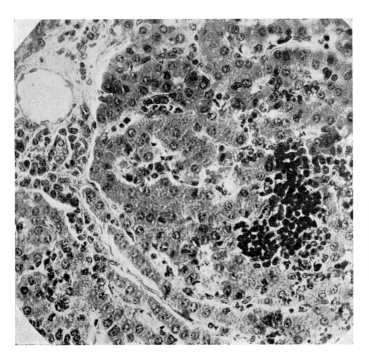

Fig. 17.28 — Hepatic lesions in nutritional anemia of a pig. Note one large and two smaller hematopoietic centers and several scattered erythrocytes. (Doyle, Mathews, and Whiting; Jour. A.V.M.A.)

## ANEMIA

In nutritional anemia of young pigs the liver is enlarged and has a mottled appearance. The enlargement is due to the presence of dense collections of erythroblasts and myelocytes — active hematopoietic centers (Fig. 17.28) — and also to cloudy swelling of the hepatic epithelium, to hemorrhages, and passive hyperemia. The passive hyperemia can be attributed partly to myocardial degeneration with the accompanying cardiac dilatation and hydropericardium. The mottled appearance of the liver is due to an intermingling of normal with degenerated epithelium (Fig. 9.8). In the liver lobules, cloudy swelling and fatty degeneration of the epithelium may have a central, an intermediate, or a peripheral location (Fig. 17.29). Sometimes entire lobules are degenerated. If recovery takes place, some degree of cirrhosis remains.

## Disturbances in Growth and Cell

### ATROPHY

**General atrophy** of the liver occurs in general nutritional diseases, cachectic diseases, old age, and in starvation. The atrophy depends upon a decrease in size of liver cells and therefore, of the lobules. The organ becomes firmer, the parenchyma decreases, and the interstitial tissue remains the same. The latter appears to be relatively increased. The borders of the lobes become sharp. **Local atrophy** of the liver is due to tumors, cysts, tuberculous and actinomycotic nodules, abscesses, and parasitic cysts (Fig. 8.2). The size of the atrophied area is dependent upon the size of the etiological factor. Unaffected portions of the liver undergo compensatory hypertrophy. In intralobular atrophy of the liver there is macroscopically no atrophy of the organ, but microscopically, the cords of the liver cells are atrophied due to pressure by chronic hyperemia or connective tissue proliferation.

### CLOUDY SWELLING

Cloudy swelling is an indication of a rather mild hepatic intoxication. The irritant may be an inorganic or organic chemical substance which is brought to the liver by the portal vein from the intestine.

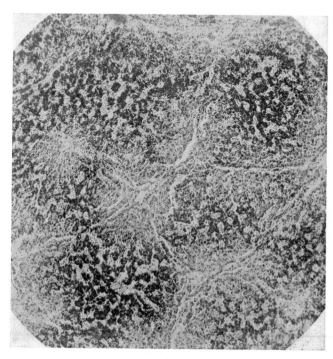

Fig. 17.29 — Hepatic fatty degeneration in nutritional anemia in a pig. Fat in the epithelial cells in the centers of the lobules is stained with Sudan III. Low power. (Doyle, Mathews, and Whiting; Jour. A.V.M.A.)

The particular chemical agent may be the salt of some heavy metal like arsenate of lead which has been ingested accidentally, or one that has been administered in excessive doses such as arsenic trioxide. On the other hand, it may be an alkaloid, a glucoside, or a saponin found in an ingested poisonous plant, or carbon tetrachloride used as an anthelmintic. Then again the irritant may be the products resulting from the growth of *Spherophorus necrophorus* and *Salmonella chloraesuis* in the cecum and colon of a pig, or those resulting from a heavy infestation of intestinal roundworms. More frequently still, hepatic cloudy swelling may result from the severe bacterial and viral intoxications in most of the acute septicemic diseases. Macroscopically, the liver is enlarged, the borders are obtuse, the consistency is soft and exceedingly friable, the color is dull grayish brown (cooked appearance), and the cut surface bulges. Microscopically, the cells are enlarged, the cytoplasm is granular, and the nuclei are often indistinct. The cells may recover, or the changes may progress to fatty degeneration and necrosis. This progressive degeneration and death of cells is often called necrobiosis.

### AMYLOID INFILTRATION

Amyloid infiltration of the liver is ordinarily said to be rare in animals, but there is some evidence that it occurs more frequently than is generally thought. The amyloid is possibly a precipitation product of an antigen-antibody reaction, although there is reason to believe that it may result from a hyperglobulinemia. It is observed in chronic pyogenic processes, chronic tuberculosis, and in horses used for serum production. If the condition is extensive, the liver is enlarged, of a firm, waxlike consistency, its color pale brown (anemic), and its capsule distended. The cut surface has a lardaceous appearance. Microscopically, in hematoxylin and eosin stained sections, there are homogeneous eosinophilic masses deposited between the cords of liver cells and blood sinuses. The process begins at the periphery of the lob-

ules and extends to the center. Pressure atrophy and anemia result and sometimes icterus. Hepatic rupture is possible.

### GOUT

In visceral gout of birds, crystals of uric acid and of monosodium urate may be deposited in the parenchyma as well as upon the surface of the liver. The cut surface has a frosty appearance.

### FATTY LIVER

**Fatty infiltration** of the liver is physiologic in animals being fattened, in pregnant females, in castrated males, and in brooding hens. Pathological fatty infiltration may be the result of increased intake and assimilation of fat as in overfeeding or fattening of animals, or decreased oxidation of fat as in disturbances of nutrition and in the early stages of certain chronic infectious diseases (tuberculosis).

An extremely fatty liver is often present in severe cases of ketosis (acetonemia) in cows and ewes. The condition occurs most often in well-nourished, high-producing cows following parturition, and in poorly fed pregnant ewes carrying twins or triplets. These animals require a high carbohydrate ration as a source of energy. If such a ration is lacking, the liver draws upon the fat reserves and converts the fat to ketone bodies. In this shift of liver functions from glycogen storage to the conversion of fat to ketone bodies, large quantities of fat are stored. The liver presents the picture of extreme fatty infiltration.

In diabetes mellitus of dogs and cats a characteristic lesion is a fatty liver. In diabetes, when glycogen is not stored in the liver, fat is transported from the fat depots to the liver and stored much as it is in ketosis.

**Fatty degeneration** of the liver usually has the same etiology as cloudy swelling. As mentioned several times previously, however, it requires a more drastic irritant to disturb the fat metabolism of cells than it does to upset the protein metabolism. Therefore, the principal difference between the etiology of these two degenerations is one of quantitative rather than of qualitative effect of the irritant. The principal injurious agents are bacterial toxins (especially toxins of the bacteria and viruses of the specific infectious diseases), organic poisons (chloroform, carbon tetrachloride, glucosides and alkaloids of certain plants such as the lupines, vetches, senecios, crotalarias), and inorganic poisons (arsenic, phosphorus, antimony). Macroscopically, the liver is about normal in size, but if there is extensive degeneration, it may be smaller than normal (Figs. 9.8 and 17.30). Microscopically, the fat is located intracellularly either peripherally, intermediately, or centrally in the lobule (Figs. 9.10 and 17.29). There is much speculation as to why the degenerative changes in some cases are located mostly peripherolobularly, in others intermediolobularly, and in still others centrolobularly. The question has not been satisfactorily answered. It is believed that the distribution of blood in the lobules, the difference in selective activity of the hepatic cells in different parts of the lobules, and variations in the chemical reactions in the different zones of the lobules may have a bearing on the explanation. Usually the fatty changes are accompanied by cloudy swelling, pyknosis, and karyolysis.

It would seem that extreme fatty degeneration of the liver should be associated with marked interference with hepatic function. In dogs fatty degeneration of the liver does not interfere with one of its activities at least, namely uric acid destruction.

## PIGMENTATION

In the study of general pathology, jaundice was considered with the other endogenous pigmentations. It was learned that jaundice is a hyperbilirubinemic condition characterized by the deposition of bile pigment in many of the tissues, particularly in the skin and mucous membranes. It was further learned that jaundice occurs in three forms: prehepatic (hemolytic), intrahepatic (toxic), and posthepatic (obstructive). The subject should be completely reviewed at this point. (See Chapter 9.)

**Prehepatic jaundice (hemolytic jaundice).** In the present discussion the prehepatic form could logically be omitted since its pathogenesis is not related to a disturbance in liver structure. Liver function, however, is speeded up and overtaxed because in this condition the undue destruction of erythrocytes floods the organ with hemobilirubin — so much of this pigment, in fact, that the liver cannot convert all of it into cholebilirubin. The result is that hemobilirubin accumulates in the blood, stains the tissues moderately, and can be demonstrated to be present in the serum by one of the reactions to the van den Bergh test. Excessive amounts of cholebilirubin are formed by the liver and excreted into the intestine (Fig. 9.17). Obviously, large quantities of urobilinogen are formed in the intestine and reabsorbed. Extra-large amounts of it are excreted in the urine and can be detected by the appropriate test. The large-molecule hemobilirubin cannot pass the renal filter and

Fig. 17.30 — Cross section of a liver of a pig with nutritional anemia to show fatty degeneration. Areas of degeneration appear as grayish-yellow mottlings through the organ. (Doyle, Mathews, and Whiting; Jour. A.V.M.A.)

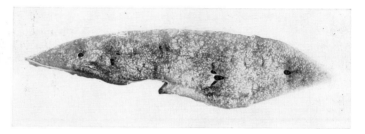

therefore does not appear in the urine. Even though hemolytic jaundice is not the result of a liver disturbance, this much pertaining to it is repeated here, principally to emphasize the clinical laboratory means by which it may be differentiated from the other two types which are associated with intrahepatic and posthepatic lesions.

**Intrahepatic jaundice (toxic jaundice).** As stated previously, two factors operate to produce toxic jaundice: First, there are degeneration and necrosis of the hepatic epithelial cells, and secondly, there is escape of cholebilirubin from the bile capillaries into the blood sinusoids. This second factor is directly related to the first; that is, the degeneration and necrosis of the hepatic cells result in rupture of the bile capillaries (Fig. 9.18). Cholebilirubin then appears in the blood as it does in obstructive jaundice. Furthermore, the damaged liver cells function below par and this results in a retention of some hemobilirubin. The presence of the retained hemobilirubin and the regurgitated cholebilirubin in the blood can be detected by the dual purpose van den Bergh test. The injured liver cells excrete less bile into the intestine. This means there is less urobilinogen formed in the intestine and consequently less of it to be reabsorbed into the blood and excreted by the kidneys.

Poisons capable of damaging the hepatic epithelium so that toxic jaundice is the result are varied. A list of them would include: phosphorus, arsenic, lead, antimony, selenium, chloroform, carbon tetrachloride, and phytotoxins of some of the lupines, vetches, and ragworts. Toxins produced in heavy ascarid and hookworm infections have also been incriminated as causes of toxic jaundice. Infections accompanied by putrefactive processes (septic infections), such as suppurative and gangrenous traumatic pericarditis in cattle and septic endometritis, occasionally have toxic jaundice as a partial manifestation. Among organisms which often cause hepatic degeneration and necrosis sufficient to lead to toxic jaundice should be listed the spirochete of leptospirosis and the virus of infectious canine hepatitis.

In most instances the gross appearance of the liver is that of a very acute nonsuppurative necrotizing inflammation. In toxic jaundice of selenium and ragwort poisoning, however, the hepatic lesion is a chronic nonsuppurative inflammation, although in the initial stages of the poisoning, degeneration and necrosis of the liver parenchyma are prominent.

**Posthepatic jaundice (obstructive jaundice)** may be due to occlusions, partial or complete, of the bile ducts by gallstones (rare), pressure upon the bile ducts by tumors, parasite cysts, and enlarged lymph nodes, and by the presence in the bile ducts of such parasites as the ascarids of pigs (Fig. 17.31), the flukes of sheep and cattle (Fig. 17.32), and the fimbriated tapeworm of sheep. It may also have for

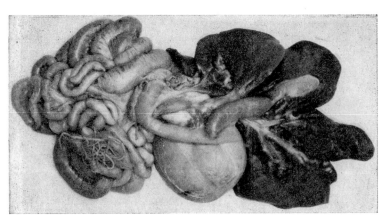

Fig. 17.31 — Invasion of the hepatic ducts and gall bladder of a pig by ascarids, a very common cause of obstructive jaundice. (Department of Veterinary Pathology, Michigan State University.)

its cause a partial or complete closure of the bile ducts by inflammatory swelling of the mucosa (cholangitis). This cholangitis may originate from an extension of a catarrhal duodenitis.

In obstructive jaundice, bile pigment (cholebilirubin) appears in the blood and urine (Fig. 9.19). If the obstruction is complete, bile does not reach the intestine, and as a result, urobilinogen is not reabsorbed and excreted in the urine. Bile salts also accumulate in the blood in obstructive jaundice.

Staining of the tissues in obstructive jaundice is intense. The yellowish pigmentation is especially noticeable in the mucous membranes, conjunctiva, unpigmented skin, connective tissue, adipose tissue, heart valves, intima of the blood vessels, and in the body fluids. It is very prominent in the subcutaneous fat of affected pigs when the median ventral cutaneous incision is made at the beginning of a post-mortem examination. In horses and in Jersey and Guernsey cattle it is easy to confuse the normal color of adipose tissue with icterus. Parts of the body that are not discolored in obstructive jaundice are the cornea, brain, nerves, and cartilage.

The pathogenesis of obstructive jaundice is as follows: The hepatic ducts or the common bile duct become obstructed either completely or partially. The bile duct system becomes distended with bile, which raises the pressure in the bile ducts and bile capillaries. As a consequence, some of the bile ducts and bile capillaries rupture and seepage of bile into the tissues of the portal sheath and into the blood sinusoids occurs. The bile pigment in this instance is cholebilirubin.

In the further development of obstructive jaundice, pressure upon the hepatic cells by the bile accumulating in the bile capillaries results in constriction of the blood sinusoids. The total effect of the pressure on the hepatic cells and upon the sinusoids is atrophy and degeneration. This is due both to pressure and hypoxia.

In the early stages of posthepatic jaundice the liver is moderately large, rather firm but not definitely hard, and the parenchyma is stained with bile. When the condition becomes more chronic, as it does when gallstones or liver flukes are the cause, the ducts not only become enlarged but also become tortuous (Fig. 17.32). An inflammatory reaction develops around the bile ducts in the portal sheaths. This reaction is characterized by cellular infiltration, edema, and fibrosis. Accompanying

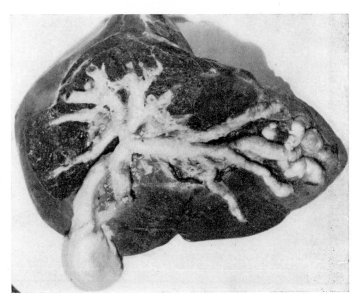

Fig. 17.32 — Chronic cholecystitis and cholangitis in liver fluke invasion in a cow. (Morrill and Shaw, Oreg. Agr. Exper. Sta.)

these changes in the portal sheaths there is moderate degeneration of the parenchyma. The liver becomes enlarged and hard. The severity of the inflammation depends upon the amount of infection present with the obstruction. Infection may be so great as to cause abscesses in the ducts.

**Carotenosis.** An exogenous hepatic pigmentation which is occasionally encountered by federal meat inspectors is carotenosis in cattle which originate in southwestern United States. The liver and hepatic nodes are stained an intense yellow or reddish yellow and show degenerative and proliferative changes. The carotene itself is not toxic, but it is thought to occur in association with a toxic agent probably derived from some plant.

**Melanosis.** Hepatic melanosis is occasionally seen in veal calves in packing houses. It has no significance from the standpoint of the health of the animals.

### Necrosis

Hepatic necrosis may have a diffuse or a focal distribution. The causes of diffuse hepatic necrosis are practically the same as for fatty degeneration, that is, toxic substances of various kinds. Whether the end result of a liver intoxication will be fatty degeneration or necrosis is dependent upon the quantity and quality of the irritant. Necrosis is the next change after fatty degeneration.

Focal hepatic necrosis is a characteristic lesion of several infections. Dull grayish, sharply circumscribed areas of coagulative necrosis are caused by *Spherophorus necrophorus* (Fig. 10.3). A quite similar focal necrosis occurs in the livers of lambs that have so-called **black disease,** a toxemia arising from the combined effects of the liver fluke *Fasciola hepatica* and the spore-forming anaerobe *Clostridium novyi*. The damage caused by the flukes in the bile ducts favors the growth of the anaerobes. A severe necrotic hepatitis results, characterized by areas of coagulative necrosis that are usually about 2 to 4 millimeters in diameter. Circular areas of coagulative necrosis with either dull gray or dark reddish brown centers, alternating

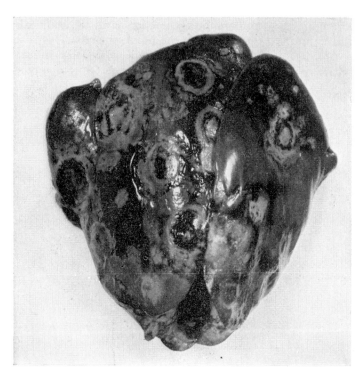

Fig. 17.33 — Focal necrosis of the liver of a turkey due to **Histomonas meleagridis,** the cause of infectious enterohepatitis (blackhead). (Durant, Jour. A.V.M.A.)

with concentric rings of these two colors, are caused by the protozoan parasite *Histomonas meleagridis* in infectious enterohepatitis (blackhead) of turkeys (Fig. 17.33). The concentric light and dark rings seem to represent periodic extensions of the necrotic process. Hemorrhage into the gray rings of coagulative necrosis changes their color to reddish brown, sometimes green. The latter color is due to disintegrating blood pigment. In the livers of some lambs that are aborted by ewes infected with *Vibrio fetus*, similar lesions of coagulative necrosis are sometimes seen. Areas of caseous necrosis occur in the centers of lesions produced by *Mycobacterium tuberculosis* in the liver. These areas are especially common and prominent in the livers of domestic fowl.

When the liver lobules are killed by an irritant that reaches all of them almost simultaneously through either the portal vein or the hepatic artery, the intralobular location of the necrosis may be peripheral intermediate central, or in irregularly distributed foci. The irregularly distributed foci of necrosis are quite likely to be due to colonies of bacteria. The other types of intralobular necrosis are more apt to be caused by inorganic or organic toxic substances. For instance, centrolobular necrosis (Fig. 17.34), which is the most common form, is associated with toxic substances occurring in various pathological conditions such as: uremia, cardiac and pulmonary infarcts, diseases of the gastro-

intestinal tract, infections, burns, severe trauma, traumatic shock, and poisoning with arsenic, chloroform, and carbon tetrachloride. Midzonal and peripherolobular necrosis have not been so regularly associated with such hepatotoxic factors.

Blood usually collects in the necrotic areas due to sinusoidal damage. Next to the necrotic areas hepatic cells show fatty degeneration, and cells still farther removed from the necrotic foci show cloudy swelling. Usually, when the changes just described occur, there is also hyperemia and the presence of leukocytes both within the lobules and in the portal canals so that the whole process is actually a hepatitis. Macroscopically, the liver is about normal in size. Its surface has a dull yellowish to grayish-brown, mottled appearance. It ceases to be friable and becomes flabby.

A centrolobular necrosis of the liver may also have its origin linked with a vascular disturbance. In hepatic passive hyperemia of sudden onset the central area of the lobules shows necrosis. Such a vascular disturbance occurs in cardiac failure. The central vein of the lobule becomes distended, the sinusoids radiating from it are dilated, and the liver cells between them undergo necrosis. The necrosis is the result of hypoxia and impaired neutralization of poisons.

In the liver necrosis caused by the specific organisms named at the beginning of this discussion of necrosis, the areas of dead tissue occur without respect to the

Fig. 17.34 — Subacute toxic liver necrosis with early cirrhosis in a pig. The lighter-colored lobules show a centrolobular necrosis. The darker lobules display hemorrhage following necrosis. Simultaneously with the parenchymal alterations the interstitial tissue is proliferating, resulting in exaggerated lobulation and pseudolobulation. (Department of Veterinary Pathology, Michigan State University.)

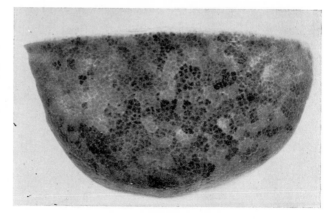

boundaries of lobules. They may originate in lobules but extend in all directions so that large areas of the liver, lobular and interlobular alike, are involved. The architecture of the liver may persist in the areas of coagulative necrosis as in necrophorus infection, but it completely disappears in large areas of caseous necrosis such as occur in tuberculosis.

In the normal liver cells of the dog, especially, the enzyme glutamic-pyruvic transaminase is very active. When the liver cells are severely injured, the amount of this enzyme in the serum becomes greatly increased. Its presence there in abnormal amounts can be used as an aid in the diagnosis of severe liver damage.

**Bacillary hemoglobinuria.** Synonyms for this disease are red water and icterohemoglobinuria. It is an acute septicemic disease of cattle, rarely of horses, swine, and sheep, occurring in the Sierra Nevada and Coast Ranges in the United States, and the Chilean Andes of South America. It is caused by *Clostridium hemolyticum* and is characterized by a sudden onset, a rapid course, high temperature, hemoglobinuria, and occasionally by intestinal hemorrhages. The disease is transmitted by the liver fluke. Recovered animals are carriers of the infection.

The lesions depend upon the presence of a hemolytic and necrotizing toxin. Hemorrhages appear in the alveolar tissue of the mucous and serous membranes and in the subcutis. Hemorrhagic infarction of the liver (Fig. 17.35) is fairly constant, likewise hemoglobinuria. Subcutaneous edema similar to that found in pasteurellosis and anthrax occurs. Icterus is present, and hydroperitoneum (hemoglobin-stained) is marked. The gall bladder is distended with dark-colored flocculent bile. The spleen, surprisingly, is not enlarged. Death occurs in 24 to 36 hours.

In California a **hepatic necrosis in sheep** has been observed for several years. The condition is peculiar because the extent and distribution of the necrosis in the organ is so unusual and because the cause of the condition remains obscure. Macroscopically, the affected livers have a characteristic mottled appearance — irregular, depressed reddish-brown areas interspersed among raised yellowish-brown areas. The organ, which remains practically normal in size, may be affected throughout. The gall bladder is distended with bile. Microscopically, the altered liver is one in which multilobular foci of necrosis are interspersed among large areas of apparently normal lobules.

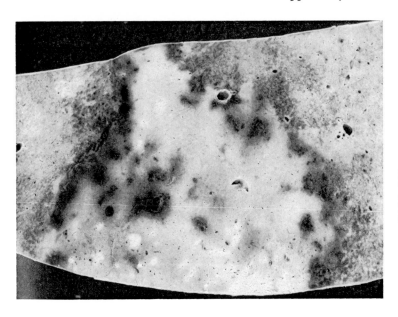

Fig. 17.35 — A large infarct of the liver, a constant lesion in bacillary hemoglobinuria of cattle. (Records and Vawter, Nev. Agr. Exp. Sta.)

## Hepatitis

### ACUTE NONSUPPURATIVE HEPATITIS

The pathological alterations in acute hepatitis can vary considerably, and as a consequence, several types can exist depending upon whether the degenerative, exudative, or proliferative changes predominate. At times it is difficult to draw the line between toxic degeneration and hepatitis. Hepatitis, however, is characterized by hyperemia, cellular infiltration, cloudy swelling, and fatty degeneration. Toxic degeneration, on the other hand, is characterized only by the degenerative changes. Hepatitis may be primary, but it is probably more often a partial manifestation of some infectious disease and toxicosis. Three outstanding examples of specific infectious diseases characterized by acute nonsuppurative hepatitis are viral hepatitis of dogs (infectious canine hepatitis), histomoniasis of turkeys (so-called blackhead), and viral hepatitis of ducklings.

Among the toxicoses are plant and mineral poisonings. Occasionally climatic conditions are such that certain toxic molds will grow on plants or grain and when consumed in sufficient quantities will cause acute nonsuppurative hepatitis. *Pencillium rubrum* and *Aspergillus flavus* have caused this lesion in swine and cattle. The macroscopic and microscopic appearance of acute hepatitis is much the same as that of toxic degeneration, except that vascular and cellular infiltrative changes are added. The result is the impairment of the several functions of the liver so that the condition has an exceedingly far-reaching effect on the health of the animal.

In acute hepatic disease, such as acute hepatitis, injury to the hepatic cells causes the cell membranes to become more permeable to the intracellular enzymes glutamic pyruvic transaminase and glutamic oxaloacetic transaminase, particularly to the former. This permits the enzymes to escape into the blood plasma. Their presence there can be detected by the clinical pathologist and used as an aid in the diagnosis of the hepatic injury.

**Infectious canine hepatitis.** This disease has been designated by the following names: contagious canine hepatitis, infectious hepatitis, canine viral hepatitis, and canine endothelitis.

The disease in the dog and enzootic encephalitis in the fox are caused by the same virus. The timber wolf, coyote, bear, and other mammals are susceptible to the virus. The lesions in the nervous system are not found in the dog as in the fox.

The virus enters the body through the digestive tract and possesses a selectivity for endothelial and hepatic cells. The incubation period varies from a few hours, when the virus is ingested, to 6 to 9 days when dogs are placed in direct contact with one another. Upwards of 75 to 90 per cent of the cases recover within 2 weeks.

The fatal fulminating type of disease presents a rather characteristic pathological syndrome. Little weight loss is evident. Icterus is occasionally present. The tonsils and lymph nodes throughout the body may be enlarged and hyperemic. Hemorrhages are frequently present in various organs and tissues of the body such as the brain and cord, meninges, thymus, heart, stomach, and intestine. Frequently, a serosanguineous fluid is found in the abdominal cavity. Fibrinous exudate may be deposited on the liver or among the loops of the intestine. The liver is slightly enlarged and usually shows small macroscopic foci of necrosis. The gall bladder generally has a thickened edematous wall.

The outstanding micropathological changes are present in the liver, usually centrolobularly, and include hyperemia, edema, hemorrhage, and necrobiosis with an infiltration of neutrophils, lymphocytes, and macrophages. These are the lesions of an acute hepatitis. Intranuclear inclusion bodies, which may be basophilic, eosinophilic, or neutrophilic, are present in the hepatic epithelium, endothelium, and Kupffer cells (Fig. 17.36). The use of stained impression films of the liver may be a useful post-mortem diagnostic aid.

The intranuclear inclusions (Cowdry's type A) are endotheliotropic with the exception of those found in the liver cord cells, and may be found in the spleen, brain, heart, lymph nodes, and less commonly in the endothelium elsewhere. With the electron microscope the inclusion bodies in the hepatic cells are observed to be composed of an amorphous matrix in which are numerous viral particles assuming three different forms — uniformly dense particles, those containing a dense central body, and those with transparent cores.

When one examines liver sections of dogs he may occasionally discover intranuclear inclusions whose occurrence is puzzling. The crystals are generally hexagonal in shape, 7 to 12 $\mu$ long by 5 to 7 $\mu$ wide. They are not soluble in the usual solutions used in routine tissue fixing and staining, and are neither acidophilic nor basophilic. They are not associated with any specific disease such as infectious canine hepatitis or canine distemper.

Due to these retrograde endothelial changes in the blood vessels, there is a tendency toward edema which may be observed in the brain, heart, lungs, gall bladder, subcutaneous tissues, with hydrothorax and hydroperitoneum occurring occasionally.

The blood picture is characterized by a fleeting neutrophilia followed by a rapidly developing leukopenia with increased sedimentation rate. Eosinophils tend to disappear from the blood entirely. The urine is characterized by high concentration and pathologic amounts of albumin and cholebilirubin.

### CHRONIC NONSUPPURATIVE HEPATITIS

Chronic hepatitis (cirrhosis) is characterized by a combination of degenerative changes of the parenchyma and proliferative changes of the interstitial tissue and accompanied usually by some regeneration of the hepatic cells. Chronic hepatitis occurs in all species of domestic animals — most frequently in swine, dogs, horses, cattle, and sheep; seldom in birds. It has been observed in animals in zoos. The cause is frequently unknown. In general it is produced by toxic agents mostly of an organic nature, bacterial toxins, and animal parasites. Among the organic toxic

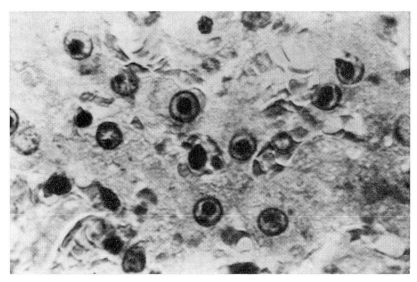

Fig. 17.36 — Intranuclear inclusion bodies in the hepatic epithelium in infectious canine hepatitis. (Department of Veterinary Pathology, Michigan State University.)

agents are poisonous plants such as some of the senecios, the crotalarias, and the seeds of yellow tarweed (*Amsinckia intermedia*), alcohol in distillery wash, and toxic substances resulting from continuous and excessive putrefaction in the intestine. Among the bacterial toxins may be mentioned those which are derived from members of the intestinal or colon-typhoid group. Prominent among the animal parasites are ascarid larvae in pigs, flukes in cattle and sheep, larval forms of tapeworms in various animals, and larval strongyles in horses.

In the western Great Plains and Rocky Mountain regions livestock often become poisoned with selenium by eating plants or grain grown on soil containing this mineral. In western Canada the narrow-leaved vetch (*Astragalus pectinatus*) and the two-grooved milk vetch (*Astragalus bisulcatus*) are the main plants which convert insoluble selenium from the soil into the soluble organic form which is capable of poisoning animals. To a lesser degree other plants, even wheat, can poison animals. The animals are said to have "alkali disease," or to have been "alkalied." One of the important lesions in this intoxication is atrophic cirrhosis of the liver.

The manner in which chronic hepatitis develops varies much, depending upon the intensity of the irritant, its location in the liver, and the period of time over which it operates. In general, degenerative changes occur first and proceed from slight disturbances of cell metabolism to complete death (necrosis), the entire progressive process being called necrobiosis. Next, or at times simultaneously, the intralobular reticulum increases in amount and eventually shrinks. Unaffected groups of the liver cells undergo compensatory hypertrophy. They also attempt to replace dead cells by regeneration.

In a more detailed description of the pathogenesis of chronic nonsuppurative hepatitis it must be stated that the irritant reaches the liver by one of three routes: (1) by the portal vein, (2) by the hepatic artery, and (3) by the hepatic ducts.

If the injurious agent comes to the lobules by the branches of the portal vein, the periphery of the individual lobules is most severely affected and mild degenerative changes of the hepatic cells come on slowly. At the same time a slight proliferation of the intralobular connective tissue occurs. Sometimes the mild irritant stimulates the production of intralobular connective tissue without causing degeneration of the parenchyma. But even when this happens, the liver cells do not escape eventual injury because the increased connective tissue results in pressure and starvation atrophy of the cords of hepatic cells. In some cases the connective tissue increase is around the central vein. In those cases there may be hindrance to the flow of blood from the lobules. This allows the irritant to remain longer in contact with the center of the lobules. If the irritant consists of immature forms of worm parasites, such as ascarid larvae in swine, which are brought to the liver by the portal vein, areas of chronic inflammation arise wherever the larvae lodge.

When the irritant reaches the lobules by the branches of the hepatic artery, the tissue of the portal canals and the interlobular connective tissue show the effects of the damage. In these places there is a lymphocytic infiltration as well as a connective tissue proliferation.

When the irritant ascends the bile passages, the inflammation extends from the interlobular bile ducts and perhaps also the intralobular bile capillaries into the surrounding tissue. The result is a connective tissue hyperplasia in and around the lobules.

Macroscopically, the liver is firm and at times extremely hard (Fig. 17.37). In advanced stages of chronic hepatitis, incision of the tissue produces a grating sound. The normal architecture of the lobules is lost. It is replaced by islands of parenchyma, varying much in size and shape, which are surrounded by newly formed connective tissue. The central veins disappear or at least are inconspicuous. The surface of the liver is rough, sometimes "hobnailed." The color varies from light grayish red, light yellow (fatty changes predominating) to intense yellow or green (icterus). The size of the liver varies. It is large if hyperplasia predominates and small if much atrophy of the parenchyma occurs.

In parasitic cirrhosis of swine caused by the migrating larvae of *Ascaris lumbricoides* the cirrhotic areas are usually circumscribed, superficial, and multiple. There is a general mottling of the surface of the liver if the areas are numerous. The white or gray areas of focal cirrhosis as a result of ascarid infection are in sharp contrast to the dark reddish-brown liver parenchyma.

Microscopically, the picture varies considerably, depending upon the nature of the irritant and the stage at which the examination is made. In general, it can be visualized from the description of the pathogenesis and gross appearance already given.

In well-advanced chronic nonsuppurative hepatitis the first thing to attract attention in viewing a section is the marked increase in connective tissue. Not only is the increase between the lobules — where it normally can be seen to a greater or lesser extent, depending upon the species of animal — but also within the lobules. The lobules appear to be subdivided by it into smaller lobules. The condition is referred to as pseudolobulation. This gives the appearance to some lobules of having no central vein. The part of the lobule which possesses the central vein may have it located eccentrically. As a result of the connective tissue proliferation, the hepatic epithelial cells are compressed and poorly nourished. They appear atrophic. Islands of them which may be less affected undergo compensatory hypertrophy. Where there has been loss of hepatic epithelial cells there also may be attempts at regeneration. The young cells look more robust and take the stain more intensely. In the newly formed connective tissue which divides the lobules into pseudolobules, there are numerous and prominent newly formed bile ducts. Where cords of liver cells remain, clumps of bile pigment are often distinct. Macrophages, lymphocytes, and plasma cells are the prominent cellular constituents of the exudate.

The effects of hepatic cirrhosis are far-reaching. Besides the impairment of the many functions of the liver, distinct organic changes occur in other viscera. Interference with the portal circulation is the most serious because it results in abdominal ascites. The factors responsible for the ascites are:

**1. A mechanical factor.** Hindrance to the flow of portal blood through the liver increases the pressure in the portal venous system (hydrostatic pressure), which in turn results in a loss of fluid through the capillary endothelium.

The effect of hindrance to the flow of portal blood becomes more apparent when one recalls that the portal venous system drains most of the blood from the gastrointestinal tract, spleen, and pancreas. In normal dogs, while the average mean pressure in the portal is more than three times that of the hepatic vein and the abdominal vena cava, in dogs with hepatic cirrhosis the pressure in the portal vein becomes increased twofold (portal hypertension).

**2. Decreased colloid osmotic pressure.** Diminished production of serum albumin by the damaged liver results in hypoproteinemia with the consequent loss of fluid from the capillaries. While increased portal vein pressure and reduced colloid osmotic pressure generally have been considered to be important contributing factors to ascites in cirrhosis, there is experimental evidence in albino rats that they do not play a significant role. The experiment, however, while discrediting the importance of these factors, has not furnished a substitute explanation for the ascites.

**3. Hormonal factor.** The impaired liver fails to inactivate the antidiuretic hormone originating in the posterior pituitary. This results in an increased quantity of

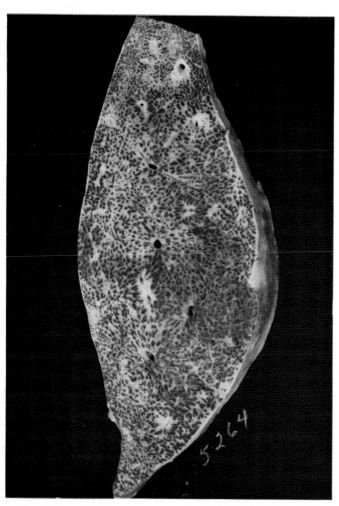

Fig. 17.37 — Hepatic cirrhosis in a 5-year-old gelding. Liver weighed 64 pounds. (Department of Veterinary Pathology, Michigan State University.)

the hormone which inhibits renal function.

The newly formed connective tissue often fills in the blood sinusoids. With fewer vascular channels to convey blood through the liver, an excessive amount of it accumulates in the portal system. This results in passive hyperemia of the stomach, pancreas, spleen, and intestine. In this state these organs are more subject to inflammation. Also with the portal hyperemia comes hydroperitoneum. Besides interfering with the portal circulation, the newly formed connective tissue encroaches upon the hepatic epithelium. The displaced and atrophied epithelium produces less albumin for the blood plasma. This decrease in serum albumin lowers the colloidal osmotic pressure of the blood and aggravates the ascites already developing as a result of the hindrance to portal circulation. Pressure of the connective tissue upon the cords of liver cells compresses the bile capillaries and impedes the flow of bile in them. The result is some degree of obstructive jaundice. Decreased bile secretion leads to digestive disturbances. Because the detoxifying function of the liver cannot be performed normally, toxins having an affinity for tissue of the central nervous system may cause degenerative changes in the brain such as are seen in the so-called walking disease of horses.

The ability of the liver to remove bromsulfathalein from the blood and excrete it within a given time after it has been injected intravenously is a function test applicable to the diagnosis of chronic diffuse nonsuppurative hepatitis of horses and cattle.

**Multiple nodular hepatic cirrhosis** sometimes occurs in domestic mammals, particularly in old dogs. The liver may be normal in size or vary either way from normal. Glisson's capsule and the peritoneum are usually normal in thickness, but the surface of the liver is very much nodulated (Fig. 17.38). The nodules vary in size up to large peas. The surface of the large nodules are flattened. In color they are mostly dull yellow. When cut, they consist of yellow or brownish-yellow soft tissue which bulges from the cut surface. The nodules are surrounded by dense, grayish connective tissue.

In man a similar condition is called Laennec cirrhosis. The histogenesis of it has been studied in detail. It is presumed that the condition in animals develops in a similar manner. It appears that the hepatic changes are the result of a prolonged vitamin B complex deficiency and a deficiency of a lipotropic factor.

The first stage in the development of nodular cirrhosis is an overloading of liver cells with fat. The liver cells are so uniformly distended with fat that the cords of cells compress the sinusoids into an almost bloodless state. The liver capsule becomes tense and the cut surface of the organ bulges.

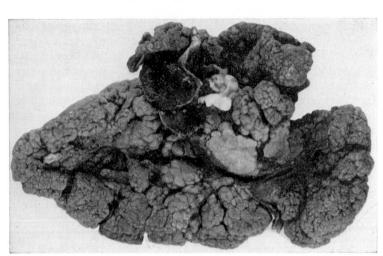

Fig. 17.38 — Nodular cirrhosis, liver of a dog. (F. W. Schofield.)

The second stage is a mild inflammation appearing in the interlobular spaces, especially in the angles of the spaces where the portal trinities are located. Signs of the inflammatory reaction are a lymphocytic infiltration together with small numbers of plasma cells and neutrophils.

In the third stage the inflammatory reaction has aged enough for a proliferation of fibroblasts to begin in the interlobular spaces. With this there is a proliferation of capillaries.

In the fourth and fifth stages, strands of the interlobular newly formed connective tissue penetrate the lobules and subdivide them into smaller lobule-like segments. Capillaries go with the strands of connective tissue and often connect with the central vein of the lobule. Some of the capillaries leave these strands of connective tissue and run independently straight through the parenchyma to a central vein.

The sixth and last stage has been going on simultaneously with these later stages. In this stage, attempts are made by the parenchyma to regenerate, but the attempts are feeble. In these attempts, adenoma-like nodules of young hepatic cells are formed. They give the organ its nodular appearance. With the proliferation of hepatic cells there is also a proliferation of canaliculi cells, but most of the canaliculi serve no purpose because they have no lumina. Furthermore they have a helter-skelter distribution in the parenchyma and even appear in the newly formed connective tissue.

In the early stages of nodular cirrhosis, when the liver is filled with fat and the connective tissue is young, the liver is hypertrophic. After much of the parenchyma has been crowded out and the connective tissue has matured, the organ becomes atrophic. The feeble attempts at regeneration do not materially change the size of the organ but they do alter its appearance; they are responsible for the nodular topography.

### SUPPURATIVE HEPATITIS

Suppurative hepatitis can be produced by any of the pyogenic bacteria. Infection results by direct introduction (primary) or by metastasis (secondary). Primary infection reaches the liver by means of foreign bodies penetrating from the alimentary tract. Often a single abscess results. Secondary infection is usually hematogenic or by extension from neighboring organs. Hematogenic infection occurs through the portal vein, the hepatic artery, or by the umbilical vein of newborn animals.

The location of liver abscesses can very well be related to the source of portal blood coming to any given area in the organ. In the dog, for instance — and it is presumed that it may be true for other mammals also — the left side of the liver receives its portal blood from the stomach, spleen, and most of the colon. The right side receives its blood mainly from the duodenum, head of the pancreas, and upper jejunum. Macroscopically, the young abscesses are sharply defined, light yellow, greenish-yellow, or dirty gray foci with pulpy or creamy centers. They are odorless or foul-smelling, depending upon the cause. Old abscesses vary much in size, are encapsulated, and may be calcified. Microscopically, the abscesses begin as mere collections of leukocytes. Later, each abscess is surrounded by an inflammatory zone, the tissue undergoes necrosis, and a connective tissue capsule forms, surrounded by a margin of leukocytes. In young abscesses numerous bacteria are present in the pus; in old ones there are few or none. The results may be death due to absorption of toxin if the suppurative hepatitis is extensive. Sometimes there is healing of the abscesses. At other times a few encapsulated abscesses cause no apparent trouble. Superficial abscesses may result in local peritonitis and adhesions. If they rupture, general peritonitis may result. Rupture of abscesses into vessels results in pyemia.

Abscesses of the liver of cattle deserve special mention because their occurrence calls for the condemnation of an alarming number of livers in packing houses. There appears to be a relationship between their occurrence and that of rumenitis and telangiectasis. It is believed that bacteria, especially *Spherophorus necrophorus*, enter the portal circulation and reach the liver because of their presence in the inflammatory lesions of the rumen. (See page 460.)

## Tumors

The most common hepatic tumors originate from liver cells and intrahepatic bile ducts. Gall bladder tumors are rare. The liver cell tumors, both the benign ones (adenomas) and the malignant ones (carcinomas, hepatomas) have their greatest incidence in cattle and sheep, and next greatest in dogs and cats. In cattle, adenomas are reported to occur most often in the right half of the liver. Benign tumors of the intrahepatic bile ducts are reported in cattle, sheep, dogs, and cats. Malignant ones (adenocarcinomas, hepatomas) occur most often in horses, dogs, and cats. In animals, reports in general indicate that the malignant tumors are more often unicentric in origin, with multiple secondary

metastasis to other parts of the liver. Less often they are multicentric in origin. Liver cell carcinomas are especially invasive into the portal blood vessels. Benign liver cell tumors (adenomas), particularly in sheep, have been described as possessing extramedullary hematopoietic characteristics. This is not considered to be a function of the neoplasm however. Hemangiosarcomas (Fig. 17.39) are occasionally observed in dogs.

Hepatic tumors composed of lymphocytes and myelocytes are frequently observed in cattle and chickens. Since, embryologically, the liver is closely related to the blood-forming organs, it is not to be wondered at that it may, in postnatal life, show definite reactions and participate in diseases of those organs. In this connection lymphosarcoma and myelocytic tumors are important.

Lymphosarcoma is often accompanied by hepatic changes. The changes are either diffuse or focal. Grossly, in the diffuse

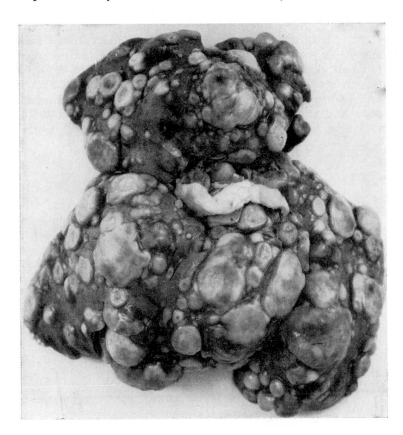

Fig. 17.39 — Hemangiosarcoma of the liver of an 8-year-old dog. Transplantations had occurred on the parietal peritoneum and mesentery. (Department of Veterinary Pathology, Michigan State University.)

form the liver is enlarged and its color is either unevenly or uniformly grayish brown or grayish white. Microscopically, there is a lymphocytic and lymphoblastic infiltration. At first this is confined to the portal sheaths and interlobular connective tissue (Fig. 17.40). Later it extends into the lobules so that the sinusoids become packed with cells which cause pressure atrophy of the hepatic cells and their eventual disappearance (Fig. 17.41). The lymphocytes are believed to originate in the liver.

In the focal form, nodules of lymphocytes appear. The nodules may vary in size up to 2 or 3 centimeters in diameter and are grayish white in color.

In myelosarcoma the gross appearance of the liver is the same as in lymphosarcoma, but obviously the microscopic appearance is different because the infiltrating cells belong to the myelocytic series.

### Agonal Changes

When one inspects an organ at a necropsy, he is aware that changes which he observes may have occurred days, weeks, months, or years before death, or just prior to death, or after death. At this point in the study of hepatopathy it is appropriate to list some changes that may occur just prior to death — changes which are said to be agonal. There are four such changes:

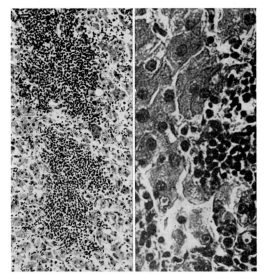

Fig. 17.41 — The liver of a horse with lymphosarcoma. Accumulations of lymphoblasts in the sinusoids caused atrophy of the cords of hepatic cells. ×110 and ×440. (Iowa State University Veterinarian.)

(1) The disappearance of glycogen from the liver cells. This is the most conspicuous change and results in deeper staining of the cytoplasm when the sections are stained in the usual manner (hematoxylin-eosin). (2) A breakup or disorganization of the cords of liver cells. (3) Centrolobular necrosis. (4) Perisinusoidal edema, which is a mechanical edema associated

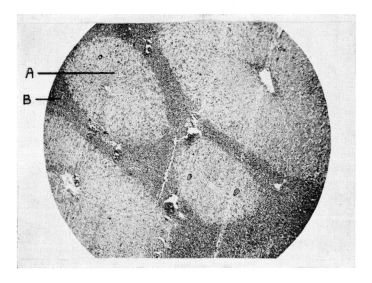

Fig. 17.40 — The liver in lymphosarcoma. Early stage.
**A,** liver lobules showing some neoplastic cells invading between hepatic cords;
**B,** interlobular tissue invaded by neoplastic cells.
×13. (Biester and McNutt, Jour. A.V.M.A.)

with cardiac failure or increased permeability of the sinusoidal wall due to hypoxemia or the presence of toxic products of bacterial growth.

## GALL BLADDER AND HEPATIC DUCTS

Accessory gall bladders are reported to be fairly common in cats. Most of the cases described have been bifid gall bladders.

**Stenosis** of the gall bladder and hepatic ducts may be complete or partial. It may be due to concretions, foreign bodies, parasites, tumors, inflammatory swelling, and strictures. **Compression stenosis** results from incarceration in hernial openings, tumors, parasitic cysts, abscesses, adhesions, hematocysts, and enlarged lymph nodes. **Foreign bodies** are occasionally encountered. Sand has been reported in the bile ducts and gall bladders of pigs. Fimbriated tapeworms and flukes are causes in sheep, and ascarids in hogs. **Hemorrhages** are common in acute septicemic disease. **Cholecystitis** and **cholangitis** appear in the same forms that involve any mucous surface. Their cause is bacteria from the duodenum whose establishment may be favored by foreign bodies, concretions, and parasites. *Escherichia coli* is a frequent causal agent.

In hyperkeratosis of cattle caused by highly chlorinated naphthalenes there may be **nodular mucoid proliferation** of the epithelium of the large bile ducts and gall bladder. There may also be involvement of the intrahepatic ducts. They undergo a proliferation which is accompanied by a fibrosis of the liver. The latter impinges upon the ducts, causing them to develop cystic dilatations which contain mucus.

**Cholelithiasis** is not an important condition in veterinary science. It is seldom that cases of gallstones are encountered. At Denver only 21 cattle out of over 2,000 examined, and at South St. Paul 23 out of 5,725, had these concretions. Very few cases have been reported in dogs and cats.

The alterations produced in the bile ducts of the liver of cattle by the fluke *Fasciola hepatica* are a combination of pathological processes. The changes are greatest along the paths of migration of the parasites and at places where they become more or less stationary. This is principally in the bile ducts of the liver. The tissue changes probably are the result of mechanical injury caused by the parasites and by the toxic products of their metabolism, or by toxic substances formed in the tissues destroyed by them. Beginning within the lumen and progressing in an outward direction, the changes are as follows: If the irritation is slight, the epithelium lining the ducts appears to undergo a general reactionary hyperplasia. The epithelial cells proliferate so much that it is necessary for the epithelium to buckle, and consequently tall, complex folds of it are pushed out into the lumen. The folds also push outwardly into the tunica propria. This causes the epithelium to have the appearance of forming compound tubular glands. If the flukes remain more or less stationary but completely fill the ducts, pressure atrophy of the epithelium or even erosion of it occurs. The walls of the bile ducts outside the epithelium are involved in a low-grade chronic inflammatory reaction shown by the presence of fibroblasts with newly formed collagenous fibers, numerous lymphocytes, and occasional areas of calcification.

Grossly, bile ducts altered by the presence of flukes become enlarged and cordy (Fig. 17.32). They are most prominent on the omasal surface of the liver where they stand out distinctly as gray or white cordlike ridges against a dark reddish-brown background of liver parenchyma. When cut transversely, their thick fibrous walls do not collapse. Flukes are not usually as numerous in the ducts as the lesions would seem to indicate.

## PANCREAS

### Functional Disturbances

Diseases of the pancreas which bring about destruction of the gland parenchyma result in a reduction in the amount of pancreatic fluid entering the intestine. The deficiency of trypsin, steapsin, and amylopsin disturbs the digestion of proteins, fats, and starch in the intestine. The animal becomes undernourished. Evidences of the failure of fat digestion appear in the feces. They become greasy because they contain neutral fat and fats only partially split. The condition is called steatorrhea.

Sometimes the same destructive influences that damage the pancreatic parenchyma may also affect the islands of Langerhans. Then sugar appears in the blood in amounts up to 0.3 to 0.8 per cent (hyperglycemia) and in the urine up to 15 per cent (glycosuria). The general condition is termed sugar diabetes (diabetes mellitus). Since in this disease there is a disturbance of glycogen metabolism, the animal undergoes a progressive emaciation.

Disease conditions of the pancreas in which there may be either destruction of the parenchyma, or of the islands, or of both are not numerous. Most important is inflammation, especially the chronic form which terminates in an increase in the connective tissue along with the disappearance of the glandular epithelium. Another but less important condition is pancreatic atrophy seen most often in aged animals. Occasionally the functions of the organ may be inhibited or arrested by occlusion of the pancreatic duct with calculi or worm parasites.

**Changes of the lumen of the pancreatic duct,** similar to the changes in the hepatic duct, may occur. Concretions are rare. When they are present, they are chalk-white, faceted much like dice, appear in large numbers, and are rather uniform in size, although the size is quite variable (2 to 15 mm.), depending upon the species of animal.

**Fat necrosis** is occasionally encountered in old hogs, in dogs, sheep, horses, and cattle. The necrosis of the fat begins in the pancreas and may extend to the adipose tissue of neighboring regions. The reasons for the escape of the pancreatic enzymes may be attributed to injuries, inflammation, circulatory disturbances, and stasis of secretion in the pancreas. The lipolytic and proteolytic enzymes gain entrance to the tissues and cause intravital self-digestion.

Pathologists have been puzzled by the occurrence of fat necrosis in the adipose tissue of the pericardium, subpleura, mediastinum, and mediastinal lymph nodes in association with pancreatitis. Experiments on dogs and cats have given an explanation. In these animals it has been discovered that the peritoneal and thoracic systems are continuous, and that when the pancreatic duct is ligated, pancreatic lipase is transported by these lymphatics to the structures mentioned. Lipase did not appear to be transported by the blood vessels.

Macroscopically, the necrotic foci vary in size from the head of a pin up to large coalescing masses which are opaque, dull white, or yellowish white and dry (cut like soap). They are surrounded by a red zone of inflammation and may show central softening. In the mesentery of cattle they are sometimes mistaken for tuberculosis. Microscopically, the fat cells lack nuclei. Some are filled with needle-like crystals (fatty acids), others with homogeneous pale, pinkish-blue material (calcium soap) when stained with hematoxylin and eosin, and still others with deep blue masses (precipitated calcium salts) (Fig. 10.8). The necrotic areas are surrounded by a zone of leukocytes in which an occasional giant cell may appear. Old foci may be encapsulated. The condition is seldom apparent clinically.

**Diabetes mellitus** is generally said to be an uncommon disease among domestic mammals. Greater attention to clinical laboratory procedures among small animal practitioners and researchers using dogs for laboratory animals has made it apparent that diabetes occasionally occurs among dogs and cats. In order to get an understanding of what happens in the body in diabetes, it is necessary first of all to review very briefly the steps that take place in the normal metabolism of substances concerned in diabetes.

Muscles and other tissues require glucose. To get it, carbohydrates are digested in the intestine and the resultant glucose is absorbed and transported to the liver by the portal vein. In the liver the glucose is stored as glycogen, and when needed, is again converted to glucose, and carried to the muscles and other organs by the blood. In the muscles it becomes a source of energy by oxidation, with carbon dioxide and water left behind as by-products.

Each step in this process, to a large extent, is regulated by hormones elaborated by the pancreas, the pituitary, the thyroid, and the adrenal cortex. In diabetes mellitus of dogs a shortage of insulin produced by the pancreatic islets seems to be the important factor. In health this hormone is active in the storage of glycogen by the liver and the release of sugar from the blood into the tissues. So well do all of the factors operate in health, that the blood sugar level in dogs remains constant at about 60 to 100 mg/100 cc of blood (Folin method). In diabetes this blood sugar balance is upset, and the glucose level raised.

In the diabetic dogs and cats which form the subjects for the few histological reports of diabetes so far recorded, it would seem that the principal cause of the trouble is a deficiency or lack of insulin production. In these animals pancreatic islets were either totally lacking or, if present, were few in number and abnormal in structure. The abnormalities in the few islets present were generally atrophy and hydropic degeneration of the islet cells, and hyalinization and fibrosis of the islets proper. In cases of spontaneous human diabetes, and in experimental cases in dogs and rabbits, it has been shown that this so-called hydropic degeneration of the islet cells (*beta* cells) is actually glycogen infiltration.

These disturbances in the islets were practically always associated with pancretic atrophy. Some of the atrophied pancreases were fibrotic, with only nodules of parenchyma remaining. Others were composed of a more uniform mixture of the deficient parenchyma and fibrotic tissue. There is a possibility that such pancreases are the result of chronic pancreatitis.

The effects of this total lack or deficiency of insulin on the animal body are dramatic. Since glucose cannot be stored or wholly utilized, it accumulates in the blood (hyperglycemia). Much of it spills over into the urine (glycosuria). This raises the osmotic pressure in the uriniferous tubules and prevents reabsorption of water which results in the passage of excessive amounts of urine (polyuria). This deprives the tissues of needed water (dehydration), and causes increased thirst (polydipsia). Furthermore, since glucose cannot be stored or completely utilized, the body is required to draw upon its fat reserves for nutrition. This causes fat and ketones to appear in the blood (lipemia and ketonemia) and ketones to appear in the urine (ketonuria). Large amounts of fat are moved from the depots to the liver (hepatic fatty infiltration). This draft upon the fat reserves, and depletion of glycogen stores, usually leaves the animal emaciated in spite of a good or even a ravenous appetite (polyphagia). The ketones in the blood neutralize the blood alkali (acidemia), and this in turn stimulates respiration (air-hunger) and terminates in coma.

Diabetes mellitus is said to be the cause of rather sudden death of feeder lambs when they are overfed on carbohydrates, especially on corn-sugar molasses which is rich in monosaccharides. It is believed that these sugars in this kind of molasses are assimilated too easily and rapidly. The sugar in cane molasses, on the other hand, is said not to be so easily assimilated and does not therefore cause diabetes mellitus so often. Descriptions of the gross and microscopic changes in this condition in lambs is lacking, but it is said that, clinically, the lambs pass into a coma and die rather suddenly.

## Pancreatitis

Pancreatic diseases of domestic animals seem to be neglected in veterinary literature. One of the few detailed reports on this subject in the dog was made at the Angell Memorial Hospital in Boston where about 70 cases were encountered among more than 1,800 necropsies.

The reason dogs do not show clinical evidences of pancreatitis more often may be due to the presence of two pancreatic ducts. In 84 per cent of the dogs examined, there were two ducts, and those two had interductal anastomoses within the pancreas. If one duct is obstructed for any reason, the other may function sufficiently to avoid the onset of signs of the obstruction.

**Acute necrotic pancreatitis** occurred in 14 dogs whose average age was 7.6 years. About three-fourths of these dogs were obese. The onset of the disease was sudden and was characterized by fever in the initial stages followed by a fall in temperature as the animal approached collapse. Death occurred in about 5 days. Abdominal pain was an important sign of the disease. In dogs that survived long enough for severe damage to occur to the islet cells there was an excess of sugar in the urine and blood (glycosuria and glycemia).

Macroscopically, the pancreas was swollen, edematous, or hemorrhagic and was flecked superficially with tiny foci of fat necrosis. The entire gland or parts of it were affected.

Microscopically, there were areas of acinar necrosis and hemorrhage accompanied by a leukocytic infiltration.

**Chronic pancreatitis** affected 19 dogs whose average age was 8 years. About half of these dogs were obese. The onset of the disease was gradual, but often a month or so previously the dog had had a digestive disturbance which was probably a mild attack of acute necrotic pancreatitis. In several of the cases the first signs of illness were polydipsia and polyuria. Usually, in spite of a ravenous appetite the dog lost weight, and there was bloat, flatus, and a diarrhea with greasy, fetid stools. In about one-third of the cases injury to the islet cells was great enough to cause glycosuria and glycemia.

Macroscopically, the pancreas itself was shrunken and distorted. In some cases the only remaining functional portions of the gland were nodules of it near the exit of the main pancreatic duct. Peripancreatic fibrosis resulting from extension of the inflammation to the adjacent peritoneum took the form of adhesions. There was fatty infiltration of the liver.

Histologically, areas of massive fibrosis had replaced portions of the destroyed gland. Remaining remnants of the organ displayed an increase of the interlobular connective tissue. Areas of both an acute and a chronic inflammation were present in some glands. The hepatic changes were a centrolobular fatty infiltration with perilobular fibrosis.

**Pancreatic fibrosis** was present in five dogs, four of which were obese. Their average age was 6.6 years, and the duration of the disease averaged 24 days. None of the dogs had signs of diabetes mellitus.

Macroscopically, there was general atrophy of the pancreas but no massive scarring or adhesions as in chronic pancreatitis.

Microscopically, periductal, interlobular, and intralobular fibrosis were prominent changes. While hyalinization of the periductal connective tissue occurred, there were no changes in the epithelium of the ducts. There was no acute inflammatory reaction. In the most severe cases the acinar tissue disappeared or only a few islands of it remained.

**Pancreatic atrophy** involved five cases. The dogs were younger — average age $1\frac{1}{2}$ years. Death did not occur until 116 days on the average. The dogs became emaciated in spite of a ravenous appetite. Stool-eating (coprophagy) was common in this group. The increased food intake together with inability to digest carbohydrates resulted in bulging abdomens, the passing of massive, dry, gray, greasy stools. There was no glycosuria or glycemia, which would indicate the persistence of some islet cells.

Macroscopically, the pancreas was exceedingly thin (1 mm. or less) and had the appearance of red lace. It was easily transilluminated.

Microscopically, there were isolated collections of acinar cells which lacked the structure of acini. The larger ducts were normal, lying in a connective tissue stroma which was infiltrated slightly with lymphocytes.

**Etiology.** Since very little research has been done on the cause of pancreatic disease in animals, one can only speculate on this subject. Naturally the origin of the cause might be enterogenous, hematogenous, or by extension from neighboring tissue or organs. Etiological agents of enterogenous origin may be foreign bodies, bacteria, or animal parasites which ascend the pancreatic duct. Such agents might cause a periductal inflammation with resulting stenosis which in turn could lead to retention of pancreatic secretion and rupture of the duct-acinar system. This tissue damage would give rise to an inflammatory reaction. In man, emphasis has been placed upon bile regurgitated by the pancreatic duct from the ampulla of Vater as a causative factor in pancreatitis. The possibility of this occurring in dogs is not great because dogs have two pancreatic ducts, and the larger and more important one of the pair does not empty into the common duodenal orifice with the common bile duct. In cats, however, it does, but reports of pancreatitis in them are even more rare than in dogs, so bile as an etiologic agent apparently is not important.

## Tumors

Pancreatic tumors are rare. The few reported have originated mostly from the exocrine cells (acinar cells). Extremely rare is one arising from the endocrine cells (islet cells). E. L. Stubbs at the University of Pennsylvania studied a tumor in a 12-year-old mongrel dog. The dog displayed signs of hyperinsulinism which were associated with the overproduction of insulin by the tumor. Although the tumor, which was located in the body of the pancreas, was only 1.1 × 1.2 cm. in diameter and was encapsulated, it caused a chain of symptoms among which were attacks of vertigo, falling over when attempting to eat, walking in a daze, and a ravenous appetite following seizures. Blood sugar before addition of sugar to the diet was 37 mg/100 cc; after treatment, 47 mg/100 cc; after surgical removal of the tumor, 61 mg/100 cc. Following surgery there were no apparent abnormal manifestations.

## PERITONEUM

**Abnormal contents. Foreign bodies and substances** may originate from without or from the organs of the abdominal cavity. They may produce local or diffuse peritonitis and death. **Ingesta** may originate from a ruptured stomach or intestine; **urine** or **bile** from rupture of the urinary bladder or gall bladder, respectively; **blood (hemoperitoneum)** from rupture of the liver, spleen, ovarian cysts, the expression of a corpus luteum, rupture of the gravid uterus, or rupture of any large abdominal vessel. In sweet-clover poisoning of cattle, in which large hemorrhages occur in the serous membrane of the abdominal cavity, hemoperitoneum may be so extensive that one to three gallons of sanguinous fluid may be present. **Eggs** may be encountered in birds (Fig. 19.16) and **fetuses** in other animals.

**Fluid (hydroperitoneum, ascites, dropsy)** occurs rather frequently, especially in dogs and cats, less frequently in sheep and cattle, and seldom in other animals. The fluid is a transudate. It may result from: (1) chronic hindrance to the outflow of venous blood from the abdominal cavity (hepatic cirrhosis, chronic inflammation of the portal vein, heartworms in dogs, chronic cardiac, and pulmonary diseases); (2) changes in the composition of the blood such that the fluid is increased and the proteins decreased (hydremia). The deficiency of proteins lowers the colloidal osmotic pressure which prevents reabsorption of fluid. This is observed in stomachworm infestation in sheep; (3) tumors of the peritoneum, especially in chickens; and (4) increased capillary permeability for fluid as occurs in edema disease of pigs, an enterotoxemia arising from a toxin produced in and absorbed from the intestine. The toxin is elaborated by a hemolytic strain of *Escherichia coli* of a particular serotype. Grossly, the peritoneal cavity contains a clear or straw-colored fluid. The maximum amount of fluid reported in horses is 170 liters; in dogs, 20 liters. In edema disease of pigs as much as 500 ml. has been found. The specific gravity is about 1.013. Coagulation is absent or slight. The peritoneum is smooth. Later, however, it may become rough because long-continued ascites acts as an irritant to the serosa and produces a mild inflammation with fibrous thickening.

**Hemorrhages** of the peritoneum are among the usual lesions of several of the septicemic and toxemic diseases, such as anthrax, pasteurellosis, and enterotoxemia of lambs. They also are common in sweet-clover poisoning of cattle. The most fre-quent location of the hemorrhages is the serosa of the diaphragm, stomach, and intestine.

**Peritonitis** is frequent in nearly all species of domestic animals. The forms are, according to the course, acute and chronic; according to the character of the inflammatory process they are serous, fibrinous, suppurative, and hemorrhagic. Peritonitis is caused by bacteria (micrococci and streptococci in horses, *Corynebacterium pyogenes* in cattle and swine, *Bacillus anthracis*, *Escherichia coli*, members of the Pasteurella group). In swine a fibrinous serositis of the peritoneum, pleura, and pericardium is sufficiently common and distinctive enough to bear the name of the man who first described it — Glasser's disease. The cause is unknown but is presumed to be an infectious agent. In visceral gout in chickens the cause is not known. The manner in which the tissue

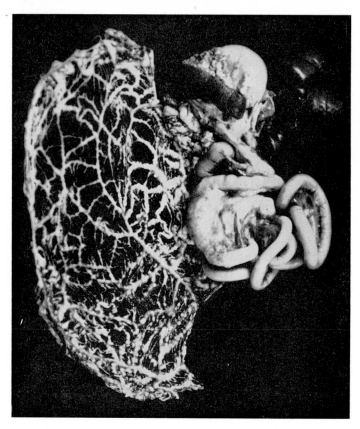

Fig. 17.42 — Lymphosarcoma of the small intestine of a cat with metastasis to the lymphatics of the omentum. The intestine was almost completely occluded by the tumor. (Department of Veterinary Pathology, Michigan State University.)

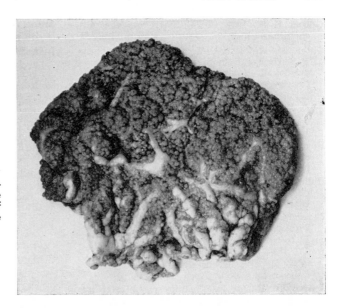

Fig. 17.43 — Transplants of an ovarian papillary adenocarcinoma to the omentum in a dog. (Department of Veterinary Pathology, Michigan State University.)

changes in peritonitis take place depends upon whether the infection is primary or secondary. In primary infection the alterations involve only the peritoneum. In secondary infection other organs are first involved (gastric or intestinal ulcers, rupture of hollow organs, abscesses in abdominal organs, foreign body perforations, specific infectious diseases such as pasteurellosis). The changes are similar to those on other serous surfaces.

**Tumors.** Tumors of the mesentery and omentum are not common, and when they do occur, they are usually secondary malignant ones which either metastasize from the intestine (Fig. 17.42), or become transplanted from other organs such as the uterus, liver, or ovaries (Fig. 17.43). A chronic inflammation in histoplasmosis of dogs may resemble tumor metastases or transplants so much that the condition may be mistaken for a neoplastic disease.

## REFERENCES

Archibald, J., and Whiteford, R. D.: 1953. Canine atrophic pancreatitis. Jour. A.V.M.A., 122:119.

Bartlett, D. E.: 1949. Procedures for diagnosing bovine venereal trichomoniasis and handling affected herds. Jour. A.V.M.A., 114:293.

Bay, W. W., Doyle, L. P., and Hutchings, L. M.: 1951. The pathology and symptomatology of transmissible gastroenteritis. Amer. Jour. Vet. Res., 12:215.

Biester, H. E., Eveleth, D. F., and Yamashiro, Y.: 1936. Intestinal emphysema in swine. Jour. A.V.M.A., 41:714.

Boughton, I. B., and Hardy, W. T.: 1934. Contagious ecthyma (sore mouth) of sheep and goats. Jour. A.V.M.A., 38:150.

Cello, R. M., and Kennedy, P. C.: 1957. Hyperinsulinism in dogs due to pancreatic islet cell carcinoma. Cornell Vet., 47:538.

Clawson, A. B.: 1934. Some symptoms and lesions produced by stock-poisoning plants. Jour. A.V.M.A., 38:179.

Collier, J. R.: 1956. Abscesses of the pharyngeal region of swine. Amer. Jour. Vet. Res., 17:640.

Cordy, D. R., and McGowan, B.: 1956. The pathology of massive liver necrosis in sheep. Cornell Vet., 46:422.

Davidson, W. B.: 1940. Selenium poisoning. Canad. Jour. Comp. Med., 6:19.

Doran, D. J.: 1955. The course of infection and pathogenic effect of *Trichostrongylus axei* in calves. Amer. Jour. Vet. Res., 16:401.

Farmer, R. K., Hughes, D. L., and Whiting, G.: 1951. Infectious enterohepatitis (blackhead) in turkeys: A study of the pathology of the artificially induced disease. Jour. Comp. Path. and Therap., 31:251.

Gibson, K. S.: 1951. Cholelithiasis and choledocholithiasis in a cat. Jour. A.V.M.A., 121:288.

Gitter, M., and Lloyd, M. K.: 1957. Haemolytic *Bacterium coli* in the "bowel oedema" syndrome. II. Transmission and protection experiments. Brit. Vet. Jour., 113:212.

Green, G. R., Ziegler, N. R., Green, B. B., and Dewey, E. T.: 1930. Epizootic fox encephalitis. I. General description. Amer. Jour. Hyg., 12:109.

Hagan, W. A., and Zeissig, A.: 1933. Six years' experience with a herd experimentally infected with Johne's disease. Cornell Vet., 23:1.

Hallman, E. T., and Witter, J. F.: 1933. Some observations on the pathology of Johne's disease. Jour. A.V.M.A., 36:159.

Hanson, L. E.: 1958. Histological lesions in ducks with virus hepatitis. Amer. Jour. Vet. Res., 19:712.

Harris, P. N., Henderson, F. G., and Chen, K. K.: 1957. Hepatic cirrhosis induced in sheep by *Senecio longilobus*. Arch. Path., 64:297.

Jensen, R., Deane, H. M., Cooper, J. L., Miller, V. A., and Graham, W. R.: 1954. The rumenitis-liver abscess complex in beef cattle. Amer. Jour. Vet. Res., 15:202.

Jones, E. W., Johnson, L., and Moore, C. C.: 1957. Torsion of the bovine cecum. Jour. A.V.M.A., 130:167.

Kernkamp, H. C. H.: 1945. Gastric ulcers in swine. Amer. Jour. Path., 21:111.

———, Roepke, M. H., and Jasper, D. E.: 1946. Orchitis in swine due to *Brucella suis*. Jour. A.V.M.A., 98:215.

McCulloch, E. C.: 1940. Hepatic cirrhosis of horses, swine, and cattle due to the ingestion of seeds of the tarweed, *Amsinckia intermedia*. Jour. A.V.M.A., 96:5.

M'Fadyean, J.: 1919. Botryomycosis. Jour. Comp. Path. and Therap., 32:73.

McNutt, S. H.: 1934. Brucella infection of swine. Jour. A.V.M.A., 37:620.

Meyer, K. F., Stewart-Anderson, B., and Eddie, B.: 1940. Canine leptospirosis in the United States. Jour. A.V.M.A., 95:710.

Moll, T., and Brandly, C. A.: 1955. Pneumonia-enteritis of the newborn calf: III. The reproduction and transmissibility of the disease. Vet. Med., 50:101.

Morgan, B. B.: 1944. Bovine Trichomoniasis. Burgess Publishing Co.

Morrill, D. R., and Shaw, J. N.: 1942. Studies of pathology in cattle produced by liver fluke (*Fasciola hepatica*). Oreg. Agr. Exper. Sta. Bul. 408.

Philip, C. B.: 1955. There is always something new under the "parasitological" sun (the unique story of helminth-borne salmon poisoning disease). Jour. Parasit., 41:125.

Pollock, S.: 1951. Slobbers in the rabbit. Jour. A.V.M.A., 119:443.

Records, E., and Vawter, L. R.: 1945. Bacillary hemoglobinuria of cattle and sheep (Red Water Disease). Nev. Agr. Exper. Sta. Tech. Bul. 173.

Runnells, R. A.: 1941. Cecal and colic artery occlusion in the horse. Mich. State Univ. Vet., 1:67.

Schlotthauer, C. F., and Miller, J. A. S.: 1951. Diabetes mellitus in dogs and cats. Jour. A.V.M.A., 118:31.

Schwartz, B., and Alicata, J. E.: 1932. Ascaris larvae as a cause of liver and lung lesions in swine. Jour. Parasit., 19:17.

Seibold, H. R., Bailey, W. S., Hoerlein, B. F., Jordan, E. M., and Schwabe, C. W.: 1955. Observations on the possible relation of malignant esophageal tumors and *Spirocerca lupi* lesions in the dog. Amer. Jour. Vet. Res., 16:5.

Sojka, W. J., Erskine, R. G., and Lloyd, M. K.: 1957. Haemolytic *Escherichia coli* and "oedema disease" of pigs. Vet. Rec., 69:293.

Syverton, J. T.: 1943. The virus of infectious feline agranulocytosis. I. Characters of the virus: Pathogenicity. Jour. Exp. Med., 77:41.

Thomsen, A.: 1934. Brucella infection in swine. Acta Path. et Microb. Scand., Suppl. 21:1.

Timoney, J. F.: 1957. Oedema disease in swine. Vet. Res., 69:1160.

Van Es, L., Cantwell, L. R., Martin, H. M., and Kramer, J.: 1929. On the nature and cause of "the walking disease" of Northwestern Nebraska. Nebr. Agr. Exper. Sta. Bul. 43.

White, B. B.: 1940. Vesicular exanthema of swine. Jour. A.V.M.A., 97:230.

# CHAPTER 18

# Urinary System

Most irritants reach the kidneys by way of the general circulation. This means that their effects may be felt first in the renal corpuscles and next in the tubules. A brief review of the functions of the kidney will emphasize the importance of the tissue changes which may occur there. In general, the function of the kidneys is to keep the composition of the blood constant by:

1. Eliminating excessive amounts of water from the blood

2. Excreting nitrogenous wastes such as urea, uric acid, allantoin, ammonia, and hippuric acid

3. Eliminating inorganic salts which are derived mostly from food

4. Removing from the blood nonvolatile, soluble foreign substances such as pigments which originate from food or which have been produced in the body.

The kidneys act in three ways to maintain this constant composition of the blood. First, the capillaries of the glomeruli function as filters for water and also for constituents of the blood plasma which can pass through the capillary wall by dialysis. The fluid which passes through this membrane contains all the constituents of the blood plasma except the colloids and the water which they are able to hold back. Secondly, as the fluid passes down the convoluted tubules, substances that are needed in the blood are reabsorbed by the epithelial cells and returned to the capillaries around and between them. Thirdly, the epithelial cells of the tubules apparently form and secrete some substances such as ammonia and hippuric acid. They also concentrate and excrete some foreign substances such as food and body pigments.

Injuries to the glomeruli and to the tubules may change these functions. When the permeability of the glomerular capillary tuft is increased due to irritation, albumin appears in the urine (**albuminuria**). The albumin content of the urine is further increased by degeneration of the epithelium of the convoluted tubules. The loss of albumin from the blood reduces the colloidal osmotic pressure of the blood which in turn results in **generalized edema.** The edema is apparently not due alone to the loss of albumin from the blood, but also to a generalized increased permeability of the capillaries which is caused by the same irritant that increases the permeability of the glomeruli. A **retention of chlorides** in the tissues of the body accompanies the edema and aggravates the condition by increasing the passage of fluid into the tissues. Hypofunction on the part of the glomeruli results in the retention of nitrogenous waste products in the blood.

The excretion of urea is a function often

upset in renal disease. Urea is the chief nitrogenous end product of protein metabolism and, along with water, is one of the two most important constituents of urine. Normally urea is excreted in the glomerular filtrate. If the renal filter is injured, as it is in some renal diseases, the amount of water passing through it is diminished and likewise the amount of urea. This results in retention of urea in the blood, and is associated with a severe intoxication called uremia. Urea is not the cause of the intoxication because it is nontoxic when present in the blood even in large amounts. Its presence in the blood, however, in increased amounts in renal disease indicates inadequate excretory function.

Indications of uremia are numerous and varied. Among them are: (1) hyperemia of the mucous membranes, (2) inflammation of the mucosa of the alimentary tract, sometimes with ulcer formation, (3) dehydration and debility associated with the lesions of the alimentary tract, (4) urinous body odor, (5) muscular twitching, and finally (6) coma, and perhaps (7) death. These are characteristics of a very severe intoxication.

In the lumen of the tubules, granular casts (Fig. 18.1) originate from particles

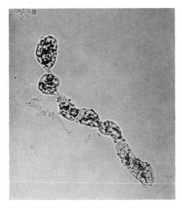

Fig. 18.1 — Portion of a cast from a uriniferous tubule of a horse kidney affected with nephritis. (Department of Veterinary Pathology, Michigan State University.)

of albumin that are fused in the glomeruli. They are also the result of extrusion of albuminous granules by the tubular epithelial cells which have undergone cloudy swelling and hyaline degeneration. Casts may also be formed of leukocytes, erythrocytes, necrotic and desquamated renal epithelial cells, and masses of hyalin. With swelling of the renal corpuscles there is a decrease in the amount of urine (oliguria). The urinometer shows this to be urine of **high specific gravity.** With an increase in the intertubular connective tissue there is an interference with the reabsorption of fluid by the convoluted tubules and with the resultant concentration of urine in them. This is evidenced by an increased amount of urine (polyuria). This urine has a **low specific gravity.** See Table 18.1 for the values of the normal specific gravity of the urine of different species.

TABLE 18.1

SPECIFIC GRAVITY OF URINE OF DIFFERENT SPECIES*

|  | Range | Average |
|---|---|---|
| Horse | 1.025–1.060 | 1.040 |
| Ox | 1.030–1.045 | 1.032 |
| Sheep and Goat | 1.015–1.045 | 1.030 |
| Pig | 1.010–1.050 | 1.012 |
| Dog | 1.016–1.060 | 1.025 |
| Cat | 1.020–1.040 | 1.030 |

* W. Ellenberger and Arthur Scheunert.

Hemorrhage of the kidneys permits blood to become mixed with the urine (hematuria). Whenever the destruction of erythrocytes is excessive, free hemoglobin is present in the blood but a normal renal filter will not permit it to pass through into the urine. A renal filter made more permeable by injury will permit hemoglobin to pass through (hemoglobinuria). Likewise hemobilirubin present in the blood in hemolytic diseases cannot pass through a normal renal filter but can through a diseased one (hemobilirubinuria). When the liver allows cholebilirubin to regurgitate into the blood, or when bile duct obstruction prevents its excretion into the intestine, it is excreted in the urine (cholebilirubinuria).

# KIDNEY

## Disturbances of Circulation

### HYPEREMIA

Acute general active hyperemia may be seen in acute interstitial nephritis produced by leptospira and other bacterial agents, and in general infections such as hog cholera, swine erysipelas, and ovine enterotoxemia. The kidneys are swollen, edematous, and have a more intense color due to the increased amount of arterial blood.

Acute focal active hyperemia involving portions of the kidney is observed in the vicinity of areas of suppurative nephritis and ascending pyelonephritis and at the borders of tumors and infarcts where inflammation is present.

Acute general passive hyperemia involving the entire kidney is observed with sudden cardiac failure as is associated with thiamine deficiency in the pig, acute pneumonia, and thrombosis of the posterior vena cava or the renal veins. If the cause of the hyperemia is located in one renal vein, the passive hyperemia will be unilateral. Both kidneys will be involved if the venous obstruction is located in the heart, lung, or posterior vena cava. The lesion causing the hyperemia has existed for only a short period of time, and there must be no deposition of connective tissue in the kidney as the result of the hyperemia. The kidneys are distended with blood, their color is a cyanotic red as the result of hypoxia, and the larger veins within the kidneys are prominent.

Chronic general passive hyperemia is associated with lesions in the heart, lung, posterior vena cava, or renal veins which persist for a long period of time so that the kidney shows some permanent alteration such as atrophy or fibrosis. Tumors of the adrenal gland or abscesses near the renal vein can produce a general passive hyperemia of a single kidney. The kidneys are noticeably swollen and the medulla is dark red due to long-standing dilatation of the expandable venous system. The escape of cellular blood components should never be confused with the lesions of interstitial nephritis.

Chronic focal passive hyperemia is not diagnosed as it has no significance and would be impossible to recognize grossly or microscopically in most instances.

### ANEMIA

General anemia (involving the entire kidney) is observed when an oligemia, oligocythemia, or oligochromemia of the entire animal exists as is produced by a hemorrhagic, hemolytic, hypochromic, aplastic, or hypoplastic anemia. While the cortex is noticeably paler, the most prominent changes are always in the medulla, and in advanced cases the renal pyramids may be practically white. The kidney can adjust to maintain reasonably normal function, but in sudden loss of blood the glomerular pressure may drop until no urine is formed (anuria).

Complete occlusion of the renal artery by a thrombus results in an infarcted and nonfunctional kidney. Accidental ligation of the renal artery occasionally occurs when dogs are spayed. In an attempt to ligate bleeding ovarian or uterine vessels, the renal artery is included in the ligation. One of the authors has observed bilateral renal artery ligation following the spaying of a dog. If only one kidney is involved and it is sterile, it undergoes necrosis and becomes calcified. If the necrotic kidney contains pyogenic bacteria, an abscess is the result.

Local anemia is seen when thrombi or emboli become established in the renal artery or its branches. Thrombi are rare in the kidney while emboli are relatively frequent; both are responsible for the development of infarcts.

Infarcts are usually wedge-shaped in the kidney. If the arciform branch of the renal artery becomes plugged with an embolus, the infarct will involve both the cortex and medulla. When only the interlobular branch is involved, only the cortex will be affected. The latter infarcts will be cone-shaped, with their base at the surface of the kidney and their apex pointed towards the pelvis. Immediately after the obstruction occurs in the artery, there is a transitory anemia of the area. As the result of the deficiency of blood, the collateral circulation from the surrounding areas of the kidney begin to pour blood into the capillary network of the infarcted area, and this stuffing with blood causes the area to become intensely red. It is therefore designated as a **red infarct.** If the collateral circulation is not adequate to maintain the life of the renal tissue, death of the area occurs. The necrosis begins in the center of the infarcted area 2 to 6 hours after the vascular obstruction occurs and progresses peripherally. The entire area of infarction has undergone necrosis in about 72 hours. Autolysis occurs in the area of infarction, and the erythrocytes liberate their hemoglobin. The hemoglobin, being very soluble in the tissue fluids, diffuses into the surrounding renal tissue, and when hemoglobin is no longer present the area of infarction lacks color and then is known as a **pale** or **anemic infarct.** After the infarct has been organized and the connective tissue has shrunken, there may be marked distortion of the kidney. The region of infarction is then firm in consistency and gray or white in color as the result of scar tissue. It is now no longer called an infarct but instead is designated as a **renal scar** or a healed infarct.

The early vascularity of the inflammatory zone adjacent to the infarct may give it a ringed, bulging appearance when viewed through the intact capsular surface of the kidney at this stage. Later, as the necrotic parenchyma is removed, it will appear depressed. The preservation of a tiny zone of parenchyma in the outer cortex over the infarct and the perirenal connective tissue prevents actual rupture of the capsule. The capsule and extreme outer cortex can establish a collateral circulation through the intact perirenal vascular system, and that is why the capsule is usually intact over an infarct. It is obvious that if the source of an embolus or the nature of the thrombus from which it came is known, the effect on the kidney will be more predictable. Living cells, such as parts of tumors or microorganisms capable of establishing themselves (for example streptococci and corynebacteria), can result in a progressive nephritis. In other cases, as in those resulting from fragments of parasites, living cells are not present, and the obstruction is strictly mechanical blockage of the vessel (**aseptic infarcts** to differentiate from **septic infarcts** of bacterial infections). Unfortunately there is the tendency for many infarcts to be multiple as in those related to bacterial endocarditis in the dog and pig, strongylosis in the horse, and heartworm in the dog. The differentiation of a progressive nephritis initiated by septic emboli from other types of focal chronic interstitial nephritis is often impossible, but the presence of healing or healed infarcts should never be overlooked. Unfortunately, the distortion may be so advanced when the lesions become extensive that one cannot identify the healed areas of infarction.

## HEMORRHAGE

Petechial hemorrhages occurring in the outer cortex but under the capsule are important in the recognition of the septicemias. In hog cholera, subcapsular hemorrhages are a result of injury to the vascular endothelium. In bovine leptospirosis and in oak tree poisoning in cattle, one can easily mistake hemoglobin or blood pigment casts in the convoluted tubules of the outer cortex for hemorrhages, particularly if both casts and hemorrhages are present in the same kidney. Hemorrhages into the pelvis, the perirenal tissue, and beneath the capsule are more diffuse in nature. In sweet-clover poisoning or when the kidney is traumatized, they may be large enough to be of the suffusion type. There is a close association of renal hemorrhage with hematuria.

## EDEMA

The most common type of edema seen in the kidney is an **inflammatory edema** associated with acute interstitial nephritis, whether the nephritis is focal or diffuse. It is also found as a component of the cellular reaction located at the borders of tumors, infarcts, or any other process that causes a destruction of existing parenchyma. It is obvious that it would be found also when there is passive hyperemia of the kidney in conditions generally classed as **noninflammatory edemas.**

In advanced cases the involved portions of the kidney — and that may include the entire kidney — are noticeably swollen and, when incised, feel soggy on their cut surfaces. The cut edges bulge, and pressure must be exerted to bring the edges together.

**Hydronephrosis.** When an obstruction to the flow of urine from a kidney develops slowly or intermittently, the kidney will eventually reach a stage where its pelvis begins to dilate and enlarge. The development is the same whether the obstruction is in the ureter, bladder, urethra, or whether it is unilateral or bilateral. Of course, in bilateral obstruction, uremia will develop before lesions of advanced hydronephrosis are seen. When obstruction is sudden and complete, there will be only a slight dilatation due to cessation of glomerular filtration and rapid degeneration of the kidney. Glomerular filtration does not cease in partial obstruction, and in a few weeks the dilatation is not reversible. Besides the dilatation of the pelvis, cysts that communicate with the pelvis develop in the medullary substance; the cortex becomes progressively thinner due to collapse and disappearance of tubules. Histologically, the failure of the glomeruli to atrophy and disappear is characteristic unless there is a complicating pyelonephritis. Pyelonephritis is not unusual because with the interference with escape of urine, infections will ascend the urinary tract.

Almost all hydronephrosis is acquired. Occasionally, malformed renal arteries or ureters can be associated with hydronephrosis in a young animal.

## Disturbances of Growth

### AGENESIS

Bilateral agenesis is incompatible with life and would result in a stillborn animal. Unilateral renal agenesis is frequently reported in all species of domesticated animals. Failure of development of all or part of the kidney, ureter, renal artery, or renal vein may be responsible. The opposite kidney usually undergoes compensatory hypertrophy.

### HYPOPLASIA

Hypoplasia of the kidney is seldom reported in domesticated animals. If congenital, one would expect the opposite kidney to undergo compensatory hypertrophy.

Congenital cyst formation is most common in the pig, both as single and multiple cysts. Multiple congenital cysts are rather frequent in dogs and cats and occasionally are seen in cattle, horses, and sheep. The condition can be designated as **congenital polycystic kidney** if extensive. These cysts may be seen in the medulla but are usually confined to the cortex. Medullary cysts should be examined carefully to see that they do not communicate with a dilated pelvis and hence actually be a manifestation of hydronephrosis. Acquired cysts as a group are characteristically smaller than the congenital variety and are related to inflammatory lesions that could account for pinching off a tubule and dilatation of its proximal end.

### HYPERPLASIA

Hyperplasia of the glomerular and tubular structures of the kidney is uncommon. Occasionally, when stimulated by toxins, they give the impression that there are more cells than normal, but it is difficult to substantiate this by comparison with control kidneys. Hyperplasia of renal white fibrous connective tissue occurs when it is stimulated by various toxic and infectious agents.

### HYPERTROPHY

Renal hypertrophy is very common in all domestic animals. Following renal glomerular or tubular injury, the remaining renal cells become larger than normal and thereby are able to compensate for the loss of renal epithelium. When one kidney is destroyed (renal artery ligation, ureteral obstruction, or bacterial infection), the remaining kidney becomes greatly enlarged and compensates for the loss of renal tissue. As far as renal function is concerned, the hypertrophic tissue may be able to achieve full compensation. The hypertrophic kidney may be as much as twice its normal size. Histologically, the hypertrophy involves the cells of the nephron unit, and the cells may be twice as large as the normal cells of the structure.

### METAPLASIA

Metaplasia of the kidney usually involves the interstitial white fibrous connective tissue only. It is usually the result of bacterial infection. Masses or plates of bone may be found in the kidney when metaplasia has occurred.

## Disturbances in Cell Metabolism

### CLOUDY SWELLING

Cloudy swelling is due to various inorganic, organic, and bacterial toxic substances. A list of them would include practically the same injurious agents which cause similar changes in other parenchymatous organs. All of these toxic agents reach the kidney by way of the blood stream. Naturally, they injure the glomeruli and convoluted tubules first and the collecting tubules next. The epithelium is highly specialized and sensitive to irritants. Therefore, protein metabolism is easily disturbed. The proximal convoluted tubules are frequently the only tubules affected, due to their high susceptibility to injury. The cells usually recover unless the changes are progressive and develop into a more severe type of injury.

**Macroscopic appearance.** Macroscopically, the kidney is swollen, has a bulging cut surface, and has a cooked appearance.

**Microscopic appearance.** Microscopically, the cells appear cloudy, their cytoplasm is granular, and they stain more intensely with eosin. Because the cells contain more fluid than normal, they are swollen and protrude into the lumen of the tubules. Post-mortem autolysis is frequently mistaken for cloudy swelling. However, in post-mortem autolysis the cells do not swell, and therefore the lumen of the tubules has a normal diameter.

### HYDROPIC DEGENERATION

Hydropic degeneration refers to tubular degeneration characterized by the formation of clear cytoplasmic vacuoles that do not contain glycogen, fat, or mucin and are presumed to be tissue fluids. There is usually little change in the nuclei of the cells, and cell recovery can be predicted on the basis of minimal nuclear injury. In overdosages of ether, chloroform, or carbon tetrachloride these vacuoles will appear and primarily affect the proximal convoluted tubules and to a lesser extent the loops of Henle and distal convoluted tubules. Experimental evidence indicates that the vacuoles form in fluid balance disturbances such as vomiting, diarrhea, and following excessive hemorrhages. This is believed related to excessive loss of potassium. Vacuoles will also appear after the administration of hypertonic sucrose. Their appearance in many animals submitted for necropsy often cannot be explained on the basis of the history and other lesions.

### GOUT

In the fowl, in which the urine is normally rich in uric acid and urates, deposits of uric acid and urates occur on the surface of the kidney, in Bowman's capsule, and in the collecting tubules. They appear as needle-like crystals microscopically. They give the kidney a white-stippled appearance. This is another manifestation of visceral gout. The etiology is not known.

Baby pigs, 1 to 9 days of age, affected with viral transmissible gastroenteritis (T.G.E.) become so dehydrated by the severe diarrhea that there is insufficient fluid for the proper elimination of renal excretion. As urine concentration occurs when the glomerular filtrate passes through the tubules, a point of supersaturation is finally reached when various salts contained within the filtrate precipitate out of solution. The salts are prominent in the renal medulla where the collecting ducts of the papillae are quite uniformly distended with an orange to white precipitate of monosodium urate and uric acid. The papillae have a streaked appearance as though pencilled with orange or white pigment. The renal pelvis, the ureters, and the bladder also contain the precipitate. The nonprotein nitrogen content of the blood is increased due to urea and uric acid. The blood urea nitrogen may be increased up to 30 times normal (normal = about 11.3 mg/100 cc blood).

## AMYLOID INFILTRATION

Amyloid infiltration of the kidneys occasionally occurs in dogs. The amyloid is deposited around the capillary loops of the glomeruli and around the intertubular capillaries. Its presence usually leads to renal failure terminating in uremia.

Andersson in Sweden has studied the so-called "large white kidneys" of cows and has discovered that they are lesions of amyloidosis. The surface of the enlarged organs, besides being grayish white to grayish brown in color, is studded with pinhead size, yellow, opaque foci which are elevated enough to give the surface a slightly granulated appearance. The amyloid is deposited around the capillary loops in the glomeruli, and forms a mantle around the capillaries in the cortex and medulla. Affected glomeruli grossly look like light homogeneous, transparent dots. In the cortex and medulla the deposits form narrow yellow streaks which parallel the uriniferous tubules and the collecting ducts. Kidneys are sometimes erroneously diagnosed as chronic diffuse glomerulonephritis.

## FATTY DEGENERATION

The disturbance of fat metabolism resulting in fatty degeneration of the renal epithelium occurs under the same conditions as it does in the heart, liver, adrenals, skeletal muscle, or wherever it can occur. In the kidney, the same as in the other organs, it is the expression of a severe injury of the kidney cells. In most cases it is the result of an intoxication. The same long list of toxic substances mentioned in connection with hepatic fatty degeneration could, for the most part, be repeated here as causative agents for renal fatty degeneration.

The injurious substances usually reach the kidney by means of the general circulation, and no part of the renal epithelium is exempt from injury. It is well to keep in mind that this type of cell disturbance is a common alteration in many of the severe acute infectious diseases, particularly those which are septicemic.

**Macroscopic appearance.** The kidneys are enlarged, swollen, have a bulging cut surface, are friable and greasy in consistency, and are white, buff, yellow, or orange in color. The color depends upon the species of animal. Cat kidneys are almost white, while the equine kidneys are nearly orange in color. The kidneys frequently have a mottled appearance. This mottling is due to variations in the amount of blood in various portions of the kidney. The blood masks the color of the fat and gives it a reddish hue. The radial striations peripheral to the arcuate arteries are due to the fat contained within the epithelium of the ascending and descending tubules. An abundance of fat is normally found in these tubules and is especially prominent in well-fed dogs. It does not represent fatty degeneration.

**Microscopic appearance.** The tubular cells, particularly the convoluted cells, contain distinct vacuoles often varying greatly in size, and the nuclei may be dark and pyknotic or show other evidence of degeneration. In the inflammatory diseases, the interstitial lesions (to be discussed later) may distort the gross and microscopic appearance of fatty degeneration and cloudy swelling. One should confirm doubtful cases by staining sections with a lipid stain and being certain that the vacuoles contain fat.

In adult dogs and cats it is normal for fat to be present in the cells of the proximal convoluted tubules. In puppies and kittens it is absent but as dogs and cats approach a year of age the stainable fat appears, and it increases in amount as the animals age. It is also present in the ascending and descending arms of Henle's loops in mature dogs and cats. Its physiologic presence in these locations must be kept in mind when looking for evidences of fatty degeneration.

GLYCOGEN INFILTRATION

Glycogen infiltration is of little significance in domestic animals. The amount of glycogen in the tubular epithelium increases in amount in diabetes.

PIGMENTATION

**Hemoglobin.** Pigmentation of the urine with hemoglobin occurs when there is excessive hemolysis of the erythrocytes. The appearance of hemoglobin in the urine is known as hemoglobinuria.

**Protozoan blood diseases** (Texas fever and babesiasis of cattle and babesiasis of dogs) cause hemolysis of the erythrocytes with a hemoglobinuria as the result. Various bacterial diseases, such as bacillary hemoglobinuria of cattle and sheep and leptospirosis of cattle, cause hemoglobinuria. **Post-parturient hemoglobinuria** frequently occurs in heavy milk-producing cows within a few weeks after parturition. It seems to be associated with feeding a ration low in inorganic phosphorus.

**Bile pigments.** A small amount of urobilinogen is normally excreted in the urine (Table 18.2). When there is hemolysis and the liver is normal, the amount in the urine is increased greatly. In toxic jaundice the amount is increased somewhat as a result of the inability of the sick liver cells to handle it or as a result of its being "regurgitated" by the liver cells.

Cholebilirubin is increased somewhat in the urine in toxic jaundice because of regurgitation by the liver cells. It is markedly increased in obstructive jaundice because it cannot be excreted by the bile passages.

**Muscle pigment.** Myoglobinuria occurs in horses in the disease called **azoturia.**

Research explains the appearance of myoglobin in the urine during this disease as follows: During periods of rest, horses store or retain large quantities of glycogen in the heavy muscles such as those of the loin, thigh, croup, and shoulder region. Violent exercise or work following the rest suddenly increases the metabolism of the glycogen with the consequent formation of excessive amounts of sarcolactic acid. This is hydrophilic, and its presence in the muscle cells causes them to swell and undergo coagulative necrosis. The necrotic change results in liberation of myoglobin with its subsequent appearance in the urine.

**Melanin.** Melanosis is seen occasionally in the renal pelvis of sheep. It has no pathological significance.

**Necrosis**

COAGULATIVE NECROSIS

Coagulative necrosis is the most common type of necrosis observed in the kidney and in most instances involves the tubular epithelium. This is to be expected since the glomerular filtrate is concentrated as it passes through the tubule, thereby increasing the toxicity of any injurious substance it might contain.

Tubular necrosis is a more advanced stage of tubular injury than fatty degeneration or cloudy swelling and is a result of prolonged administration of toxic substances or the administration of compounds that are extremely irritating to the renal tubules. Some of the latter irritants produce necrosis in a few minutes or hours and are usually chemical agents that gain entry into the blood stream and are conveyed to the kidney. Ether and chloroform will sometimes produce necrosis of the

TABLE 18.2
BILE PIGMENT EXCRETION IN HEALTH AND IN JAUNDICE

|  | Normal | Hemolytic (Prehepatic) | Toxic (Intrahepatic) | Obstructive (Posthepatic) |
|---|---|---|---|---|
| Urobilinogen......... | + | +++ | ++ | ................ |
| Cholebilirubin........ | ................ | ................ | + | +++ |

proximal convoluted tubules in excessive overdoses rather than the hydropic degeneration mentioned earlier. As might be expected, the proximal convoluted tubules show the earliest and most severe damage, and often this damage extends rapidly to the loops of Henle and the distal convoluted tubules. One should expect to find hemorrhages, edema, and cellular inflammatory infiltrations in the nearby interstitial tissues. These changes should not be confused with interstitial nephritis where the tubules are not primarily affected and the more advanced lesions appear in the interstitial tissues rather than in the tubules.

One can designate these advanced tubular lesions as **tubular nephrosis** but never **nephrosis** unless convinced that there is equal damage to the glomeruli. Since the term nephrosis is used in describing human diseases and includes chronic diseases of the glomeruli and sometimes tubules where there is excessive loss of protein, it is well to avoid similar generalities in describing animal diseases.

**Mercury** poisoning with its characteristic tubular necrosis is of great economic importance in cattle, horses, and swine due to its rather frequent occurrence and the high resulting mortality. One must remember that it is the mercury salts that are toxic and that in therapeutic agents the mercury is stabilized so that only in excessive oxidation is it ever toxic. Metallic mercury is highly insoluble and hence not toxic. The treatment of oats with a mercurial fungicide and the later feeding of leftover oats to livestock probably is the most common history of poisoning with this group of compounds. The kidneys are markedly enlarged in terminal fulminating cases and usually gray or pale in color. The coagulative type of necrosis appears in the proximal convoluted tubules usually on the first day of the illness, with the nuclei disintegrating and the cytoplasm becoming granular. Eosin-staining droplets of protein are seen in the tubules in the second and third days and are probably protein that has passed through the glomerular filter and is trapped in the blocked tubules. A little later, leukocytes — particularly neutrophils — appear in the tubules and interstitial tissues. Casts of leukocytes and hyaline and granular material frequently appear in the tubules. After a week, regeneration of tubules begins even though at this time calcium may be found in the basement membranes of these new cells and in the debris and casts in the tubules. By the third week, regeneration is usually complete. Glomeruli do not appear to be damaged in any stage of the disease.

**Oak tree** poisoning is another excellent example of a rather common tubular necrosis and is seen primarily in cattle. It also occurs in sheep, horses, and wild ruminants. It appears after the oaks are beginning to leaf out in the spring and is frequently seen when the grass is slow to appear. If other feed is not available in other seasons, animals may strip the scrub oak trees in range country and become ill. Constipation followed by a diarrhea that may be hemorrhagic, evidence of kidney damage together with a history of available oak trees, lack of feed, and sudden death in one to several days are the complaints that are most helpful in diagnosing the disease. At necropsy one sees large pale kidneys containing subcapsular petechial hemorrhages and the visible pigment casts mentioned earlier in the discussion of hemorrhages. The necrosis of proximal convoluted tubules is usually very extensive and of the coagulative type, with an early loss of the nuclear and cell outlines so that the limits of necrotic epithelium may not be apparent. Hemoglobin and other types of casts frequently are present and appear to fill the lumens of many of the damaged proximal convoluted tubules.

Other compounds capable of producing tubular nephrosis when ingested are ethylene glycol and diethylene glycol (antifreezes) and dichromate solutions. Antifreeze poisoning has been observed in small animals confined in garages where the antifreeze solution has been drained from the radiator and left in an open container. The drinking of a relatively small amount of the solution caused the renal degeneration and the appearance of crystals of calcium oxalate in the lumen of the convoluted tubules and collecting ducts.

Overdosages of sulfonamides and the ingestion of certain oxalate-containing plants (*Halogeton glomeratus*) produce a tubular necrosis. In these necroses, crystals of the sulfonamides and oxalate are deposited in the tubules in such quantity that some researchers believe the crystals are responsible for a mechanical obstruction of many of the nephrons. Calcium oxalate crystals are also deposited in the tubules in diethylene glycol necrosis due to oxidation of the glycol. Hemoglobinuria is commonly seen in the sulfonamide necroses and is believed to be related more to hemorrhages from the interstitial tissues than leakage through the glomeruli. As might be expected, deep-staining casts, believed to be hemoglobin casts, as well as masses of erythrocytes are seen in the tubules.

## Nephritis

Inflammation of the kidneys is a complex process for the following reasons: (1) Individual parts of the organ are intimately associated with one another; a glomerulus with its uriniferous tubule constitutes an inseparable unit; injury to a glomerulus sympathetically affects the tubule and vice versa. (2) Degenerative-necrotic changes of the tubular epithelium stimulate the intertubular connective tissue (interstitial tissue) to proliferate. (3) Chronic inflammatory processes may later become overshadowed by a more recent acute reaction. (4) Various nephritis-producing agents may cause the same type of inflammation, or an individual irritant may produce different types. (5) From the standpoint of pathogenesis, nephritis may originate hematogenically or urinogenically. Further, it may be suppurative or non-suppurative. The reaction may involve principally the glomeruli and the tubules or the interstitial tissue, and may be diffuse or focal. Based on these facts nephritis can be classified as follows:

A. Hematogenic
  1. Glomerulonephritis
    a. Acute
    b. Subacute
    c. Chronic
    d. Subclinical
    e. Sclerosing nephropathy
  2. Interstitial nephritis
    a. Acute
    b. Focal suppurative
    c. Chronic

B. Urinogenic ascending pyelonephritis

### GLOMERULONEPHRITIS

The mistaken identification of subclinical glomerulonephritis and scattered focal glomerular lesions (that we prefer to call sclerosing nephropathy) for acute and subacute glomerulonephritis by veterinary pathologists at necropsy is due in part to the extreme rarity of glomerulonephritis in the domesticated animals. Bell has pointed out that in man proliferative glomerulonephritis of varying intensity develops in a notable percentage of infections and toxic diseases and that it is only when capillary obstruction becomes severe that symptoms arise which are recognized as those of acute glomerulonephritis. He further states that glomerulonephritis should be considered as an extreme degree of a very common reaction to injury on the part of the glomerular endothelium.

Domesticated animals fortunately do not exhibit commonly more than the mildest type of reactions to a toxic or antigenic agent. In fact, a mild, persistent subclinical glomerulonephritis is so rare that it is confusing to the veterinary clinician, and in the living animal is apt to be regarded as a manifestation of interstitial nephritis when simple laboratory tests of the urine establish the existence of lesions. About the only clue may be the persistence of a bacterial infection at some other body site, and then the final correlation must be made at necropsy. It is necessary to be aware of changes in representative areas in both kidneys to make an unqualified diagnosis of glomerulonephritis. In suspected cases, one must take adequate blocks of each in order to inspect an adequate number of nephrons. There should not only be evidence of damage in nearly every nephron examined but it should be severe damage. Secondary glomerular damage in subacute and chronic interstitial nephritis is always patchy in distribution, and there should be no difficulty in its differentiation.

While a few reports are made of glomerulonephritis in dogs and horses, one cannot find adequate descriptions of its occurrence in other domesticated animals.

**Acute, subacute, and chronic glomerulonephritis.** Although reports suggest that glomerulonephritis is rather common in horses injected with bacterial cultures or toxins for the production of immune serums and antitoxins, investigations have found this not to be true. Horses may die suddenly in the first few weeks following injections, but their death is usually directly related to the inoculations and cannot be attributed to a secondary diffuse glomerulonephritis. Isolated cases of glomerulonephritis in the horse and the dog are seen, and the majority of these animals are under 3 years of age. There have been no adequate bacteriologic investigations to incriminate the streptococci, which are believed to be a trigger to the

acute episodes in man. However, streptococcic diseases are so very common in the young horse that one would want good documentation to rule out this association. In man, in the acute type, a slightly swollen kidney with petechial hemorrhages scattered throughout the cortex is seen which develops into **the large white kidney** of the subacute stage. These large white kidneys are described in dogs and horses, and with them, faded petechial hemorrhages are noted scattered in the cortex. The kidneys are enlarged up to 2 times their normal size and bulge on being sectioned. The cortex is widened up to $1\frac{1}{2}$ its normal thickness and is yellow-gray in color. With the exception of 1 case of acute glomerulonephritis in the dog, the 4 cases in the horse and the 7 in the dog that were reviewed by the authors were in the late subacute or early chronic stage. In these cases, the kidneys were distinctly gray rather than brownish red, only slightly smaller than normal, noticeably firmer than usual, and often with scattered tiny cysts in the cortex. Signs of nephritis were evident by failure to concentrate urine by 5 of the 7 dogs (i.e. specific gravity under 1.012), marked albumin in the urine, urinary casts, high blood urea nitrogen, and evidence of uremia.

The single case of acute glomerulone-

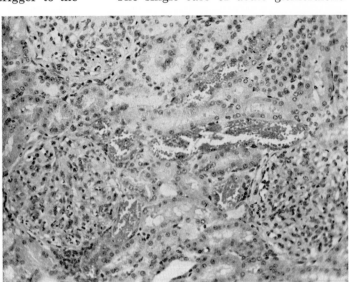

Fig. 18.2 — Acute glomerulonephritis in a dog, showing several swollen cellular glomeruli. ×185. (AFIP Acc. 210753).

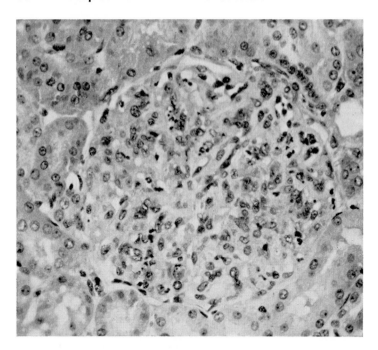

Fig. 18.3 — Acute g l o m e r - ulonephritis in a dog, show- ing the glomerular lesion. The glomerulus is swollen, nearly avascular, and fills Bowman's capsule.   ×210. (AFIP Acc. 210753).

phritis studied in a 9-year-old mixed spaniel dog is believed to be very rare in domesticated animals, and its relation to generalized malignant lymphoma also present in the animal is not understood. It is included in this discussion to show what one might expect to find if making that diagnosis (Figs. 18.2 and 18.3). The glomeruli are swollen, nearly avascular, and fill Bowman's capsule. Numerous large endothelial cells and neutrophils obstruct the lumen of the glomerular capillaries and would seem to be responsible for the glomerular ischemia. In this case, large deposits of hemosiderin were present in the renal tubules.

Differences between the subacute and chronic stage microscopically are slight and may be represented only by increased numbers of almost completely hyalinized or collapsed glomeruli and more evidence of cystic dilatation of scattered groups of tubules in the cortex. There is an active proliferation of the epithelial cells of Bowman's capsule, and this proliferation (Fig. 18.4) results in adhesions between the glomerular tuft and the parietal layer of Bowman's capsule in both stages. Some-

times the proliferation also forms distinct crescent-shaped masses in the glomeruli that are called **epithelial crescents.** Endothelial cells are also actively proliferating in most glomeruli in this stage. The proliferations close off many capillaries, and the occluded capillaries appear as cellular hyaline masses in the tufts. At this stage of development, fatty degeneration of the proximal convoluted tubules may be seen, or they may appear slightly atrophic, be dilated and atrophic, or appear to be unaffected.

Although there have been histories of bacteriologic or possible bacteriologic infections of several months' duration in several subacute and chronic cases in dogs, there have not been conclusive bacteriologic studies done to make definite associations. Histories of tonsilitis, bronchitis, endocarditis, myocarditis, splenic abscess, and pneumonia are suggestive.

**Subclinical glomerulonephritis.** As indicated earlier, subclinical glomerulonephritis refers to those cases of mild persistent nephritis in which distinct glomerular lesions are noted. The authors have only seen this disease in dogs, and in the few cases studied have again, as in the more severe and diffuse types of glomerulonephritis, associated it with chronic bacterial infections (tonsils, lymph nodes, skin, and prostate gland). These dogs do not have a terminal nephritis. At the time of death, they are still concentrating urine, are not uremic, and do not exhibit urea retention. Appreciable quantities of albumin in the urine and moderate numbers of urinary casts can be demonstrated.

There is no interstitial scarring or infiltrations of reactive cells to indicate an interstitial nephritis. However, there is a noticeable thickening and sometimes dilation of the glomerular capillaries. Endothelial cells are slightly increased in number and noticeably increased in size. However, erythrocytes are still seen in the capillary tufts. Proliferation of epithelial cells of Bowman's capsule in relation to capillary change is not excessive as one might expect to see in glomerular lesions secondary to an interstitial nephritis. Sometimes the glomeruli appear lobulated, and when the tissues are stained for fat,

the foci of epithelial proliferation that give the lobulated appearance are related to fat deposits.

## SCLEROSING NEPHROPATHY

Sclerosing nephropathy is common in old or mature dogs and to a lesser extent in older cattle, cats, swine, and horses. It is represented by small scattered microscopic lesions involving the Bowman's capsule, the glomerular capillaries, and the juxtaglomerular apparatus. These changes are not extensive enough or sufficiently advanced to justify a diagnosis of glomerulonephritis, and neither the appearance of the kidneys nor the history will support the existence of more than a mild nephritis. It appears that glomerular emboli that do not have viable bacteria in them can account for some of these lesions (Fig. 18.5). Many of the others, particularly those with exaggerated proliferations of the Bowman's capsule, can well be the results of an interstitial nephritis that has healed and left only slight scarring (Fig. 18.6).

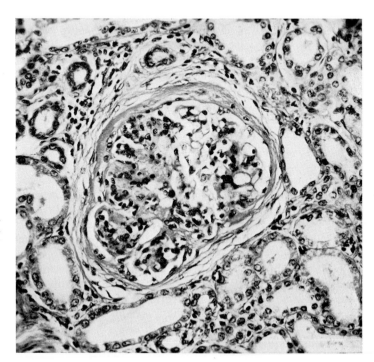

Fig. 18.4 — Subacute glomerulonephritis in a male Doberman pinscher. ×275. (AFIP Acc. 266753).

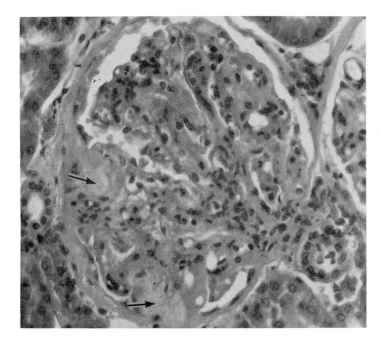

Fig. 18.5 — Sclerosing nephropathy in a 12-year-old male mongrel. Large quantities of fat are present in the glomeruli in this case and are most prominent in the epithelial proliferations which o f t e n form adhesions between the glomerular capillaries and Bowman's capsule (arrow). × 315. (AFIP Acc. 283588).

A prominent juxtaglomerular apparatus is seen in many dogs, and it sometimes is associated with slight thickening of the glomerular loops. Most of the capillaries are only narrowed, and erythrocytes can be seen in their lumina. In some instances, the juxtaglomerular apparatus is represented by several vascular channels, and each is surrounded by a hyalinized mass which is sparsely interspersed with nuclei resembling those of epithelial cells. The hyaline material does not resemble amyloid. These areas contain many lipid granules as shown by the oil-red O stain. The fat is not birefringent and stains blue with the Nile-blue sulfate stain. The presence of fat in these tufts and in some of the thickened Bowman's capsules is not surprising, as the presence of fat is associated with many chronic diseases.

Except for replacement of scattered groups of tubules in the cortex and medulla with minor interstitial scarring, occasional scattered dilatations of tubules, and some minor infiltrations of plasma cells and lymphocytes, there are no other significant lesions in these kidneys. When the latter changes are established, it

further supports the idea that preceding interstitial inflammatory lesions are responsible for some cases of mild glomerular damage.

### INTERSTITIAL NEPHRITIS

No method of division of the interstitial nephritides is completely satisfactory. If one includes all of the relatively mild lesions of a focal or generalized nature that are found, he soon finds himself dealing with subclinical lesions. It should be realized that the kidney has remarkable ability to recover from interstitial nephritis. In many cases of interstitial nephritis resulting from a systemic disease, there should be a healing of the kidney lesions along with other manifestation of a return to good health. Naturally, this is most apt to occur if the lesions are not suppurative and have not become organized. Even the persistence of leptospira in dog, cattle, and swine kidneys for periods of months after the disease was recognized does not imply that, in that disease, chronic interstitial nephritis is apt to develop in more than a few isolated cases. There may be only a few animals that show more than relatively mild manifestations. There is often a limited nephritis associated with many of the viral diseases, and this is believed to be more of a renal reaction to secondary invaders than to the virus. We believe that a focal suppurative nephritis precedes many of the cases of chronic interstitial nephritis in our domesticated animal.

## ACUTE AND SUBACUTE NONSUPPURATIVE NEPHRITIS

Acute nonsuppurative nephritis can lead to uremia if it is of a diffuse nature and if there is sufficient damage to nephrons. The presence of albumin in the urine, low specific gravity of urine, and sometimes hematuria may be found either with or without uremia.

In advanced cases, the kidneys may be noticeably swollen. Small hemorrhages are present in the parenchyma in some cases. On section, grayish streaks or foci are noted at the corticomedullary junction zone and, in advanced cases, may be scattered throughout the cortex and outer medulla. Histologic examination reveals many tiny foci of lymphocytes, plasma cells, and mononuclear cells in the inner cortex between the tubules. Neutrophils may be present in this cellular exudate but are not prominent. Cloudy swelling, fatty degeneration, and even necrosis with beginning regeneration of tubular epithelium may be seen. Casts frequently occlude tubules.

While many generalized infections result in an acute nephritis, by far the most common one, and one that can be specifically associated with it, is canine leptospirosis. It is sometimes possible in these cases to demonstrate, with appropriate silver stains, tightly coiled argentophilic leptospirae with the characteristic hooked end in the convoluted tubules of the cortex.

In leptospiral infections in swine the acute lesions seen are usually focal and not as extensive in the cortex as those seen in

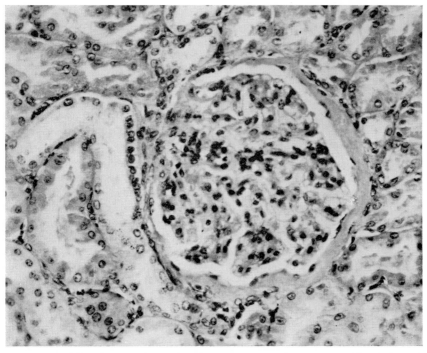

Fig. 18.6 — Sclerosing nephropathy. Bowman's capsule is noticeably thickened. ×276. (AFIP Acc. 234712).

dogs. In cattle the reaction can be as severe as in dogs and is characterized by more neutrophils in the interstitial tissues and free or in casts in the involved tubules.

In the dog a subacute stage of leptospirosis that follows the acute syndrome in 4 to 8 weeks can be seen in carrier animals. Only a few of a small group of carriers from an outbreak will show this, as in most the lesions are minimal even where leptospirae can be demonstrated in tubules. The textbook kidney in these cases appears only slightly atrophic or fibrous on section and has an adherent capsule. Large white or grayish nodular masses in the outer medulla and adjacent cortex can easily be seen. This tissue mass extends as radial streaks through the entire cortex in these kidneys (Fig. 18.7). Since this corticomedullary zone also is extensively in-

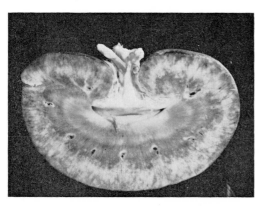

Fig. 18.7 — Subacute leptospirosis. Many irregular gray foci are present in the cortex and outer medulla and are most prominent at the corticomedullary junction. (AFIP Acc. 198982).

volved in acute leptospirosis, it can be assumed that there is progressive development of these lesions. Microscopically, the nodular masses are composed of histiocytes, mononuclear cells, and in more severe cases a few neutrophils. They distort the interstitial tissues and replace groups of tubules. Sometimes there are smaller infiltrations of plasma cells and lymphocytes between the larger masses.

No one has demonstrated that there are significant lesions of leptospirosis beyond this subacute stage.

Many cases called **white spotted kidney** in calves (Fig. 18.8) are actually an acute to subacute nonsuppurative nephritis associated principally with navel infection, pneumonia, and enteritis. Often the calves outwardly recover and are sent to slaughter, and the healing kidney lesions may be all that the meat inspector can see in his limited post-mortem inspection. Most of these kidneys are in the subacute stage, and the grayish to white zones of infiltration can easily be seen through the intact capsule. Sometimes these scattered areas of infiltration appear to replace over half of the cortical area of the kidney, but there is not the acute inflammatory changes that we associate with a fulminating nephritis. There are usually only a few scattered neutrophils in these lesions or in adjacent tubules.

Calves may also show lesions of focal suppurative nephritis, or there may be both a suppurative and nonsuppurative nephritis in the same kidney.

It is usually difficult to isolate any bacteriologic agents from these kidneys, and it is quite possible that any pathogenic microorganisms have already been eliminated in this recovery stage.

## FOCAL SUPPURATIVE NEPHRITIS

This type of nephritis is important in all species of domesticated animals and is capable of progressing in a period of months to a stage of chronicity that can be designated as chronic interstitial nephritis. Much controversy exists as to importance of many other kidney lesions including leptospiral lesions in regard to the development of a later chronic interstitial nephritis. This can never be resolved until careful research is done on the problem.

Many of the focal suppurative lesions are associated with specific pyogenic infections (in foals, _Shigella equirulis_, streptococci, and _Escherichia coli_; in cattle, _Corynebacterium pyogenes_, streptococci, and _Escherichia coli_) which reach the kidneys via the blood stream. A smaller group of infections reach the kidneys by ascending the urinary tract and are desig-

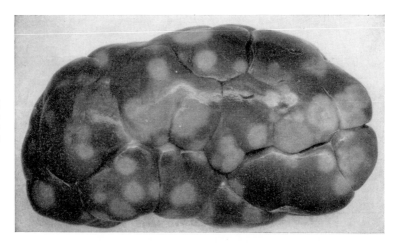

Fig. 18.8 — White spotted kidney in a calf. (Department of Veterinary Pathology, Michigan State University.)

nated as an **ascending pyelonephritis.** They are always accompanied with urinary bladder, ureter, and kidney pelvis lesions and will be discussed separately even though they produce similar damage in the kidney. Endocarditis, traumatic pericarditis in cattle, navel infections, and endometritis are examples of infections that may become generalized and lodge in the kidney. Sometimes they appear as septic emboli in the glomerular tufts or in other small capillaries of the kidney as miliary abscesses. These abscesses may enlarge rapidly and infiltrate large areas in an affected kidney.

**Macroscopic appearance.** Kidneys with suppurative nephritis may vary greatly in appearance. Often irregular yellow or gray areas are seen under the surface of the capsule, and when superficial they may be either raised or depressed. Areas of hyperemia or hemorrhage may surround the lesions in their early stage and later may be replaced by a distinct capsule. On section, the lesions may be linear or circumscribed and may involve scattered areas in the medulla as well as the more common location in the cortex. There may be much more severe involvement of one kidney than the other. The linear lesions may extend through the entire cortex and medulla as the infection follows the tubules and eventually may result in **pyelitis** (inflammation of the pelvis). When pyelitis is established, there is often free pus in the

pelvis, and care must be exercised not to confuse it with an ascending pyelonephritis. In advanced cases with involvement of the ureters and urinary bladder, it may not be possible to determine conclusively whether it was originally an ascending or descending infection.

**Microscopic appearance.** On histologic section, it is evident that the inflammatory reaction is much more severe than in most of the nonsuppurative nephritides. The most striking lesion is the widespread infiltration of polymorphonuclear leukocytes. This cellular exudate is either slightly or completely encapsulated or assumes a linear pattern which fills and distends the intertubular spaces. Necrosis and liquefaction are most prominent in the larger lesions in which the parenchyma is either greatly distorted or has disappeared. Mononuclear cells resembling lymphocytes, plasma cells, and histiocytes are observed at the borders of the lesions or intermixed with the polymorphonuclear cells in the linear infiltrations. The replacement of damaged parenchyma with connective tissue is evident. It is not unusual to see polymorphonuclear leukocytes within tubules. Often the tubules in the involved areas are collapsed or dilated and filled with acidophilic homogeneous casts. Indentations of the capsule in association with the appearance of scars in sections in which the acute lesions are still present suggest the development of the contracted, pitted kidney. In the medulla there are frequently large areas in which loss of medullary tubules is associated with interstitial infiltration of a finely granular eosinophilic material resembling lymph. Usually only a few polymorphonuclear leukocytes and histiocytes are seen in these areas. The hypertrophy and dilatation of the remaining medullary tubules are proportionate to the degree of medullary damage as evidenced by the loss of tubules. In a few cases where abscesses protrude from the surface of the kidney, cellular infiltrations, including neutrophils and lymphocytes, are present in the perinephric tissues as well as in the parenchyma of the kidney. Attempts to identify the more chronic stages of the disease should be aided by the fact that the parenchyma between lesions is altered only by secondary changes in the acute stages. In the discussion of chronic interstitial nephritis it will be pointed out that lesions in less advanced cases are similarly separated by only a slightly distorted parenchyma.

Multiple focal abscesses are seen in the cortex of the kidney of market pigs, older sows, and boars. Like the **white spotted kidney** of calves, it is probably in most instances secondary to some pre-existing primary infection. No specific microorganism has ever been consistently incriminated to be the cause of the condition, and usually the abscesses appear to be sterile.

Animals with suppurative nephritis may be quite ill, and it is often difficult to determine to what extent the kidney lesions contribute to the illness. However, the existence of hematuria, albuminuria, a lowered specific gravity, and, in some instances, symptoms of uremia are indicative of damage to the kidney.

## CHRONIC INTERSTITIAL NEPHRITIS

Chronic interstitial nephritis is not nearly as important clinically in the dog as many writers have indicated in published reports. Many of the lesions of chronic interstitial nephritis seen at necropsy are well compensated for in the dog before death. There is no justification for listing the lesions as a cause of death unless they are quite extensive or there is supporting clinical data. This does not mean that uremic deaths do not occur in association with chronic interstitial nephritis. Undoubtedly many do, but it does not add up to a high percentage. There may be albuminuria and low specific gravity of the urine also, but one does need this information before assuming that the dog has a terminal chronic interstitial nephritis. In pigs, cats, horses, cattle, and sheep it is also seen rather frequently. Next to the dog, pigs and cats seem most susceptible.

The kidneys with these more chronic lesions are usually small, firm, and pale, and one kidney may be more contracted than the other. The surface is often irregularly or uniformly nodular, with some of the nodules so small that they give the kidney a granular appearance. In some kidneys, cysts directly beneath the capsule are visible macroscopically. The kidneys are fibrous and cut with resistance. On section, the cortex is narrowed and the normal markings are completely or partially obliterated. The medulla is reduced proportionally in width. In pigs, kidneys often appear very pale and retain a proportionately larger size than in other animals. Histologically, the fibrosis appears very late in these porcine kidneys, and hence the kidney with a diffuse nephritis is slow to progress to a contracted state. In the dog tiny cystic spaces are noted and are usually in the outer medulla at the base of the medullary pyramids. Minute or linear cysts are scattered also through the cortex, but these are usually smaller than those in the medulla. The cysts in the outer medulla on histologic examination are found to be hyperplastic tubules, glandlike in appearance and frequently dilated (Fig. 18.9). Hyaline casts are often seen in these tubules, and the dilated tubules frequently extend into the cortex together with thin-walled, atrophic tubules.

Histologically, in most cases of chronic interstitial nephritis definite fibrotic bands

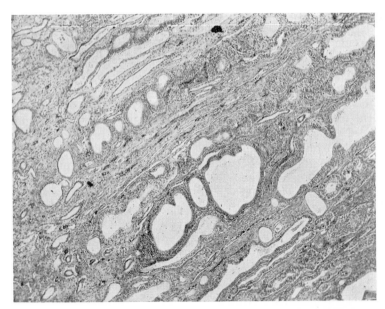

Fig. 18.9 — Chronic interstitial nephritis (canine). Hyperplastic tubules are frequently quite dilated in the medulla. ×48. (AFIP Acc. 200570).

extend irregularly throughout the entire cortex and medulla. It is these linear fibrotic zones that are most characteristic of this type of nephritis. Partial replacement of the cortical parenchyma by this connective tissue results in atrophy, collapse, and obliteration of tubules and glomeruli. It should be emphasized again that nephrons in the areas between these fibrotic zones appear intact, and this parenchyma shows little degenerative change. Glomeruli and tubules near the linear zones often become quite cystic, probably due to partial damage to nephrons.

In the extremely small contracted kidney a definite fibrotic band separates the cortex and medulla; it seems to form in segments that become continuous. Some of the irregularly nodular kidneys have wedge-shaped areas of fibrosis which suggest the complication of a healed infarct.

### ASCENDING PYELONEPHRITIS

In most domesticated animals ascending pyelonephritis is occasionally seen. In prostatitis in dogs, in tumors of the urinary tract that cause obstruction and in association with urinary calculi, one can expect a partial stasis of urine and the probability that pyelonephritis will develop. Histologically, the pelvis and medulla should be more severely involved than when there is a descending infection as we have already discussed. Ureters, urinary bladder, and sometimes the urethra show secondary inflammatory changes in this disease. Economically, in swine and cattle, urinary calculi and a specific corynebacterium infection are of major importance.

A specific infectious pyelonephritis (Figs. 18.10 and 18.11) which occurs most often in cows and sows is caused by *Corynebacterium renale*. It is generally believed that the infection enters the lower urinary tract after parturition and ascends to the kidney. If the distribution of lymphatics in the ox and the pig is the same as in the rabbit and the dog, the lymphatic network in the wall of the bladder and ureter is connected with a similar network in the renal hilus and also a network in the pelvic organs. With such a distribution of lymphatics it is easy to understand how the infection can be an ascending one.

**Macroscopic appearance.** Macroscopically, both kidneys are enlarged (Fig. 18.10). The capsule is easily removed except, perhaps, in spots. The kidney surface shows grayish-white foci resembling those in focal interstitial nephritis. It can be differentiated upon incision. Upon incision of the kidney the most striking lesions appear at the tips of the papillae which project into the minor calyces. It can be seen that the process is extending from the tips of the papillae up into the medulla. The renal calyces are dilated with slimy exudate containing numerous small, irregular concretions (Fig. 18.11). The wall is eroded, dirty gray in appearance, often bleeding. The papillae have either disappeared, leaving ulcer-like depressions in the pyramids, or are present but necrotic, and when incised from the apex toward the capsule show gray radiating streaks. A distinctly red zone is at the border of the necrotic tissue. Both the minor and major calyces are distended with slimy, often blood-tinged, exudate. The pelvis is absent in the bovine kidney, so it is incorrect to say that the animal has a pyelitis, but usage has firmly established this name. The lesions in the ureters are similar. Occlusion of the ureters may result in extreme stasis of urine in the pelvis, which in turn produces pressure atrophy of the renal tissue. The lobes may become pus sacs (pyonephrosis).

**Microscopic appearance.** Microscopically, there is leukocytic infiltration of the renal corpuscles and periglomerular tissue. Usually, numerous bacteria are seen here. Cellular casts in the tubules become more numerous as the pelvis and major and minor calyces (in cows) are approached. Necrosis of the tubular wall may result. In the papillae the inflammatory process is similar, and in addition, there is marked intertubular inflammatory edema with large collections of bacteria. At the apex of the papillae there is complete necrosis. The necrotic areas are bounded toward the cortex by a hyperemic zone. Later, along this zone appears granulation tissue. The necrotic portion of the papillae may slough off, leaving scar tissue.

The urine from a kidney showing this infection contains much stringy, viscid, dirty grayish exudate in which are often microconcretions. There is also hematuria. Smears made from the pus stained with the ordinary dyes reveal the diphtheroids.

### Tumors

With a few exceptions, renal tumors of domestic animals are not very common. Even those that are encountered most frequently do not occur often. Sarcomas, except lymphosarcomas, are very rare.

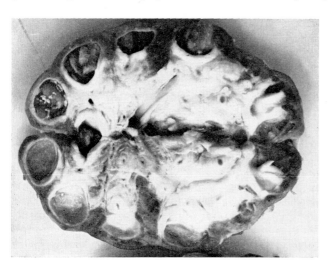

Fig. 18.11 — Lesions of infectious pyelonephritis in the kidney. Eroded papillae result in enlarged calyces. Calyces contain slimy blood-tinged exudate and calculi. (Department of Veterinary Pathology, Michigan State University.)

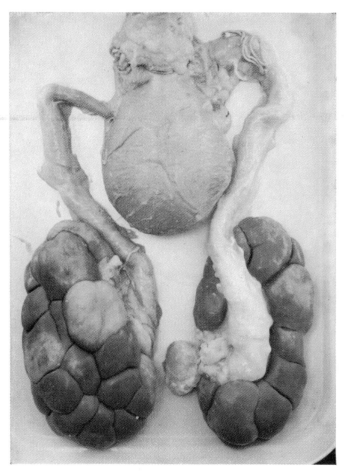

Fig. 18.10 — Specific infectious pyelonephritis and ureteritis in a 7-year-old Angus cow. (Department of Veterinary Pathology, Michigan State University.)

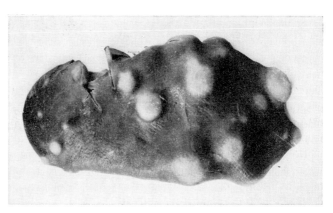

Fig. 18.12 — Lymphosarcoma of a kidney of a 7-month-old hog. Similar tumors appeared in the other kidney, liver, lungs, parietal pleura, and left prepectoral region. (Feldman, Jour. A.V.M.A.)

Lymphosarcomas (Fig. 18.12), however, attract attention in pigs and cats. In cats they appear to be a manifestation of a visceral lymphosarcoma. Epithelial tumors, adenomas, and adenocarcinomas are seen occasionally in all species.

Of special interest is the **embryonal nephroma** (nephroblastoma) which is a mixed-cell tumor arising from the tissues in and near the nephrogenic ridge of the embryo (Fig. 18.13). It is the most frequent renal tumor of swine in the United States, but it has been reported in practically every species of domestic animals, including chickens. The embryonal nephroma is located either within the renal capsule at one of the poles of the kidneys or nearby anteriorly or posteriorly. If it is located within the capsule, it consists of a single or a few grayish-white nodules projecting from the surface of the organ. An extremely large nephroma consists of a grayish-white lobulated mass that dis-

places most of the organ or may project from it (Fig. 18.13). The tumor is practically always well encapsulated, which probably accounts for the rareness of metastasis. In 125 cases studied in Colorado, metastasis occurred in only 9.

Histologically, the nephroma is a heterogeneous mixture of tissue elements among which connective tissue and epithelium predominate. From the well-developed capsule of connective tissue, strands of this tissue permeate the parenchyma of the tumor, subdividing it into masses of various sizes and shapes. The parenchyma in some areas has the appearance of a fibrosarcoma, in others of an adenoma. The cells of the sarcomatous areas are round, ovoid, or spindle. The cells of the adenomatous portions seem to be attempting to form alveoli and irregular, branching blind tubules, and occasionally renal corpuscle-like bodies. The cells forming alveoli and tubules are cuboidal or columnar. Those

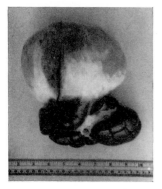
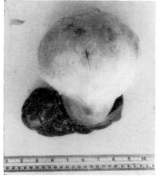

Fig. 18.13 — Embryonal adenomyosarcoma (nephroma) of the kidney of an 18-month-old heifer. (Department of Veterinary Pathology, Michigan State University.)

forming renal corpuscle-like bodies are flat or cuboidal. To complicate the pattern of the tumor, sinuses and crypts filled with blood or hyaline-like material may be mixed with the other elements. Occasionally, smooth and striated muscle and, very rarely, cartilage and bone may be present also. Some of the epithelial cells usually are in a state of mitosis.

**Lymphosarcomas** of the kidney are either focal or diffuse. Focal lesions on the surface of the organ consist of grayish-white nodules, variable in size, which project above the surface of the kidney. When the organ is incised, they appear distributed throughout the renal substance. Their cut surface is gray, smooth, and rather shiny. In the diffuse form the kidney has a uniform grayish discoloration.

In both the focal and diffuse forms the intertubular tissue is infiltrated with rather large, somewhat embryonic lymphocytes. In the focal form they collect in such large numbers around the tubules that they completely displace the renal tissue (Fig. 18.14). In the diffuse form they cause pressure atrophy of the tubules and glomeruli. Eventually both the tubules and glomeruli may disappear. Hemorrhages are often prominent (Fig. 15.8).

## RENAL PELVIS AND URETERS
### Dilatation of the Pelvis

Dilatation of the pelvis may be caused by concretions (Fig. 12.2), tumors, parasites, and urine (hydronephrosis). Dilatation due to the first three is not very common. An increasing number of reports of the presence of specimens of the giant kidney worm (*Dioctophyma renale*) in the pelvis of dogs are appearing in the literature. Most of the worms, however, escape from the pelvis and are found free in the abdominal cavity or in the perirenal tissue. Dilatation of the pelvis with urine (hydronephrosis) due to this worm is of frequent occurrence.

Dilatation of the pelvis may be congenital or acquired. Congenitally, it is due to atresia of the ureter. This is rather frequent in pigs, less so in calves. Acquired hydronephrosis is caused by concretions in the ureters, tumors of the bladder, and hypertrophy of the prostate (dogs). Outside of the urinary tract the cause may be abdominal tumors or a pregnant uterus compressing the ureters. In pigs the conformation of the bladder predisposes it to hydronephrosis. The predisposing factors are its large size, long neck, and the fact that the ureters enter the bladder posteriorly in the

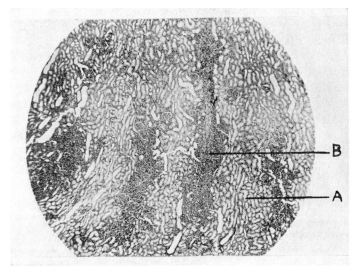

Fig. 18.14 — Kidney of a pig with lymphosarcoma.
A, renal tubules undergoing degenerative changes;
B, fields of infiltrating neoplastic cells.
× 13. (Biester and McNutt, Jour. A.V.M.A.)

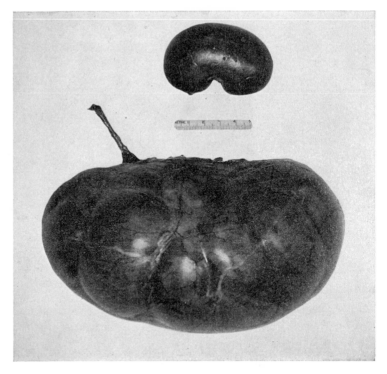

Fig. 18.15 — The hydronephrotic and the normal kidney of an 18-kg. dog. The hydronephrotic kidney weighed 1,200 gm. and contained 1,100 cc. of turbid, yellow-brown fluid. (Weight of normal organ, 53 gm.) Cause of hydronephrosis was apparently atresia of ureter. (Carl Olson, Jr.)

region of its neck. As a consequence, when the bladder is filled, it hangs down into the abdominal cavity. The long neck is then pressed against the acetabular branch of the pubis, and urination is interfered with.

Macroscopically, the papillae of the medulla undergo atrophy and finally disappear. Later, even the cortex may atrophy, so that all that remains is the connective tissue which separates the lobules, and the blood vessels that course through the interlobular connective tissues (Figs. 18.15 and 18.16). The result is a large loculated sac filled with urine or serous fluid. At times the cysts are separated by remnants of renal tissue.

In the microscopic picture two changes predominate — atrophy of the parenchyma and a chronic inflammatory reaction of the interstitial tissue. The former is characterized by atrophy of the renal tubular epithelium and collapse of the glomeruli. Later, the renal corpuscles become hyalinized. Simultaneously with these changes there occurs a fibrosis and lymphocytic infiltration of the interstitial tissue. There is hypertrophy of the remaining isolated normal parenchyma.

The results of hydronephrosis depend upon whether the alterations affect one or both kidneys. Frequently it is unilateral. When this is the case, the other kidney compensates. If the condition is bilateral, renal insufficiency and uremia occur. This may be postponed, however, by islands of functional tissue which may show compensatory hypertrophy. Occasionally, the large saclike kidney may rupture. Death then occurs as a result of peritonitis and uremia.

### Circulatory Disturbances

The most important circulatory disturbances are pelvic hemorrhages. They occur in various septicemic diseases but are of especial diagnostic value in acute hog cholera. Both petechial and diffuse hemorrhages appear.

### Pyelitis and Ureteritis

The mode of origin of these conditions may be hematogenic (descending) or

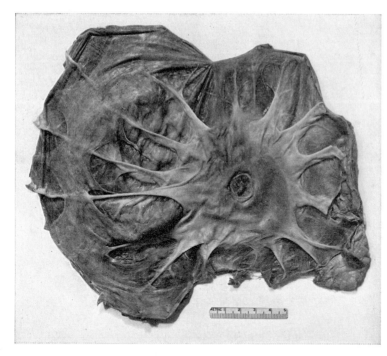

Fig. 18.16 — Interior of the hydronephrotic kidney shown in previous illustration. Wall of the hydronephrotic sac consisted of greatly atrophied k i d n e y parenchyma and connective tissue. (Carl Olson, Jr.)

urinogenic (ascending). The most important form is that produced by *Corynebacterium renale* in cattle. Catarrhal pyelitis may accompany chronic interstitial nephritis in dogs. In old male dogs prostate enlargement may predispose to pyelitis and ureteritis. In horses and dogs pyelitis usually occurs with pelvic calculi.

## URINARY BLADDER

**Changes of position.** Most important of the displacements is inversion associated with prolapse through the urethra into the vulva. Usually this happens only in pregnant animals or following parturition. It is seen mostly in cows but sometimes in sows and mares. The results depend upon the duration of the condition because circulatory disturbances arise at once. If the passive hyperemia persists, necrosis of the prolapsed bladder occurs. In dogs, straining due to enlarged prostate and to constipation may lead to perineal hernia. The displaced bladder becomes dilated and inflamed, and uremia usually causes death.

**Concretions.** Calculi are most frequent in horses, cattle, and sheep. They are less frequent in dogs (Figs. 18.17 and 18.18), and occur only occasionally in hogs. In ruminants, calculi are believed to be due to potassium salts in wheat bran, white corn, cane hay, beet pulp, and beet-sugar molasses. In small amounts these salts are mild diuretics, but their ingestion over long periods is reported to cause nephritis and cystitis resulting in calculi formation. Experiments to prove this have not been entirely conclusive. In Alberta and Montana, where there is a high incidence of urolithiasis in range calves in winter months, the concretions form in both sexes but are more serious in the male.

In the southern Great Plains, urinary calculi are associated with the fattening of steers on grain sorghums. Urolithiasis can be reduced considerably by feeding threshed sorghum (milo) rather than the heads. This is especially true if the milo is supplemented with phosphorus (bone meal). When corn is used as a source of carbohydrate, the lithiasis is further reduced or prevented. The reason for this is not known.

In lamb-feeding sections of the United

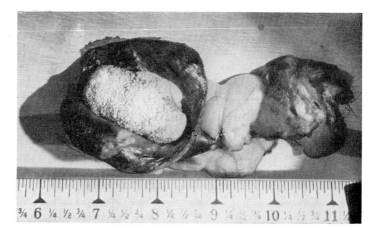

Fig. 18.17 — Urolith in the bladder of a dog. (Smith, Jour. A.V.M.A.)

States and Canada, urinary calculi occur in a rather high percentage of the wethers in certain feed lots. Wethers with calculi are inclined not to eat, often stand with arched backs, and attempt to urinate frequently but only dribble urine or pass no urine at all. Death usually does not occur until the bladder or ureters rupture. The escaped urine then distends the abdomen and gravitates into the tissues, eventually collecting in the subcutis along the sheath and ventral surface of the belly. Sheep feeders call this stage of the condition water belly. Since the calculi may lodge in the sigmoid flexure of the urethra, perforation of it may occur and the escaping urine may likewise seep out into the surrounding tissues. If the calculi lodge in the processus urethrae, perforation of it may give temporary relief.

Uroliths in sheep consist of a variety of minerals (calcium and aluminum phosphates, calcium carbonate, and aluminum silicate with urates).

**Changes of the lumen.** Dilatation of the bladder may be due to inflammation of the lumbar portion of the cord (canine distemper), urethral calculi or strictures, enlarged prostate, and cystitis.

**Disturbance in continuity.** Rupture may occur in a normal or already diseased bladder. It may be the result of occlusion of the urethra by calculi, or be due to trauma or inflammation.

**Circulatory disturbances.** Hemorrhages occur under the same conditions as those in the pelvis. Along with hemorrhage in other parts of the body and a suitable history, they are considered important among the lesions of hog cholera.

In northwestern United States and in British Columbia an idiopathic condition among cattle called **endemic hematuria** has for its chief lesions hemorrhages and mild inflammation of the bladder mucosa. In the later stages of the disease in the hemorrhagic areas, vascular channels are formed which eventually become hemangiomas. Two types of these blood-vascular tumors are described: First, one in which the vascular channels are thin-walled and

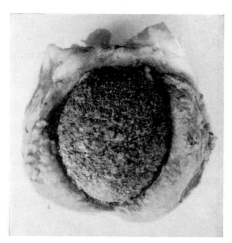

Fig. 18.18 — Urolith about 5 cm. in diameter in the chronically inflamed bladder of an 11-year-old dog. (Department of Veterinary Pathology, Michigan State University.)

supported by connective tissue stroma. This one has the appearance of a benign hemangioma. Second, one in which the endothelial cells of the newly formed, thin-walled vascular channels undergo extensive proliferation. As a result, the endothelial lining of the channels becomes several layers thick. Finally, these cells form cords or whorl-like masses which invade the surrounding stroma. The cords may extend through the mucosa into the muscularis and give the appearance of a hemangiosarcoma.

## Cystitis

This is of frequent occurrence. A common cause is *Escherichia coli* in the presence of stagnated urine. Streptococci are another frequent cause. Corynebacteria seem to be of increasing importance in cows and sows. The infection of the bladder may be ascending or descending. The ascending type occurs in cows with suppurative endometritis and vaginitis. Sometimes its origin may be the result of catheterization. Occasionally, in calves and foals the infection enters by way of the urachus. The descending type of the infection appears in animals which have suppurative nephritis and pyelonephritis.

### ACUTE CYSTITIS

In the **catarrhal** form of acute cystitis the mucosa is red and swollen and the urine cloudy. Microscopically, there is desquamation of the epithelium, subepithelial hyperemia, and pronounced leukocytic infiltration. There are few or no hemorrhages. If hemorrhage is marked, the designation is changed to **hemorrhagic cystitis.** In **purulent cystitis** there is a heavy infiltration of the submucosa, and even the muscularis, with leukocytes. The latter wander through the epithelium into the lumen. The **fibrinous** and **fibrinonecrotic** forms occur in all animals but particularly in cats, cattle, and swine. The superficial form is fibrinous, the deep form fibrinone-

crotic. In the former the membrane is more easily removed than in the latter.

### CHRONIC CYSTITIS

The **catarrhal** form of chronic cystitis is usually associated with calculi. Macroscopically, the mucosa is thickened, normally colored or lighter than normal (gray), occasionally red. Microscopically, there are desquamation of the epithelium, subepithelial lymphocytic infiltration, connective tissue hyperplasia, and muscle hypertrophy. A **polypoid** form is seen occasionally in cattle, and a **follicular** form is said to be frequent in dogs. In the latter the entire mucosa shows miliary, gray nodules which microscopically are like lymph nodes. The etiology is unknown.

## URETHRA

**Foreign bodies.** Those encountered mostly are calculi and broken catheters. Urethral calculi are reported to occur most frequently in steers that were castrated when very young. In Montana it has been determined by measurement of the diameter of the lumen of the urethra that there are marked average minimal differences in the sizes of the lumen in calves castrated at 1 month, 3 months, and in the uncastrated bull calves when these animals reach 10 months of age. The measurements were taken in February, which is the time of the year when the incidence of urinary lithiasis is usually at its peak in Montana. The study indicated that a bull calf at 10 months of age should be able to pass a stone 44 per cent greater in diameter than a calf of the same age castrated at 1 month, and a calf castrated at 3 months should pass a stone 13 per cent greater than a calf castrated at 1 month. The calculi obstruct the urethra at the sigmoid flexure. Calculi are encountered quite generally in bucks and wethers in the lamb-feeding sections of the United States. The calculi lodge in the sigmoid flexure and in the processus urethrae of the penis. The results depend upon the duration of lodgement. There may be dilatation, paralysis and rupture of the bladder, and a severe urethritis with necrosis and gangrene.

**Changes in the lumen.** Stenosis of the urethra is caused by external pressure (enlarged prostate in dogs, abscesses, tumors) or by strictures (fibrosis resulting from calculi and faulty catheterization). Strictures in male dogs may arise from exostosis of the os penis.

**Inflammation (urethritis).** This is very common in animals. It is most commonly associated with the presence of urinary calculi. Urethritis is observed in ascending and descending suppurative infections of the urinary tract. It is a very common lesion of *Corynebacterium renale* infections in cows.

## REFERENCES

Andersson, A.: 1936. On amyloidosis of the kidneys in cattle. Skand. Vet., 241.

Bell, E.: 1943. Hyperplasia of the pulmonary alveolar epithelium in disease. Amer. Jour. Path., 19:901.

Brodey, R. S.: 1955. Canine urolithiasis: A survey and discussion of fifty-two clinical cases. Jour. A.V.M.A., 126:1.

Ehrenford, F. A., and Snodgrass, T. B.: 1955. Incidence of canine dioctophymiasis (giant kidney worm infection) with a summary of cases in North America. Jour. A.V.M.A., 126:415 and 127:246.

Hemsley, L. A.: 1956. *Leptospira canicola* and chronic nephritis in cats. Vet. Rec., 68:300.

Madsen, L. L., Earle, I. P., Heemstra, L. C., and Miller, C. O.: 1944. Acute uremia associated with "uric acid infarcts" in the kidneys of baby pigs. Amer. Jour. Vet. Res., 5:262.

Monlux, A. W.: 1953. The histopathology of nephritis of the dog. I. Introduction. II. Inflammatory interstitial diseases. III. Inflammatory vascular diseases of the kidney. Amer. Jour. Vet. Res., 14:425.

Newsom, I. E., Tobiska, J. W., and Osland, H. B.: 1943. The effect of rations on the production of urinary calculi in sheep. Colo. Agr. Exper. Sta., Tech. Bul. 31.

Platt, H.: 1951. Chronic canine nephritis. III. The skeletal system in "Rubber Jaw." Jour. Comp. Path. and Therap., 61:197.

Plummer, P. J. G.: 1944. Histopathology of enzootic bovine haematuria. Canad. Jour. Comp. Med. and Vet. Sci., 8:153.

# CHAPTER 19

# Genital System

## Part I: Female

### FUNCTIONAL DISTURBANCES

Diseases of the female generative organs directly interfere with ovulation, fertilization of the egg, and the development of the fetus. Some of these diseases lead to premature expulsion of a living or dead fetus, others to temporary or permanent sterility.

The functions of the female reproductive organs can also be impaired indirectly by abnormal conformation of the pelvic girdle, by painful diseases of the abdominal muscles at the time of parturition, and by diseases of the spinal cord. When such conditions exist, there is either a mechanical hindrance to the normal function or a decrease in nervous irritability of the organs which also interferes with their normal activities.

Diseases of the ovaries usually disturb the whole sex life of the animal. Even with the involvement of only one gland this may appear. Such conditions as cystic ovaries, ovaritis, ovarian tuberculosis, and neoplasms are frequently accompanied by symptoms of stimulated sexual desire (nymphomania). It is believed that this is partly due to the continuous formation of estrin.

Formerly it was believed that in inflammation of the vagina, the cervix, and the uterus the exudate had a deleterious effect on the spermatozoa so that they could not remain viable long. In the cow at least, if inflammation of these parts prevents conception, it is not because the pathologic process alters the pH of the vaginal fluid. Recent experiments indicate that retained placentae and metritis do not materially affect the constancy of the pH values of the fluid. The normal pH value for the cow is approximately 7, with the vast majority of the variations falling between 6.5 and 7.5.

### OVARY

**Disturbances of circulation. Hemorrhages.** Slight hemorrhage occurs at the time of ovulation. Exceptionally, it can be extensive, especially in the hen. Mechanically produced hemorrhage may result from expressing cysts or corpora lutea in the treatment of sterility in cattle. Follicular hemorrhage occurs in pullorum infection of hens.

**Ovaritis or oophoritis** is rare in animals. There are no histological reports of exudative oophoritis. There are a few reports of a chronic indurative process. Abscesses of the ovaries are occasionally reported, usually in connection with metritis. They are probably the result of an ascending infection.

**Cysts** occur in all animals, but especially in cows, sows, and mares. Cysts originate principally from two sources: follicles that have not ruptured (follicular cysts) and persistent corpora lutea (lutein cysts).

In a study of cystic ovaries in 352 dairy

cows in New York the location of the cysts were: in left ovary 23 per cent, right ovary 33.2 per cent, and both ovaries 43.8 per cent. More than 73 per cent of these cows were nymphomaniacs, and over 26 per cent failed to have estrum.

**Follicular cysts** are the most frequent form. Macroscopically, they are single or multiple, involving one or both ovaries. In size, they are minute up to that of a fist. Their wall is thin, usually tense. The cysts contain a clear, serous fluid of low albumin content. Microscopically, the ovum is absent. The membrana granulosa has shrunk and is represented by a layer of flat cells which lines the inner wall of the cyst (pressure atrophy). At times it disappears entirely.

There is evidence that cystic degeneration of the ovaries of dairy cows is related to a structural and functional disturbance of the pituitary, and that this in turn is associated with recent pregnancy and high milk production. In these animals, follicles develop but do not rupture, and as a consequence, corpora lutea do not form. Some of these cows remain in constant heat (nymphomania); others do not.

In many cases of cystic ovarian degeneration the cervix and uterus become enlarged due to glandular hyperplasia of the mucosa. The hyperplastic glands secrete an excessive amount of mucus and are transformed into retention cysts. Mucus accumulates in the uterus along with cell debris, and simulates pus. Upon palpation the enlarged flabby uterus may be mistaken for one affected with endometritis.

The pituitary becomes enlarged, and cytologic changes, which are reported to be pathognomonic, occur in the anterior lobe. Chief among these cytologic changes is the presence of abnormal forms of the basophilic cells. These cells develop large nuclei with large nucleoli, their chromatin pattern becomes irregular, and their cytoplasm becomes homogeneous, hyalin-like, and acidophilic (pink with eosin).

It is suggested that these abnormal cells may produce large amounts of the follicle-stimulating hormone. Why these cells become altered is not known, but the circumstantial evidence is that severe functional strain on them following pregnancy and during the height of lactation may be an etiologic factor. Heredity may play a part also. Functionally these cells, to some extent at least, seem to have lost their ability to cause ovulation and luteinization.

**Lutein cysts** are rare and of little significance except in purebred, high-producing dairy cows. Both the follicular and lutein cysts in cattle are usually associated with diseases of the uterus, especially endometritis. Endometritis in turn may be a manifestation or sequela of brucellosis. The nature of this association of uterine diseases with ovarian cysts has not been determined. The cysts may result in pressure atrophy of the ovary, prevention of ovulation, and nymphomania.

**Tumors.** Epithelial tumors are of most significance. **Adenoma** and **carcinoma** have been reported. Both may be solid (Fig. 19.1) or cystic. **Cystic teratomas** and **dermoid cysts** also occur (see Chapter 13).

Fig. 19.1 — Tumor derived from the cells of the stratum granulosum of the Graafian follicle of a 2-year-old heifer. It would be classed as an adenoma. (Department of Veterinary Pathology, Michigan State University.)

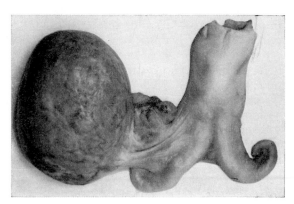

## FALLOPIAN TUBE

**Salpingitis** is seldom recognized macroscopically, but it may be of more frequent occurrence than is generally thought. In cows it appears to be almost exclusively an ascending infection in connection with endometritis. In ducks it is due to flukes. In hens a descending infection occurs in connection with *Salmonella pullorum* infection of the ovaries. The degree of pathological alteration varies from a very slight to a very pronounced inflammatory reaction. It may terminate in stenosis of the tube. If a collection of serous exudate results, the condition is designated hydrosalpinx, and if pus accumulates, pyosalpinx. The extreme rarity of salpingitis in mares may be explained on the basis of the anatomical structure of the union of the tube and the uterine horn.

In Wisconsin a study of repeat breeder cows showed that lesions of the oviduct interfere with conception. The lesions most often encountered were hydrosalpinx, chronic interstitial salpingitis, and pyosalpinx, in the order named.

Histologically, sections of hydrosalpinx cases have a very distinctive appearance. The distended lumen of the tube looks like a multilocular cyst, which indeed it is. Cystic cavities are separated by branching atrophic mucosal folds. The folds are lined by squamous or low cuboidal epithelium devoid of cilia. The cysts contain pale pink granular material and some cell debris.

The microscopic appearance of chronic interstitial salpingitis is about as one would imagine. There is extensive cellular infiltration of all layers of the tube. The cells are chiefly lymphocytes and plasma cells.

In pyosalpinx the entire wall of the tube is infiltrated with leukocytes, with neutrophils particularly prominent but with lymphocytes and plasma cells also present. The leukocytic infiltration is heaviest in the lamina propria. Cytoplasmic projections of the epithelial cells may be present and resemble those occurring in the post-estral phase of the normal virgin heifer. The lumen is filled with purulent exudate.

## UTERUS

**Displacements.** The most important displacements of the uterus are inversion alone or with prolapse and torsion. The causes of the first two are incomplete involution after parturition, relaxation of the broad ligament, and lying with the hind quarters inclined downward. The predisposing cause of torsion is a relaxed broad ligament. The fundamental pathology is like that of similar conditions in the intestine.

A less frequently occurring uterine displacement in bitches is herniation either into the thoracic cavity through the diaphragm or through the inguinal canal (metrocele). Metrocele is reported to occur more frequently in older bitches. Diaphragmatic hernia of the uterus may result from severe abdominal contusion. In either case a fetus may be contained in the herniated portion of the uterus.

An extensive study of vaginal and uterine prolapse has been made in Hereford cows, a breed which is said to be especially susceptible to this uterine displacement. The condition occurs only while the cervix is relaxed. This is during a period beginning at parturition and extending to about 72 hours post partum. This displacement is extremely rare in dry cows. Vaginal prolapse occurs more than three times as frequently as uterine prolapse.

**Foreign substances.** Among these may be pieces of obstetrical equipment, antiseptic solutions, dead fetuses, remains of fetal membranes, exudate, blood, and gas.

**Disturbance in continuity.** Perforations and ruptures of the uterus may be traumatic (common) or spontaneous (rare). Their pathology is similar to that of other perforations and ruptures. They usually result in fatal peritonitis. Occasionally, the uterus contracts, and healing occurs by scar formation. Of particular interest are spontaneous uterine ruptures in cows which occur during labor. The uterine rupture is accompanied by rupture of the fetal membranes. The calf lies in the fetal fluid in the peritoneal cavity. The cord and placental attachments may remain intact so that the calf may be delivered alive by caesarian section.

**Local disturbances of metabolism. Melanosis** occurs frequently in the uterine mucosa and oviducts of ewes. The deposits are confined almost entirely to the cotyledonary areas in the uterus. They may extend into the tubes or into the cervix. The condition has no physiological or pathological significance. It was formerly thought to be a hematogenous pigmentation and to have a relationship to the reproductive cycle, but it occurs in virgin ewes as well as in those that have borne lambs.

**Disturbances of circulation. Hemorrhage** of the uterus is physiologic in the course of the estrual cycle. It is pathologic in some acute septicemic diseases (petechiae) and in dystocia where there is trauma of the uterus. **Thrombosis** is seen in the uterine veins in the course of septic metritis. The thrombosis may extend to the posterior vena cava. Septic emboli may originate and produce lesions in remote organs (lungs, spleen, kidneys).

## Metritis

Metritis occurs rather frequently in all species of animals. It most often follows parturition. The causes are bacteria (*Corynebacterium pyogenes*, streptococci, staphylococci, *Escherichia coli*, *Spherophorus necrophorus*, *Brucella abortus*), chemical agents (irritating antiseptics), thermic influences (hot douches), and mechanical injury (obstetrical instruments, projecting fetal bones as a result of embryotomy). For mares, *Klebsiella genitalium*, *Streptococcus zooepidemicus*, and *Salmonella abortivoequina* should be included. The avenue of infection is usually by way of the vagina but is hematogenic in Brucella infection.

## ACUTE CATARRHAL ENDOMETRITIS

This must not be confused with the condition of the uterus at estrum and during involution after parturition. Macroscopically, the uterus externally shows no apparent alterations. Upon being opened, it presents a cloudy, dark or light chocolate-colored, viscid fluid (Fig. 19.2). The mucosa is swollen and hyperemic. The surface is rough. There are large and small

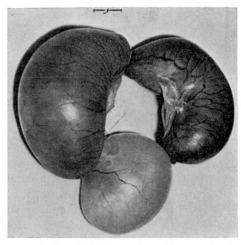

Fig. 19.2 — Hydrometra and cystic right ovary of a cat. Both horns of the uterus were distended with thin, watery mucous exudate. (Iowa State University Veterinarian.)

necrotic shreds lying loose in the uterine lumen or attached to the mucosa. If the shreds are removed from the mucosa, a defect occurs. The alterations are confined to the mucosa and lumen. Microscopically, the capillaries and arterioles are distended with blood. There is hemorrhage with extensive leukocytic infiltration in the mucosa. Frequently, superficial necrosis of the epithelium is present. The uterine glands may be filled with leukocytes and also show a periglandular leukocytic infiltration. Thrombosis of the small vessels of the mucosa is frequent.

## CHRONIC CATARRHAL ENDOMETRITIS

This is characterized by an increase in the thickness of the endometrium due to

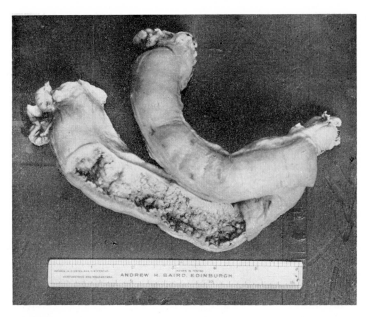

Fig. 19.3 — Chronic diffuse cystic endometritis in a dog. Portion of uterine wall has been removed to show mucosa. (Kennedy and Baird, Jour. A.V.M.A.)

a proliferation of fibroblasts and infiltration with plasma cells. The thickening may not occur uniformly on account of the gland ducts, which are more or less fixed. Therefore, polypoid thickenings occur (**chronic polypoid endometritis**). As time goes on, superficial connective tissue proliferation may cause closure of the gland ducts. The secretion accumulates in the glands, resulting in cysts (**chronic cystic endometritis**) (Figs. 19.3 and 19.4). This is seen especially in the dog. In other cases, neither polyps nor cysts develop, but instead the mucosa is uniformly thickened, later contracts, the glands atrophy, the mucosa becomes a thin, fibrous membrane (**chronic atrophic endometritis**).

### ACUTE PURULENT METRITIS

The disease is the result of a severe puerperal infection with pyogenic bacteria. Since this infection follows parturition, the involutionary process has not been completed. This may cause some difficulty in determining just which tissue changes are physiologic and which are pathologic. Externally, the serosa shows an inflammatory process. It is dull and covered with a fibrinous exudate. There is an edematous infiltration of the serosa. The uterine wall is easily torn. The musculature appears thickened, is friable, and dirty gray in color. In the uterus there is a large quantity of turbid, putrid exudate. The mucosa is thickened, and its surface is dull, rough, and covered with fine shreds. Microscopically, there is extreme leukocytic infiltration of the whole uterine wall and extensive inflammatory thrombosis of the uterine vessels. Focal necrosis of the mucosa and degeneration of the muscle fibers are marked. Edema and leukocytic infiltration of the subserosa are prominent. The condition results in thrombosis of the veins in the broad ligament. This gives rise to septic emboli which lodge in distant organs (septicemia and pyemia).

**Brucellosis** (Bang's disease, or infectious abortion of cattle) is a chronic infectious disease caused by *Brucella abortus* and characterized by inflammatory lesions of the uterine mucosa, of the fetal membranes, the fetus, and frequently resulting in premature expulsion of the fetus, and frequently terminating in chronic metritis leading to sterility. Since abortion is only one manifestation of Brucella infection in cattle, and even then not a constant one, the name "infectious abortion" is inadequate for this disease. In considering large numbers of infected cows, it has been determined that only about 65 per cent abort, and of these about 65 per cent abort only once and about 23 per cent twice. A much smaller percentage abort more than twice. Signs of the disease which may be just as evident are retained fetal membranes, decreased milk production, weak calves, calf pneumonia, and calf diarrhea. It is quite probable that 40 to 50 per cent of the infected cows eventually become disqualified as breeders due to the sequelae of the disease.

The portals of entry of the infection are the digestive tract, the conjunctiva, and the skin. Even unbroken skin, experimentally at least, has been shown to be an avenue of entrance. Formerly, the vagina was considered an important invasion point. There is evidence that this avenue of entrance of *Brucella abortus* may be of importance. Verified cases have been reported in which the infection was transmitted by artificial insemination when the semen of infected bulls was used.

When the bacteria enter the mucosa of the digestive tract, they are carried first to the mesenteric lymph nodes, where they may multiply or be completely destroyed. If they survive, they are probably carried by the thoracic duct to the blood stream. In the blood stream, it is now believed, a bacteremia develops which terminates in 3 to 4 weeks. During this bacteremia there are no clinical manifestations of the disease. In cows, at the termination of the bacteremia, the organism remains localized in the pregnant uterus in the fetal and maternal placentae, in the mammary gland and lymph nodes of the mammary gland, and perhaps also in the lymph nodes of the uterus. In bulls the localization is principally in the genital organs. In both cows and bulls it occasionally localizes in the joints and tendon sheaths. In a few instances the infection has been reported localized in the spleen and in the mediastinal lymph nodes of cows, and in the

Fig. 19.4 — Chronic diffuse cystic endometritis in a dog. **Right:** Showing portion of a large cyst occupying half of picture and containing blood, and several cysts of smaller size. ×60. **Left:** Cysts containing cell debris and mucoid material. Cyst walls are plicated, and there is interstitial lymphocytic infiltration. ×60. (Kennedy and Baird, Jour. A.V.M.A.)

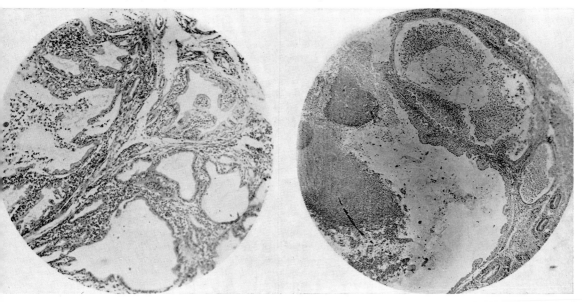

mesenteric lymph nodes of calves which have been fed infected milk.

Nonpregnant uteri are not suitable for the growth of *Brucella abortus*, but the organism usually does not appear in the uterus until after 4½ months of pregnancy. If, however, the organism enters the mucous membrane of the pregnant uterus by way of the lymph and blood circulation, it multiplies principally in the covering epithelium of the chorionic tufts, and spreads between the chorion and the uterine mucous membrane (intercotyledonary spaces). As a result, the chorionic tufts undergo degeneration, autolysis, and necrosis. On their surface a fibrino-purulent exudate forms and gradually loosens the fetal placenta from the maternal placenta. At the same time, the organisms penetrate into the connective tissue layer between the chorion and the allantois, the navel cord and the body of the fetus (by the blood circulation or by swallowing amniotic fluid). In all these places the organisms produce a serous infiltration. In the digestive tract of the fetus a more pronounced inflammatory process may be induced. Loosening of the connection between the fetal and maternal placentae results in a gradual separation of the fetal membranes and finally, in most cases, expulsion of the fetus and its coverings. Sometimes the fetus dies, but the membranes remain attached, in which case a mummified fetus results. *Brucella abortus* usually disappears from the uterus within 6 to 8 weeks. It has been reported that one cow harbored the organism in the uterus for 7 months after abortion.

When the organism can no longer be found in the uterine exudate, it may be found in the **udder** and **supramammary lymph nodes,** where it localized either prior or subsequently to abortion. The incidence of mammary gland infection is 30 to 50 per cent of the infected cows. The organism apparently produces a subacute or chronic focal inflammatory reaction here. If another conception occurs, the organism may again be conveyed to the developing fetal membranes, resulting in repetition of the above processes. Pregnancy in some cases terminates at full term in spite of the infection in the fetal membranes and udder. In some of these cases only retained fetal membranes or diarrhea or pneumonia in the newborn calf are evidences of infection. If the calf lives, it rapidly eliminates the infection unless fed infected milk, in which case it harbors the infection as long as the contaminated milk is fed. Agglutinins, however, may persist for as long as 5 months. The period of incubation is variable. Axel Thomsen says, "The younger the fetus, the longer is the period of incubation." He found that when he infected cows at the time of service, the average period of incubation was 225 days, but when he infected heifers seven months after service, the period was only 53 days.

In the uterus of the cow there is acute necrotic placentitis, or subacute or chronic placentitis (the predominance of one over the other probably depends upon the number and virulence of the organisms or the resistance of the tissues). There is often retention of the fetal membranes, which is probably due to inflammatory swelling of the villi (chorionic tufts) and the walls of the crypts (uterine cotyledons), and to an accompanying fibrosis (Fig. 19.5). Acute necrotic cotyledonitis and endometritis are of frequent occurrence. Normal fetal membranes are thin and translucent. As a result of Brucella infection they become diffusely thickened and leathery, or thickened only in small foci so that small elevations project above the surface. Normal maternal and fetal cotyledons are dull red in color. In brucellosis they become partially or entirely yellowish brown or brown in color and may show areas of caseous necrosis.

In calves there may be fetal pneumonia (focal bronchopneumonia) and enteritis, which, while probably not primary disease processes due to *Brucella abortus*, are frequently associated with this infection. Pneumonia due to *Brucella abortus* has been observed in newborn calves.

In the udder of cows there is evidence

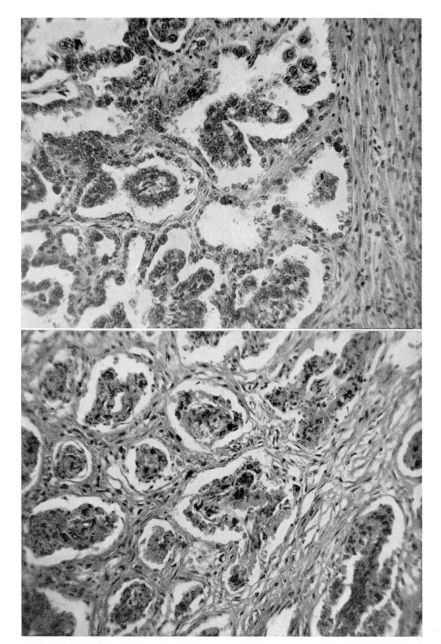

Fig. 19.5 — **Above:** Portion of a normal cotyledon of a cow at fifth month of pregnancy. **Below:** Portion of a cotyledon of a pregnant cow infected with **Brucella abortus.** The changes associated with the chronic placentitis contribute to the death of the fetus and retention of fetal membranes. (Department of Veterinary Pathology, Michigan State University.)

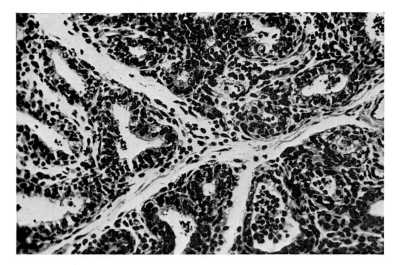

Fig. 19.6 — Chronic mastitis in a cow. Note interacinal connective tissue increase and lymphocytic infiltration, atrophy of the acini, absence of secretion, and relatively small amount of exudate. ×200. (Department of Veterinary Pathology, Iowa State University.)

that the Brucella produces a subacute or chronic focal mastitis which is characterized by focal infiltration of the interalveolar tissue with lymphocytes and neutrophils (Fig. 19.6). The tiny areas of leukocytic infiltration eventually become foci of fibrosis. The alveoli in these areas become atrophic. In other foci the alveoli are involved in a more acute inflammatory process characterized by the presence of a highly cellular exudate (mostly neutrophils) in their lumina, and by degeneration and necrosis of their epithelial cells (Fig. 19.7). As a result of these changes, the quality of the milk is changed because it contains inflammatory exudate. It is characterized by an increase in leukocytes,

chlorides, and alkalinity. The leukocytic content of the stripping milk is of more significance than of the foremilk.

In the bull, inflammatory disturbances in the testicles, epididymis, and seminal vesicles have been observed occasionally (Fig. 19.8). Arthritis occasionally occurs in both cows and bulls.

In **swine**, brucellosis is a chronic infection caused by *Brucella suis* and characterized by localization of the organism in various parts of the body, with the production of low grade inflammatory processes sometimes accompanied by suppuration. Clinically, porcine brucellosis may be characterized by abortion, emaciation, lameness, and a rather high rate of mortality.

Fig. 19.7 — Acute mastitis in a cow. Many of the acini are filled with inflammatory exudate instead of milk. ×100. (Department of Veterinary Pathology, Iowa State University.)

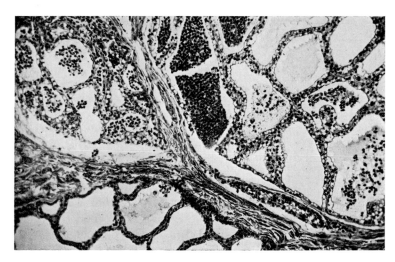

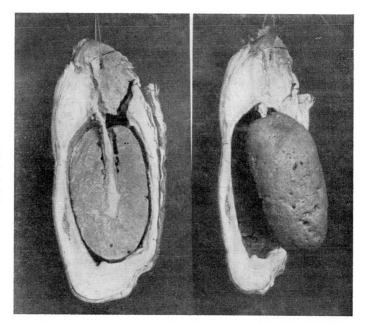

Fig. 19.8 — Chronic suppurative orchitis in a bull due to **Brucella abortus.** There is also chronic periorchitis, epididymitis, and funiculitis. The abscess cavity was between the testicle proper and the tunica albuginea and contained 1½ pints of pus. (Barnes and Brueckner, Jour. A.V.M.A.)

Experimentally, infection can be transmitted by way of the digestive tract, the conjunctiva, and the vagina. Transmission by the boar by way of the vagina is presumed to be of greatest importance. Abortions occur as early as the twenty-second to thirtieth day of gestation, but litters may be carried full-term even when the uterus is infected. At first, the organism probably causes a very insignificant bacteremia. Later, it localizes in various parts of the body where it produces small foci of chronic inflammation which often undergo suppuration. *Brucella suis* is strongly pyogenic in some locations.

The histological changes produced by *Brucella suis* are fairly constant, but the location of the lesions is not. The lesions have been reported in various organs of swine such as the uterus, testicle, epididymis, seminal vesicle, various bones, joints, bursae, lymph nodes, spleen, kidney, liver, and brain. See Figures 8.3, 11.27, 7.5, 19.9, 19.10, and 19.11 for illustrations of lesions.

In general, the lesions are those of a chronic inflammation with considerable induration. In practically all organs that become infected there is an increase in the interstitial tissue together with a leukocy-tic infiltration of this tissue. In glandular organs the tubules may degenerate, or atrophy, or become dilated. The dilatation may be the result of retained secretions so that the glands are cystic. Other glands may be distended with desquamated epithelial cells and leukocytes. Some of these glands become converted into abscesses. These changes are very prominent in the endometrium. In the brain *Brucella suis* produces foci of necrosis which are variable in size. There is a sharp line of demarcation between these necrotic areas and the surrounding tissue. Around these foci of necrosis the parenchyma of the organ is replaced by a rather wide vascular zone of cellular infiltration. The infiltrating cells are a mixture of lymphocytes, neutrophils, eosinophils, macrophages, and fibroblasts. Most of the descriptions of lesions in the brain, as well as in other organs, emphasize the relatively large number of eosinophils in this zone and in the vessels at the periphery of the necrotic centers.

These lesions have some of the characteristics of the tubercles caused by *Mycobacterium tuberculosis*. The caseous centers may undergo some calcification, and just outside their border in the cellular

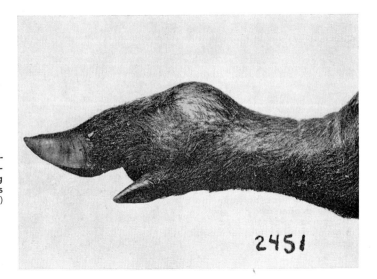

Fig. 19.9 — Suppurative arthritis of the metatarsal-phalangeal articulation of a pig due to **Brucella suis.** (James and Graham, Jour. A.V.M.A.)

zone there may be a few giant cells. Like tubercles these lesions may heal by granulation. Two characteristics make them different from tubercles: first, the presence of so many eosinophils in the cellular zone, and secondly, the tendency of the caseous centers to suppurate.

Retention of the fetal membranes following abortion due to *Brucella suis* is not common in sows. The uterine mucosa is usually markedly inflamed, and the organ contains a thin purulent exudate after a sow aborts.

**Bovine genital trichomoniasis.** This is thought to be primarily a venereal disease of cattle caused by *Trichomonas foetus.* The occurrence of *T. foetus* has been reported in virgin bulls and heifers. *T. suis* can also infect heifers and then be transmitted from heifer to heifer.

Most frequently the infection is transmitted to the cow by the bull during coitus, or vice versa. It may be transmitted by semen containing the protozoa in the case of artificial breeding. In the bull, the preputial cavity is the most common site of

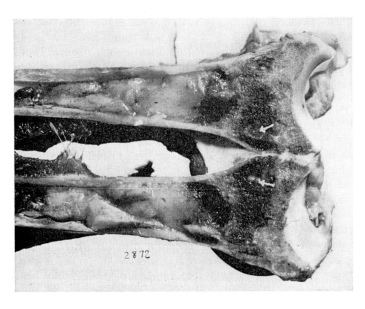

Fig. 19.10 — Suppurative osteomyelitis of the tibia of a pig due to **Brucella suis.** Arrows indicate abscesses containing creamy yellow pus. (James and Graham, Jour. A.V.M.A.)

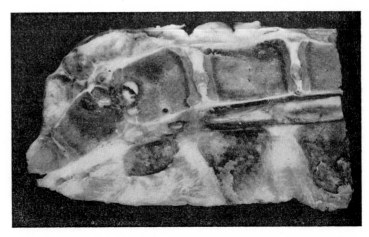

Fig. 19.11 — Spondylitis in a pig due to **Brucella suis.** The process involves the adjacent epiphyses of the bodies of the last lumbar and first sacral vertebrae. The ventral surfaces of the diseased vertebrae are underlaid by an excessive amount of new bone tissue, 1.5 cm. thick. (Feldman a n d O l s o n, A.V.M.A.)

infection with the highest number of organisms on the portion of the glans penis not including the galea. Some workers have reported organisms in the epididymis, ampullae of the ductus deferens, and seminal vesicles. Although trichomonads may not be demonstrated, the organisms may be regularly transmitted to breeding females. An untreated infected bull very rarely recovers from the disease.

Trichomonads may remain in the vagina or migrate through the cervix to the uterus. Abortions may take place any time during the gestation period, but early abortion (1 to 16 weeks after the last breeding) is the rule. Recovery may take place spontaneously.

Destruction of the placental attachments often results in abortion accompanied by the discharge of large quantities of pus. On the other hand, the fetal membranes may be retained and a chronic catarrhal or purulent endometritis (pyometra) may occur. Marked destruction of the uterine mucosa may render the animal hopelessly sterile. The fetus may be retained and undergo maceration with the accumulation of pus in the uterus.

Inflammatory swelling of the prepuce accompanied by a mucopurulent discharge may be observed in acutely infected bulls. Trichomonads may be demonstrated readily during the acute stage which frequently subsides within 10 to 14 days.

**Staphylococcosis.** In dairy cows which have been artificially inseminated, *Staphylococcus albus* occasionally causes acute purulent endometritis which results in abortion. A combination of factors appears to be associated with this infection — semen contaminated by the organism and deep penetration of the female genital organs by the inseminating instrument, usually to a point anterior to the internal orifice. The origin of the contamination may be the bull. In one instance, in a 7-month period 37½ per cent of the pregnancies resulting from the semen of a certain bull terminated in purulent endometritis with abortion. Abortion occurs late in pregnancy. There is necrosis of the cotyledons, and a copious grayish-tan exudate is present.

**Vibrionic abortion** is an enzootic infectious disease of ewes and cows caused by *Vibrio fetus.* Most outbreaks have been confined to ewes on certain farms in widely separated parts of the country. Since it is primarily a disease of sheep in the United States, the description of the disease given here will be mostly for that species. In ewes the infection appears and disappears suddenly. Usually it does not attack the same flock in successive years but may skip a few years and then reappear. The reason for this has not been explained.

Transmission of the vibrio in cows is chiefly by coitus and in ewes probably by the ingestion of contaminated food even though the organism may be present in semen. Experimentally, ewes can be infected easily per orum in the third, fourth, and fifth months of gestation. As many as 40 to 50 per cent of the lambs may be lost. In cows uterine vibriosis may be responsible for repeat breeding.

The principal symptom of this vibrionic infection is abortion, which occurs most often about 6 weeks prior to the normal lambing time. Because of this it is presumed that the period of incubation under natural conditions can be measured in weeks. Experimentally, the period of incubation is 13 to 113 days.

The pathogenesis of vibrionic abortion has not been fully determined. The vibrios are known to accumulate in the capillaries where the maternal and fetal placentae come in contact. As a result of their presence in the capillaries, the nutritive transfer between the mother and fetus is interfered with and the fetus dies. The death of the fetus in turn leads to its premature expulsion. A bloody, mucoid discharge from the vulva may precede the abortion.

Gross lesions of ovine vibriosis occur in the fetal membranes and placentae as well as in the endometrium and fetus. There are areas of edema in the fetal membranes. The endometrium is covered with dark brown fluid containing partly clotted blood. The placentae, which normally are firm and glistening in appearance, become dull and soft. They are swollen and have dark centers with dark streaks radiating to the periphery. Usually the fetus is dead and decomposed when abortion occurs. The stomach of the fetus contains reddish-brown, slimy fluid with flakes suspended in it. The body cavities contain blood-tinged fluid. Sometimes in the livers of these fetuses there are necrotic areas ranging in diameter from 1 mm. to 1 cm. which have some resemblance to the liver lesions caused by *Histomonas meleagridis* in infectious enterohepatitis (blackhead) of turkeys.

Microscopically, the ovine endometrium is involved in a rather mild inflammatory reaction. There is a small amount of cellular exudate in the glands and a mild serocellular infiltration of the lamina propria. Neutrophils are prominent. In the placentae both the fetal villi and maternal crypts are affected. The space between their epithelia contains blood and some giant cells which are probably the same type of cells that are present in the maternal epithelium. Necrosis of the epithelium of both the villi and crypts occurs, and also hyperemia and edema of their stroma.

In the bovine the vibrio is present in the fetal membranes, fetus, and uterine discharges of aborting cows. The membranes are flecked with thickened, opaque, leathery areas, and yellowish foci are present in the cotyledons. These are areas of inflammation and necrosis. These lesions are not materially different from those occurring in brucellosis. In experimentally induced bovine vibriosis, salpingitis, endometritis, and extensive generalized inflammatory edema of the fetal membranes occur. Abortion, however, generally occurs earlier in vibriosis than in brucellosis — 5 months as against 7 months. In Western Australia vibriosis is reported to be the immediate cause of at least 75 per cent of the infertility in dairy cows.

**Infectious abortion of mares** is an acute localized disease of mares characterized by metritis and cervicitis which lead to abortion and may finally terminate in sterility. It has been found that *Salmonella abortivoequina* and *Streptococcus genitalium,* either alone or together, or in association with other bacteria, are frequent causes of this disease.

Pathological changes in the uterus are quite constant and in many respects characteristic. *Salmonella abortivoequina* produces an acute endometritis and cervicitis in which there is little damage to the tissues, while *Streptococcus genitalium* causes an acute inflammation with extensive degenerative changes. The exudate produced is a thick mucocellular mass of a dark-red or brownish color. The quantity, character, and color of the exudate are reported to be of diagnostic value.

Barring complications, the affected mare

recovers promptly from the *Salmonella abortivoequina* infection. With the *Streptococcus genitalium* infection, however, metritis persists for a long time, and recovery, as a rule, does not occur without treatment.

### CHRONIC PURULENT ENDOMETRITIS

The disease occurs in cows, sows, and bitches. In cows the protozoan parasite, *Trichomonas foetus*, in association with pyogenic bacteria, has been found in some cases to be the cause. In a smaller per cent of the cases the condition has been found in the absence of pyogens. The uterus is distended with pus which varies in color with the particular pyogenic bacteria causing the inflammation. Sometimes the pus is liquid and flows readily out of the cervix and vagina (leukorrhea). At other times it is more or less inspissated. In trichomoniasis in cows a macerated fetus and fetal membranes may be present in several liters of fairly thin, grayish, purulent exudate.

In dogs chronic purulent endometritis is usually a disease of older animals, 11 to 12 years of age, occurring 40 to 90 days post estrus. If the cervix is open, the horns rarely become more than 3 cm. in diameter, the wall is thick, and only a small amount of mucopurulent exudate is present in the uterus. Two histological changes are prominent in the lamina propria of the endometrium: fibrosis and an infiltration of lymphocytes and plasma cells. These changes are accompanied by a minor degree of atrophy of the endometrium. When the cervix is closed the uterus becomes extremely distended (pyometra). The wall is very thin, and the normal architecture has disappeared. Glands are very rare, and the epithelium of the endometrium frequently undergoes squamous metaplasia. Only a few collagen fibers remain between the endometrium and the myometrium. The myometrium is also atrophic, and its stretched smooth muscle cells stain poorly. *E. coli*, staphyloccocci, and streptoccocci are usually present in the exudate.

In dogs with chronic purulent endometritis the number and kinds of leukocytes in the peripheral blood are changed to such an extent that a blood-cell examination is important in making a diagnosis. No hard and fast rule can be made for the blood picture because it is variable, depending upon whether the cervix is open or closed. Generally, however, the number of leukocytes ranges from 20 to 80 thousand with an average of about 40 thousand. The cases having closed cervix usually fall in the upper half of this range. Neutrophils increase most. A variable number of these are immature forms. In cases that run unfavorable courses the total leukocyte count may run above the average while at the same time there are few immature forms. In favorable cases immature neutrophils constitute 10 to 40 per cent of the total, and lymphocytes do not exceed 40 per cent. Anemia is not a characteristic of the condition. Erythrocyte sedimentation rate is variable — 8 to 40 mm. per hour. It is highest in cases with a closed cervix. Blood urea ranges from 30 to 160 mg./100 ml.

Clinical signs in cases which have an open cervix are vaginal discharge and slight inappetence, but cases with a closed cervix may show marked general symptoms such as vomiting, increased thirst, and prostration.

Whether chronic purulent endometritis of bitches is a part of the hormone-induced complex of cystic hyperplasia and pyometra is uncertain because it has not been reproduced experimentally as have the three manifestations of this complex. There is a strong possibility, however, that chronic purulent endometritis may be the end result of repeated acute attacks of the complex. In a study by Dow in Scotland, most of the cases had a previous history of postestral genital disease.

Besides the altered blood picture (leukocytosis) there may be other changes in the body associated with chronic purulent endometritis of bitches. Some degenerative changes of the solid organs would be expected in very severe cases in which large amounts of toxic material are absorbed. In such a pyogenic infection, metastatic abscesses are also occasionally to be expected.

### ACUTE NECROTIC METRITIS

Necrotic metritis is caused by *Spherophorus necrophorus*. The pathology is similar to that of necrophorus infection in other parts of the body.

### CHRONIC NECROTIC ENDOMETRITIS

This disease occurs mostly in sows. A staphylococcus has been reported as the cause. The mucosa becomes enormously thickened and extensively necrotic. The lumen becomes a tiny fissure.

### CYSTIC HYPERPLASIA-PYOMETRA COMPLEX IN THE BITCH

The bitch, and sometimes the cat, is subject to a peculiar combination of uterine changes characterized by a cystic hyperplasia of the epithelium of the endometrium, excessive mucus production by the hyperplastic glands, and often by an acute purulent inflammation superimposed upon this already much altered epithelium. According to an extensive study of this condition made by Dow in Scotland, the age of the affected bitches is 7 to 8 years; only a small per cent of the animals are less than 6 years of age. A high per cent of the bitches in his study had never whelped. While infection was present in many, but not all, of the uteri, the condition appears not to be primarily an infection. The microbial invaders are the pyogens *E. coli,* staphylococci, and streptococci.

Clinically the complex is associated with certain phases of the estrus cycle. Most cases appear 5 to 90 days post estrus, which is the luteal phase of the cycle. In the study by Dow all clinical cases had persistent corpora lutea so it has been theorized that the hormone progesterone may be the cause of the primary endometrial hyperplasia and that the presence of the pus in the uterus is a secondary condition resulting from the invasion of the pyogens. This belief is substantiated by experiments in which a condition quite similar to this complex has been produced by injections of progesterone (luteal-body hormone) into ovariectomized bitches. This belief is further substantiated by the fact that ovariectomy of affected bitches brings relief in 5 to 15 days. It should be mentioned in this connection that Dow also observed other ovarian lesions in some of his dogs such as proliferation of the tubules of the rete ovarii, cystic follicles, and granulosa cell tumors.

Clinical signs of the complex are concerned chiefly with the estrus cycle, which becomes completely upset. In addition, in the cases in which the pyogens have been active and in which the pus has been retained in the uterus (pyometra), there are general symptoms such as increased thirst, listlessness, depressed appetite, and even vomition. The most common indications of disturbed sexual cycles are irregular estrus, abnormal duration of proestrus and estrus, bleeding throughout proestrus and estrus, vaginal discharge of mucus or pus if the cervix is open, swollen vulva, and pseudo-pregnancy (phantom pregnancy, pseudocyesis).

**Lesions.** This complex is characterized by three types of lesions, all of which have been reproduced experimentally.

1. Many of the bitches have **uncomplicated cystic hyperplasia** of the endometrium with excessive production of mucus which flows from the vagina. This may occur at any stage of the estrus cycle. The uterus is enlarged; the endometrium is thickened and contains mucus-cysts up to 1 cm. in diameter. The cysts are distributed uniformly throughout the entire length of the body and horns. In about one-fourth of Dow's cases in this category, *E. coli* was present in the mucus. No inflammatory cell infiltration is associated with the cystic endometrial hyperplasia in these cases.

2. A smaller number of bitches have cystic hyperplasia of the endometrial epithelium **complicated by a plasma cell in-**

filtration of the lamina propria and by polypoid proliferations of the endometrium. These changes result in a very thick endometrium. Were it not for the fact that the cervix is usually open in these cases, the excessive mucus secreted by the hyperplastic epithelium would distend the uterus. Usually, however, the uterus is seldom more than 2 cm. in diameter. *E. coli* is present in the mucus of most of these cases. The affected dogs usually never have whelped, and the lesions occur between 35 and 70 days post estrus.

3. More than half of the bitches affected with this hormonally induced complex have a variable amount of cystic hyperplasia **complicated with acute purulent inflammation** of the endometrium. Between and around pus-filled cystic glands the lamina propria is infiltrated chiefly with neutrophils. The inflammatory reaction often extends into the myometrium. If the cervix remains closed, the uterus and horns become greatly enlarged (pyometra). The horns are elongated and involved in a series of annular constrictions alternating with dilatations (ampullae). These constrictions and dilatations give the uterus the appearance of being gravid. The uterine wall is thick at the constrictions and thin at the ampullae. The endometrium is rough due to pus-filled cysts, focal hemorrhages, and ulcers. The color of the uterine exudate is yellow to green tinged reddish-brown, the variations in color being due to hemorrhage. The three pyogens already mentioned are often present in the exudate. Toxicosis from pus retention in the cases with closed cervix causes pronounced general symptoms. This form of the complex occurs 5 to 85 days post estrus. Almost two-thirds of the bitches have abdominal distension.

Clinical laboratory examination is an aid in the diagnosis of this third form of the complex. The leukocyte count may be increased up to 145 thousand, usually exceeding 40 thousand if the cervix is closed. As many as 35 per cent of the neutrophils may be immature. Neutrophils are abundant in vaginal smears. The erythrocyte sedimentation rate increases to between 10 and 55 mm. per hour. A rate in excess of 30 mm. per hour is associated with high mortality or slow postoperative recovery. Blood urea levels of 65 mg/100 ml or more point towards poor surgical risk. Radiographically the uterine ampullae simulate the appearance of midpregnancy.

## VAGINA AND VULVA

**Changes in form** of the vagina and vulva are due principally to cysts. The **canals of Gartner (remnants of Wolffian ducts)** may persist in cows and present a double or single row of cysts on the floor of the vagina from the external os to the external urethral orifice. They contain clear fluid or gray gelatinous masses and are lined with simple epithelium. The **glands of Bartholin (glandulae vestibulares majores),** located in the lateral walls of the vulva, may become cystic as a result of an inflammatory process which produces strictures of the ducts, leading to an accumulation of secretion.

**Disturbances in continuity** (lacerations) are of frequent occurrence during normal parturition or as a result of unskillful obstetrical manipulation. Occasionally they occur during copulation. The results depend upon whether or not infection occurs.

### Vaginitis and Vulvitis

The etiology of vaginitis is the same as that for inflammation of other mucous surfaces, i. e., mechanic, thermic, chemic, and infectious agents. Infectious agents of most importance in this connection are *Spherophorus necrophorus* (mostly in cows), an unidentified microorganism in infectious granular vaginitis of heifers and cows, the *protozoan* parasites *Trypanosoma equiperdum* in dourine of mares, and *Trichomonas foetus* in cows.

In bred heifers and cows a nodular vaginitis or granular venereal disease usually called **infectious granular vaginitis** is widespread. The cause has not been established but it appears to be a pleomorphic microorganism. Exudate from an infected heifer transferred to the vulva of a healthy heifer will give rise to an inflammation in a week. In 2 or 3 weeks nodules appear in the mucosa, and in 2 to 4 months they reach their maximum development and gradually subside. These nodules in the inflamed mucosa are hyperplastic lymph nodules which may protrude through the overlying epithelial covering (Fig. 19.12).

In the Corn Belt a **necrotic vulvitis** occasionally affects several heifers in the same feed lot (Fig. 19.13). The cause has not always been determined; in some instances these cases have been due to *Spherophorus necrophorus,* which has been transmitted by "nosey" pigs while the heifers were lying in the feed lot.

In the Corn Belt during certain years a **vulvovaginitis** occurs among young gilts. The etiology is unknown, but a correlation apparently exists between the occurrence of the disease and the feeding of poor corn. There has been speculation as to whether

estrogenic substances present in forage plants may initiate the condition. Such substances have been reported to cause vulval and vaginal hyperemia in ewes. The macroscopic appearance of this condition as seen in Iowa is, first of all, a swelling of the vulva as occurs during estrum. It is smooth, firm, and swollen. The lips separate and display a hyperemic vaginal mucosa. The condition may progress to prolapse of the vagina. Prolapse results in passive hyperemia. The prolapsed portion may extend out 6 inches with a diameter of 4 inches. It is easily injured and becomes hemorrhagic and eroded. If infected, it becomes purulent. In sections, hyperemia, edema, and cellular infiltration are the primary alterations. The condition results in prolapse of the rectum in 5 to 10 per cent of the cases and prolapse of the vagina in as high as 30 per cent of the gilts in some herds. Death usually does not result except in cases of prolapse and then only from secondary causes (hemorrhage, septic cystitis, uremia, constipation, and septicemia).

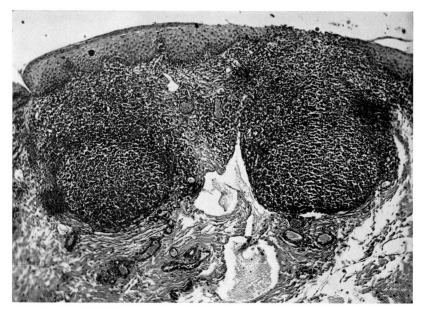

Fig. 19.12 — Two lymph nodules in vulval mucosa of a cow with infectious granular vaginitis. One nodule normal, the other hyperplastic and breaking through epithelium. (Department of Veterinary Pathology, Michigan State University.)

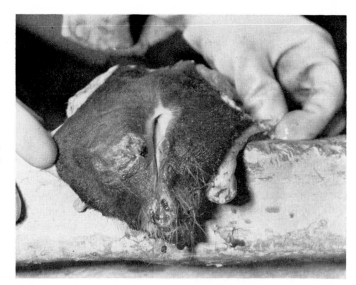

Fig. 19.13 — Necrotic vulvitis in the bovine as the result of bites inflicted by swine.

Infectious pustular vulvovaginitis of cows is an uncommon viral disease in the United States in which small foci of epithelial degeneration develop in the vulva and vagina. The degenerating epithelial cells may contain intranuclear inclusion bodies and necrose. The necrotic foci become infiltrated with neutrophils. Adjacent necrotic foci may coalesce and form ulcers. Fever and neutropenia characterize the infection, which runs a short course but may be severe enough to cause an endometritis. Vulval nodules following the infection may consist of solitary lymph nodules whose surface epithelial covering did not regenerate.

In California an **infectious catarrhal vaginitis and cervicitis** of cows similar to one occurring in South Africa has been shown to be due to a virus.

### Tumors

Various kinds of tumors occasionally occur in the vagina and vulva. Among them are vaginal fibromas and fibropapillomas of cows, vaginal fibromas (Fig. 19.14), fibroleiomyomas, and leiomyomas of bitches, and histiosarcomas of both sexes of dogs. Most important, however, are the fibropapillomas of cows and the histiosarcomas of dogs.

The **transmissible fibropapilloma** (papilliform fibroma), is a wartlike tumor occurring on the vulva of young cows and on the penis of young bulls. These tumors regress spontaneously. They are caused by the same virus which causes infectious cutaneous papillomas of cattle. The tumor usually appears as a single neoplasm on the penis or in the vulva or vagina. These tumors are variable in size and have a cauliflower-like appearance. Practically all of the tumors, to some degree, have an ulcerated surface, probably as a result of trauma. The cut surface is pink or grayish white and glistening. Large tumors have necrotic centers; most have broad bases.

Histologically, fibropapillomas consist of connective tissue covered with stratified squamous epithelium of varying thickness. Young tumors have the appearance of fibrosarcomas because the connective tissue is composed of young fibroblasts, and mitotic figures are common. In older tumors the connective tissue has matured, mitosis has ceased, and collagen fibers become prominent. Among the collagen fibers, however, extra large fibroblasts remain whose nuclei contain one or more glassy, weakly stained eosinophilic bodies. The connective tissue growth is covered by stratified squamous epithelium 10 to 50 cells thick. Long narrow projections of this epithelium extend into the main connective tissue mass. Surface ulceration follows a vacuolar degeneration of the epithelial cells accompanied by a leukocytic infiltration into the vacuoles.

The **histiosarcoma** of dogs is a most unusual tumor among domestic mammals for two reasons. First, it is transmitted from one sex to the other by coitus. Second, the animal having the tumor implants the neoplastic cells into the genital mucosa during the coital act. More female than

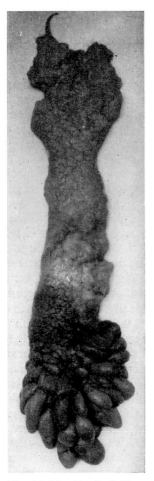

Fig. 19.14 — Vaginal fibromas in a 7-year-old dog. (Department of Veterinary Pathology, Michigan State University.)

male dogs, however, are reported to have the tumor. It is a neoplastic disease of young dogs, 1 to 6 years of age, the age at which sexual activity is greatest. While the condition seems to have almost world-wide distribution, its incidence seems to come and go. In one decade, areas in which it is prevalent may be practically free from it in another decade. This may be due to the fact that dogs develop resistance to the tumor. In affected animals the tumor regresses and the individual is resistant to the tumor thereafter. At the Mayo Clinic 32 per cent of the dogs used in an experiment with this tumor had natural resistance to the tumor cell.

Grossly, the histiosarcoma varies greatly in the number of tumors present in an individual and in the size, shape, and consistency of the growth. The most constant gross characteristic is the anatomical location, which may be any part of the vagina, vestibule, or labia in the female, and on the penis or parietal surface of the prepuce in the male — occasionally on the scrotum or perineal region. The tumors are more likely to be covered by mucosa in the female and more likely to be ulcerated in the male because in the latter they are more exposed to trauma.

Histologically, the tumor cells are large and either round, polyhedral, or slightly ovoid but generally uniform in size. The nuclei are large, round, and vesicular but hyperchromatic with prominent nucleoli. There is usually abundant but poorly stained cytoplasm with the usual hematoxylin and eosin stain. Mitosis is prominent. The cells look rather highly malignant, but metastasis seldom extends farther than the regional lymph nodes. The rather closely packed diffuse masses of cells may be separated by strands of connective tissue in two ways: (1) Delicate strands of the tissue may push the tumor cells into pseudoalveolar groups. (2) Stronger bands of the stroma may cause the tumor cells to be arranged in cords. If the tumor has been traumatized, inflammatory cells are present. The origin of the neoplastic cells has not yet been determined with certainty. Various investigators have considered them to be derived from the following cells: lymphoblasts, reticuloendothelial cells, and histiocytes. Those who believe that the parent cell is the histiocyte call the tumor **histiosarcoma**.

## GENITAL ORGANS OF THE FEMALE BIRD

In the ovary, **follicular cysts** are occasionally encountered. **Degenerative changes** are seen in a high percentage of hens having *Salmonella pullorum* infection (Fig. 17.18). Somewhat similar changes also appear in laying hens that have been suddenly thrown out of egg production. **Hemorrhage** may occur in connection with ovulation. The most frequent **tumors** of the ovary are the lymphosarcomas. Cystadenomas (Fig. 19.15), and adenocarcinomas also occur.

The oviduct may undergo **torsion** or **prolapse**. It may rupture and permit eggs to accumulate in the abdominal cavity (**stone butt**) (Fig. 19.16). Rather frequently a remnant of the right oviduct may persist and give rise to one or more **retention cysts (water butt)**. **Foreign bodies** such as roundworms, flukes, and ingesta may ascend the tube. Concretions occasionally form in the tube. One or more eggs may become lodged in it (**egg bound**). **Salpingitis** has been reported in pullorum disease of pullets and in fluke infestation of ducks.

In the egg may appear **blood spots (liver spots)** or **foreign bodies** that have ascended the oviduct. The yolks may be **double** or **discolored**. Occasionally, an egg is **yolkless**. Some eggs appear **laminated**. Sometimes there occurs an **egg within an egg**. Frequently eggs are **soft-shelled**.

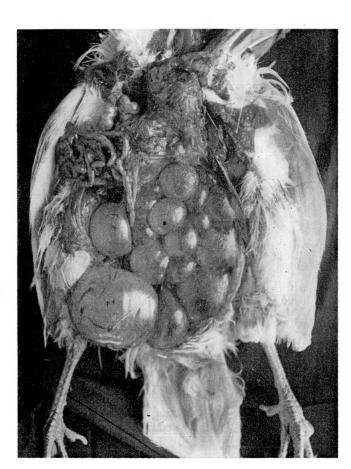

Fig. 19.15 — Cystadenoma of the ovary of a hen. (Records and Vawter, Nev. Agr. Exp. Sta.)

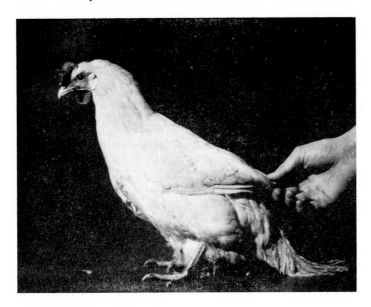

Fig. 19.16 — Rupture of oviduct with accumulation of eggs in abdominal cavity. Note duck-like posture. (McKenney, Jour. A.V.M.A.)

## MAMMARY GLAND (UDDER)

### Functional Disturbances

The function of the mammary gland is primarily to supply milk for the offspring. In the cow and the goat this function has been greatly extended to that of supplying milk also for human consumption. For this reason disturbances of the function of the mammary gland of these animals have an added importance. Diseases of this gland alter its function by changing the quantity and quality of its secretion. Pathologic conditions responsible for this may be located in the parenchyma and interstitial tissue, or in the ducts. The most devastating process which can involve this gland and alter its function is inflammation. When the gland becomes inflamed, the secretion of milk diminishes or may even cease. The milk which is secreted is mixed with inflammatory exudate so that it contains a much larger number of leukocytes than is normal. The greatest increase is in neutrophils. The presence of excessive numbers of leukocytes can be detected by the Whiteside and California mastitis tests. Desquamated epithelial cells become more abundant. Blood chlorides and alkali present in the inflammatory edema appear in the milk. Hemorrhage gives rise to erythrocytes in the secretion. The temperature of the udder and the suitableness of milk as a medium for the growth of microorganisms furnish ideal conditions for the development of mastitis-producing bacteria. Mastitis-producing streptococci can be detected by the Hotis test. In the udder, bacteria behave just as they do in test tubes in the laboratory — they coagulate the milk and may also digest the curd. Part of the curd digestion is carried on, however, by proteolytic enzymes of the neutrophils. When the curd is forced out of the teat canal through the teat sphincter, it has a stringy or ropy appearance. In chronic inflammation there is proliferation of connective tissue so that the udder becomes fleshy or meaty in consistency.

**Acquired changes of form.** Cystic dilatation of the lactiferous ducts may occur as a result of constrictions in the ducts due to chronic inflammatory processes. The secretion accumulates above the constriction, resulting in a cyst. In the teats, chronic inflammation may result in cicatrization, strictures, and polypoid proliferations.

**Pigmentation. Melanin** is common in gilts of the colored breeds. In packing houses its presence in bacon bellies is designated seedy **bellies, seedy bacon,** or seedy cut (Fig. 9.15). The pigment also appears in lard prepared from belly fat. The pigmentation is due to a dipping-in process of the melanoblasts during fetal development of the mammary gland. The melanin is scattered along the gland ducts. **Hematogenous pigmentation** is rather common in gilts reaching sexual maturity and in pregnancy. It is called **red seed.**

**Circulatory disturbances. Active hyperemia** occurs physiologically before and after parturition and occurs pathologically in mastitis. **Edema** occurs physiologically along with hyperemia before and after parturition. **Hemorrhage** occurs during mastitis, and as a result of trauma, especially in pendulous udders. The occurrence and pathogenesis of **embolism** and **thrombosis** are similar to those in the uterine veins. They result in infarction and necrosis of the region supplied by the affected vessel. The condition may affect a whole quarter. It is rather frequent in cows. The infarcted area becomes marked off by an inflammatory zone. The dead tissue separates from the living. If it is deep in the udder, it becomes encapsulated and is called a sequestrum; if superficial, it may rupture at the surface and completely slough away.

## Mastitis of Cattle

Mastitis or mammitis is caused by mechanical injury, toxic agents that have been injected into the udder or possibly those which have been produced within the body and excreted in the milk, and bacteria (staphylococci, streptococci, *Escherichia coli, Corynebacterium pyogenes, Pseudomonas aeruginosa, Brucella abortus, Mycobacterium tuberculosis, Actinomyces bovis, Actinobacillus lignieresi, Nocardia asteroides,* and *Serratia marcescens*). Retained fetal membranes and metritis may furnish the source of the infectious agents.

**Role of mechanical milking in etiology of mastitis.** A contributing factor in the cause of mastitis may be the mechanical milker. At the Storrs Agricultural Experiment Station a group studied the effects of variations in vacuum levels (10, 13, and 17 inches of mercury) when the pulsations were 48. They also varied the duration of milking. The project was conducted on first-calf heifers which were considered mastitis-free. Mild inflammatory foci occurred in both the teats and glands without relation either to vacuum level of the machine or duration of milking.

At the California Agricultural Experiment Station a project demonstrated that the negative pressure (vacuum) used in mechanical milking can injure the tissues of the teat and lactiferous sinus. Injury is likely to occur when the teat cups are left on after the milk flow has ceased, especially if they "crawl," or when pulsators, pulsator hoses, or rubber liners have become defective. Trauma, together with milk as a culture medium, provides a perfect situation for the growth of pathogens.

**Pathogenesis.** The manner in which the udder becomes infected is not fully known. Experiments indicate that it is easy to produce mastitis when pathogenic streptococci are introduced directly into the teat canal. Exposure of the intact and scarified udder to infection has not caused mastitis. Blood stream infection by way of the mammary artery has not been successful unless the number of streptococci used was far in excess of that which would appear in the blood stream under natural conditions. Infection by way of the digestive tract has not occurred when 200 cc. of streptococcic culture have been fed daily for three weeks even when intestinal irritants were also administered. When, however, the teat orifice was congenitally malformed, or when it was injured in various ways, infection of the gland by exposure of the tip of the teat to streptococci was easy to accomplish. Even these experiments, however, leave the question unsolved because they do not explain why several animals in a single herd may develop mastitis during a relatively short period of time when no apparent teat injury occurs.

**Relation of cause and effect.** A very extensive and thorough study of the pathology of mastitis of dairy cows was made in

Connecticut by Helmboldt, Jungherr, and Plastridge on udders collected during a 20-year period in a herd which was free from Brucella infection. The study is especially valuable because they studied the bacteriology as well as the pathology of the 130 udders which formed the basis of their project. They included an additional 8 udders from other sources.

The microorganisms responsible for the mastitis in their study were streptococci (*Str. agalactiae, dysgalactiae,* and *uberis*), staphylococci (hemolytic and nonhemolytic), coliforms (*E. coli, A. aerogenes* and members of the Klebsiella group), and *Corynebacterium pyogenes.*

In general these organisms produce an acute mastitis — very seldom a chronic form. The acute changes vary from mild to severe and from practically no loss of tissue to considerable necrosis. Neutrophils are always present in the exudate, usually in numbers greater than 500,000 per ml.

The inflammatory reaction is not a single continuous one but multiple, scattered, progressive ones. In an affected quarter at a particular time, foci of inflammation of variable size and age may be scattered widely. Some are in the early stages of development, others are well along, and still others have reached the terminal stage. Because of this the inflammatory process has a long course but the histological changes at any moment are in the acute stage. This sort of course leads the clinician and the milk sanitarian to diagnose the disease as chronic mastitis, whereas the tissue alterations indicate that it is actually a continuing series of very acute reactions.

The investigators classified their acute cases as slight, moderate, and marked. To simplify the material for instruction purposes the authors have grouped the slight and moderate cases under the heading "mild" and the marked cases under the heading "severe." They also have included chronic mastitis in their classification.

To make it easier to understand the relationship of the etiological bacterial agents to these forms of mastitis the authors have briefly summarized some of the information.

1. Generally streptococci cause moderate acute rather than chronic mastitis as is generally supposed. There is no difference in the changes produced by the three varieties of streptococci.

2. The mild acute inflammation caused by the coliform organisms is like that caused by the streptococci, but the coliforms are more likely to produce a severe acute mastitis which is more destructive than the severe acute form caused by the streptococci. Indication of this is the larger amount of replacement connective tissue in coliform mastitis. Furthermore, in severe coliform mastitis, macrophages and lymphocytes predominate over neutrophils in the alveoli.

3. Staphylococci cause mild acute, severe acute, and chronic mastitis. The mild acute form resembles the mild acute form produced by the streptococci and the coliforms. Most cases of staphylococcic mastitis are mild acute.

4. *C. pyogenes* causes severe acute mastitis with more tissue destruction than caused by the coliforms, and death may result.

### MILD ACUTE MASTITIS

In mild acute mastitis the anatomical extent of the individual lesions in a quarter vary greatly. In the mildest cases a focus of inflammation includes only a part of a lobule or at most a whole lobule. In more severe cases a focus consists of a whole lobule or more. The foci of the same age have the same structure, but since foci of different ages are present simultaneously, the histological picture in a quarter is quite varied.

**Pathogenesis.** Bacteria localize in a lobule and begin to incite an inflammatory reaction. Neutrophils leave the capillaries in the interalveolar tissue. The alveolar epithelium swells (cloudy swelling) and becomes vacuolated (fat). Some cells slough. The interalveolar and periductal tissue thickens due to accumulation of exudate and proliferation of connective tissue. The exudate, besides the neutrophils, includes lymphocytes, macrophages, and plasma cells. Besides infiltrating the interalveolar and periductal tissues, exudate appears in the lumina of the alveoli. Later the affected alveoli and interlobular ducts atrophy (involute). Secretion of milk in this area ceases. The lymphocytes disappear from the interalveolar and periductal connective tissue. The bacteria leave the involuted area by way of the ducts and invade other areas. The inflammatory process in this manner becomes continuous and progressive in the affected quarter. The involuted area does not likely function again during that particular lactation period.

**Histological appearance.** The earliest histological changes are observed in the alveolar and ductal epithelium of portions of lobules. The cells swell (cloudy swelling) and are usually unduly vacuolated (fat). The secretion mixed with exudate in the alveoli is clotted and attached to the alveolar lining by pseudopodia-like processes. Bacteria are not seen at this stage. Free epithelial cells are in the clot. Between alveoli and around the ducts a few neutrophils are present. The inflammatory reaction may terminate here or progress to a little more severe form in which the foci enlarge to include whole lobules or more.

In this slightly more extensive, moderate form of acute mastitis the epithelial changes are like those in the milder form, but atrophy of the epithelium, an indication of the oncoming involution, may already begin to appear. There is more extensive desquamation of the epithelium. Neutrophils are very numerous in the alveoli. The other leukocytes are not as conspicuous. At this time in the inflammatory reaction the milk sanitarian would generally record more than 500,000 leukocytes per ml. of milk. If coliform organisms are the cause, macrophages and lymphocytes may predominate in the alveoli. The clotted secretion in the alveoli contains all the cellular elements including desquamated epithelium. Corpora amylacea, free in alveoli or embedded in atrophied alveoli, may be common.

The periductal tissue is hyperemic, edematous, and infiltrated with leukocytes. Even the lining of the cistern is in a state of irritation as indicated by a leukocytic infiltration of the lamina propria, proliferation of fibroblasts, epithelial metaplasia (stratified squamous), and epithelial desquamation. An incidental finding is corpora amylacea embedded in the accessory glands of the lining of the teat cistern.

Acute mastitis progressing this far is the most common form. Bacteria which cause it are streptococci, staphylococci, and coliforms. The authors would add *Brucella abortus* to this list.

### SEVERE ACUTE MASTITIS

Whereas in mild acute mastitis the inflamed areas are seldom much more than a lobule in size, in severe acute mastitis the affected areas are large, sometimes occupying a part of a quarter. In the less extensive cases the condition may subside in a few days, but in the extensive ones the course is usually much longer. Fundamentally the changes are the same as in the mild acute form. In severe acute mastitis, however, necrosis may overshadow these changes. There is loss of normal architecture. The great amount of destruction may be the result of extension of the inflammation to the walls of blood vessels where thrombi then result and lead to infarction. The infarcted areas become abscesses or give rise to areas of gangrene. Repair occurs by the formation of granulation tissue which becomes scar tissue.

Microorganisms responsible for the cases of severe acute mastitis in the Connecticut study were hemolytic staphylococci (7 cases), coliforms, *C. pyogenes* (2 cases), *Str. agalactiae* (1 case), and beta-hemolytic streptococcus (1 case).

### CHRONIC MASTITIS

If the damage in severe acute mastitis is not as great as that just described, a state of equilibrium may develop between the etiological agent and the tissue defenses with neither able to overcome the other. This results in a long drawn-out inflammatory process in one focus resulting in much fibrosis. This is truly a chronic inflammation. While the Connecticut researchers found this to occur very seldom in their herd, this is not the rule in ordinary herds. When it did occur, there were colonies of bacteria present in a quarter and these were surrounded by granulation tissue. The adjacent udder was not particularly affected except that it was compressed by the mass of developing granulation tissue.

Microorganisms which caused chronic mastitis were mostly hemolytic staphylococci (7 cases).

## GANGRENOUS MASTITIS

In describing acute diffuse mastitis it was mentioned that one termination of the condition may be gangrene. In that instance the gangrenous inflammation is secondary. Gangrene here is a sequel to thrombosis of the vessels of the affected quarter. There are instances, however, when gangrene is primary. In such cases the condition appears sporadically in certain herds, and may affect lactating and non-lactating cows. It usually comes on suddenly and affects one or more quarters. Signs of gangrene usually appear within 24 to 48 hours. The teats and udder become cold and bluish, and are insensitive to pain. There may be emphysema of the udder. The cow shows a marked systemic reaction, important signs of which are fever, anorexia, dullness, and reluctance to move. Death may come in 3 to 4 days, or if the animal survives, the affected tissue sloughs and healing may occur.

Organisms which have been isolated are *Staphylococcus aureus, Corynebacterium pyogenes,* and *Clostridium perfringens,* but experimental inoculations of udders with the staphylococcus and the corynebacterium have not produced a type of mastitis like that seen in spontaneous cases.

## CRYPTOCOCCIC MASTITIS

An uncommon form of mastitis due to a yeast, *Cryptococcus neoformans,* is becoming important not only because of its increasing prevalence but also because of the public health implications of the presence of this organism in the udder, and therefore in the milk. In one instance there was circumstantial evidence that the infection was introduced into udders as a result of a routine practice of the dairyman to infuse all quarters with a penicillin mixture at the end of each milking period.

In the acute stages of cryptococcic mastitis, liquefactive necrosis of the udder parenchyma is prominent, but the interstitial tissue is almost unaffected. There is little or no inflammatory reaction incited by the presence of the yeast at first. Later — that is, in the chronic stages of the infection — there is such massive proliferation of macrophages and fibroblasts that pressure atrophy of the udder parenchyma occurs. Many of the macrophages contain cryptococci.

## NOCARDIAL MASTITIS

Mastitis caused by *Nocardia asteroides* is an uncommon condition, but in a California herd it affected 18 per cent of the cows. This microorganism, like a few other soil fungi, is capable of becoming an animal pathogen. As such it causes chronic focal reactions which take the form of nodules.

### Mastitis of Ewes

Among ewes a very severe, acute diffuse mastitis frequently occurs. It is designated blue bag by sheepmen. At times this form of mastitis becomes widespread in a flock. It is characterized by necrotic, gangrenous processes and is apparently caused by bacteria among which staphylococci are prominent. In Montana a member of the Pasteurella group has been isolated from cases. Macroscopically, the udder is enlarged and dull blue in color. From the teats a dirty, often bloody, foul-smelling secretion may be obtained. The cut surface is dark brown, almost black in color, sometimes partly greenish, and shows areas of softening.

### Tumors

Tumors of the mammary glands of dogs and cats are of greatest importance. In dogs a fairly benign mixed-cell tumor is quite common in bitches 9 to 13 years of age. In cats 8 to 12 years of age adenocarcinomas which metastasize to the axillary and inguinal lymph nodes, and sometimes internally, are fairly frequent.

The so-called mixed tumors of the bitch are of special interest principally because they are usually composed of a variety of tissues and are generally benign. They consist of epithelial, fibrous, and mucoid connective tissue, often with islands of hyaline cartilage and spongy bone. Some pathologists believe the epithelial components are derived from the mammary gland myoepithelium. The presence of cartilage and bone suggests a metaplasia among the mesenchymal components of the tumor. Probably not more than 10 per cent of these tumors become malignant. When they do, they metastasize first to local lymph nodes. Since the majority of these tumors involve the posterior glands, metastasis occurs to the inguinal nodes more often than to the axilliary nodes.

Rather critical observations have been made which seem to indicate that these mixed tumors of the mammary gland are associated with a hormonal disturbance in bitches. The tumors have frequently been found in bitches that had ovarian cysts, multiple corpora lutea, and endometrial hyperplasia. This belief is substantiated by the fact that spayed bitches seldom have these tumors. It is reported also that if ovariectomy is performed when a mixed mammary gland tumor first appears, it often decreases in size or disappears.

True adenocarcinomas in bitches are relatively rare. Occasionally the spongy bone components of a mixed tumor become malignant and transform a mixed tumor into an osteosarcoma.

Tumors of the udder parenchyma of cows are extremely rare. In the routine examination of the udders of 13 million cows by federal B.A.I. inspectors, no neoplasms were found. A polyp-like fibroma occasionally originates at the fold between the teat and gland cisterns of dairy cows. In some cases it may be the result of trauma from milking practices.

# Part II: Genital System - Male

## FUNCTIONAL DISTURBANCES

Diseases of the male generative organs may interfere with the production of spermatozoa, the secretion of suitable alkaline fluid for their preservation in the vagina, and the depositing of the spermatozoa in the vagina and cervical canal. A male that fails in his part of the reproductive process is said to be impotent.

Stallions whose testicles have not descended into the scrotum either unilaterally or bilaterally from the abdominal cavity (cryptorchidism) frequently show indications of increased sexual urge (satyriasis), and become vicious and unmanageable. If the cryptorchidism is bilateral, the animal is impotent.

The secretion of the prostate and also of the seminal vesicles in animals that possess them provides a vehicle to carry the spermatozoa. The volume of this fluid which is ejaculated is large so that the spermatozoa are distributed over a wide area. Diseases of these accessory sex glands may therefore disturb their functions, and consequently the quantity and quality of their secretions, sufficiently to hinder reproduction as far as the male animal is concerned.

## TESTICLE AND EPIDIDYMIS

**Local disturbance of metabolism.** The epithelial cells of the seminiferous tubules, especially the developmental stages of the seminal cells, are very sensitive and easily undergo degeneration. The degeneration leads to **atrophy** of the testicle. The testicle becomes small and firm. Microscopically, it can be noted that the spermatogenesis ceases. There may be hyalinization of the membrana propria of the tubules and an increase in the interstitial connective tissue. These changes probably occur most frequently in the dog. They may appear in the course of a general disease or occur as a senile change. In research laboratories testicular atrophy, often accompanied by scrotal hernia, has been reported in mice that were fed a ration which was contaminated with stilbestrol. The feed was contaminated by milling equipment which had just previously been used to prepare a feed supplement for cattle. **Calcification** of the testes of bulls is fairly common. The condition often affects the seminiferous tubules of both testes and is not associated with age. Even though multiple foci of calcification may be present, the animal usually does not become sterile. **Melanosis** of the testicles often occurs in roosters and gobblers.

**Circulatory disturbances. Petechiae** may occur during the course of the acute infectious and intoxicative diseases in which hemorrhages usually appear in other parts of the body. **Passive hyperemia** occurs in connection with torsion of the spermatic cord.

**Orchitis and epididymitis.** The causes of inflammation here are trauma and infection. The latter may originate by extension or by way of the blood stream. Infection is due to the same varieties of microorganisms that are associated with genital infections in the female. *Brucella suis* appears to be a common cause of orchitis in boars (Figs. 8.3 and 7.5), *Brucella abortus* in bulls (Fig. 19.8), and *Corynebacterium ovis* in rams. The results of orchitis and epididymitis are principally those described for atrophy.

In Australasia, Slovakia, and California **epididymitis of rams** is of great economic importance. In a survey in California it occurred in 27 per cent of 5,000 rams examined. It results in reduced fertility. The cause is a bacterial agent which has not been completely classified.

Grossly, the tail of the epididymis becomes enlarged up to 4 or 5 times the normal size. The consistency is firm and the contour irregular. The tunica albuginea is thickened. In some cases in the thickened tunic there are solitary or multiple out-pouchings of the epididymis (spermatoceles) containing creamy-tan inspissated pus. Usually adhesions bind together the parietal and visceral layers of the tunica vaginalis at the tail of the organ. Similar adhesions are present between the tail of the epididymis and the distal pole of the testis. These adhesions are usually due to rupture of spermatoceles. At times the entire epididymis is enlarged due to distention of the tubules with spermatozoa that are retained by constrictions of the tubules. Along with these changes the testis may undergo atrophy and fibrosis.

Histologically, the inflammatory reaction begins with a mild, widely distributed perivascular edema and lymphocytic infiltration of the interstitial tissue. As the reaction increases in intensity plasma cells and neutrophils appear. The epithelium of the tubules also becomes involved. It undergoes hyperplasia accompanied by foci of intra-epithelial edema which constitute microcysts. Epithelial cells adjacent to the cysts undergo hydropic degeneration. As the intra-epithelial microcysts increase in size and numbers the lumen of the tubules becomes constricted and obliterated. What remains of the lumen is filled with exudate. Proximal to such constrictions spermatozoa may accumulate and distend the tubules of the body and head of the epididymis. The accumulated sperms sometimes incite a chronic inflammatory reaction of the tubule lining and wall. The cellular alterations are characteristic of this type of inflammation including giant cells. As the epididymitis continues, the early serocellular inflammatory reaction of the interstitial tissue gives way to fibrosis and cicatrization. The reaction may extend to the testis causing atrophy, foci of sperm stasis with an intratubular chronic inflammatory reaction, calcification, and peritubular fibrosis.

**Cysts** may be acquired or congenital. Acquired cysts result from inflammatory constrictions of the tubules of the epididymis (accumulation of secretion). Congenital cysts originate in the vestiges of Gartner's (Wolffian) and Müller's ducts.

**Tumors.** Testicular tumors have been studied more extensively in dogs than in the other domestic mammals. The reasons for this are: (1) Opportunities and facilities for studying them are greater than in other animals because dogs are used so frequently for laboratory purposes. (2) The individuals using them in laboratories have a special interest in the study of neoplasms of all kinds. (3) Small animal practitioners, by the nature of their practice, have a greater interest in laboratory diagnosis and more frequently submit tumors for histological examination. (4) Dogs are kept long enough to reach the "tumor age."

Primary tumors may originate from any of the tissues composing the testes. The most important ones, however, arise from the following cells: (1) Germinal epithelium of the convoluted tubules (**seminomas** or germinomas). (2) Sertoli cells. (3) Interstitial or Leydig cells. The latter two are simply designated **Sertoli-cell tumors** and **Leydig** or **interstitial cell tumors.** Because the tissue of origin in all three instances is glandular — either exocrine or endocrine — these tumors are, strictly speaking, either adenomas or adenocarcinomas depending upon whether they are benign or malignant. All three classes, however, often have cytological characteristics of malignancy, but only a few of them metastasize. The average age of dogs having these tumors is 8 to 12 years. In dogs of this age a nodular hyperplasia of the interstitial cells is common but is not considered to be a neoplastic disease. It is usually bilateral in occurrence.

Some testicular tumors of dogs cause the animals to undergo certain anatomical and behavioral changes. Sertoli-cell tumors generally contain sufficient estrogen to produce symptoms of hyperestrinism. Anatomically there is atrophy of the opposite testis. The epithelium of the prostatic portion of the urethra, together with that of the ducts and acini of the prostate, undergoes metaplasia, i.e., becomes a stratified squamous type. The prostate usually undergoes atrophy. A hyperplasia of the ducts and alveoli of the mammary glands causes these organs to enlarge. There is swelling of the prepuce and loss of hair. Change in behavior is manifested by depressed libido, and the affected dog attracts other male dogs like a female in estrum.

Some of the anatomical changes occurring as the result of excessive estrogen secretion by Sertoli-cell tumors are explained as follows:

Atrophy of the unaffected testis when the opposite testis is neoplastic is due to the inhibitory action of estrogen on the gonadotrophic hormones which influence the size and functional activity of the organ. Degeneration of the spermatogenic epithelium results.

Estrogen causes enlargement of the nipples, multiplication of the lactiferous ducts, and proliferation of the lining epithelium (gynecomastia).

The loss of hair (alopecia) is associated with the atrophy of hair follicles and sebaceous glands caused by the estrogen.

**Teratomas** of the testes are uncommon. Two types have been reported: (1) dermoid cysts and (2) solid teratomas. The former have been reported in horses and the latter in roosters. The authors have seen a feather-containing dermoid in the testis of a gander. Occasionally, in the solid teratomas where all three germ layers are represented, one tissue may predominate over all others, and the tumor will appear to be an osteoma, chondroma, leiomyoma, or any other type of benign tumor. There is always the possibility that such a tumor may become malignant.

## SCROTUM

**Hydrocele** is uncommon in animals. It occasionally occurs in stallions in connection with inguinal hernia. **Periorchitis** originates from trauma, by extension, or hematogenically. In bulls and boars it may be due to Brucella organisms. Other specific forms are tuberculous and actinomycotic.

## SPERMATIC CORD

Funiculitis is frequent in barrows, geld-ings, and steers. After castration the stump of the cord becomes infected through the open castration incision. The condition is often referred to as scirrhous cord. In bar-rows the condition described here is prob-ably more often an inflammation of the scrotum and surrounding tissues than it is of the cord. In barrows the cord is usually cut short. High castration incisions, how-ever, favor the scrotal infection.

Funiculitis may be caused by *Staphylo-coccus aureus, Spherophorus necrophorus, Actinomyces bovis, Actinobacillus lignier-esi,* and *Mycobacterium tuberculosis.* Spirochetes may be the etiological factor in many cases in swine (Fig. 19.17). By special staining with silver nitrate, they can be demonstrated in the necrotic tissue of the chronic inflammatory reaction which characterizes this condition (Fig. 16.6).

The inflammatory process is of a chronic proliferative, suppurative, necrotic nature (thick-walled abscesses, often with fistula formation). Macroscopically, the tumor-like formations vary from 2 ounces to $22\frac{1}{2}$ pounds. In the early stages the mass is firm. Later, fluctuating areas develop. These rupture and form fistulous tracts to the outside, and emit a foul-smelling fluid. Microscopically, the wall of the abscess consists of granulation tissue (Fig. 11.11). The center of the abscess is necrotic and gangrenous. In the wall adjacent to the central necrotic mass, the vessels are plugged with thrombi and leukocytes. Great numbers of spirochetes appear in this area.

## SEMINAL VESICLE

Spermatocystitis or seminal vesiculitis. Both nonspecific and specific forms occur. The condition is especially important in bulls of the dairy breeds. The same bac-teria that are responsible for other genital infections are present.

## PROSTATE

Inflammation (prostatitis) is most fre-quent in dogs (Fig. 11.8), but occasionally it occurs in bulls.

Hypertrophy of the prostate occurs very frequently in old dogs (Fig. 19.18). It oc-curs in 60 per cent of uncastrated dogs. Considerably over half of these dogs were aged. All house-trained dogs have lesions, but less than half of the farm dogs show them. The cause of the condition is not known, but environment may be signifi-cant since hypertrophy occurs mostly in dogs that are subject to forced urine re-tention. It may be a compensatory hyper-trophy accompanying senile atrophy of the gland. A similar process occurs frequently in other organs (testicles, liver, spleen, pancreas, adrenals) of aged dogs. Another theory is that the glandular hyperplasia of the prostate is due to an excess of male hormone.

Macroscopically, the prostate is en-larged. Its surface is smooth or nodular. The cut surface shows distinct lobulation. The nodules are surrounded by a heavy connective tissue stroma. Frequently there are cysts. The proliferative process causes compression of the urethra, which leads to stasis of urine and compensatory muscular hypertrophy of the urinary bladder wall.

Microscopically, the glandular epithe-

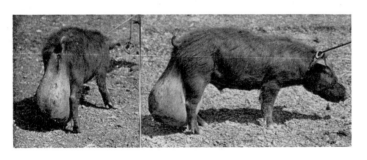

Fig. 19.17 — Chronic funicu-litis (scirrhous cord) in a bar-row in the region of castra-tion wounds. This tumor-like formation weighed $22\frac{1}{2}$ pounds after surgical remov-al. (Howarth, Jour. A.V.M.A.)

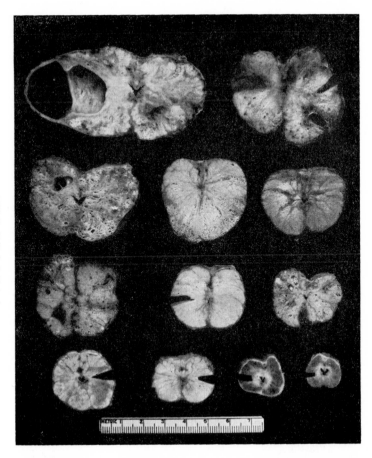

Fig. 19.18 — Hypertrophy and hyperplasia of the prostate of dogs. Cross-section views of several glands obtained from dogs of various ages. Note different degress of hypertrophy and urethral obstruction. The two small glands in lower right corner are essentially normal. (Schlotthauer, Jour. A.V.M.A.)

lium and interstitial tissue both share in the enlargement of the gland. The relative amount of increase of either varies much, but there is no true tumor formation (Fig. 19.19). At times the gland tubules become greatly dilated (cysts) and fuse with other dilatations to form larger cysts. The cysts are lined with atrophied epithelium. These changes resemble a cystadenoma. In other places the epithelial cells proliferate, which results in the epithelium being thrown into folds. The prostate then has the appearance of a papillary adenoma. Foci of inflammatory cell infiltration are almost always present (probably of secondary origin).

Calculi of the prostate in animals have seldom been reported in the literature. In man such calculi apparently arise from corpora amylacea, but these bodies are very rarely seen in animals, which may account for the rarity of calculi. In a case in a dog reported by Lumb the greatly enlarged prostate contained two cysts in which were 35 calculi ranging in size up to 10 mm. They were smooth, discoid, moderately hard concretions. Their color was variable — white, mottled, or streaked with brown. Chemically they consisted mostly of triple phosphate. The wall of the cyst which contained the calculi was thin and involved in a mild inflammatory reaction. The cyst lining was metaplastic, composed of cornified, stratified squamous epithelium which was papillated. Listlessness, dysuria, fever, and leukocytosis (48,750 per cm., mostly neutrophils) were prominent signs of this lithiasis.

Tumors. In dogs, primary adenocarcinoma is of greatest importance.

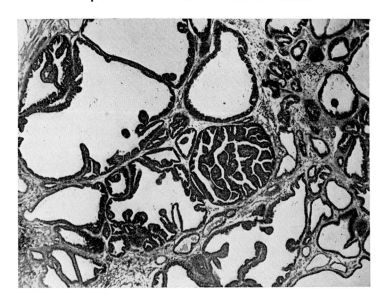

Fig. 19.19 — Cystadenomatous hypertrophy of the prostate of a dog. ×50. (Schlotthauer, Jour. A.V.M.A.)

## PREPUCE AND PENIS

**Edema.** Stasis-edema of the sheath in geldings and stallions appears in cachectic diseases. If of long duration, induration of the tissues may occur.

**Foreign bodies.** Concretions of smegma and inorganic salts are often observed in stallions and geldings.

**Prepucitis and penitis.** These are frequent in the dog and pig. The prepucial opening may be closed (phimosis). Pressure upon the prepuce results in the dripping of a yellowish, purulent fluid. The mucosa of the penis and prepuce is in a state of catarrhal inflammation. Solitary lymph follicles in the mucosa are enlarged. The urethral orifice is usually not involved.

There is no specific cause. If the penis becomes protruded and held out by the swollen prepuce, the condition is called paraphimosis.

**Tumors.** The most important tumor of the external genitals of the horse is the squamous-cell carcinoma of the glans penis. It is a tumor of low malignancy occurring chiefly in geldings. There is some experimental evidence that it may be incited by the accumulation of smegma. In young bulls a papilliform fibroma of the prepuce and penis is due to a virus. This tumor also occurs in the vagina and vulva of the heifer (see page 565). In the dog the most important external genital neoplasm is the histosarcoma (see page 566).

# REFERENCES

Barker, C. A. V.: 1956. Some observations on testicular calcification in bulls. Canad. Jour. Comp. Med., 20:37.

Creech, G. T.: 1935. Organic lesions in swine caused by *Brucella suis*. Jour. A.V.M.A., 39:211.

Dow, C.: 1958. The cystic hyperplasia-pyometra complex in the bitch. Vet. Rec., 70:1102.

Durrell, W. B.: 1949. Infectious vaginitis in cattle: a review with additional notes. Canad. Jour. Comp. Med., 13:32.

Fitch, C. P., Boyd, W. L., Bishop, L. M., and Kelly, M.: 1939. Localization of *Brucella abortus* in the bovine uterus. Cornell Vet., 29:253.

Garm, O.: 1949. Investigations on cystic ovarian degeneration in the cow with special regard to etiology and pathogenesis. Cornell Vet., 39:39.

Goodpasture, E. W.: 1942. Virus infection of the mammalian fetus. Science, 95:391.

Hadlow, W. J., Grimes, E. F., and Jay, G. E.: 1955. Stilbestrol-contaminated feed and reproductive disturbances in mice. Science, 122:643.

Helmboldt, C. F., Jungherr, E. L., and Plastridge, W. N.: 1953. The histopathology of bovine mastitis. Storrs Agr. Exper. Sta., Bul. 305.

———, Mochrie, R. D., Plastridge, W. N., Eaton, H. D., Easterbrooks, H. L., and Hale, H. H.: 1954. Effects of abnormal machine milking on the histopathology of udders of first-calf heifers free of mastitis. Amer. Jour. Vet. Res., 15:15.

Hofstad, M. S.: 1940-41. The changes produced by *Brucella abortus* in the milk and udder of cows infected with Bang's disease. Report of N. Y. State Vet. Coll., 138.

Innes, J. R. M., Seibold, H. R., and Arentzen, W. P.: 1952. The pathology of bovine mastitis caused by *Cryptococcus neoformans*. Amer. Jour. Vet. Res., 13:469.

Kendrick, J. W., Gillespie, J. H., and McEntee, K.: 1958. Infectious pustular vulvovaginitis of cattle. Cornell Vet., 48:458.

Kennedy, P. C., Frazier, L. M., and McGowan, B.: 1956. Epididymitis in rams: Pathology and bacteriology. Cornell Vet., 46:303.

Kernkamp, H. C. H., Roepke, M. H., and Jasper, D. E.: 1946. Orchitis in swine due to *Brucella suis*. Jour. A.V.M.A., 98:215.

Lumb, W. V.: 1952. Prostatic calculi in a dog. Jour. A.V.M.A., 121:14.

McEntee, K.: 1950. Fibropapillomas of the external genitalia of cattle. Cornell Vet., 40:304.

McNutt, S. H.: 1934. Brucella infection of swine. Jour. A.V.M.A., 37:620.

———, Purwin, P., and Murray, C.: 1928. Vulvovaginitis in swine (preliminary report). Jour. A.V.M.A., 26:484.

Marsh, H.: 1932. Mastitis in ewes caused by infection with a *Pasteurella*. Jour. A.V.M.A., 34:376.

Pattison, I. H.: 1958. The progressive pathology of bacterial mastitis. Vet. Rec., 70:114.

Pier, A. C., Gray, D. M., and Fossatti, M. J.: 1958. *Nocardia asteroides*: A newly recognized pathogen of the mastitis complex. Amer. Jour. Vet. Res., 19:319.

Plastridge, W. N., Williams, L. F., Easterbrooks, H. L., Walker, E. C., and Beccia, R. N.: 1951. Vibriosis in cattle. Storrs Agr. Exper. Sta., Bul. 281.

Schalm, O. W.: 1944. Gangrenous mastitis in dairy cows. Vet. Med., 39:279.

Simmons, G. C., and Kittall, W. T.: 1953. Epididymitis of rams. Australian Vet. Jour., 29:33.

Simon, J., and McNutt, S. H.: 1957. Histopathological alterations of the bovine uterus. I. Studies with *Vibrio fetus*. Amer. Jour. Vet. Res., 18:53.

Spencer, G. R., and McNutt, S. H.: 1950. Pathogenesis of bovine mastitis. II. The pathologic alterations in twenty-five mammary glands. Amer. Jour. Vet. Res., 11:188.

Talanti, S.: 1959. Observations on pyometra of dogs with reference to the hypothalamic-hypophyseal neurosecretory system. Amer. Jour. Vet. Res., 20:41.

Thomsen, A.: 1934. Brucella infection in swine. Acta Path. et Microbiol. Scand., Suppl. 21:1.

# CHAPTER 20

# Nervous System

## FUNCTIONAL DISTURBANCES

Diseases of the nervous system throw the body or its parts out of adjustment with the environment either in relation to conditions which exist outside of the body or within the body. Since the nervous tissue consists primarily of neurons linked together in conduction paths, disease processes which upset the adjustment of the body to its environment must affect these nerve cells and the conduction paths formed by them. Functional disturbances of the nervous system become all the more apparent if it is realized that when a neuron is destroyed it cannot be replaced. If functional disturbances of any one part of the brain deserve emphasis over those of other parts, they should be those which have their seat in the brain stem. Here lie the conduction paths between the higher parts of the brain and the spinal cord, the sensory and motor nuclei of most of the cranial nerves, the correlation neurons between these nuclei, much of the central mechanism of the postural reflexes, the reflex centers which control the heart rate, respiration, vasomotor tone, and also the reflex centers for the regulation of the motor and secretory activities of the alimentary canal.

Irritants which alter the colloids of the nerve cells and their fibers disturb the ir-ritability and electromotor force of these structures. The direct result is a disturbance in the functions of the nervous system, and the indirect effect is an alteration in the activities of the organs. Naturally, if the central nervous system is the place of attack, the functional disturbances may be numerous and widespread throughout the body. Not only may the mental state of the animal be affected but also its body movements, its gland secretions, and its reflexes. What has just been said should be qualified to some extent because focal alterations in the central nervous system may not produce general manifestations but only local ones in rather circumscribed areas of the body. Functional disturbances which owe their existence to alterations in the central nervous system are said to have a central origin. In contradistinction to this, those having their origin in diseased nerves are peripheral.

When the nervous system fails to perform its duties, there must be present alterations in structure. Sometimes the deviations in structure can be easily seen, even with the unaided eye. For instance, one may have no difficulty in viewing a cerebral hemorrhage, a glia-cell tumor, an encysted parasite, a brain abscess, an area of encephalomalacia, or a thrombus of a vessel of the brain. In other cases no changes can be detected grossly, but microscopic alterations involving the neurons, the glial cells, the leukocytes, and the blood vessels explain the disturbed nervous function. As a basis for still other altered functions, not even microscopic changes can be demonstrated. In these cases it seems reasonable to attribute the abnormal nervous activity to physiochemical alterations in the make-up of the neurons and fibers because changes in their function can be produced experimentally by injecting into animals certain chemicals such as phosphoric acid and the salts of sodium, potassium, and magnesium.

We previously mentioned that the various activities of the brain can be upset by disease. These changes are loss of consciousness, nervous depression, and increased nervous irritability.

Loss of consciousness may be due to the effect of various toxic agents upon the brain. This mental state appears in many of the intoxications — mineral, plant, bacterial, and parasitic. It is attributable in part to changes in the neurons and fibers which are demonstrable microscopically and to others which are not, but which are believed to be due to chemical changes in the protoplasm of the nerve cells and fibers. Of a different nature is the loss of consciousness caused by stunning. Here injury to the delicate dendrites of the nerve cells is supposed to interfere with the passage of impulses along the conduction paths.

The degree and duration of loss of function of the central nervous system depend upon the cause and extent of the injury. Slight damage may result in only temporary insensibility. If the medulla is involved, there may be paralysis of the body and legs, and serious disturbance of respiration and circulation. If the loss of consciousness is complete, a state of coma is said to exist. In coma the animal lies outstretched and motionless; its reflexes are gone; the pupils of the eyes do not react to light stimulus; respiration is slow and at times irregular; the pulse and heartbeat are weak, and the skin cool. Death may occur in a few minutes or after several days.

A second type of change of mental state is nervous depression. Underlying this condition is pressure upon the brain. The origin of the pressure may be hemorrhage within the cranial cavity, a brain tumor, collection of fluid within the ventricles, and inflammatory exudate in the meninges or in the brain. The signs of brain pressure are loss of feeling, diminished cerebral reflexes, partial or nearly complete loss of consciousness, sleepiness and muscular incoordination. The animal stands in a stupor, leans its body against objects, hangs its head, and rests it upon objects where possible. The eyelids droop, and the pupils are dilated. It may remain standing for hours in the same place, sometimes with a pair of its legs crossed or with the front legs flexed in a kneeling posture. At other times the animal may walk about with uncertain gait, frequently running into objects. Sometimes it may turn in circles. It does not respond to calls, to commands, or to being struck. No attempt is made to fight flies even though they bite savagely. The animal rarely attempts to eat, but if it does, it simply holds the food in its mouth without attempting to masticate. It pushes its nose deeply into water placed before it. The ears seem to be lifeless and the lips may hang in a flaccid condition. Circulation and respiration are slow. These are the classic signs of disturbed nervous function in equine encephalomyelitis.

The primary causes of the increased cranial pressure — the ones listed above — bring on two important secondary causes, namely, venous hyperemia and lymph stasis. Whenever the brain swells, the outflow of venous blood and the cerebrospinal fluid is hindered. The extreme pressure upon the neurons apparently results in the depression.

The third change in the mental state due to pathological conditions of the brain is nervous excitement. It results from congestion and inflammation of the brain and its coverings, from thermic influences, and from the effects of certain toxins. The manifestations of excitement are variable. The chief symptoms are those of delirium and mania. The animal abruptly ceases to be docile. It becomes extremely antagonistic to the usual means of restraint, fights, and in the fighting may injure itself since it deliberately runs into objects used to restrain it. Climbing over objects, throwing itself, crying out, biting the attendant or other animals, and frothing at the mouth are all signs of nervous excitement. Furthermore, the eyes have a starey or wild look, and the conjunctiva is red. The animal may finally fall in convulsions. Rabies is a disease in which these are the signs of disturbed nervous function.

Disturbances in nervous function also occur in muscles. In general there are two types of disturbances: one characterized by increased muscular activity (spasm), and the other by loss of contractility (paralysis and paresis). Underlying each there are usually alterations in innervation.

Muscle spasms are characterized by sudden, violent, involuntary contractions. The contractions may be persistent, that is, continuous (tonic spasms), or intermittent (clonic spasms). A mild form of spasms confined to groups of muscles is called tremor. It appears in epidemic tremor of chicks, a filtrable viral disease. In tremor the involuntary contractions follow one another in close succession. When muscle spasms become so widespread that they involve the whole body, including the limbs, the condition is designated convulsions. Convulsions often occur in puppies infested with ascarids. An attack of alternating tonic and clonic spasms accompanied by loss of consciousness is termed epilepsy. Strong continuous contractions of large areas of the voluntary musculature of the body are characteristic of tetanus — the nervous intoxication produced by the exotoxin, tetanospasmin, of *Clostridium tetani.*

The few illustrations already given of agents which cause muscle spasm indicate that we have some knowledge of the etiology of conditions displaying this type of disturbed function. There are several other known causes such as strychnine, ergotine, lead, carbon dioxide, and tremetol, the toxic principle in white snake root (*Eupatorium urticaefolium*). Toxic substances produced in the body, such as urea or its precursor, should be included also. Diseases of the parathyroids or removal of these glands result in tetanic muscle spasms referred to as tetany. These glands are an important part of the mechanism which regulates the amount of calcium in the blood. When the parathyroids cease to function, the calcium level of the blood falls. Calcium is then removed from the muscles. Their lowered calcium content is manifested by increased neuromuscular irritability (tetany). A heritable defect in pigs is characterized by tremor, but the cause is unknown. It is well known that the tetanospasmin of *Clostridium tetani* unites chemically with the protoplasm of nerve cells in the medulla and produces its damage. In some cases the exact nature of the injury done by the irritant which causes the spasms is not known.

The results of spasms on the body are governed by the location of the increased muscle irritability. If the contractions are of short duration, the injury is slight. If of longer duration, there may be muscle atrophy. Spasms of the respiratory muscles naturally interfere with respiration and may result in asphyxia. This is common in tetanus. Spasms of the masseters and related muscles may result in starvation.

The second form of neuromuscular functional disturbance is paralysis (the complete immobility of a muscle) and paresis (the incomplete loss of motion). An alteration in muscle function which has some resemblance to paralysis is ataxia. In it, however, the muscle has not lost its mobility but its movements are uncertain, awkward, and not coordinated. There is apparently some interference in the conduction of nervous impulses to the muscle.

Among the causes of paralysis the one of concern at the moment is defective innervation of the muscle. The disturbance in innervation may have its location in the motor centers or in the conduction paths. Regardless of where it is, the movement of the motor impulses is inhibited and immobility results. The injuries to the nerve cells and fibers which give rise to the loss of muscle function may be due to degeneration of the nerve cells produced by poisons such as bacterial toxins and lead salts. The injuries to the nerves may be due to stretching, bruising, pressure, or may be associated with certain nutritional deficiencies such as occur in blacktongue of dogs and goose-stepping of pigs. Anatomically, the place of injury can be in any of the motor centers of the brain, in the cord, or in the peripheral nerves. Paralysis arising in the brain cortex and in the peripheral nerves is usually unilateral (hemiplegia). A bilateral paralysis of the posterior part of the body and hind limbs resulting most often from injury to the cord is called paraplegia.

The results and termination of paralysis are governed by the duration of the condition, the extent of body involvement, the importance of the function of the muscles affected, and by the cause of the lost muscular action. When one recalls the functions of the various muscles of the body and then considers the effects of their loss of function, he will have little difficulty in listing the possible terminations of paralysis.

## REACTION OF NERVOUS TISSUE TO INJURY

In studying the reaction of tissues to injury, the reader will have become increasingly aware that four factors in the reaction have been considered to be very fundamental. These factors are (1) tissue susceptibiliy to injury, (2) tissue ability to regenerate, (3) ability of the connective tissue to fill the gap left by the destruction of the highly specialized parenchyma cells, and (4) the relative usefulness of the substituted tissue to the organ. It has been noted that, in general, these factors vary greatly with the different tissues. To be specific, let us consider them briefly as applied to cardiac muscle and hepatic epithelium, and then in greater detail as applied to nervous tissue.

Cardiac muscle is moderately susceptible to injury, has no ability to regenerate, is readily repaired by substitution, and is able to function very well in the presence of the less specialized tissue. Hepatic epithelial cells on the other hand are easily destroyed, have unusual ability to regenerate, are often replaced by connective tissue if the injury is long-continued and mild, but may atrophy because they are compressed and poorly nourished as a result of the presence of this connective tissue.

Nervous tissue is quite susceptible to injury. Destroyed neurons cannot be replaced by healthy remaining neurons. Repair by substitution with connective tissue is not the rule, and when it does occur, it is often a liability rather than an asset. Since the central nervous system is not composed of structural units like lobules, but is a system in which special functions are under the control of particular areas, it is apparent that injury of these areas may result in much more alarming effects than the destruction of a few units of a lobulated organ. In studying the reaction of nervous tissue to injury, it is essential to examine separately the reaction of the neurons and the glial cells.

**Neurons.** For the most part, neurons are damaged by hypoxic, toxic, and traumatic influences. Hypoxic injury occurs in cardiac failure and in pneumonia, toxic injury in infectious diseases, particularly the neurotropic viral diseases, and traumatic injury in severe concussion. In cats in which fever has been induced experimentally and in cats from whom food and water have been withheld prior to death, nerve-cell bodies (cytons) shrink, the chromidial substance undergoes progressive changes, and glycogen is depleted. One must keep this in mind when examining the brains of animals which have gone through a period of fever, dehydration, and starvation before death.

Because the cytons are large, it is relatively easy to study the microscopic signs of injury in them. The nuclei may become displaced to the periphery of the cells, swell or contract, and undergo karyolysis or karyorrhexis. The nucleolus may enlarge and shift to the periphery of the nucleus. In the plasma, lipochrome and fat become more prominent. The Nissl bodies undergo fragmentation and dissolution (chromatolysis). This change, however, must not be confused with the disappearance of the Nissl bodies which occurs after long periods of work. With the disappearance of the Nissl bodies, vacuoles appear in the plasma of the nerve cells. Sometimes the Nissl bodies undergo a condition similar to pyknosis of nuclei instead of fragmentation and chromatolysis. The neurofibrils display changes last. They may take basic stains, undergo fibrolysis, or become thicker and capable of intense impregnation with certain agents.

Up to a certain point a degenerating cyton can recover. Just what that point is has not been determined, but it is probably dependent upon the severity of the nuclear injury. When the protoplasmic changes pass this point, the nucleus dies. Along with these degenerative changes in the cytons there may also be signs of injury to the nerve fibers. Most prominent among these are swelling of the fibers and degeneration of the myelin sheath (demyelination). The destroyed fibers in the central nervous system do not regenerate.

It is often difficult to differentiate between post-mortem autolytic changes and ante-mortem cyton degeneration because they have close resemblance. Aids in distinguishing ante-mortem degeneration are changes in the surrounding tissue which usually accompany cyton degeneration — such changes as hyperemia, edema, and phagocytic response. Even these changes, however, can occur within the last few hours before death and can be said to be agonal. The matter is further complicated because in some cases the neurons can be killed almost instantly before the surrounding tissues can react.

**Neuroglia.** The supporting tissue of the central nervous tissue is composed of glial cells and their fibers. These cells are the astrocytes, oligodendroglia, and microglia. The astrocytes form the bulk of the matrix.

In hypoxic and toxic conditions they are stimulated to proliferate. Their increase is designated gliosis. The same stimulus that will kill neurons will often cause gliosis. If the distribution of the causative agent is uniform throughout the brain, the gliosis is diffuse. If, however, the brunt of the injury is borne by localized areas, the gliosis is focal. Proliferating astrocytes cannot fill in defects like young vascular connective tissue.

It should be said here that defects in the central nervous system are seldom repaired by connective tissue. When they are, the connective tissue usually originates from the adventitia of blood vessels. In brain abscesses the connective tissue may form a thin capsule around the pus. Astrocytes proliferate outside the capsule. Because astrocytes cannot fill in a defect in brain tissue, such an area becomes a cyst bordered by astrocytes.

Microglia are the brain histiocytes and as such belong to the reticuloendothelial system. In an area containing degenerated nerve cells they increase in number and show marked amoeboid movement and phagocytic activity. They phagocytize hemosiderin from hemorrhages and fat from necrotic nervous tissue, especially from disintegrating myelin sheaths. They cannot digest the fat very well and as a consequence often become large "foam cells."

When cytons begin to degenerate, both microglia and oligodendroglia move in around the sick cells. They are said to be satellites of the neurons. This congregating of the glial cells is designated satellitosis. When cytons die, these glial cells phagocytize them, a phenomenon termed neuronophagia or neuronophagy.

In hematoxylin-eosin-stained sections only the nuclei of glial cells are stained. The microglia look like mononuclear phagocytes. The astrocyte and oligodendroglia nuclei are larger. Astrocytes and microglia are most numerous in the gray matter and oligodendroglia in white matter. Degenerative bodies (corpora amylacea) sometimes form in astrocytes. When the astrocytes die and disappear, the corpora amylacea remain free in the brain tissue.

## THE CEREBROSPINAL FLUID IN NEUROPATHOLOGY

The ventricles of the brain, the spinal canal, and the subarachnoid space contain most of the cerebrospinal fluid. It serves as a medium for metabolic exchange and as a cushion for the central nervous system. The principal part of the fluid is probably formed by the choroid plexus in each of the four ventricles. The flow of the fluid appears to be from the lateral ventricles through the foramina of Monro into the third ventricle, from the third ventricle through the aqueduct of Sylvius into the fourth ventricle, and from the fourth ventricle out through the foramina of Luschka and Magendie into the subarachnoid space which is continuous from one end of the central nervous system to the other.

Of special significance in neuropathology is the communication of the subarachnoid space with lymph spaces or sheaths of the blood vessels of the brain and similar spaces or sheaths of the cranial nerves,

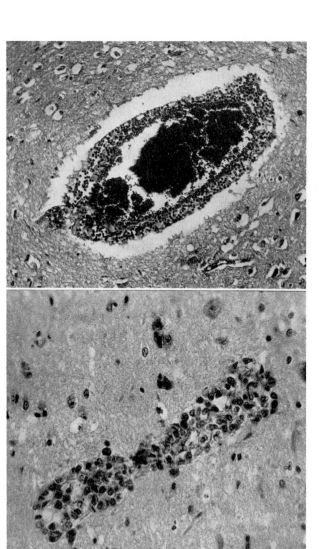

Fig. 20.1 — Acute nonsuppurative encephalitis.
**Above:** Perivascular cuffing with leukocytes in a horse brain.
**Below:** Similar process in the cerebrum of a guinea pig.
(Doyle, Jour. A.V.M.A.)

particularly of the olfactory nerve. The communication originates in the following manner: The pia and arachnoid invest the vessels of the brain for a considerable distance into the brain substance. This means that the subarachnoid space also extends down into the brain tissue with these vessels.

The subarachnoid space therefore has a perivascular relationship to the vessels and is called the space of Virchow-Robin. The inner lining of the space is a continuation of the arachnoid membrane and blends with the adventitia of the vessels. The outer layer of the space — the layer which is in direct contact with the brain tissue — is the pia. The flow of lymph in the perivascular space is from the brain tissue towards the subarachnoid space. The significance of the perivascular space is that in brain infections it becomes a collecting place for inflammatory exudate (Figs. 20.1 and 20.2).

The subarachnoid space also communicates with the lymph spaces of the cranial nerves. This is of importance with respect

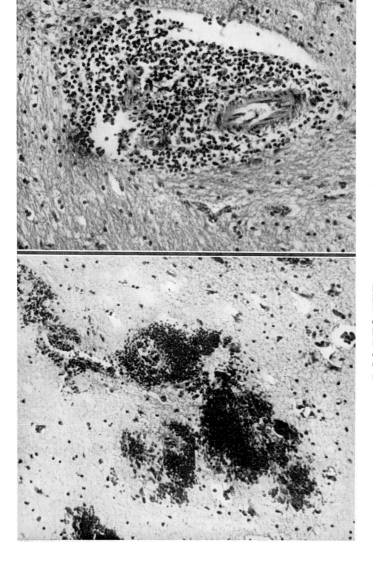

Fig. 20.2 — **Above:** E q u i n e infectious encephalomyelitis. Brain showing perivascular cuffing. ×200.
**Below:** Moldy corn poisoning. Brain showing hemorrhage and necrosis.
(Schwarte, Biester, and Murray; Jour. A.V.M.A.)

to the olfactory nerve because nasal infec-tions may ascend this lymph sheath to the subarachnoid space and incite an inflam-mation of the meninges which has the pos-sibility of extension to the brain proper by retrograde passage up the perivascular spaces of the brain (Figs. 20.3 and 20.4). This is believed to happen in equine en-cephalomyelitis and at times in strangles.

The principal structures for the outflow of the cerebrospinal fluid are the arachnoid villi. These tiny organs are simply thin-walled outpouchings of the arachnoid membrane into intradural and subdural venous sinuses.

Normal cerebrospinal fluid of the dog is clear, colorless and of a watery consis-tency. Biochemically the content of globu-lin is never more than 10 mg/100 ml, uric acid 0.3 to 1.8 mg/100 ml, and the leuko-cyte count is very low. In disease the quan-tity and quality of fluid may change. In ca-nine distemper, for instance, the fluid may increase in quantity and become cloudy, occasionally sticky. If the fluid is blood tinged, it is red or pale yellow. Biochemi-cally, the globulin increases up to 130 to 1,500 mg/100 ml, uric acid up to 1.1 to 4.7 mg/100 ml, and lymphocytes and some-times neutrophils become numerous.

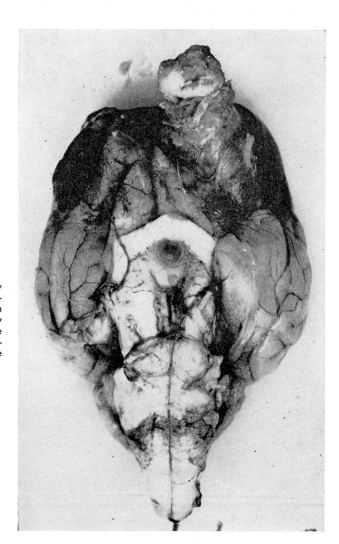

Fig. 20.3 — Abscess of the olfactory lobe of a ewe resulting from the ex-tension of a purulent inflammation from the ethmoid region, probably by way of the lymph sheaths of the olfactory nerve. (Department of Vet-erinary Pathology, Michigan State University.)

## CENTRAL NERVOUS SYSTEM
### Disturbances of Circulation

HYPEREMIA

Acute general active hyperemia is present when bacterial or viral diseases involve the entire central nervous system (rabies, viral equine encephalomyelitis and hog cholera).

Acute focal active hyperemia is seen in the vicinity of abscesses, tumors, and infarcts, where focal brain injury has occurred or where repair is taking place.

Chronic general passive hyperemia occurs if there is a passive hyperemia resulting from a lesion in the heart or lung or an obstruction to the flow of blood from the brain such as thrombosis of both jugular veins. The histological evidence of chronicity is based on the presence of an increased number of glial cells throughout the brain and spinal cord.

Chronic focal passive hyperemia occurs if a tumor or abscess presses upon a vein or a thrombus forms within a vein causing a reduction in the flow of blood from a local area of the brain. The chronicity of the lesion is based on the degree of glial cell proliferation in the area. This vascular disturbance is seldom diagnosed in animals because vascular disease is relatively uncommon as compared to man and because good venous anastomoses occur in most parts of the brain.

HYPOSTATIC OR POST-MORTEM CONGESTION

Hypostatic congestion (post-mortem congestion) is commonly observed in the central nervous system and is frequently confused with the hyperemia of inflammation. The poorly supported blood vessels in the meninges, brain, and spinal cord become engorged with blood if the head is lower than the rest of the body. This is

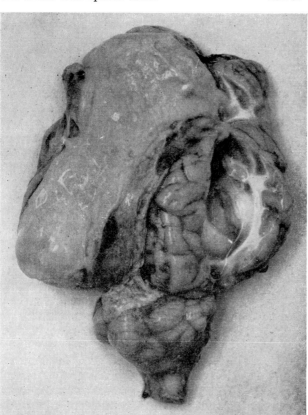

Fig. 20.4 — Purulent meningitis in a ewe. (Department of Veterinary Pathology, Michigan State University.)

often observed in the dog when the head is allowed to hang over the edge of the post-mortem table for a period of time prior to necropsy examination.

## ANEMIA

**General anemia** of the entire brain and spinal cord is present when anemia involves the entire individual. It is seen in infectious viral anemia of the horse, parasitic anemia accompanying gastrointestinal parasitism, excessive hemorrhage, and the anemias associated with a deficiency of iron, copper, and the vitamin B complex.

The brain and spinal cord are whiter than normal, and the blood vessels contain a decreased number of erythrocytes and are correspondingly less prominent. Microscopic and sometimes macroscopic areas of liquefactive necrosis as well as gliosis and neuron degeneration may be present if the anemia persists for a long period of time. Areas of necrosis are common in the human but are seldom observed in animals. These alterations are the result of a deficiency of oxygen.

**Local anemia** or ischemia occurs as the result of a deficiency of arterial blood in a local area of the brain or spinal cord. Thrombosis and embolism are the two principal causes of ischemia.

**Thrombosis** occurs when the endothelium of a vessel is injured. It is observed in hog cholera, traumatic injury associated with skull fractures, abscesses or tumors invading the wall of a vessel, and in arteriosclerotic diseases in which the intima of the blood vessel is damaged.

**Embolism** is a common cause of local anemia. The emboli consist of agglutinated bacteria, portions of a thrombus, parasites, tumor cells, or agglutinated erythrocytes. The emboli usually originate from lesions in the lung or in the left atria or ventricle of the heart but may also originate from lesions in the carotid artery and its branches.

If the blood supply is not adequate to supply the nutritive and oxygen require-ments of the area, **infarction** occurs. The infarcted area may be pale or red depending on the number of erythrocytes and the amount of hemoglobin present. The result of infarction is liquefactive necrosis of the involved area.

## HEMORRHAGE

Hemorrhage in the brain and spinal cord is most frequently associated with septicemic diseases such as hog cholera, anthrax, pasteurellosis, malignant edema, and leptospirosis in the dog as well as the invasion of the central nervous system by various pyogenic bacteria such as staphylococci, streptococci, salmonella, corynebacteria, and pleuropneumonia-like organisms. Invasion of blood vessels by tumors will also result in hemorrhage.

Hemorrhage occurs as the result of traumatic injury following automobile accidents or gunshot wounds. Hemorrhages may result from arteriosclerotic diseases of the brain and spinal cord. However, this is very uncommon in domestic animals, but is reported to occur in old parrots and ostriches. Hemorrhage is often present in the brain of the newborn as the result of traumatic injury during birth.

## EDEMA

Edema of the brain and spinal cord occurs when local or general passive hyperemia is present. It is also observed when an increased permeability of the vascular endothelium exists as occurs in shock and antu poisoning. The edematous fluid is observed in a perivascular location in the Virchow-Robin space.

A special form of edema in the central nervous system is known as **hydrocephalus**. If the fluid accumulates in the subdural and subarachnoid spaces, it is known as **external hydrocephalus**. If the fluid is found in the ventricles of the brain, it is designated as **internal hydrocephalus** (Figs. 20.5 and 20.6). The accumulation of fluid in the spinal canal is called **hydromyelia**. In most instances this fluid is a secretory substance and not a true transudate.

The cause of hydrocephalus is basically an interference with the flow of cerebrospinal fluid from the choroid plexuses of the lateral ventricles through the ventricular system and into the subarachnoid space where the fluid is absorbed by the arachnoid villi. In most instances it occurs as the result of a malformation in the central nervous system during the development of the embryo. The septum pellucidum may be incomplete so that the fornix is not supported. The unsupported fornix acts as a valve preventing fluid from entering the interventricular foramen. The interventricular foramen, the third ventricle, or the fourth ventricle may be incomplete so that the flow of fluid is restricted or prevented. The leptomeninges of the cerebellum may be continuous with the leptomeninges of the medulla oblongata, and as a result the cerebrospinal fluid cannot flow from the fourth ventricle into the subarachnoid space. The distortion of the skull of the brachycephalic breeds of dogs interferes with the flow of cerebrospinal fluid from the fourth ventricle into the subarachnoid space. The arachnoid villi may be imperfectly formed or may be absent and, as a result, the cerebrospinal fluid will not be absorbed.

Hydrocephalus can be a hereditary disease and is often lethal. Both recessive and dominant types are described. In some herds of cattle the incidence of the abnormality is so high that considerable economic loss is experienced by the owner and drastic changes in the bloodlines must be carried out. In most instances the introduction of selected males from other families will prevent additional losses without too great a disruption of the herd breeding program. It is observed in bulldog calves in

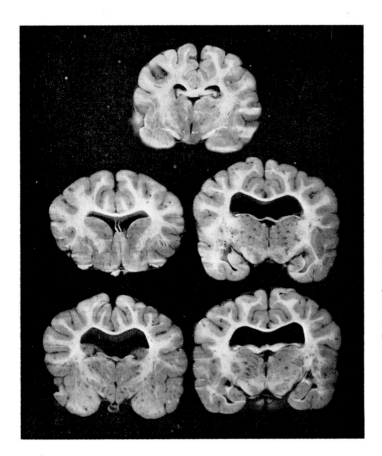

Fig. 20.5 — **Above:** Cross section of normal brain of a dog. **Below:** Four cross sections of brain of dog showing internal hydrocephalus. Both brains were obtained from fox terriers of similar age and size. (Schlotthauer, J o u r . A.V.M.A.)

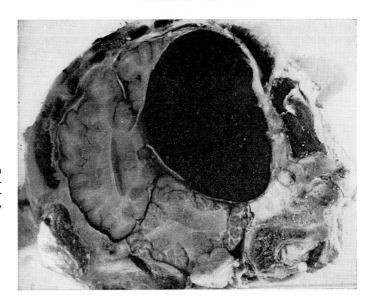

Fig. 20.6 — Porencephally in a calf. Most of left hemisphere of brain has undergone pressure atrophy. (Sholl, Jour. A.V.M.A.)

many breeds of cattle, but especially in the Dexter breed. It is also seen in the Holstein-Friesian, Jersey, Shorthorn, Hereford, and Telemark breeds. In the canine it is observed most frequently in the boxer, Boston bulldog, English bulldog, dachshund, and Chihuahua.

Acquired hydrocephalus occurs when tumors, abscesses, or parasite cysts compress some portion of the ventricular system so the cerebrospinal fluid cannot pass. It may also occur if clotted blood, exudate, parasites, or cholesteatomas are found within the lumen of the ventricular system and cause obstruction to the flow of fluid.

Whatever the cause of the hydrocephalus with its increased intracranial pressure, a resulting complication occurs. The cerebellum and medulla are forced posteriorly into the foramen magnum. As the pressure is increased, the fourth ventricle is stenosed until cerebrospinal fluid cannot pass into the subarachnoid space, and as a result it accumulates in the ventricular system anterior to the fourth ventricle.

External hydrocephalus is usually the result of rupture of the thin dorsal wall of the third ventricle which allows the fluid to escape into the subarachnoid space between the cerebral hemispheres and the cerebellum.

Hydromyelia may occur when the pressure cone resulting from intracranial pressure interferes with the free flow of cerebrospinal fluid into the subarachnoid space but allows it to enter the anterior opening of the spinal canal. Hydromyelia may also occur if the anterior opening of the spinal canal is stenosed by the pressure cone resulting from increased intracranial pressure, or if clotted blood, exudate, parasites, or tumors obstruct the spinal canal.

The result of hydrocephalus is compression atrophy of the surrounding nervous tissue causing depression, incoordination, ataxia, and death. If hydrocephalus occurs before ossification of the skull bones takes place, enlargement of the cranium may occur, the fontanelles are open, and the sutures between the cranial bones are broad and membranous. If ossification of the cranial bones has taken place before the hydrocephalus occurs, the enlargement of the skull is not present.

### Disturbances in Growth

APLASIA

Aplasia of portions of the brain and spinal cord are observed in young animals. If the aplasia interferes with the locomotion of the animal, the individual dies from starvation or is destroyed by the owner.

Small areas of aplasia that do not cause locomotor disturbances are usually not observed.

## HYPOPLASIA

Since the anomalies and malformations of the central nervous system are frequently examples of hypoplasia, the more common disorders of growth will be mentioned briefly under this heading. It should be remembered that the alterations, even though described only in one species, may occur in other species of animals as well.

**Congenital posterior paralysis in calves** occurs in Norwegian Red Poll and Red Danish breeds of cattle. A similar disease is observed in other breeds as well. The animals have a paralysis of the posterior limbs and may show muscle tremors. Lesions are present in the anterior portion of the thalamus.

**Congenital posterior paralysis in swine** is described in the Cornwall, Landrace, and Large White breeds. A similar disease is encountered by swine practitioners in other breeds. Paralysis is present at birth. Lesions are found in the cerebrum, cerebellum, and spinal cord.

**Spastic paresis in cattle** is observed in the Holstein-Friesian and Simmental breeds. It is observed in calves and is characterized by rigidity of one or both gastrocnemius muscles. **A periodic spastic paresis** is observed in older cattle and is characterized by sudden contraction of the muscles of one or both rear legs. This disease occurs in several breeds of cattle. Opinion varies as to the etiology. Some claim it is a congenital hereditary defect while others have attempted to associate it with a phosphorus deficiency.

**Congenital tremors in swine** is observed in several breeds. The symptoms appear at birth or shortly thereafter, and as many as one-third of the pigs may show symptoms. The muscular tremors and rigidity of the skeletal muscle interfere with the movement of the pigs, and starvation may occur. Many pigs will recover in 3 to 4 weeks. The etiology is not clear. Intrauterine viral infections, deficiency diseases, and hereditary diseases have been

suspected. The vaccination of sows for hog cholera will produce neurological symptoms of this type in the newborn.

**Congenital muscle spasms in goats** has been observed for many years and was first described in Texas in 1904. These animals, because of their peculiar reaction to sudden noise, are frequently shown in carnivals. When the goats are startled by a sudden noise their limbs become rigid and they are unable to move about. No lesions have been described in the central nervous system. It is believed the site of the abnormality is in the muscle fiber.

**Spinal muscular atrophy in the canine** is a hereditary lethal disease. It is observed in the great Dane, Saint Bernard, and in great Danes crossed with bloodhounds. The basic lesion is necrosis of the motor neurons in the spinal cord which results in atrophy of the muscles of the posterior limbs.

**Cerebellar hypoplasia** and even aplasia are observed in pigs, dogs, cats, lambs, goats, and calves. There is considerable variation in the extent of the hypoplasia that is present. Hereditary forms of the disease are described. Kittens with cerebellar hypoplasia are often unable to stand, and roll in a lateral direction in an attempt to gain their feet. Transplacental viral infections of the fetus may result in this malformation in the cat. In cattle the disease is most frequently observed in the Jersey, Hereford, Guernsey, and Holstein-Friesian breeds.

## HYPERTROPHY

Hypertrophy of the brain and spinal cord may occur, depending on the cell that is involved. The neuron does not increase in size even though there is considerable locomotor or mental activity. The glia do increase in size when stimulated by various irritants, and this would cause some enlargement of the brain and spinal cord. The microglia show the greatest degree of hypertrophy.

## HYPERPLASIA

Hyperplasia of the central nervous system occurs when there is an increase in the number of glia. The glia, especially the microglia, increase in number when the brain is exposed to hypoxia and various gastrointestinal intoxications. Hyperplasia of the neurons does not occur.

### METAPLASIA

Metaplasia within the central nervous system involving the nervous tissue proper does not occur. Metaplasia may occur in the connective tissue of the meninges and blood vessels, and when this occurs, cartilage and bone may be found.

### ATROPHY

Atrophy of the brain and spinal cord is frequently observed. Atrophy of the cerebrum is very well demonstrated in cases of hydrocephalus in which the cortex may be less than 5 mm. in thickness. Pressure atrophy (Fig. 20.6) also occurs in the vicinity of tumors, abscesses, hematocysts, depression fractures of the skull, protruding herniated intravertebral discs, and in areas of ischemia.

Senile atrophy of the brain as observed in the human is seldom observed in domestic animals. The explanation for this is that the arteriosclerotic diseases responsible for the atrophy in man are not present in domestic animals. In addition, animals seldom live long enough to reach the stage of senility when central nervous system changes would be expected. Even in severe cachexia the animal usually dies before any visible alteration of the brain occurs. Atrophy is often described with infectious diseases, but evaluation of the cellular reaction usually indicates it is a disturbance in cell metabolism or necrosis rather than atrophy.

## Disturbances in Cell Metabolism

### CLOUDY SWELLING

Cloudy swelling occurs in the cells of the brain and spinal cord, especially in the neurons, as the result of hypoxia or the irritation produced by toxic substances or infectious agents. It is the first response of the cell to injury. The neurons or the glia become larger than normal and the cellular outline more round as fluid accumulates in the cell cytoplasm. In addition, the cellular structures are not as distinct as normal. There are no gross alterations that would indicate cloudy swelling is present.

### FATTY DEGENERATION

Fatty degeneration of the cells of the brain and spinal cord appears as fat droplets in the cytoplasm of the cells. The alteration is observed in the neurons. Great care should be taken in diagnosing fatty degeneration in the glia since some of the glia, especially the microglia, are phagocytic, and their cytoplasm will contain lipoid droplets that have been phagocytosed.

### HYDROPIC DEGENERATION

Hydropic degeneration may occur in the brain and spinal cord. It is a continuation of cloudy swelling in which droplets of edematous fluid are observed in the cytoplasm of the neurons and glia. Special staining technics must be used to differentiate these droplets from fat and other cytoplasmic inclusions.

### AMYLOID INFILTRATION

Amyloid infiltration does not occur in the central nervous system of most domestic animals. Para-amyloid infiltration of the spinal nerve roots has been recognized as a clinical entity for some time in Shetland colts in Maryland and Virginia. The animals show posterior incoordination that resembles the symptoms shown by wobblers.

### GLYCOGEN INFILTRATION AND GOUT

Glycogen infiltration does not occur in the central nervous system. How frequently **gout** involves the central nervous system is not clear because the brain and spinal cord are seldom examined.

### PIGMENTATION

Pigmentation is commonly observed in domestic animals. **Melanin** is most frequently found in the pia mater of the anterior one-fourth of the brain. It is especially common in heavily pigmented animals such as Angus and Jersey cattle and Hampshire sheep. Focal areas of melanin are found in other portions of the meninges and at times within the brain and spinal cord. The pigment does not produce a local inflammatory reaction, and there are no clinical symptoms associated with its presence.

Hemoglobin and its derivatives may impart color to the tissues. Imbibition of the tissues with blood results in a **pink** or **red** color and is found when post-mortem changes have taken place or when hemorrhage into the central nervous system has occurred and the erythrocytes have undergone autolysis.

**Yellow** or **green** colors may be observed in the vicinity of hemorrhage when hematoidin diffuses into the tissues.

A **brown** color is seen when hemosiderin is found in an area where hemorrhage has occurred.

**Black, gray,** and **green** coloration is observed when putrefaction has taken place.

In older individuals a **brown** pigment is frequently observed in neurons, glia, and ganglion cells. It is referred to as wear-and-tear pigment. The pigment does not give the Prussian blue reaction for iron, absorbs the common fat and lipoid stains, and is fuchsinophilic. Because of its fuchsinophilic properties it is frequently mistaken for a Negri body.

CALCIFICATION

Calcification within the central nervous system is frequently observed but is more commonly found in the meninges than in the brain and spinal cord proper. The two antecedents of calcification — degenerating or dead tissue and faulty circulation — must be present before calcium is deposited. For that reason it is found in abscesses, infarcts, parasite lesions, sites of old hemorrhage, in masses of exudate, and in necrotic neurons.

Calcification and siderosis of the globus pallidus is frequently observed in the equine and occasionally in the bovine. The minerals are deposited in the walls of the blood vessels and in the neurons. Although degenerative and necrotic changes are observed in the area, clinical symptoms are seldom shown even when the alterations are extensive.

**Necrosis**

COAGULATIVE NECROSIS

Coagulative necrosis involves the neurons and the glia. It occurs as the result of severe injury to the cells produced by hypoxia, chemical poisons, bacterial or viral toxins, or the invasion of a cell by a viral agent.

No macroscopic alterations are observed. Microscopically, the cells are swollen and approach a more globular shape, the Nissl substance becomes less prominent and may entirely disappear (tygrolysis or chromolysis), the cytoplasm stains more intensely with eosin, and the nucleus shows karyoschisis, karyorhexis, karyopyknosis, or karyolysis. The necrotic neurons may have microglia accumulating around them, a process that is known as **satellitosis.** When the microglia phagocytose the necrotic neuron, the process is called **neuronophagia.**

Some neurons appear shrunken, and the Nissl substance stains more intensely with hematoxylin. This alteration is quite common and does not represent necrosis. If the cells are dead, satellitosis and neuronophagia should be present.

The necrotic change does not involve just the body of the neuron but is also observed in the axon and dendrite of the necrotic cell as these structures extend through the central nervous system, and especially in the axons that are grouped together in tracts. The axis cylinder as well as the medullary sheath shows the same swelling and increased eosin staining as does the body of the neuron. The myelin of the sheath is extremely unstable and disintegrates into a lipoid substance. The process is known as lipoid degeneration. On cross section the swollen axis cylinders are often designated as "myelin balls," which is incorrect as longitudinal section reveals them to be columns or the altered axis cylinder. The necrotic axon is surrounded and infiltrated with microglia which remove the dead tissue by phagocytosis.

The lipoid in the degenerating myelin

can be stained with various fat stains such as osmic acid, but the staining is extremely fickle and unreliable and must be carefully controlled if erroneous interpretations are to be prevented.

Focal areas of coagulative necrosis are observed in any portion of the brain when *Spherophorus necrophorus* is brought to the brain by the blood stream from lesions in other parts of the body. The necrotic tissue is sharply demarked from the surrounding tissue just as it is in other organs.

## LIQUEFACTIVE NECROSIS

Liquefactive necrosis is a common alteration in the brain and spinal cord because of the unstable nature of the lipoidal substance of which the central nervous system is composed. Necrosis of the brain is practically always of the liquefactive type. The reason that liquefactive necrosis occurs in the brain instead of the coagulative and caseous types is that the nervous tissue contains little coagulable albuminous material but is rich in lipoids. When a portion of the central nervous system undergoes death, the autolytic enzymes quickly bring about the disintegration of myelin into a liquid mass that consists primarily of lipoid.

Liquefactive necrosis is also observed when the central nervous system is invaded by pyogenic microorganisms. The enzymes of the neutrophils bring about rapid liquefaction of myelin and other structures.

Infarction is one of the common causes of liquefactive necrosis. The infarct may occur as the result of an embolus composed of tumor cells, a portion of a thrombus, or parasites, or it may occur as the result of thrombosis of an artery. The location and the extent of the infarction depend on the type of injury and the size of the vessel obstructed. Infarcts are most frequently found in the cerebrum.

Infarction is often observed in the dog following injury from an automobile when the head is traumatized. Frequently, the dog appears to have recovered from the initial injury, but 3 weeks to 6 months later, neurological symptoms return and at necropsy a large area of liquefaction is observed in the brain, usually in the cerebrum and particularly in the vicinity of the motor center.

**Moldy corn disease (cornstalk disease).** Liquefactive necrosis frequently occurs in equines that have consumed moldy corn or cornstalks for a period of at least 30 days. This is called moldy corn disease or cornstalk disease. The necrotic areas are found in the white matter of the cerebrum and cerebellum but are best demonstrated in the white matter between the motor centers of the cerebral cortex and the corpus striatum. The lesions may be macroscopic or microscopic in size. Gross lesions are observed in about 50 per cent of the cases. Sometimes the necrotic area has a yellowish color as compared to the surrounding white brain. At other times, especially if the necrotic area is large, hemorrhage occurs into the necrotic tissue so that the area is readily discernible (Fig. 20.7). When the larger areas are incised, the necrotic tissue flows from the brain, leaving a cavity that is often spanned by the remains of blood vessels. The pathogenesis of the lesion has never been explained.

**Thiamine deficiency.** Some fur-bearing animals (foxes, mink, and ferrets), when fed continuously a ration containing certain frozen fish such as carp, Great Lakes herring, Atlantic herring, Pacific mackerel, mullet, northern pike, smelt, and suckers, display the following symptoms: anorexia, weakness, emaciation, diarrhea, and paralysis terminating in death. Because the symptoms of paralysis are so prominent, and because the disease was first recognized on the Chastek Fur Farm in Minnesota, the disease is usually referred to as **Chastek paralysis.** The species of fish named above are not deficient in thiamine but they contain, in some but not all parts of their bodies, an enzyme which destroys the thiamine before the fish are fed. If the fish are ground, the enzyme is distributed throughout all of the meat and the enzymatic action can take place more quickly.

A similar disease is described in cats fed a ration consisting exclusively of canned fish. The cats show ataxia, convulsions, paralysis, coma, and death.

The macroscopic lesions in fur-bearing animals and cats consist of bilaterally symmetrical focal areas of hemorrhage and liquefactive necrosis in the periventricular gray matter and are most consistent and severe in the inferior colliculi. The microscopic examination reveals much more extensive hemorrhage and necrosis than was seen on macroscopic examination.

A thiamine deficiency occurs in horses feeding on *Equisetum arvense*. This plant contains a heat-labile, thiamine-destroying factor that inactivates the thiamine normally found in the intestinal tract of the horse. Hemorrhages and neuron degeneration are found in the cerebrum, caudate nucleus, corpora quadrigemina, and cerebellum.

As a result of a thiamine deficiency,

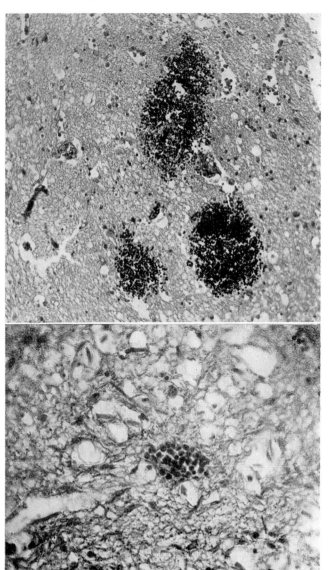

Fig. 20.7 — **Above:** Minute hemorrhages of the brain of a horse. **Below:** Focal infiltration of lymphocytes in brain stem of a horse. (Doyle, Jour. A.V.M.A.)

ataxia, muscle tremors, and convulsions occur in **calves** and **lambs** fed exclusively a milk diet. Thiamine is ordinarily synthesized in the rumen of cattle and sheep by the bacteria that are present. If the proper thiamine-producing flora are not present, this synthesis will not occur. A thiamine deficiency is particularly apt to occur if sulfonamide drugs or antibiotics are administered, as these drugs will destroy the rumen flora that is capable of producing thiamine. A similar deficiency can occur in pigs and horses.

**Vitamin E deficiency.** Liquefactive necrosis often occurs as the result of a vitamin E deficiency in the ration of chicks and poults. The disease is known as **encephalomalacia.** The necrotic areas are most frequently observed in the white matter of the cerebrum and the cerebellum. Hemorrhage into the necrotic area is quite common, and because of the presence of the blood, the necrotic areas can often be seen on macroscopic examination.

**Copper deficiency.** A copper deficiency, locally known as swayback, is a disease of sheep in England, Africa, Australia, South America, and the United States. In the United States it is found in Montana and Colorado. It is observed in other ruminants such as the alpaca and llama.

The incidence of the disease varies from year to year depending on climatic conditions and food availability. The disease is observed in newborn lambs. The ewes show no symptoms or lesions. The severity of the disease varies a great deal from those cases that show only a slight locomotor disturbance to those that are so paralyzed they are unable to stand or move about. Some animals are blind. The lambs die from starvation since they are unable to stand to nurse or to move about and follow the ewe. Many lambs can be kept alive for long periods of time if they are bottle fed.

The lesions are located in the white matter of the cerebrum. There is considerable variation in the degree of injury that is present. In mild cases, only microscopic lesions are observed, while in more severe cases the entire white matter of the cerebrum may undergo liquefactive necrosis. The lesions are bilaterally symmetrical. The areas of necrosis may be yellow or amber in color and gelatinous in consistency or they may be fluid in nature and contain blood which gives them a red color. The gray matter of the brain is not involved. Secondary degeneration of nerve tracts is observed in the middle and posterior portions of the brain as well as in the spinal cord.

**Blue tongue.** Liquefactive necrosis of the white matter of the cerebrum occurs in lambs whose mothers had been vaccinated for blue tongue while they were pregnant.

**Focal symmetrical spinal necrosis** involving both ventral horns of the spinal cord is observed in sheep in the Rift Valley of Kenya. The lesions are found in the cervical and lumbar portions of the cord. There is progressive incoordination and paralysis.

### CASEOUS NECROSIS

Caseous necrosis occurs when the brain is invaded by *Mycobacterium tuberculosis*. The necrotic area appears as a dry, crumbly, yellowish-white mass that may contain areas of calcification. Microscopically, no cellular or architectural structures are visible in the necrotic tissue. The area is surrounded by a zone of glia, lymphocytes, and macrophages and contains acid-fast bacteria.

### GANGRENE

Gangrene of the central nervous system is the result of the invasion by saprophytic microorganisms. They are introduced by traumatic injuries of the skull or as septic emboli from areas of gangrene in the lungs. A special form of gangrene (malignant edema) occurs when members of the clostridium group of organisms invade the central nervous system.

## Inflammation
### TERMINOLOGY

**Encephalitis** — inflammation of the brain.
**Myelitis** — inflammation of the spinal cord.

**Encephalomyelitis** — inflammation of the brain and spinal cord.

**Meningitis** — inflammation of the meninges.

**Pachymeningitis** — inflammation of the dura mater.

**Leptomeningitis** — inflammation of the pia mater.

**Meningoencephalomyelitis** — inflammation of the meninges, brain, and spinal cord.

### SEROUS ENCEPHALITIS AND MYELITIS

Serous encephalitis and myelitis occur when a mild irritant involves the central nervous system. They are characterized by the cardinal signs of inflammation and increased amount of cerebrospinal fluid. Since the amount of cerebrospinal fluid is difficult to ascertain in the necropsy specimen, this diagnosis is seldom made because it must be based on the character and the amount of the exudate.

### FIBRINOUS ENCEPHALITIS, MYELITIS, AND MENINGITIS

Fibrinous encephalitis, myelitis, and meningitis are observed in sheep and cattle when the central nervous system is invaded by pasteurella. They are characterized by the cardinal signs of inflammation and the abundance of fibrin in the subarachnoid and Virchow-Robin space, in the ventricles of the brain, and in the spinal canal. Fibrinous inflammation is also observed in sporadic bovine encephalitis and pleuropneumonia-like infection in swine.

### SUPPURATIVE ENCEPHALITIS, MYELITIS, AND MENINGITIS

Suppurative encephalitis, myelitis, and meningitis are observed in all species of animals. They are characterized by the cardinal signs of inflammation, and the principal constituent of the exudate is pus. The inflammation is focal or diffuse. If it involves the meninges, it is usually diffuse, and when it involves the brain or the spinal cord, it occurs as focal or multiple focal areas of inflammation.

The pyogenic organisms are usually staphylococci, streptococci, corynebacteria, pasteurella, listeria, and pleuropneumonia-like organisms. These bacteria enter the brain by direct extension from a suppurative otitis, suppurative ophthalmitis, suppurative inflammations of the nasal passages and the cribiform plate, and suppurative inflammation of the tail following docking or perforating wounds of the skull. The organisms also reach the brain through the lymphatic channels that accompany the nerves or by way of the blood stream. Multiple abscesses in the brain and spinal cord are found when a septicemia is present. A suppurative inflammation often gains entrance to the central nervous system by way of the atlanto-occipital joint. In these cases there is a suppurative polyarthritis that often originates from an umbilical infection, pneumonia, or an infection with pleuropneumonia-like organisms. The injury produced by the suppurative inflammation will depend on the location of the lesions, the number of abscesses, and whether the inflammation is focal or diffuse.

**Listeriosis.** *Listeria monocytogenes* produces a suppurative meningoencephalomyelitis in the bovine and ovine. The disease is infectious but apparently not contagious. The character of the organism suggests it is a soil type and probably grows free in nature. Outbreaks of the disease are frequently associated with the feeding of silage, particularly pea silage.

The route of invasion of the organism into the central nervous system is not known. In rodents and birds, where a septicemia with multiple abscesses is present, it is easy to explain how the organism invades the central nervous system. However, in sheep and cattle, a septicemic form of the disease is apparently not present and the organism is usually found only in the central nervous system. It has been suggested that the organism gains entrance to the cranial cavity by way of the cranial nerves or through the cribiform plate from the nasal cavity. At the National Institute of Animal Health in Japan the results of an interesting research project indicate that the organism invades the oral or nasal mucosa and travels along the trigeminal nerve to the brain stem where the most important lesions of listeriosis are located. There is some evidence that a virus may accompany and assist the organism in producing the infection.

There are no macroscopic alterations in the brain or spinal cord. The most characteristic lesion is the presence of multiple microabscesses in the caudate and lenticular nuclei, thalamus, corpus quadrigemina, medulla oblongata, cerebellum, and to some extent in the spinal cord. This should be kept in mind when bacteriological or histological examinations are made.

In the early stages of the disease the microabscesses contain numerous neutrophils and occasional eosinophils and glia. As the disease progresses and recovery begins to take place, the neutrophils decrease in number, and finally the area contains only phagocytic glia. Liquefactive necrosis occurs in the region of the microabscesses. Degenerative and necrotic alterations are observed in the neurons and tracts in the vicinity of the areas of inflammation.

In addition to these alterations there are active hyperemia, perivascular cellular cuffs composed of lymphocytes and neutrophils, and a general gliosis of the brain and spinal cord. Examination of the blood does not reveal the monocytosis observed in the rabbit.

The lesions, particularly in recovering cases of listeriosis, are quite similar to those of sporadic bovine encephalomyelitis.

Bacteriological staining methods reveal that the organism is located in the microabscesses. Usually the bacteria are few in number. Since these microabscesses are often located at rather wide intervals in the brain stem, large amounts of brain material must be cultured or inoculated into experimental animals if an isolation is to be accomplished. Large plugs of tissue are removed from the thalamus, pons, medulla oblongata, and ventral portions of the cerebellum. These are ground in a mortar and pestle with sterile saline until a thick fluid mixture that may be drawn into a pipette or syringe is obtained. The material is then added to four blood agar pour plates in one gram, one-half gram, one-quarter gram, and one-eighth gram amounts. The plates are incubated at 37.5° C. for 48 hours. The growth appears as small colonies surrounded by a zone of hemolysis. It is absolutely essential that large amounts of brain material be cultured if the organism is to be isolated with any degree of accuracy.

The placing of the brain in the refrigerator for several days or weeks to increase the number of organisms present is not satisfactory from a diagnostic point of view because the diagnosis is so delayed that it is of little value to the farmer or the practitioner. In addition, in routine postmortem material the specimen is often contaminated and, as a result, if the brain is held in the refrigerator, it becomes so overgrown with proteus and coliform bacteria that a bacteriological isolation is difficult or impossible.

A very satisfactory method of isolation is to inoculate mice intracerebrally with brain material. Mice are quite susceptible to infection, and the organism is present in large numbers in the brain of mice succumbing to the disease.

**Sporadic bovine encephalomyelitis.** Sporadic bovine encephalomyelitis is a disease of cattle caused by a pleuropneumonia-like organism. It begins as a fibrinous pleuritis, peritonitis, pericarditis, arthritis, and tendovaginitis followed by neurological disturbances. When the arthritis involves the occipital joint, the infection may extend into the central nervous system. Although many of the animals in a herd may show stiffness, abdominal tenderness, increased respiratory rate, and swollen joints and tendon sheaths, it is only in a few animals that the organism invades the central nervous system. It is for this reason that the central nervous lesions are sporadic and that the disease has been named sporadic bovine encephalomyelitis.

The lesions of the central nervous system consist of an acute diffuse meningoencephalomyelitis in which the inflammatory exudate consists primarily of lymphocytes and macrophages intermixed with neutrophils. In some animals the neutrophils are very abundant. Perivascular cuffing is present, and the Virchow-Robin space is filled and sometimes distended with lymphocytes, macrophages, and neutrophils. The meningitis is usually most severe in the vicinity of the brain stem and the cerebellum. Focal cell accumulations composed of lymphocytes, macrophages, microglia, and neutrophils are found throughout the brain but are most numerous in the brain stem and the cerebellum. In addition, there is a general gliosis, neuron degeneration, and necrosis and myelin degeneration.

The lesions are similar to those observed in listeriosis. The major differences are: (1) Fewer neutrophils are present in the cellular infiltration in sporadic bovine encephalomyelitis, especially in the focal cellular accumulations in the brain and spinal cord. (2) In sporadic bovine encephalomyelitis, the macrophage is much more prominent and the meningeal cellular reaction is more pronounced. (3) Gram-positive bacteria can be demonstrated in the focal lesions in listeriosis while the pleuropneumonia-like organisms cannot be demonstrated in sporadic bovine encephalomyelitis.

**Suppurative encephalitis in sheep.** An acute diffuse suppurative meningoencephalomyelitis is observed in sheep in England. A delicate hemolytic Gram-positive organism has been isolated from the exudate. It occurs during the summer months, and the morbidity and mortality are low.

Macroscopic lesions consist of the cardinal signs of inflammation and a tenacious green pus on the meninges of the brain stem and the cerebellum. The microscopic lesions consist of a typical suppurative inflammation of the meninges, brain, and spinal cord.

A diffuse fibrino-suppurative meningo-encephalomyelitis is occasionally observed as isolated cases or as a flock problem in the United States. *Pasteurella multocida* is isolated from the exudate.

EOSINOPHILIC ENCEPHALITIS IN SWINE

Eosinophilic meningoencephalomyelitis is observed in swine that have consumed excessive amounts of salt (NaCl). Swine are not poisoned by salt if water is available. If they have consumed large amounts of salt in the feed or in the brine from pickling vats, salt poisoning may occur if they cannot obtain sufficient water to dilute the salt. The encephalitis is apparently due to the sodium ion as similar lesions can be produced with other sodium salts such as sodium lactate.

Clinical examination of the animals reveals recurrent convulsive seizures, blindness, rigidity, normal temperature, and the tendency to back up when the tetanic and convulsive seizures appear. The posterior weakness, twisting, and swaying observed in hog cholera are not present.

Macroscopic lesions are not observed in the central nervous system. The microscopic lesions consist of a diffuse meningoencephalomyelitis that is most severe in the cerebrum and especially in the cerebral cortex. The most prominent lesion is the presence of large numbers of eosinophils in the exudate. The eosinophils are prominent in the perivascular cuffs and in the meninges. Degenerative changes may be observed in the neurons. There is a slight general gliosis.

HEMORRHAGIC MENINGOENCEPHALOMYELITIS

An infectious hemorrhagic encephalomyelitis, apparently caused by a viral infection, has been described in France and Germany. A specific disease characterized by a hemorrhagic meningoencephalomyelitis does not occur in the United States. Many descriptions of hemorrhagic encephalomyelitis are probably just hemorrhage or liquefactive necrosis with hemorrhage into the necrotic tissue.

Occasionally inflammation of the central nervous system is characterized by large amounts of blood in the exudate so that a diagnosis of hemorrhagic inflammation may be made. This type of lesion is observed in anthrax, blackleg, malignant edema, strangles, hog cholera, salmonellosis, pasteurellosis, and infections with pleuropneumonia-like organisms in cattle and swine.

### LYMPHOCYTIC MENINGOENCEPHALOMYELITIS

Lymphocytic meningoencephalomyelitis is the most important form of central nervous system inflammation in animals. It is characterized by the cardinal signs of inflammation, and the lymphocyte is the principal constituent of the exudate. Viruses are the main cause of lymphocytic inflammation. It is a prominent lesion in infectious viral encephalomyelitis of the horse, epizootic fox encephalitis, rabies, hog cholera, canine distemper, epidemic tremors of chicks, and Newcastle disease.

**Macroscopic appearance.** Macroscopically, in most cases there are no changes, or only uncharacteristic changes. Often, there is only hyperemia of the pia mater, the brain, and cord, slight edema of the pia mater, and slight increase of the ventricular fluid. Rarely, there are petechiae. A macroscopic examination cannot be depended upon as a means of diagnosis. A microscopic examination is more dependable, but even here it must be remembered that in the early stages the extent of the lesions is limited, and careful and painstaking search of several areas of the brain and cord must often be made before changes are disclosed.

**Microscopic appearance.** Microscopically, the changes involving the blood vessels are the most striking. While the degenerative changes of the parenchyma are less easily demonstrated, they are certainly no less important, and from the clinical standpoint the effect of them is even more manifest. The vascular change is hyperemia, which results in perivascular edema and is accompanied by an infiltration of the adventitia and perivascular lymph-sheaths with lymphocytes (so-called perivascular cuffs) (Figs. 20.1 and 20.2). These changes occur in both the

white and gray matter, and in varying degrees in the pia mater. The nerve cells and fibers undergo degenerative changes. As a result of these changes, focal miliary softening may occur. The vascular and perivascular changes give rise to pressure, which in turn is partly responsible for the grave clinical manifestations of encephalitis. Reparative processes begin early and are characterized by a proliferation of the larger glial cells (gliosis). The degenerated and necrotic cytons are surrounded by microglia cells (satellitosis) and eventually phagocytosed by them (neuronophagia). Death of the animal usually occurs, but if it survives, permanent injury remains and is manifested clinically by paresis or paralysis as in canine distemper and encephalomyelitis of horses.

Several of the diseases mentioned above are characterized by the presence of cell-inclusion bodies (rabies, canine distemper, fox encephalomyelitis). These bodies are round or oval and are capable of being stained with specific dyes. Their nature is unknown. By some they are considered to be the infective agent, by others as a coating around the infective agent produced by the infected cells, and by still others as products of cell degeneration.

**Rabies** is an acute viral disease transmitted from animal to animal or from animal to man by the bite or scratch of a rabid individual. The incubation period varies from about 8 days to 3 months or more. Probably some animals that become infected are carriers and do not show clinical symptoms. Clinically, it is characterized by locomotor disturbances, irritability, aggressiveness, the tendency to chase moving objects such as chickens, a hoarse bellow, and paralysis.

It is caused by a virus, *Formido inexorabilis*, which is found in the central nervous system, the salivary gland and its secretions, and at times in other tissues and organs such as the lacrimal, mammary, and pancreatic glands, and the blood. The route of the virus from the point of inoculation to the brain is not known. It has been suggested the virus travels through the body along the nerve axons but others contend it is disseminated through the body by way of the blood and lymphatic systems.

There are no characteristic macroscopic lesions in the brain or any other organ. Traumatic injury and general passive hyperemia are seen in many individuals. It is often said the presence of foreign bodies in the gastrointestinal tract is commonly observed in rabies. The authors have not been able to substantiate this in the many cases of rabies they have observed.

The microscopic lesions consist of a very diffuse and severe meningoencephalomyelitis. In general it can be said to be the most severe lymphocytic inflammation observed in the central nervous system of domestic animals in this country. It is true that cases of rabies do occur in which the lymphocytic inflammation is moderate or mild in degree, but great care should be exercised in these cases before a diagnosis is made, and above all a viral isolation and identification should be accomplished.

Perivascular lymphocytic cuffing is present. There are both focal and diffuse gliosis. The focal glial nodules are frequently called Babes nodules. They are indicative of rabies but are not diagnostic as similar nodules are found in other viral diseases. Coagulative necrosis of neurons and glia is present as well as satellitosis and neuronophagia. In addition, there is a diffuse lymphocytic meningitis.

The most characteristic alteration is the presence of an intracytoplasmic inclusion body that is known as the **Negri body** (Fig. 20.8). When the tissue is stained with basic fuchsin and methylene blue, the inclusion body appears as a purplish-red body in which centrally-located blue granules are found. One or more Negri bodies can be found in a single cell. The Negri bodies are most numerous in the ganglion cells of the hippocampus and to a lesser extent in the Purkinje cells of the cerebellum. They vary in size from 1 to 20 microns in diameter. Negri bodies are not

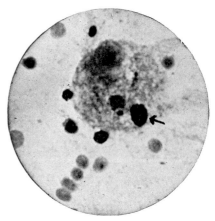

Fig. 20.8 — A Purkinje cell of a cow with 3 distinct Negri bodies. ×450. (Department of Veterinary Pathology, Iowa State University.)

present in about 25 per cent of rabid animals and in many of the remaining 75 per cent they are so few in number as to be easily overlooked.

To complicate the diagnosis of rabies, there are pseudo-Negri bodies in the brain that are often extremely difficult or impossible to differentiate from true Negri bodies. These **pseudo-Negri bodies** are most frequently observed in puppies, cats, and rodents. In all animals the number of pseudo-Negri bodies increases with autolysis and putrefaction.

Mitchell (unpublished research at Iowa State University) prepared a series of cat brain impression smears from rabid and non-rabid cats in which Negri bodies and pseudo-Negri bodies were present. When these slides were submitted to a number of individuals engaged in rabies control work, it was found that these individuals could not differentiate the Negri body from the pseudo-Negri body.

It is our opinion that if only an impression smear of the brain is made, no greater than 50 per cent accuracy in rabies diagnosis can be obtained. It is absolutely imperative that animal inoculation, viral isolation and identification, and histological examination be made of all brains suspected of having rabies if an accurate diagnosis is to be made. It must also be remembered that the rabies virus is not as resistant to adverse surroundings as we are often led to believe. It is destroyed by putrefaction, freezing and thawing, exposure to room temperature, and improper diluents. Normal physiological saline is extremely toxic to the virus.

**Pseudorabies** is an infectious viral disease of cattle, swine, dogs, cats, and rabbits. The viral agent is designated as *Scelus suillum*. Clinically, it is characterized by a rapid course (12 to 36 hours), intense itching at the site of inoculation, incoordination, and paralysis. It is usually said that furor is absent, but some individuals having pseudorabies are just as aggressive as rabid animals.

The virus apparently enters the body in feed and water contaminated with urine, mucus, and saliva from infected animals and by cutaneous inoculation at the site of traumatic injury. The virus is disseminated through the body by way of the nerves and the blood stream.

Macroscopic lesions are not observed in the central nervous system. Microscopic lesions apparently vary with the species of animal in which the disease occurs. A diffuse lymphocytic meningoencephalomyelitis as well as coagulative necrosis of the ganglion cells is observed in the rabbit and pig. The encephalitis is mild in pigs and they usually recover. However, the central nervous system symptoms and lesions must be differentiated from hog cholera by animal inoculation since no pathognomonic lesions are present.

A meningoencephalomyelitis apparently does not occur in cattle in pseudorabies. The lesions consist of coagulative necrosis of the ganglion cells and neurons. These necrotic changes are particularly prevalent in the ganglion cells and neurons at the spinal ganglia and cord level corresponding to the area of pruritis if it is present.

**Malignant head catarrh.** Although much has been written about malignant head catarrh in cattle in the United States and many cases have been diagnosed, no proven cases are on record. Since the virus has not been isolated and identified in the United States, it can rightfully be said that the disease does not exist. Other diseases will simulate malignant head catarrh, and unless a viral isolation is made, the diagnosis cannot be substantiated. A mucopurulent rhinitis and conjunctivitis in addition to an encephalitis do not constitute a diagnosis.

The lesions in the central nervous system consist of a diffuse lymphocytic meningoencephalomyelitis, and perivascular lymphocytic cuffing is prominent. Diffuse gliosis is present, and focal accumulations of microglia are found throughout the brain. Coagulative necrosis of the neurons is present and is most pronounced in the vagus and glossopharyngeal nuclei. Stenius in Finland described acidophilic cytoplasmic inclusion bodies in 50 per cent of the brains affected with malignant head catarrh in the neurons of the medulla oblongata, brain stem, spinal cord, and less frequently in the pyramidal cells of the cerebral cortex when stained with Mallory's phloxine-methylene blue.

Sheep are said to be carrier hosts of the disease. No lesions are found in the central nervous system of sheep.

**Hog cholera encephalitis.** An acute diffuse lymphocytic meningoencephalomyelitis is observed in hog cholera in 80 to 90 per cent of the animals in which the disease is allowed to run its course. In the United States it is the only diffuse lymphocytic meningoencephalomyelitis that occurs in swine as a herd problem and in which there is a high morbidity and mortality rate.

All parts of the meninges, brain, and spinal cord are involved. Perivascular lymphocytic cuffing is prominent. Degeneration and necrosis of the neurons are observed. Multiple petechial hemorrhages and occasionally larger hemorrhages are found throughout the brain. Some strains of virus produce considerable endothelial damage that results in thrombosis of the smaller blood vessels.

Similar lesions are observed in the central nervous system of swine affected with **African swine fever.** Thrombosis of the blood vessels of the central nervous system tends to be more prominent in African swine fever.

A similar inflammatory reaction may be observed in pseudorabies in swine. However, in pseudorabies the morbidity and mortality are low and, in addition, the inoculation of rabbits with brain material results in typical symptoms of pseudorabies while the hog cholera virus will not affect the rabbit.

**Enzootic porcine viral encephalitis (Teschen disease).** Enzootic encephalomyelitis produces a typical lymphocytic inflammation of the central nervous system of swine. It does not occur in the United States. The lesions are found in the gray matter of the spinal cord, the medulla oblongata, cerebellum, pons, and thalamus. The cerebrum is only slightly involved. The lesions are most severe in the gray matter of the spinal cord, especially in the ventral horns. Neuron degeneration and necrosis are prominent lesions.

Although not found in the United States at the present time, it can be differentiated from hog cholera by the distribution of the lesions. Hog cholera is a diffuse meningoencephalomyelitis involving both the gray and white matter of the brain. Enzootic encephalomyelitis is a disease found in Europe. The lesions are limited to the gray matter of the medulla oblongata, pons, thalamus, and especially that of the spinal cord.

**Canine distemper encephalitis.** Much confusion exists about the lesions of canine distemper in the central nervous system. The reason for this is that several viral agents have been isolated from the brain of the dog. These agents have not been sufficiently studied to establish them as being distinct from the distemper virus, *Torpeia canis.*

The virus produces a typical diffuse lymphocytic meningoencephalomyelitis. There are no macroscopic lesions. Not all dogs affected with distemper develop central nervous system symptoms and lesions. The incidence of encephalitis varies with the outbreak. Sometimes only 10 per cent of the distemper-affected dogs show encephalitis while in other outbreaks the incidence is much higher. Likewise, the intensity of the reaction varies from dog to dog. In some animals the lesions are slight while in other dogs in the same litter or outbreak, a very severe diffuse encephalitis is present.

The most typical microscopic lesions of canine distemper in the central nervous system are found in the cerebellum and medulla adjacent to the ependyma or meninges in the vicinity of the fourth ventricle. Usually the most intense reaction will be found just below the ependyma or the meninges and becomes less intense deeper in the surrounding brain tissue.

The lesions in the vicinity of the fourth ventricle consist of perivascular lymphocytic cuffing, myelin degeneration, hyperplasia of the capillary endothelium, gliosis, and phagocytosis of the degenerating myelin by the microglia. Acidophilic intranuclear inclusion bodies are usually present in the glia in this area of inflammation. The inclusion bodies are difficult to find in other portions of the brain. The canine distemper inclusion bodies are differentiated from rabies inclusion bodies by their intranuclear location in the glia, while the Negri body is found in the cytoplasm of the neurons, particularly in those of the hippocampus and the Purkinje cells of the cerebellum.

Since canine distemper and infectious canine hepatitis occur in young dogs and may occur in the same dog at the same time, it has been reported that the hepatitis virus produces an encephalitis. However, it has been well demonstrated that the encephalitis is caused by the distemper virus and that the hepatitis virus does not produce an encephalitis in the dog.

**Disseminated encephalomyelitis in mature dogs.** A disseminate type of encephalomyelitis has been described in older dogs (usually 2 to 7 years). Isolation of an infectious agent or transmission of the disease have not been accomplished.

The dogs appear to be "dummies" and although apparently oblivious to their environment, they are able to eat and drink. The animals show motor incoordination as evidenced by swaying, weaving, and wobbling, whether standing or in motion. They frequently fall when they attempt to change direction or shake themselves. Many stand with crossed legs, some circle constantly, others push against solid objects, and still others show a decided "hackney gait." Although they are not blind, there is a disturbance of vision. Paralysis and convulsions are not observed.

No macroscopic lesions are observed in the central nervous system. The microscopic lesions are a typical diffuse lymphocytic meningoencephalomyelitis. Perivascular cuffing is the most outstanding lesion, and frequently the cuffs are several times the diameter of the blood vessel. Neuron degeneration is observed but is not confined to any particular area. Both diffuse and focal gliosis are present. No inclusion bodies are found. The extensive demyelinization observed in canine distemper is not present. The lesions are most severe in the cerebrum, particularly in the motor centers, somewhat less severe in the thalamus and pons, moderate lesions in the cerebellum, medulla oblongata, and corpus striatum, and slight lesions in the spinal cord.

**Infectious meningoencephalomyelitis of foxes.** An acute diffuse lymphocytic meningoencephalomyelitis caused by *Tortor vulpis* is observed in foxes. The only macroscopic lesions consist of multiple petechial hemorrhages that are most pronounced in the medulla oblongata and the spinal cord.

The microscopic lesions consist of focal hemorrhage, meningitis, perivascular cuffing, capillary endothelial hyperplasia, diffuse and focal gliosis, and neuron degeneration and necrosis. Intranuclear acidophilic inclusion bodies are found in the endothelial cells of the capillaries. The intranuclear location of these inclusion bodies in the capillary endothelium is of value in differentiating this disease from canine distemper and rabies. The disease can also be differentiated from canine distemper by the use of a ferret. The ferret is susceptible to canine distemper but not to fox encephalitis.

Although the virus of fox encephalitis is identical with infectious canine hepatitis, no encephalitis is observed in the brain of dogs affected with this virus.

**Neorickettsial meningitis.** Mild nonsuppurative leptomeningitis is a constant lesion of so-called salmon poisoning of dogs, an infectious disease incident to the Pacific coast from northern California to southern Washington. This meningitis is unusual because it partakes of the characteristics of a mild chronic inflammatory reaction. The participating large mononuclear cells seem to arise from the arachnoid cells. The reaction is most pronounced in the leptomeninges of the cerebellum where the large mononuclears accumulate in the subarachnoid space. Some of the macrophages contain bodies resembling rickettsias. These may be the rickettsia *Neorickettsia helminthoeca*, which is believed to be the cause of salmon poisoning. Other cells prominent in the inflammatory reaction are lymphocytes and plasma cells.

**Infectious viral equine encephalomyelitis.** This disease, commonly called sleeping sickness by the layman, is an acute viral disease of horses and mules occurring in epizootics, and characterized by an inflammation in the brain (encephalitis) and cord (myelitis), and terminating fatally in about 50 per cent of the cases. The disease usually makes its appearance in July or August, declines in the fall, and disappears in winter. It is caused by a filtrable virus, *Erro equinus*, of which there appear to be two strains in the United States, so-called **western** and **eastern strains.** There is evidence that some of the waterfowl may serve as reservoirs of the infection. One of the gophers (*Citellus richardsoni*) has also been incriminated. In the latter case a tick, *Dermacentor andersoni*, was the vector. The period of incubation in field cases is 3 to 8 days or more.

The probable natural modes of infection are: (1) by insect transmission (mosquitoes and possibly flies and ticks), (2) by the nares, and (3) by oral abrasions. The virus remains in the blood stream during the earlier stages. It has an affinity for the nervous tissue.

There are no pathognomonic macroscopic lesions in the brain, spinal cord, or the other organs of the body. There is a general passive hyperemia as is shown by the splenic swelling. At times a complicating pneumonia and cutaneous gangrene are present. The pneumonia is the result of hypostatic congestion and the inhalation of food because of throat paralysis. The cutaneous gangrene occurs as the result of pressure necrosis of the skin in animals that are recumbent for long periods of time. Examination of the mucous membranes reveals a muddy color that is said to be icterus; however, the icteric index does not substantiate this clinical observation.

The microscopic lesions consist of a typical diffuse lymphocytic meningoencephalomyelitis with perivascular cuffing, diffuse and focal gliosis, neuronal degeneration and necrosis, satellitosis, and neuronophagia. Intranuclear inclusion bodies have been described but it is rather doubtful if they do exist; at least they are not distinct enough to be of any value in routine diagnostic work. The lesions are predominantly in the gray matter of the brain and spinal cord and are most severe in the cerebral cortex and the thalamus. The eastern strain of the virus produces much more severe and extensive lesions than does the western strain.

The most characteristic alteration of this disease is the presence of a large number of neutrophils in the meninges, perivascular cuffs, and intermixed with glia in foci throughout the brain. The presence of the neutrophils is an unusual reaction of the equine brain to viral infection. Usually the presence of neutrophils is indicative of a bacterial infection. The cellular exudate is very similar to that of listeriosis in sheep and cattle. However, the distribution of the lesions is different.

The viral encephalomyelitis and the leukoencephalomalacia occurring in moldy corn poisoning have much in common with regard to symptomatology but differ in etiology, seasonal occurrence, and tissue and blood chemical reactions. Differentiation of the two diseases, from the standpoint of gross and microscopic pathology, and chemistry of the blood are of concern here. In viral encephalomyelitis, perivascular cuffing with leukocytes, and neuronophagia are characteristic microscopic lesions mostly in the gray matter, but these changes are not present in moldy corn poisoning. Instead, in the latter there are in the white matter gross lesions which are yellowish areas of edema and soft, creamy foci of liquefactive necrosis associated with perivascular hemorrhages and neuronal degeneration. In the viral encephalitis there is a hypomagnesemia and in moldy corn poisoning a hypocalcemia and a hypermagnesemia.

The virus is also infectious for birds and has been recovered from ring-necked pheasants, pigeons, egrets, prairie chickens, and other wild birds. The domestic chicken may be infected experimentally but seems to have more resistance than other birds. Serious outbreaks of the disease also occur in the human and in other mammals.

**Borna disease** is an acute diffuse viral meningoencephalomyelitis of the horse in Europe and especially in Germany. It has not been described in the United States. Under experimental conditions it is infectious for sheep and various laboratory animals.

There are no macroscopic lesions. The microscopic lesions are typical of a viral encephalomyelitis. The lesions are most severe in the gray matter of the brain, especially in the hippocampus, thalamus, and caudate nucleus, in other words in the vicinity of the ventricular system.

Intranuclear and cytoplasmic acidophilic inclusion bodies, known as Joest bodies, are found in the ganglion cells, particularly in the cells of the hippocampus and the spinal ganglia. These bodies are round, ovoid, or diplococcic in shape, do not possess an internal structure (as in the Negri body), and are surrounded by a clear zone. They are considered to be pathognomonic of Borna disease. Fresh material is necessary for their demonstration since they disappear with autolytic and putrefactive alterations.

**Viral infectious anemia encephalitis in the horse.** A lymphocytic encephalomyelitis is observed in the horse with infectious anemia. The characteristic lesions consist of multiple small focal areas of liquefactive necrosis that are surrounded by macrophages, giant cells, and lymphocytes. The endothelium of the blood vessels shows degeneration and necrosis and, as a result, perivascular hemorrhage is present. Macrophages containing hemosiderin are found in the vicinity of the hemorrhages. Diffuse and focal gliosis are present. Neuron degeneration and necrosis are observed. The lesions are probably the result of the persistent anemia and are not pathognomonic for the disease.

**Louping ill** is an acute diffuse viral meningoencephalomyelitis of sheep in Scotland, England, and Ireland. It is characterized by excitability, ataxia, and paralysis and is transmitted by a tick (*Ixodes ricinus*). It does not occur in the United States. Young sheep or older sheep brought into an infected area are affected. It is also infectious for man, monkeys, mice, and pigs.

There are no macroscopic lesions. Microscopically, it is a typical lymphocytic meningoencephalomyelitis, but neutrophils are quite numerous in the cellular exudate. Although all portions of the brain and spinal cord are involved, the most extensive lesions are found in the cerebellar cortex. There is necrosis of neurons and

Purkinje cells, satellitosis, neuronophagia, focal and diffuse gliosis, and perivascular cuffing. No inclusion bodies have been demonstrated.

**Scrapie** is a disease of sheep that is characterized by intense pruritis, progressive incoordination, paralysis, and death. It is a disease of Suffolk sheep in Scotland, Germany, France, Canada, and the United States.

Although it is said to be an infectious viral encephalitis, there is nothing to indicate this is true. It cannot be called an encephalitis since no inflammation of the brain is present. No lesions have been described in the central nervous system. The vacuoles and inclusion bodies described in the neurons are found in normal sheep as well as sheep with other diseases, and for this reason they have no diagnostic significance.

The disease is apparently a hereditary defect of the central nervous system that appears in sheep over two years of age.

**Spinal myelitis in New York sheep** is observed as a lymphocytic myelitis involving the gray matter of the spinal cord of sheep. When these animals are startled and made to move suddenly, the rear legs collapse and the animals fall, then rapidly regain their feet and finally run off showing no additional locomotor disturbance. Animals observed for several years following the acute disease retain the tendency to fall when startled.

No macroscopic lesions are observed in the central nervous system. Microscopically, there is an acute diffuse lymphocytic myelitis of the gray matter of the spinal cord with perivascular cuffing, gliosis, and neuron degeneration. The lesions are most severe in the lumbar portion of the cord. Those animals that recover show atrophy and disappearance of the neurons of the spinal cord in the lumbar region.

**Trembles of sheep** is an infectious disease of the sheep and goat in France. It is a mild, subacute lymphocytic encephalomyelitis of the gray matter of the brain and is located primarily in the spinal cord, medulla oblongata, pons, and thalamus. There is extensive degeneration of the ganglion cells.

**French ovine encephalomyelitis.** An encephalitis has been described in French sheep and goats. At present it is not clear if this is a distinct viral disease of sheep or if it is Borna disease.

**Avian viral meninoencephalomyelitis.** This disease is popularly known as epidemic tremors. It is an infectious viral disease of chicks that is transmitted through the egg. The symptoms may appear at the time of hatching or may not appear until the chicks are 6 weeks of age, and consist of a distinct rapid tremor of the head, neck, and sometimes the tail together with ataxia. Usually no new cases develop after the birds are 6 to 8 weeks of age. The morbidity is from 5 to 50 per cent and the mortality from 1 to 65 per cent. The disease is only infectious for birds, thus differing from viral equine encephalomyelitis.

There are no macroscopic lesions in the central nervous system, which differentiates it from vitamin E deficiency in the same age bird. Microscopic lesions consist of a diffuse lymphocytic inflammation of the entire central nervous system. There is a diffuse and focal gliosis, perivascular cuffing, and degeneration of the neurons. No inclusion bodies are present. The lesions are not pathognomonic but are typical of a viral infection.

**Pneumoencephalitis of poultry (Newcastle disease)** is a viral disease of chickens, pheasants, turkeys, and other birds caused by *Tortor furens*. Neurological disturbances are observed in addition to the respiratory symptoms. The affected birds show incoordination, depression, twisting of the head and neck into abnormal position, paralysis, and death.

There are no macroscopic lesions in the central nervous system. Microscopic examination reveals a diffuse lymphocytic meningoencephalomyelitis. Perivascular cuffing is prominent. There is diffuse as well as focal gliosis. Neuron degeneration is observed. There are no inclusion bodies.

The central nervous system lesions of pneumoencephalitis, avian viral meningoencephalomyelitis, and equine viral meningoencephalomyelitis in birds cannot be differentiated from each other by histological examination.

**Transplacental viral infections.** Malformations, degenerations, and necroses may occur in the central nervous system of fetuses whose mothers have been infected with various viral diseases.

Fetal malformations, trembling, incoordination, and paralysis have been described in pigs from sows vaccinated with hog cholera virus from the tenth day to the fourth week of pregnancy.

The vaccination of ewes with bluetongue vaccine results in stillborn, incoordinate, blind, and paralytic lambs. Necropsy examination reveals massive areas of liquefactive necrosis of the white matter of the cerebrum.

Viral infections of the pregnant cat results in hypoplasia of the cerebellum of the fetuses.

## CHRONIC MENINGOENCEPHALOMYELITIS

**Tuberculous meningoencephalomyelitis.** The lesions of tuberculosis in the central nervous system consist of focal caseo-calcific encephalitis, myelitis, or meningitis. The finding of these lesions indicates that a generalized tuberculosis is present. The acid-fast organisms usually reach the central nervous system by way of the blood stream.

In the meninges the lesions are usually observed in the pia mater. Occasionally, a diffuse infection of the meninges may occur. Lesions are found in both the gray and white matter of the brain and are most frequently encountered in the cerebellum and the cerebrum. In the spinal cord the lesions are most common in the lumbar portion. The size of the lesion varies from miliary to as much as 5 centimeters in diameter.

Microscopically, the lesion consists of a central area of caseous necrosis which may be partially calcified. The necrotic tissue is surrounded by a zone of macrophages, giant cells, lymphocytes, and glia. Perivascular cuffing is observed around the vessels in the immediate vicinity of the lesion. Pressure atrophy of the surrounding nervous tissue is present.

**Cryptococcosis** is caused by a yeast, *Cryptococcus neoformans*. It is a disease of cattle, swine, cats, dogs, and many other mammals. The organism has a special affinity for tissue of the central nervous system. Although the primary lesion is usually in the skin or the lung, the organism eventually reaches the brain. The clinical symptoms consist of depression, incoordination, paralysis, and death. The clinical manifestations are not constant as the symptoms will depend on the part of the brain that is involved.

The macroscopic alterations in the central nervous system consist of a chronic meningitis. The thickened meninges have a translucent edematous appearance. The infection extends from the meninges into the brain along the blood vessels. As a result, multiple cystic spaces, containing a rather clear gelatinous material, are observed in the brain adjacent to the meninges.

Microscopically, the meninges and the cystic cavities contain numerous ovoid or spherical, budding yeastlike structures that measure 5 to 20 microns in diameter. These are surrounded by a thick gelatinous capsule. The capsule consists of glycogen as indicated by its staining reaction with the periodic acid-Schiff technic.

The extension of the infection into the brain occurs in the Virchow-Robin space around the blood vessel. The cellular inflammatory reaction consists primarily of macrophages. In the central region of the foci of macrophages and particularly in the vicinity of the yeasts, a few neutrophils can be observed. A few lymphocytes are found in the vicinity of the blood vessels within the foci of inflammation.

The character of the lesions varies considerably depending upon the rapidity of growth and the virulence of the infection. The central portion of some lesions consists of a mass of organisms surrounded by a zone of macrophages. These lesions have a definite cystic appearance. At other times, few yeasts are present in the area of inflammation. Then the area consists of a dense mass of macrophages, and the lesion does not have a cystic appearance.

The inflammatory reaction of the nervous tissue is slight considering the great destruction of the brain that takes place. The inflammatory reaction is primarily a meningitis that extends into the brain in the Virchow-Robin space and is outside of the nervous tissue proper. There is a little perivascular cuffing and a slight gliosis in the vicinity of the areas of inflammation. Apparently the organism is not irritating or toxic to the nervous tissue, and the reaction is more a pressure atrophy that results from the gradual enlargement of the cysts and the accumulation of organisms and exudate in the Virchow-Robin space and in the meninges.

## Parasitic Encephalomyelitis

### MYIASIS

*Hypoderma bovis* larvae may be found in the fat of the vertebral canal in as many as 60 per cent of cattle in areas where this parasite is found. It is thought that the larvae, while migrating to the backs of cattle, come in contact with the spinal nerves, and since the route of the nerve is a path of least resistance through the tissues, the larvae follow the nerve into the vertebral canal.

Occasionally the larvae invade the spinal cord or the brain. At times they enter the ventricular system of the brain and can be found in the lateral ventricles. The route of migration of the larvae through the brain can be seen grossly as a winding streak of hemorrhage in the path of the parasite.

*Hypoderma lineatum* (third instar) has been observed in the left corpus striatum of the brain of a horse.

The larvae of *Oestrus ovis* have been reported to invade the brain. It is doubtful if this occurs. Probably the larvae from the nasal passages or sinuses contaminate the brain when the skull cap is removed.

We have not observed an invasion of the central nervous system with this parasite. Neither have we found a publication describing this parasite in the brain in which histological preparations have been made of the tissue in the vicinity of the parasite. Inflammation must be present if the parasite were there before the death of the animal.

CESTODIASIS

**Tapeworm cysts** are quite common in the central nervous system of the animals in some parts of the world. The cysts of *Multiceps multiceps, Taenia solium, Taenia inermis, Taenis pisiformis* and *Taenia echinococcus* are the ones that are usually encountered. The ova of the tapeworms are consumed by the intermediate host, and in the digestive tract the larvae escape from the ova and enter the wall of the intestine and then migrate and are carried by the blood stream to various locations within the body. Some of these larvae, particularly those of *Multiceps multiceps*, reach the brain and there they encyst.

*Multiceps multiceps* larvae are most frequently encountered in the brain of sheep but can occur in all domestic animals. The reason for this is that the definitive host is the dog. Since sheep are in close contact with sheep dogs, they are easily infected if the dog is eliminating tapeworm ova. The grass and the water of the sheep become contaminated with ova and are ingested when the animals graze or drink. The cysts are most frequently located in the brain, particularly the cerebrum, and are also, at times, found in the spinal cord. The larvae, after leaving the capillaries in the central nervous system, may migrate through the tissue. The path of migration can be seen macroscopically. At first the route of the parasite appears as a red streak as the result of hemorrhage. Later, as the erythrocytes disintegrate, the path becomes yellow or brown.

The fully developed cyst measures 3 to 7 cm. in diameter. As the cyst enlarges there is pressure atrophy of the surrounding nervous tissue. As a result of the irritation, there is a chronic lymphocytic meningitis, encephalitis, or myelitis, depending on where the parasite is located. When large numbers of larvae enter the central nervous system there is an acute diffuse lymphocytic meningoencephalomyelitis, and the animal dies as the result of the overwhelming infection. As the cysts enlarge and press on the skull, pressure atrophy of the bone may occur. When the parasite dies the cyst wall and its content become calcified.

Cysts involving the spinal cord are usually located in the lumbar portion of the cord. Pressure atrophy of the cord occurs, and the result is incoordination and paralysis of the posterior extremities.

Although infestations with the larvae of *Taenia solium* are not as common as those of *Multiceps multiceps*, they can be very serious, especially in the human. The cysts of *T. solium* are most frequently observed in the brain of swine and dogs. The cysts measure about 1 centimeter in diameter. They do not attain the large size observed with *M. multiceps*, and only one scolex is observed in each cyst. Pressure atrophy of the nervous tissue occurs in the vicinity of the cyst.

NEMATODIASIS

Various **nematode** larvae are found in the central nervous system. Strongyle larvae are frequently found in the horse. The route of migration of the strongyle can be seen as a narrow winding line through the tissue. The path appears red or pink, later brown or yellow, as the result of hemorrhage in the area of injury.

The larvae of ascarids, strongyloides, and hookworms may be found in the capillaries or in the nervous tissue of the brain and cord. The microfilaria of *Dirofilaria immitis* are frequently observed in the capillaries of the brain, spinal cord, and meninges. *D. immitis* larvae apparently cause no injury to the brain.

A chronic lymphocytic inflammation occurs in the vicinity of ascarid, strongyloides, hookworm, or strongyle larvae that are present in the nervous tissue outside of the blood vessels. Macrophages, giant cells, and eosinophils may be present at times in the vicinity of the parasite. Numerous microglia actively engaged in removing the necrotic tissue, fibrin, and erythrocytes are found along the route of migration of the parasite.

NEUROFILARIASIS

Neurofilariasis is observed in sheep, deer, and moose in the United States.

*Setaria digitata* infections of the central nervous system have been described in goats, sheep, and horses in the Far East (Japan, Korea, and Ceylon). S. *digitata* infection of the horse is known as **Kumri** in India, Ceylon, Burma, and Assam. A similar disease may occur in the United States.

In Japan approximately 6 per cent of the sheep are affected. The disease is seasonal because the larvae of S. *digitata* are transmitted by the mosquito. The animals affected show motor weakness, incoordination, and paralysis.

Macroscopic lesions are found anywhere in the brain or spinal cord and may be single or multiple depending on the number of parasites present. The lesions consist of narrow tortuous tracts extending through the nervous tissue. They begin in the pia mater and extend obliquely into the nervous tissue.

The microscopic alterations consist of a traumatic lesion following the path of migration of the parasite. A space may be found in the center of the tract where the parasite has progressed through the tissue. This is surrounded by tissue that has undergone degenerative alterations and liquefactive necrosis. If blood vessels have been injured, hemorrhage occurs into the tract. The tract is surrounded by phagocytic microglia, lymphocytes, and eosinophiles. The blood vessels in the vicinity of the lesion show perivascular cuffing. The surrounding tissue a short distance from the tract is normal. The nerve fibers severed by the wandering larvae undergo degeneration and necrosis, and the damaged axis cylinders are greatly swollen and appear as balls or columns depending on whether the cylinder is observed in cross section or longitudinal section. Careful examination of the brain and cord as well as the cerebrospinal fluid and the formalin in which the brain was fixed will result in the finding of the larvae responsible for the lesions.

Similar traumatic lesions may be produced experimentally if needles are inserted into the tissue of the central nervous system and then retracted and several days allowed to elapse before the tissues are examined.

*Elaphostrongylus tenuis* is the cause of neurological symptoms in sheep in New York State. The sheep show motor incoordination and paralysis of the extremities, particularly the tail and rear legs.

Macroscopic examination reveals a few irregularly arranged brown areas up to 1 millimeter in diameter throughout the gray and white matter of the brain and spinal cord.

The microscopic lesions consist of multiple focal areas of meningoencephalomyelitis. These focal areas consist of a central sinuous tract that represents the path of the parasite as it migrated through the tissue. This tract contains blood as the result of the rupture of blood vessels by parasitic trauma. The tract is surrounded by an area of demyelinization and axis cylinder degeneration. Astrocytes and microglia are numerous in this area of traumatic injury. Portions of the parasites are found in some of the tracts. The meningeal cellular exudate and the perivascular cuffs consist of lymphocytes and eosinophils.

EQUINE WOBBLERS

The "wobbler" is observed among young horses and mules. Usually the animals are 1 to 2 years of age. The disease is most frequently encountered in the thoroughbred but may occur in other breeds, even draft animals.

The animals have difficulty in moving and tend to sway from side to side as they move, thus the name wobbler. Although not paralyzed, there is serious impairment of the gait, and the animals may fall if backed or turned suddenly.

Macroscopic examination usually reveals narrow tortuous tracts of liquefactive necrosis and hemorrhage in the spinal cord. The lesions are most frequently observed in the cervical portion of the cord. At times, microscopic examination of the cord is necessary to demonstrate the lesions.

Microscopic examination of the area reveals liquefactive necrosis, hemorrhage, demyelinization of nerve tracts in the area, the accumulation of microglia in the vicinity of the injury, and slight perivascular cuffing.

Although the etiology of the disease has not been demonstrated in this country, it has been pointed out that the clinical and post-mortem alterations are identical with those of Kumri (cerebrospinal nematodiasis), a disease of the equine in the Far East. All evidence indicates that this observation is probably correct, and all cases should be examined very carefully for migrating larvae in the lesions, in the cerebrospinal fluid, and in the formalin in which the brain was preserved.

### PROTOZOIASIS

**Toxoplasmosis and encephalitozoonosis.** *Toxoplasma gondi* and *Encephalitozoon cuniculi* are two protozan parasites found in the central nervous system of domestic animals. The two parasites are very similar morphologically but can be differentiated by serological methods. *E. cuniculi* is a disease of the brain of the rabbit, while *T. gondi* infects not only the rabbit but other species as well and in addition invades the visceral organs. There are no macroscopic lesions in the brain or spinal cord.

The infection reaches the central nervous system by way of the blood stream and produces a focal embolic type of lesion. The toxoplasma lesions are found throughout the brain and cord, while the encephalitozoal lesions in the rabbit are usually located dorsal to the third ventricle. The focal lesions consist of a central area of coagulative necrosis surrounded by a zone of microglia and neu-

trophils. A zone of myelin degeneration is present in the periphery of the foci.

In these foci the small pear-shaped toxoplasma or encephalitozoon can be seen occurring singly or in cysts. The most severe reaction is observed when the parasites are found singly or in small cysts. When present in large cysts the reaction is slight, and quite frequently no cellular or vascular alterations are found around them. Apparently the large cystic form is not irritating or toxic.

In addition to the focal lesions there is a lymphocytic meningitis, lymphocytic perivascular cuffing, and a slight general gliosis.

Toxoplasma infections are most frequently found in birds, cats, and rabbits. In some areas it appears that the majority of rabbits dying during the winter months have either a primary or a complicating toxoplasmosis.

In a survey of 100 cats submitted for rabies examination, Mitchell (Master's thesis, Iowa State University) found that 5 had a toxoplasma encephalitis. An equal number (5) of these 100 cats had rabies. In Iowa, toxoplasmosis and rabies are the only two specific infectious diseases of the central nervous system of cats.

**Mastigophorosis.** A chronic lymphocytic inflammation of the brain and spinal cord is found in mal de caderas of the horse, nagana of the dog, trypanosomic sleeping sickness in the horse, and leishmaniasis in the dog.

### NEUROLOGICAL SYMPTOMS ASSOCIATED WITH SYSTEMATIC PARASITISM

**Coccidiosis** and less frequently **nematode infections** of the gastrointestinal tract result in symptoms of a central nervous system disease. The animals manifest depression, weakness, incoordination, clonic spasms, and convulsions. The neurological disturbances are most frequently observed in cattle and less commonly in sheep. In the ovine the symptoms are particularly severe in the karakul.

If a complete necropsy examination is made, the gastrointestinal parasitism should be observed. There are no macroscopic or microscopic lesions in the central nervous system. The clinical manifestations are the result of a toxemia. Probably lesions in the central nervous system could occur if the severe toxemia were maintained for a long period of time.

Neurological disturbances are observed in cattle, lambs, ducks, geese, and dogs infested with **ticks.** No macroscopic or microscopic alterations are found in the central nervous system.

## Allergic Encephalitis

Allergic encephalitis can be produced when normal sterile brain is injected into the central nervous system. It produces a diffuse lymphocytic meningoencephalomyelitis and apparently can occur in all domestic animals. In experimental work it is very important that this type of encephalitis be recognized; otherwise it may be confused with viral encephalitis of various types.

## Postvaccinal Encephalitis

Postvaccinal encephalitis sometimes occurs in the dog following rabies vaccination. Fortunately the number of dogs showing this reaction is small. The disease appears 2 to 3 weeks after vaccination. The lesion in the central nervous system is a lymphocytic meningoencephalomyelitis similar to that observed in allergic encephalitis. No rabies virus is present in the brain or spinal cord.

One should not confuse postvaccinal encephalitis with rabies. If improper rabies vaccine is used, rabies may occur as the result of vaccination. Rabies following vaccination is most frequently observed in the feline and bovine.

## Postinfective Encephalitis

Postinfective encephalitis following various infectious diseases does not occur in domestic animals. It does occur in the human following measles, chickenpox, mumps, and smallpox, but no similar entity has been described in animals.

Post-distemper encephalitis is fre-

quently diagnosed, but this is an error. The encephalitis associated with the virus of Carre is part of the disease, and the diagnosis of postinfective distemper encephalitis should never be made because it does not exist.

## Metabolic Diseases and Neurological Disturbances

A group of metabolic diseases such as parturient paresis, hypoglycemia, hypomagnesemia, grass tetany, and railroad sickness frequently show neurological disturbances described as restlessness, unsteady gait, staggering, paresis, muscle spasms, and coma. No macroscopic or microscopic lesions are found in the central nervous system. The differential diagnosis will depend on a careful evaluation of the history, symptoms, and necropsy lesions.

## TOXICOSES

### Commercial Poisons

Many of the commercial poisons used in agriculture produce symptoms of a central nervous system disease. Few of them produce central nervous system lesions, and these are not pathognomonic. Since the symptoms duplicate those shown by other diseases, it is very important that toxic substances be considered in differential diagnosis.

**Lead** and **arsenic** are two very common poisonous elements found on most farms. Passive hyperemia and a few petechial hemorrhages have been described in the central nervous system of animals poisoned with these substances. Neuron degeneration has been said to be present, but the authors have not observed these changes in the animals they have examined. There is an increase in the number of glia but it is not significant enough for a definite diagnosis.

**Nitrate** poisoning results in a chocolate-colored blood because of the methemoglobinemia and, as a result, the brain will have a brown color.

The **chlorinated hydrocarbon insecticides** (benzene hexachloride, toxaphene, chlordane, aldrin, dichloro-diphenyl-tri-chloroethane, rothane, and methoxychlor) and the **organic phosphorus compounds** (parathion and malathion) used extensively in agriculture produce no macroscopic or microscopic lesions in the central nervous system.

**Mercury** poisoning has been described in swine that have ingested seed oats treated with mercurial fungicide. The principal symptoms consist of glossopharyngeal paralysis, blindness, locomotor disturbances, recumbency, and death.

No **macroscopic lesions** are observed. **Microscopic lesions** consist of degeneration and coagulative necrosis of the neurons of the cerebral cortex and the brain stem. Satellitosis occurs around the injured neurons. In addition, hyperemia and occasional small focal hemorrhages are observed.

CANINE HYSTERIA

For many years in the United States **nitrogen trichloride** (agene) has been used as a bleaching agent in the milling of wheat flour. Also during this period some dogs have been subject to a peculiar nervous disorder called **running fits, canine hysteria,** or **fright disease**. The cause was attributed to the lack of an essential amino acid, to a hypoglycemia immediately following severe exercise, to an infection with B-hemolytic streptococcus associated with intestinal roundworm infestation, and to other factors.

The condition has been experimentally produced by feeding growing dogs flour that has been bleached with nitrogen trichloride (agenized flour). Bleaching improves the appearance and baking qualities of the flour and the product is not toxic for man. When bread or biscuits made from this flour are fed continuously to dogs however, even with other feed, fits develop in some but not all of the dogs. It is theorized that the toxic product is the result of the interaction of agene with the essential amino acid methionine.

**Macroscopic lesions** in the brain are not observed. **Microscopic lesions** are found throughout the brain. Areas of liquefac-tive necrosis are found in the cerebral cortex. Degeneration and necrosis of the neurons are found in the cerebellum (Purkinje cells), medulla oblongata, pons, thalamus, hippocampus, and cerebral cortex. Although gliosis is present it is not as prominent as would be expected considering the amount of tissue damage present.

**Neurological Disturbances Associated With Clostridium Toxins**

BOTULISM

Botulism is a disease of domestic animals that occurs when food containing the toxin of *Clostridium botulinum* is ingested. This extremely potent toxin, acting on the nervous system, produces symptoms of paralysis. These symptoms consist of disturbances in vision, ptosis or drooping of the eyelid, difficulty in locomotion, paralysis of the tongue and throat, depression, respiratory paralysis, and finally death. Birds have difficulty in controlling the muscles of the neck, and as a result of the paralysis of the neck muscles and the inability to hold the head and neck erect, the disease has been called **limberneck**. In cattle the disease is sometimes called **lamsiekte** or **loin disease**.

The disease is encountered in many species of animals, but the susceptibility to the toxin varies greatly and especially to the type of toxin that is involved. Dogs, sheep, and pigs are very resistant to botulism, and under natural conditions it is doubtful if these animals are ever affected. The disease has been described in the horse, but undoubtedly it is an uncommon disease in the United States. Botulism is encountered along the Gulf Coast of Texas where it is known as loin disease of cattle. In other portions of the country a diagnosis of botulism in cattle should not be made unless the toxin is actually isolated. In the United States the disease is most commonly encountered in chickens, ducks, and waterfowl in general. The toxin is obtained from decomposing carcasses and from decaying vegetation that is found in ponds and pools during the hot summer months.

Many diseases are characterized by depression, locomotor disturbances, and paralysis. These symptoms alone, even though decaying organic matter is present in the area, do not constitute a diagnosis of botulism. The toxin must actually be demonstrated in the ingested food before such a diagnosis can be made. Fortunately, in most areas of the United States, botulism is no problem in domestic animals, and for that reason a diagnosis of botulism should not be made unless the toxin is actually shown to be present.

There are no **macroscopic lesions** in the brain or spinal cord. **Microscopic examination** reveals slight alterations in the neurons of the central nervous system. It is questionable if these alterations are actually due to the botulism toxin since similar cell alterations can be produced with various respiratory disturbances in which hypoxemia is present. The alterations in the neurons are quite likely the result of respiratory failure rather than the action of the toxin.

### TETANUS

Tetanus or lockjaw is an acute infectious disease resulting from an intoxication of the nervous system with the exotoxin of *Clostridium tetani*, and characterized by persisting spasmodic contractions of the entire body musculature or of single groups of muscles, without impairment of consciousness.

**Pathogenesis.** Spores enter wounds (puncture wounds preferably) in company with foreign bodies and pyogenic organisms, and in the presence of necrotic tissue or extravasated blood. These factors interfere with the action of leukocytes and also aid in providing anaerobic conditions for the tetanus organism. The organisms multiply rapidly and produce an exotoxin. The toxin (tetanospasmin) is carried from the wound by the blood and lymph vessels to all parts of the body in the same way all other toxic substances are. Special mention should be made of the part played in this transport of the toxin by lymphatics and interstitial spaces in nerve trunks. The action of the toxin on the spinal cord resembles that of strychnine. It suppresses all types of synaptic inhibition. In generalized tetanus there is general suppression of synaptic inhibitory action as the toxin spreads throughout the whole nervous system. This effect can be seen to best advantage when one moves quickly or makes a noise in the presence of an animal with tetanus. The animal goes into a state of continuous muscular rigidity.

The time elapsing between the introduction of the tetanus spores into a wound and the appearance of symptoms may be as short as 24 hours but it is usually 1 to 2 weeks.

There are no **macroscopic lesions** in the central nervous system. Death of the individual is the result of asphyxiation due to interference with the respiratory and cardiac functions during long periods of muscle contraction. As the result of the hypoxemia, the blood is cyanotic in color, coagulates poorly, and a few hemorrhages may be found.

**Microscopic lesions** have been described in the central nervous system. The lesions consist of slight degenerative alterations in the neurons of the brain and spinal cord. However, similar alterations may be produced as the result of hypoxemia, and therefore, since the animals actually die from asphyxiation, it is quite probable that the neurological alterations described are the result of hypoxemia rather than the action of the toxin.

### ENTEROTOXEMIA

Neurological disturbances such as incoordination, opisthotonus, weakness, paralysis, and bellowing have been described in cattle, sheep, and swine when the toxins of *Clostridium perfringens* and *Clostridium welchii* have been absorbed from the digestive tract.

No **macroscopic** or **microscopic lesions** have been described in the central nervous system. Probably the animals die so quickly that the tissues of the brain and spinal cord, following contact with the toxin, have not had time to develop degenerative and necrotic alterations. It is extremely important to remember that in all neurological diseases a lapse of time must exist following injury to allow nuclear and cytoplasmic alterations to take place.

### Central Nervous System Lesions in Ruminant Indigestion in Iowa Cattle

Strafuss (unpublished Master's thesis at Iowa State University) has described a neurological disturbance in cattle following overfeeding, improper feeding, or excessive administration of sulfonamides by mouth. The animals show anorexia, depression, salivation, staggering, blindness, asthenia, rumen atony, diarrhea, clonic spasms in the muscles of the shoulder and flank region, and paralysis. Once paralysis appears and the animals go down, they do not recover. The disease is usually seen in cattle that are 4 months to 1 year of age and is most commonly observed in the early fall shortly after the animals are placed in the feed lot. The duration of the illness is usually less than 72 hours. There are no macroscopic lesions in the brain or spinal cord.

Microscopic examination of the brain reveals that the severity of the lesions depends on the length of time the animals live. In the early stages of the disease, gliosis, satellitosis, capillary hyperplasia, and neuronophagia are observed. After 48 to 72 hours the lesions become more prominent, and neuron degeneration and necrosis are observed. In those animals that survive 2 weeks or longer, there is extensive capillary hyperplasia, severe diffuse and focal gliosis, slight perivascular cuffing, focal areas of myelin degeneration, and a vasculitis. The lesions are most prominent in the motor areas of the cerebral cortex, corpus striatum, corpus quadrigemina, thalamus, and medulla oblongata. No focal areas of liquefactive necrosis and hemorrhage are observed in the cerebral cortex as described in polioencephalomalacia.

### Polioencephalomalacia

This disease occurs in feed lot and pastured cattle. Clinically, the animals show muscular tremors, convulsions, and impairment of vision, and push against solid objects such as a fence or corner post.

**Macroscopic examination** reveals areas of liquefactive necrosis in the motor centers of the cerebral cortex. In those animals that recover, cysts containing necrotic brain tissue and disintegrating blood are found in this area.

**Microscopic examination** reveals that, in addition to the areas of necrosis in which hemorrhage occurs, there are necrosis and degeneration of the neurons and glia adjacent to the necrotic areas. The capillaries in the vicinity of the necrotic areas show hyperplasia. Microglia, engaged in the process of removing the dead tissue, are numerous in the periphery of these areas and are loaded with lipoid and tissue debris.

### Hepatic Disease and Neurological Disturbances

Just because an animal shows neurological disturbances does not necessarily mean the primary lesion is in the brain. It is frequently found that animals with severe alterations in the liver show very marked central nervous symptoms. Because of the association of liver lesions and neurological disturbances, it is very important that histological preparations of the liver be made to determine the extent of liver injury.

It is unfortunate that the central nervous system of animals showing neurological disturbances as the result of hepatic disease has usually not been studied in detail, particularly in the chronic cases where the effect of the toxin might have time to produce alterations indicating its presence.

The association of hepatic lesions with neurological disturbances is most frequently observed in the equine and less commonly in the bovine. It may occur, but not as frequently, in other species of animals.

#### EQUINE HEPATIC DYSTROPHY

In the equine there is a specific disease occurring during the late summer and early fall that is characterized by liver damage and neurological disturbances. It may also occur about 90 days following the administration of a biological product or the administration of blood. Better methods of biological production have reduced the incidence of the disease following the administration of sera and vaccines.

The equine shows severe neurological disturbances that resemble the symptoms of viral equine encephalomyelitis. There are forced movements, continuous walking in a circle or straight line, incoordination, paralysis, and death.

The history, morbidity, course, symptoms, and lesions indicate it is a viral hepatitis, yet difficulty has been experienced in demonstrating an infectious agent.

The necropsy examination reveals a large swollen liver that shows passive hyperemia, extensive fatty degeneration, and some coagulative necrosis. No **macroscopic** or **microscopic lesions** are observed in the brain or spinal cord. The neurological symptoms are apparently the result of an intoxication as the result of liver damage.

### Poisonous Plants

There are a number of plants such as senecio, astragalus, crotalaria, and alsike clover that produce hepatic disease. Apparently the hepatic damage interferes with the ability of the liver to destroy toxins from these substances. The toxic agents acting on the central nervous system produce the neurological disturbances. Lesions in the central nervous system as the result of these plant poisons have not been described.

#### THISTLE POISONING

Focal liquefactive necrosis is observed in the brains of horses that have consumed the yellow star thistle *Centaurea solstitialis* for 31 to 81 days.

The disease is locally termed chewing disease because of the tendency of the drowsy animals to stand for periods of time making chewing movements. In addition, there is impairment of eating and drinking, aimless walking, circling, and stiffness and slowness of gait.

Focal bilaterally symmetrical areas of liquefactive necrosis are observed in the globus pallidus and substantia nigra.

## NEOPLASMS

Neoplasms of the central nervous system are fairly common if the brain and spinal cord are examined. The incidence of primary (Fig. 20.9) or secondary brain tumors varies with the species of animal.

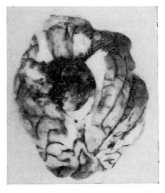

Fig. 20.9 — Glioma in the right ventricle of the brain of a 10-year-old dog. (Department of Veterinary Pathology, Michigan State University.)

They are most common in the dog and are least common in the pig and sheep. In routine necropsy material the incidence in the dog is about 2 per cent.

If neoplasms are to be found in the central nervous system, the entire brain and spinal cord must be fixed in 25 per cent formalin and then cut with a sharp knife with minimum distortion at right angles to the long axis. The slices should not be more than 5 millimeters in thickness. Each slice should be carefully examined for abnormal shape or color, and all abnormalities should be examined histologically. Even though abnormalities are not observed, routine portions of the corpus

striatum, thalamus, pons, medulla oblongata, and cerebellum should be examined by histological methods.

Since tumors are much more common
in the brachycephalic breeds, all brains
from dogs of this type should be examined
routinely. Tumors are especially apt to be
found in the boxer breed, and for this reason all dogs of this breed should be carefully examined. Quite often dogs with tumors of the central nervous system, particularly the boxer, have an increased sexual desire.

Metastatic tumors in the brain may occur in those dogs affected with neoplasms
in other organs. They are especially apt to
be found if the primary or secondary tumors are present in the lungs. For additional information on tumors consult
Chapter 13.

## PERIPHERAL NERVES

**Degeneration.** Any irritant w h i c h
causes degeneration of the nerve cells
likewise affects the nerve fibers of those
cells. This is called descending degeneration. However, degeneration may begin
in the nerve fiber and progress toward the
nerve cell (ascending degeneration). Microscopically, the degeneration frequently
involves the axis cylinder and the myelin
sheath simultaneously (total degeneration) (Fig. 20.10). Changes in the neurofibrils of the axis cylinder usually occur
first, but changes may occur in the myelin
sheath without changes in the former (in
blacktongue of dogs).

The loss of the myelin substance is such
a prominent change in degenerating nerve
fibers that special pains are taken to look
for it when studying diseases of the peripheral nerves. Myelin is a combination
of lipoids which undergoes degeneration
and dissolution when either the cell body
(cyton) or the nerve fiber is injured. At
times the degeneration occurs when there
is no apparent injury to either the cyton or
fiber as in pantothenic acid deficiency
(goose-stepping) of pigs. Loss of the myelin substance is called demyelination.

Special staining technic is necessary to
demonstrate this nerve sheath alteration.

**Regeneration.** Whereas nerve fibers in
the central nervous system regenerate
very poorly, those in the peripheral nerves
regenerate quite readily. Regeneration
may occur either after processes characterized by degeneration and inflammation
or after complete severing of the nerve,
provided healing is not prevented by an
extensive separation of the nerve endings,
or by the presence of a suppurative inflammation or formation of dense scar tissue.
If the neurilemma is intact, as it may be
in the first case, the axis cylinder and myelin sheath simply regenerate. If the nerve
is completely severed, as in the second
case, the defect is filled in by granulation
tissue originating from the three connective tissue coverings of the nerve and its
bundles. Newly formed neurilemma cells
originate at both stumps and join. There
is some question about the manner in
which the axis cylinder and myelin sheath
regenerate. The granulation tissue becomes differentiated into epi-, peri-, and
endoneurium. Occasionally, after an amputation or neurectomy has been performed, a so-called amputation neuroma
develops. This is not a true neoplasm but
simply a mass of unorganized connective
tissue and axis cylinders resulting from an
unsuccessful attempt at regeneration.

## Neuritis

The etiology is practically the same as
for degeneration: chiefly infectious and
toxic agents such as the virus of rabies and
canine distemper, the trypanosome of
dourine, and inorganic poisons such as arsenic and lead. Vitamin deficiencies such
as in beriberi and polyneuritis ($B_1$ avitaminosis) of birds, and blacktongue of dogs
are causes of a different character. The
toxic agents may reach the nerves by way
of the blood stream, lymph stream, or by
direct extension from neighboring tissues
of infected wounds, phlegmon, and abscesses. Neuritis may be acute or chronic.

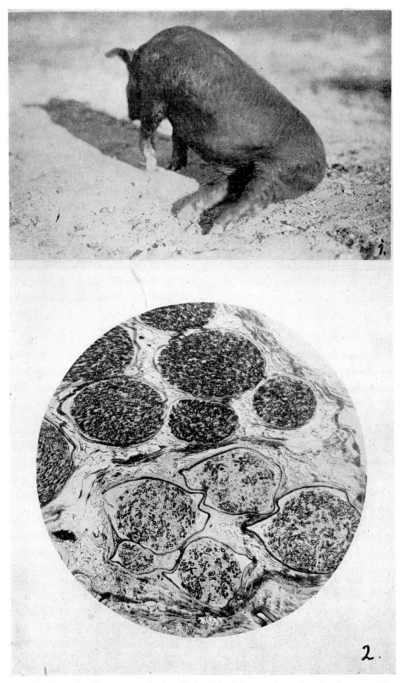

Fig. 20.10 — **1.** Motor paralysis of the hind legs of a pig. **2.** Cross section of a sciatic nerve of a pig with posterior paralysis. The five lowermost fasciculi show degeneration of the nerve fibers (Weigert-Pal stain). (Wehrbein, Jour. A.V.M.A.)

CHRONIC NEURITIS OF THE CAUDA EQUINA OF THE HORSE

This disease is characterized clinically by paralysis and atrophy of the muscles of the tail, anus, vulva, and perineum. The

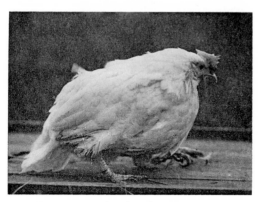

Fig. 20.11 — Neural lymphosarcoma (range paralysis) in a hen. (Iowa State University Veterinarian.)

etiology of the condition has not been determined, but traumatic injury appears to be the most plausible explanation. The lesion is frequently overlooked because the cauda equina is not examined.

Early in the course of the disease, hyperemia and hemorrhage are observed in the cauda equina. Organization of the hemorrhage occurs, and with it there is the deposition of connective tissue. Lymphocytes and macrophages are found in the cellular exudate. As the connective tissue accumulates and then contracts with maturity, pressure atrophy of the nerves of the cauda equina is the result.

NEURAL LYMPHOSARCOMA

In chickens from about 3 to 11 months of age a transmissible disease occurs which is characterized by the infiltration of many of the larger nerves with cells which appear to be lymphocytes. The nerves most commonly involved are the brachial, splanchnic, sciatic, intercostals, vagus, and optic. Lesions are especially prominent in the brachial, splanchnic, and lumbosacral plexuses. The plexuses and nerves become enlarged and change in color from the normal white to grayish. Furthermore, they become opaque instead of partially transparent. As a consequence, the normal zig-zag course of the nerve fibers in the nerve trunk is not apparent. The parts supplied by the nerves become partially or completely paralyzed (Fig. 20.11). Microscopically, the nerves are infiltrated with small and large lymphocytes. Pressure by the collections of lymphocytes causes nerve fiber degeneration.

# CHAPTER 21

# Organs of Locomotion

## Skeletal System

### Hyperemia

**Acute active hyperemia** of bone is seen in periostitis, endostitis, and osteomyelitis. The vascular change is observed primarily in the periosteum and the bone marrow since blood vessels are more numerous in these areas.

**Acute passive hyperemia** may be local or general depending upon the location of the obstruction in the venous system. If the obstruction persists, chronic passive hyperemia is the result.

**Chronic passive hyperemia** may be local or general and is preceded by the acute type. Chronic passive hyperemia causes hyperplasia of the periosteum and endosteum. The fibroblasts in these structures proliferate when stimulated by lack of oxygen and nutrient and the accumulation of waste materials from metabolic activity. Later, metaplasia takes place and the connective tissue is changed into bone. The result is an enlarged and irregularly shaped bone. The hyperplasia and metaplasia are most pronounced in the distal end of the bone because it is in this portion of the bone that passive hyperemia is most severe. These are the lesions seen in chronic pulmonary osteoarthropathy in the canine in which the cause of the chronic passive hyperemia is located in the heart or lung.

### Anemia

**Ischemia** of bone occurs if the local arterial blood supply is damaged. As the name indicates, the anemia involves only one bone or a portion of a bone. This is most frequently associated with trauma, especially a fracture of a bone.

**General anemia** of bone occurs when anemia involves the entire individual. It is prominent in vitamin B and iron deficiencies in swine and in hookworm anemia in the dog.

The **result** of ischemia or general anemia of bone is hypoplasia and atrophy in growing animals and atrophy in mature individuals. Severe or complete ischemia of bone results in necrosis.

### Hemorrhage

**Local hemorrhage** of bone is most frequently associated with trauma and is most severe when bone has been fractured. The hemorrhage is observed primarily in the periosteum, endosteum, and in the marrow cavity, and the extravasated blood accumulates in the tissue spaces of these structures. Hemorrhage in compact bone is slight because the dense osseous nature of bone does not allow the blood to accumulate. Local inflammation of bone may produce focal hemorrhage.

**General hemorrhage** of bone implies

that the lesion involves all bones of the body and is not confined to a local area. Hemorrhages of this type are petechial or ecchymotic in size. They are associated with various infectious diseases characterized by a septicemia and in diseases of the blood when the clotting time is prolonged, as in trichloroethylene poisoning in the bovine.

## DISTURBANCES OF GROWTH

### Atrophy

Atrophy may be local or general. Local atrophy is associated with a local disturbance in bone nutrition. General atrophy involves the bones throughout the individual and is most frequently the result of malnutrition or senility.

When pressure is applied to bone, the resulting loss in bone volume is termed pressure atrophy. The pressure causes ischemia, and as a result there is a lack of oxygen and nutrient in the area. Because of the impaired circulation, atrophy of bone takes place. The pressure may be in the form of **constricting** devices such as sutures, ligatures, or harnesses. It is also observed in the vicinity of **tumors**, especially when neoplasms are located in the bone marrow. **Parasite cysts** pressing against bone produce pressure atrophy as is observed in sheep infested with *Multiceps multiceps* larvae. The enlarging tapeworm cyst in the brain of the sheep exerts pressure on the adjacent osseous tissue, and atrophy of the bones of the skull is the result.

**Disuse** atrophy occurs when a limb is not used as the result of a **fracture** or **luxation**. The stimulus of work is needed to maintain normal metabolic activity in bone, and when this is not provided, atrophy takes place. Inactivity results in a decreased blood supply to the limb. Oxygen and nutrient are not brought to the part, and the waste materials of metabolism are not removed. When the normal metabolic activity is not maintained, the cells and tissues decrease in size.

**Neurotrophic** atrophy occurs when the nerve innervating a bone has been injured. This may occur when nerves have been crushed or severed as the result of trauma. When nerves are invaded by **tumors,** as occurs in neurolymphosarcomas of the chicken, or when pressed upon by enlarging **tumors, cysts,** or **abscesses,** atrophy of the bone supplied by the nerve can result.

**Nutritional** atrophy of bone occurs when **ischemia** is present. General nutritional atrophy of bone is observed as the result of a quantitative or qualitative lack of **food** in which the nutritional requirements of bone are not provided.

**Physiological** atrophy of bone occurs in the laying hen and in lactating mammals when the constituents of bone are withdrawn to supply the needs of **egg production** and **lactation.** If this type of atrophy becomes excessive, as occurs in **malnutrition,** it should then be considered as nutritional atrophy.

**Senile** atrophy of bone is associated with the ageing of an individual. Since it occurs in all individuals that reach old age, it is considered as a form of physiological atrophy. It is thought to be the result of a deficiency of growth-stimulating hormones produced by the endocrine system.

### Aplasia and Hypoplasia

When bone does not form, it is a disturbance of growth known as aplasia. Hypoplasia indicates that the bone did grow but did not reach its normal adult size. Either of these disorders may be the result of a **hereditary defect.** More frequently it is the result of an accident in the **fetal development** of the individual. The cells designated to form a certain bone may fail to grow normally or may die. At other times defects of the nervous or vascular systems may prevent the proper **nutrition** of the osteoblasts and thus the development of bone does not take place.

The most common cause of hypoplasia of bone is **malnutrition.** In malnutrition the necessary components of the ration required for the normal development of the individual are not present and as a result the individual does not grow. Hypoplasia of bone is also seen in heavily parasitized individuals or in those animals whose general growth has been retarded by various diseases such as bacterial infections.

## Hypertrophy

Hypertrophy of bone is an increase in the size and weight of an osseous structure without an increase in the number of osteoblasts or osteocytes. Hypertrophy is seen in animals in which calcium, phosphorus, and other minerals are being stored in the skeleton during a good state of nutrition. This can best be demonstrated in the bones of the non-laying hen in which the trabeculae and the shaft of the bone become so thick that the marrow cavity is almost obliterated.

## Hyperplasia

Hyperplasia of bone occurs when there is an increase in the size of the bone together with an increase in the number of osteoblasts and osteocytes. The enlargement of the bone is due to the proliferation of the cells of the periosteum and endosteum. The growth of new bone that occurs at the site of a healing fracture is an example of hyperplasia.

There is a hyperplasia of the periosteum and endosteum in chronic pulmonary osteoarthropathy. The hyperplasia is most pronounced in the distal portion of the individual bones of the legs. The disease is found in all animals but appears to be more common in the dog. The hyperplasia is the result of a chronic general passive hyperemia and edema. The cause of the passive hyperemia is found in the lungs or heart. In most instances the basic lesion is a chronic pneumonia as is produced by tuberculosis. Large abscesses or tumors in the lung may also be responsible for the passive hyperemia.

The periosteum and endosteum are quite sensitive to hypoxia, lack of nutrient, and the accumulation of waste materials as seen when passive hyperemia and edema occur. When exposed to these adverse conditions, these structures are stimulated and proliferate. Hyperplasia of the perios-

teum and endosteum is most prominent in those areas where passive hyperemia and edema are most severe. Due to the influence of gravity, the passive hyperemia and edema are most pronounced in the ventral portion of the bones, and likewise it is in the ventral portion of the bones that the hyperplasia is observed. The articular surface of the bone is usually not involved because it has a different blood supply. At times the periarticular hyperplasia becomes so excessive that it interferes with the movement of the joint.

Hyperplasia of bone is seen in the chicken in leukosis, an infectious viral neoplastic disease. The bone alterations observed in this disease are designated as osteopetrosis gallinarum.[1]

All bones of the skeleton may be involved, but the lesion is most pronounced in the metatarsus. Clinical observation of affected birds reveals a gradual enlargement of the bones. The lesions are bilaterally symmetrical. The articular surfaces are not affected. Bone growth occurs from both the periosteal and endosteal surfaces. As a result, the bone enlarges peripherally, and at the same time the marrow cavity is reduced in diameter and may be obliterated. The new growth of bone is poorly ossified, but with time more and more ossification takes place until extremely firm, dense bone is the result. The greatest bone hyperplasia and oldest lesions are seen in the distal or ventral portions of the involved bone.

Experimental and field evidence indicates that this bone disease is associated with leukosis. Tumor cells can be found in the internal organs, nerves, and blood. Because of the tumor growth, general passive hyperemia, anemia, and edema exist. The location of the lesion in the bones as well as the type of bone alteration indicates that the basic reason for the hyperplasia of the bone is a circulatory disturbance and, as indicated above, these are general passive hyperemia and edema. Passive hyperemia and edema cause bone hyperplasia, and it is in the distal and

---

[1](Jungherr and Landauer...Storrs Agr. Exper. Sta. Bul. 222, 1938).

ventral portions of the bone that the passive hyperemia and the accompanying edema are most pronounced. So it follows that it is in these areas that the hyperplasia of bone would be more apparent.

Hyperplasia of the bones of the forelimbs is observed in **newborn pigs**. Most of the hyperplasia involves the periosteum of the radius and ulna. Because of the peripheral laminated deposition of osseous tissue, there is an increase in the diameter of the bone. The tissues of the forelimbs are quite edematous, suggesting the cause of the lesion may be a vascular disturbance. It is considered a **lethal hereditary disease**. A similar bone change has been reported in newborn pigs from sows fed a ration deficient in **thiamine** and **riboflavin**.

Chronic **fluorine** poisoning causes hyperplasia of bone. The hyperplasia involves the periosteum primarily, and the new growth is arranged in concentric layers. This concentric deposition is associated with the periods when bone alterations are taking place, and represents differences in the rapidity of hyperplasia.

The alterations in the bone depend on the dosage, the type of fluorine salt consumed, the age of the animal, and the duration of the exposure. In young animals bone development is retarded. Moderate to large doses in older animals over a short period of time cause osteomalacia. Adult animals exposed to small amounts of fluorine over a long period of time develop the hyperplastic type of periosteal and endosteal growth. The bones of the legs and the mandible show the most extensive lesions.

## DISTURBANCES OF CELL METABOLISM

**Cloudy swelling, fatty degeneration,** and **hydropic degeneration** can be observed in the osteocytes, osteoblasts, and the cells of the periosteum and endosteum. **Amyloid** and **glycogen infiltration** of bone are of no importance in domesticated animals.

### Pigmentation

**Gray, black,** and **green** pigmentation of bone is observed as the result of putrefaction. Color is produced when the iron con-

tained in the blood, muscle, and other tissues combines with the sulfides formed by bacteria. The resulting iron sulfide is black and gives the decomposing cadaver its characteristic color. Various shades of **red, blue, yellow,** and **green** are observed in bone when dyes, such as methylene blue, are used therapeutically. A **black** color is observed when carbon compounds (Higgins ink) are administered intravenously. A **gray** pigmentation occurs if silver compounds are administered. Pigmentation may occur when certain plants are consumed. *Rubia tinctorum*, a plant of southern Europe that contains alizarin red, imparts a **red** color to bone.

### MELANIN

Melanosis of bone may occur as the result of misplaced melanoblasts or the invasion of bone by melanotic tumors. This pigmentation has a focal arrangement and is seen most frequently in heavily pigmented individuals or in bone invaded by metastatic melanosarcomas.

### HEMOGLOBIN AND ITS DERIVATIVES

Hemoglobin staining of bone occurs as the result of imbibition of blood associated with post-mortem putrefaction and autolysis. Hemoglobin stains the bone **pink** or **red** depending on its concentration.

In icterus the **hemobilirubin** and **cholebilirubin** will stain bone a **yellow** color.

A **brown** pigmentation of bone occurs when **hematoporphyrins** are deposited in bone. This pigmentation is called **osteohemochromatosis**. The color varies from tan to brownish black depending on the amount of pigment present and the density of the bone. The dense, compact bone shows less coloration than does the spongy bone. Histologically, there is a diffuse brown staining of the bone. The pigment is seen in the bone marrow as brown granules in the macrophages. The pigment does not give the Prussian blue reaction for iron, and it fluoresces with ultraviolet light.

### NECROSIS

**Coagulative necrosis** of bone occurs when ischemia involves a bone. It is most frequently observed in comminuted fractures where portions of bone are deprived of their blood supply. The osteocytes show the typical cellular alteration of coagulative necrosis. The bony matrix loses its distinct histological appearance and resembles macerated bone.

The necrotic bone is a mild irritant and is soon surrounded by a zone of connective tissue, blood vessels, and leukocytes as the body attempts to remove the dead tissue. Giant cells are quite numerous in the cellular reaction. Because of the dense nature of the necrotic bone, removal by the body defenses is slow.

**Liquefactive necrosis** occurs when bone is invaded by pyogenic microorganisms. The enzymes of the neutrophils are responsible for the liquefaction. It is most frequently observed in compound comminuted fractures, especially in the equine. Healing of the necrotic area is delayed because of the difficulty in removing the compact bone. The necrotic bone must be removed if healing is to take place.

Liquefactive necrosis is frequently observed in the lumbar vertebrae of swine as the result of the localization of *Brucella suis* in this region.

**Caseous necrosis** of bone occurs in tuberculosis. The lesion is most characteristic in the spongy portion of the bone and is most frequently observed in the chicken.

**Gangrene** of bone results when necrotic bone is invaded by saprophytic bacteria. The death of the bone is usually brought about by ischemia. It usually involves the bones of the tail and legs of animals subjected to freezing, ergot and fescue poisoning, constricting bandages or rubber bands placed around the extremity, or traumatic injury.

Gangrene of the tail of many species occurs when a diarrhea is present. The tail becomes covered with feces, and as the feces dry and contract on the tail they act as a constricting device that impairs the circulation. As the result of the faulty circulation, necrosis of the coccygeal vertebrae of the tail occurs.

Bite wounds of the tail are a common cause of necrosis of bone as the result of the vascular damage. It is a common condition in laboratory rats and mice because of injuries obtained in fighting or when a cannibalistic individual is present in the group. Tail cannibalism is also observed in swine.

Bacterial or viral diseases, such as erysipelas in swine and pox in mice, may damage the skin or the blood vascular system of the tail and cause necrosis of bone.

## FRACTURE OF BONE

A fracture is a break in the continuity of an osseous structure as the result of trauma.

Fractures may be simple or compound. A **simple fracture** is a disturbance in the continuity of bone in which the skin is not broken. A **compound fracture** is a disturbance in the continuity of bone in which the skin is broken and bacteria may gain entrance to the site of the break through the cutaneous defect.

A number of terms are used to describe the various fractures that involve bone. The more common types are illustrated in Figure 21.1.

Associated with a fracture of bone, there is a tearing of the tissues around the site of the break, and hemorrhage occurs in this area. The amount of hemorrhage will depend on how much vascular damage has taken place and whether major vessels have been damaged. Fatal hemorrhage can occur. Fracture of the skull can cause massive hemorrhage into the cranial cavity, resulting in compression of the brain.

**Healing** of the fracture occurs through the process of organizing the mass of blood between the ends of the broken bones. Fibroblasts and angioblasts begin to grow into the mass of blood from the surrounding tissue by using the fibrin network of the clot as a supporting structure and a stimulating medium in which to grow. The angioblasts form capillaries and the capillaries bring nutrient and leukocytes into the area needed for the organization of the extravasated blood. This invasion of the clot continues until all of

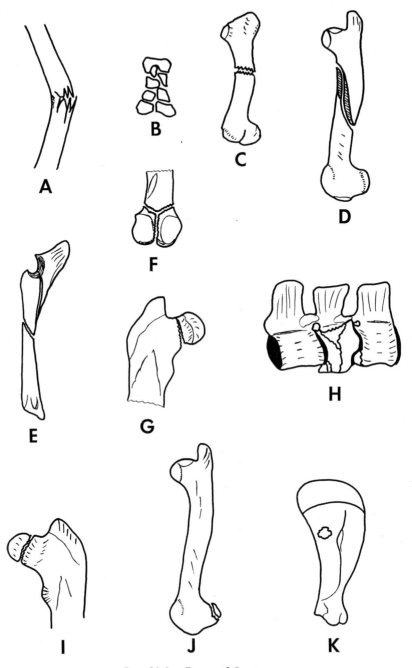

Fig. 21.1 — Types of Fractures.

A, Greenstick;   B, Comminuted;   C, Transverse;   D, Spiral;

E, Oblique;   F, T-fracture;   G, Transcervical;   H, Impacted;

I, Epiphyseal;   J, Condylar;   K, Perforating.

the blood elements deposited in the area as the result of hemorrhage have been removed.

At the same time that peripheral organization of the clot is taking place, the periosteum and endosteum begin to proliferate and grow into the clot from the ends of the broken bones. The cells of the endosteum and periosteum differentiate into osteoblasts, and osteoid tissue is deposited in the area.

The formation of osteoid tissue is well under way by the fourth or the fifth day after the fracture of the bone. Metaplasia of the connective tissue may occur, and the fibroblasts in the area will become osteoblasts and form osteoid tissue. Likewise, the capillary endothelial cells are capable of becoming osteoblasts, and they too form osteoid tissue. Finally, the entire area of hemorrhage is infiltrated with blood vessels, connective tissue, and osteoid tissue. Calcium salts have been infiltrating the osteoid tissue and converting it into osseous tissue.

**Osteoid tissue** is a mineral-deficient protein matrix formed by the osteoblast. When the osteoid tissue is mineralized it becomes **osseous tissue.** The process of mineralization of osteoid tissue is called **ossification.**

When a large gap exists between the broken ends of the bone, metaplasia of the fibroblasts in the area may result in the formation of cartilage. If this occurs, **endochondral ossification** takes place in the area.

The mass of partially ossified tissue at the site of the fracture is known as the **soft callus** or the **provisional callus,** and although ossification is not complete, it will usually support limited use of the bone 6 weeks after the fracture has occurred.

After several months the osteoid tissue is well infiltrated with mineral salts, and the area is as strong if not stronger than it was before the fracture occurred. This is known as the **hard callus** or the **definitive callus.** Even though the callus will support the activities of the bone at this time, there is no orderly arrangement of the

bone in this area. However, constant rearrangement and alteration of the bone take place in the area according to the stresses and strains placed upon the bone. With time the shape of the bone returns to what it was prior to the break, and after several months or years it may be difficult to detect the site of the fracture.

The callus associated with the periosteal tissue is called the **external callus.** The callus bulging into or occupying the marrow cavity is designated as the **internal callus.** The portion of the callus between the ends of the broken bone is termed the **in-line callus.**

There are many factors that interfere with the healing of bone. A deficiency of calcium, phosphorus, or other minerals may be present so that complete mineralization of the soft callus does not take place. Starvation, metabolic diseases, or infectious diseases may have so altered the metabolic activity of the individual that neither the soft nor the hard callus will form. The presence of bacteria in the area of injury attracts neutrophils, and liquefactive necrosis or gangrene may occur thus preventing healing from taking place. Sheets of fascia, muscle, or fat may be present between the broken ends of bone, preventing the union of the bone. Excessive movement may cause repeated fractures of the provisional callus so that complete union does not take place. When healing does not occur and bending of the limb is possible in the area of fracture, a **false joint** or **pseudoarthrosis** is said to exist. Healing may also fail to take place if the traumatic injury is not severe enough to stimulate tissue activity. Portions of bone removed under sterile surgical procedures with high-speed oscillating saws may leave so little trauma and hemorrhage in the area that bone stimulation with resulting healing does not take place or is incomplete. If a **sequestrum** (a piece of necrotic bone) is present in the area, healing will be delayed. The piece of necrotic bone causes inflammation, and this reaction prevents the formation of osteoid tissue and ossification. If the individual is old, healing may not take place because the regenerative ability of old individuals is often inadequate.

## DEFICIENCY DISEASES OF BONE

Deficiency diseases of bone are very common and are becoming more frequent as refined rations are fed and animals are pushed for maximum production in the shortest possible period of time.

### Deficiency of Minerals

The mineral deficiencies of bone vary greatly according to the geographic location of the animals and the type of ration fed. Soil deficiencies exert great influence on the incidence of bone disease. In areas in southwestern United States the soil and vegetation are deficient in phosphorus, and as a result bone diseases occur. Animals that are fed a concentrate ration are subject to a calcium deficiency since concentrate feeds are low in calcium and high in phosphorus.

In the mineral metabolism of bone a rather precise ratio between calcium, phosphorus, magnesium, fluorine, zinc, sulfur, and other minerals must exist if bone diseases are to be prevented.

A deficiency of either calcium or phosphorus results in **hypoplasia** of bone in young animals. The bones are small in all dimensions and are soft because of the lack of mineral. They can be cut with a knife or bent when force is applied. In older animals the bones undergo atrophy, a condition designated as **osteomalacia**. The shaft of the bone and the trabeculae decrease in size as the mineral is withdrawn. The bones become very fragile (**osseous fragility**) and fracture easily when subjected to trauma.

### Osteodystrophy

**Definition.** Osteodystrophy is a general term used to indicate defective bone growth. The bones may be shorter in length, bent, twisted, bowed, soft, unusually hard, or there may be improper development of trochanters and condyles.

The **etiology** is any factor that will alter bone growth. It may be a congenital anomaly, an injury, a circulatory disturbance, a mineral or vitamin deficiency, an improper ratio of minerals, or a debilitating parasitic or infectious disease. When bone is not properly formed, the weight of the individual and the traction of muscles and tendons cause unusual bone conformation.

A good example of an osteodystrophy caused by a number of factors is a disease known as **perosis** in the chicken and turkey. It is caused by an improper ratio of calcium, phosphorus, magnesium, and manganese together with a deficiency of choline and biotin. It is usually observed in birds fed excessive amounts of grain, particularly corn, in which the ration contains too much phosphorus.

The bones in perosis are short and thick, a common characteristic of improper bone growth. The weight of the bird causes the poorly ossified bone to bend laterally in its mid-portion. At the same time the condyles of the proximal end of the metatarsus show hypoplasia, and the inter-condyloid space through which the tendon of Achilles glides is shallow. Impairment of tendon and muscle growth does not occur, and as a result the tendon and muscle are longer than the length of the bones of the leg. Because of the proportionately long tendon of Achilles and the shallow inter-condyloid space, the tendon slips either medially or laterally, and a broad deformed hock is the result. The erect position of the bird requires great development of the tendon of Achilles and muscles of the leg necessary for the rapid movement of the bird, and therefore, the condyles become of very great importance in fixing the position of the tendon.

Leg weakness, poor development of the leg bones, and early symptoms of perosis are observed in broiler production in birds pushed for maximum growth in the shortest possible period of time and in confined or caged laying hens. The greater the effort made for maximum performance in these birds, the greater is the incidence of locomotor disturbance. The greater the production, the more critical is the nutritive requirement of bone and the greater is the danger of an osteodystrophy. In addition, these birds are restricted in their movement. Hypoplasia and atrophy of bone occur when movement is restricted. The hypoplastic bones and joints have difficulty in properly supporting the increasing body weight, and as a result symptoms of leg weakness are observed.

## FIBROUS OSTEODYSTROPHY

**Definition.** Fibrous osteodystrophy is an alteration in bone characterized by a decrease in the amount of osseous tissue and an increase in the amount of white fibrous connective tissue. The involved bone may or may not show an increase in width or diameter. It is a disorder of the entire skeleton involving all parts of the bone and is an indication of a general disturbance in bone metabolism.

Osteodystrophy is basically a demineralization of the bone. As the result of the lack of mineral, the bones become soft and rubbery. The traction of the muscles and tendons, as well as the weight of the individual, causes a bending, twisting, and distortion of bone. In an attempt to provide strength to the bone and in response to the irritation produced by the bending and twisting of bone resulting from the animal's movements, connective tissue proliferation takes place in the bone. As the condition progresses, there is noticeable peripheral enlargement of the bone caused by periosteal hyperplasia. The amount of connective tissue in the bone is related also to the age of the lesion. The longer the demineralization of the skeleton has been present, the greater will be the opportunity for connective tissue to form. In addition, the amount of connective tissue will depend on the species of animal in which the bone disease is found. The connective tissue of the horse responds more quickly and more excessively to irritation than does the connective tissue of other animals, and for this reason the lesions of fibrous osteodystrophy are best demonstrated in the equine.

Focal accumulations of a lymphlike fluid are observed in some animals. This fluid represents areas of edema and lymphatics distended with lymph.

Hemorrhage into bone causes a ballooning of the soft bone, and cystic masses of blood are the result. A similar ballooning may occur in those bones in which there is active bone marrow growth. In these bones the blood pressure within the marrow cavity causes a dilatation of the soft bone, and areas distended with blood and bone marrow are the result (telangiectasis).

Fibrous osteodystrophy is usually caused by renal disease, parathyroid hyperplasia or neoplasia, and mineral deficiencies.

In the dog it is most frequently associated with **chronic interstitial nephritis.** In nephritis, phosphorus retention by the kidney results in an increase in the amount of serum phosphorus. In an effort to balance the high serum phosphorus, calcium is withdrawn from the bones and demineralization of the skeleton takes place. To accomplish the demineralization of the bone there must be hyperactivity of the parathyroid. Parathyroid hyperplasia provides the required parathyroid hormone. As demineralization continues, the bones become softer and softer, and finally they can be cut with a knife or bent with relative ease. This softening of the bones is often designated as rubber bones. All bones of the body are involved, but the disease is often first observed when distortion or fracture of the mandible takes place. Many malpractice suits have been initiated following the fracture of the mandible of a dog when a veterinarian has attempted to examine the mouth of a canine having a stomatitis caused by renal disease.

**Hyperplasia** or **neoplasia** of the parathyroid, as well as the experimental administration of parathyroid hormone, will result in demineralization of the skeleton and fibrous osteodystrophy.

A deficiency of **phosphorus** may also result in fibrous osteodystrophy as is frequently observed in South Africa and in southwestern United States. This demineralization or incomplete mineralization of the skeleton is seen predominantly in cattle and horses. Connective tissue is deposited in the bone in response to the irritation and stress associated with musculoskeletal movement. If circulatory disturbances, such as passive hyperemia or edema, that may be associated with malnutrition and parasitism are also present, the connective tissue hyperplasia of the bone becomes more pronounced. Stress from movement, plus the circulatory disturbances and the effects of gravity, causes the lesion to be most pronounced in the legs and head. The alterations in the skull are often called big-head or mandible disease in the horse.

At times fibrous osteodystrophy shows a laminated peripheral deposition of bone and connective tissue. This lamination represents periods when bone repair has taken place. Peripheral laminating hyperplasia of bone may also represent a complicating **fluorine poisoning** in phosphorus-deficient areas. Sources of phosphate, such as rock phosphate, often contain toxic amounts of fluoride. If phosphate sources high in fluoride are fed, hyperplasia of the periosteum and endosteum will occur in a laminated manner.

A deficiency of **calcium** may also produce fibrous osteodystrophy, but it is not encountered as frequently nor are the lesions as severe as with a deficiency of phosphorus. A **magnesium** deficiency will cause fibrous osteodystrophy in swine.

### Vitamin D Deficiency

Vitamin D deficiency causes a disease known as **rickets.** The term rickets is used incorrectly as a synonym for osteopathy when actually it has very characteristic tissue alterations that differentiate it from other bone diseases. Most cases of so-called rickets are deficiencies of calcium and phosphorus rather than a deficiency of vitamin D. For example, it is ridiculous to diagnose a vitamin D deficiency in white-skinned hogs on green pasture exposed to the ultraviolet rays of the sun. The hogs are usually being fed a concentrate ration that is deficient in calcium, and it is the calcium deficiency that is causing symptoms of bone disease.

Rickets is a disease of man, apes, birds, and rats. Rickets has never been described in swine. Fifteen cases of rickets in calves have been described in Sweden. Examination of this work indicates the characteristic bone alterations in these

animals. Rickets is not a disease of domestic mammals in Germany.

The authors have attempted to demonstrate rickets in domestic farm mammals for more than 20 years and have not been able to do so. Clinical cases of rickets in dogs and cats have not been described. The so-called rickets in dogs and cats comprises a miscellaneous group of calcium and phosphorus deficiencies, hereditary bone and cartilage diseases, and skeletal deformities that result from other diseases such as canine distemper (see page 635). In swine the bone alterations often diagnosed as rickets are actually vitamin A deficiency, mineral deficiencies, arthritis, and the bone lesions of hog cholera or hog cholera vaccination (see page 634).

Rickets is frequently diagnosed in the canine, but the lesions of rickets are not present at necropsy examination. X-ray examination is of little value in determining the nature of the bone disease and has caused many clinical errors in diagnosis.

The enlargement of the ends of the bones of many of our breeds of dogs is the result of chondrodystrophy which is characteristic for the breed. Excessive distortion of the bone should be blamed on the hereditary cartilage deformity and not on a dietary deficiency. This is most frequently observed in the dachshund, beagle, basset, Pekinese, and bulldog breeds.

Most species of domestic animals have at birth passed the stage of bone growth during which rickets occurs. In man, rats, apes, and a few other species in which the fetus is underdevloped and not capable of moving about at the time of birth, the stage of bone growth is such that rickets may occur.

**Macroscopic lesions.** The most apparent signs of vitamin D deficiency in young animals are retarded growth, stiffness, enlargement of the ends of the bones, hypoplasia of the bones, bending and distortion of the bones, and a suppresion of the calcification of cartilage and the ossification of bone. The enlargement of the costochondral junctions, because of its resemblance to a row of beads, is often referred to as a rachitic rosary. This beading of the ribs should not be confused with the enlarged costochondral junctions that are considered normal for hereditarily deformed dogs such as dachshunds, beagles, and bassets, nor with the alterations associated with a deficiency of vitamin A or the changes that occur in the ribs with hog cholera and other disease (see page 634).

Examination of the ends of the long bones of a rachitic individual reveals a broad epiphyseal plate that consists of osteoid tissue and cartilage. The diaphyseal and epiphyseal surfaces are irregular in contrast to the flat surfaces in the normal individual. The epiphyseal plate and the adjacent diaphyseal and epiphyseal tissues have been compressed by the weight of the animal because they are soft due to insufficient mineralization. They protrude laterally, resulting in a peripheral enlargement of the ends of the bones in the vicinity of the epiphyseal line.

**Microscopic lesions.** Histological alterations characteristic of rickets are the presence of numerous capillary buds and endothelial cells invading the lacunae of the epiphyseal plate, numerous osteoblasts on the walls of the cartilaginous lacunae and the osseous and cartilaginous trabeculae, and an abundance of osteoid tissue that has not been ossified.

The first essential tissue change necessary for growth in length of a long bone is a proliferation of the epiphyseal plate of cartilage. As long as this plate is present and proliferation occurs, growth will take place. When the plate of cartilage ceases to grow or is no longer present, bone growth does not occur.

The proliferating cells of the epiphyseal plate are found in the central plane of the cartilage. This area is called the **zone of proliferation.** The more mature cells are found closer to the diaphysis or epiphysis of the bone. These more mature cells arrange themselves in longitudinal rows parallel with the long axis of the bone. As the diaphysis or epiphysis is approached, the parallel rows of cartilage become more distinct. This area is designated as the **zone of columns.** With still more maturity

the arrangement of the cartilage cells into columns becomes more distinct. In addition, broad zones of matrix exist between the columns of cells. At the same time the lacunae become larger and larger, and the cartilage cells within the lacunae begin to show degeneration. Because of the large lacunae arranged in columns, the area where they are found is referred to as the **vesicular zone.**

While changes involving the cartilage cells proper are taking place, the matrix between the cartilage cells is undergoing calcification. The concentration of mineral in the cartilage is least near the zone of proliferation and greatest in the vesicular zone near the diaphysis or epiphysis. The presence of mineral gives rigidity and strength to the cartilage. This is needed particularly in the zone of vesicles where the cartilage is no longer dense and compact.

The amount of mineral deposited in the cartilage is under the influence of the parathyroid gland and is dependent upon the amount of mineral and vitamin D available. Diseases of the parathyroid or deficiencies of minerals or vitamin D in the ration result in a low mineral content of the cartilage.

The cartilage nearest the epiphysis or diaphysis is in contact with the capillaries of the bone marrow. Those capillaries adjacent to the cartilage show active hyperemia, indicating great metabolic activity in this area. In addition, the endothelial cells are hyperchromatic and hyperplastic, indicating rapid growth potential. These hyperplastic endothelial cells in the walls of the capillaries in contact with the cartilage accomplish decalcification and solution of the cartilage matrix through alterations in the hydrogen ion potential and enzyme activity. In this manner the walls of the lacunae nearest the bone marrow are destroyed, and the capillary bud invades and fills the lacunae. Since there is less matrix to be removed in the columns of cartilage cells than between the rows of cartilage cells, the invasion of cartilage is more rapid in the columns of cartilage cells. As a result, cartilaginous trabeculae remain between the columns of cartilage cells that are being invaded by the capillary buds. These cartilage columns, strengthened by calcification, are essential if the continuity of the bone and cartilage is to be maintained and a separation along the epiphyseal plate is to be prevented.

The endothelial cells of the capillary buds are potentially capable of forming capillaries, white fibrous connective tissue, and osteoblasts. When the cartilage lacunae are invaded, the endothelial cells pave the walls of the lacunae. Metaplasia occurs, and some of the endothelial cells become osteoblasts and deposit osteoid tissue on the walls of the lacunae.

While metaplasia of some of the endothelial cells is taking place, other endothelial cells are forming capillary buds. These are removing the cartilaginous wall of the next maturing cell in the cartilage cell columns of the zone of vesicles, and the process of invasion of the lacunae is repeated. In this manner progressive growth of bone takes place.

In normal bone the newly formed osteoid tissue is mineralized — a process known as **ossification** — and firm dense bone is the result. The cartilage in these developing osseous trabeculae is gradually absorbed. Finally a network of bony trabeculae (called spongy bone) is present in the diaphysis and epiphysis.

In rickets the rate of cartilage growth is approximately normal unless the animal shows considerable debility, in which case the rate of growth is suppressed. Calcification of cartilage is retarded in the absence of vitamin D, and as a result the normal rigidity and strength of the cartilage is not present. This is particularly evident in the matrix columns in the zone of vesicles. As a result, bending, twisting, compressing, and fracturing of these columns occur. The poorly mineralized cartilage can no longer support the weight of the individual, cannot withstand the traction of the muscles, nor can it withstand the torque placed on this area as the animal moves about.

Capillary invasion of the cartilage continues at a normal or near normal rate unless other deficiency diseases are producing general debility of the individual. The conversion of endothelial cells into osteoblasts continues, and osteoid tissue is deposited on the distorted trabeculae. The osteoid tissue, however, is not properly mineralized, and the trabeculae of osteoid tissue are not able to support the stresses and pressures, just as was observed in the cartilage. As a result, bending, twisting, compressing, and fracturing of the osteoid trabeculae occur.

Because of faulty mineralization, a broad zone of distorted and compressed cartilaginous and osteoid trabeculae can be observed both macroscopically and microscopically in the region of the epiphyseal plate. As a result of the compression, lateral protrusion of tissues in the region of the epiphyseal plate occurs, causing a peripheral enlargement of the bone in this region.

The periosteal bone growth also shows alterations. The osteoblasts derived from the periosteum produce osteoid tissue at a normal or near normal rate. However, the newly formed osteoid tissue is not properly ossified and normal osseous tissue is not produced. As a result, the shaft of the bone is soft and may bend or become distorted. The attachment of tendons, ligaments, and muscles to the soft bone is insecure, and when stress is applied a separation of these structures from the bone may take place.

The bone marrow shows normal hematopoiesis and development unless the ration is deficient in other minerals and vitamins necessary for bone marrow metabolism.

### Vitamin A Deficiency

The rate of cartilage growth in vitamin A deficiency is approximately normal unless other deficiency diseases exist. Calcification of cartilage takes place at a normal rate so that the normal rigidity and strength of the cartilage are maintained. The bending, twisting, compressing, and fracturing of the matrix columns so prominent in vitamin D deficiency do not occur.

Vitamin A is very essential for bone growth as it is vitally concerned with the metabolism of the endothelial cells. When vitamin A is not available, proliferation of endothelial cells of the capillaries does not occur, capillary endothelial cells are not converted into osteoblasts, and the few osteoblasts that are present are unable to produce osteoid tissue.

With a deficiency of vitamin A the capillaries in the bone marrow adjacent to the epiphyseal plate do not show the degree of active hyperemia seen in a deficiency of vitamin D. This indicates that great metabolic activity is not taking place in this area. In addition, the capillary endothelial cells do not show hyperchromasia and hyperplasia. Because of this hypoactivity in endothelial cell metabolism, the capillaries in contact with the cartilage do not accomplish decalcification and solution of the cartilage. The capillary endothelium is unable to break down the wall of the lacunae nearest the bone marrow, and because of this the capillary bud cannot invade the lacunae of the cartilage. Since cartilage invasion by the capillaries is not taking place or is retarded, cartilage disintegration is not able to keep pace with cartilage formation and maturation. As a result, the zone of columns and vesicles becomes excessively broad.

The conversion of endothelial cells into osteoblasts is suppressed or does not occur, depending on the degree of vitamin A deficiency. Because of this, only a small amount or no osteoid tissue is deposited on the cartilaginous trabeculae that may have formed. The osteoid tissue that is formed is mineralized. Since the osteoid tissue is inadequate in amount, it is not able to support the stresses and strains placed upon it. Twisting, bending, compressing, and fracturing of the trabeculae occur in the spongy bone next to the epiphyseal plate.

The junction between the cartilage and bone is often very irregular and undulating. The reason for this is that if hemorrhage or a cavernous space filled with blood and lined with endothelium exists at the junction of the cartilage and the bone, no further cartilage breakdown occurs in this area because the capillaries are no longer in contact with the cartilage. No bone formation occurs in this area. When this inhibition of cartilage breakdown occurs at focal points along the bone and cartilage junction, an irregular rate of bone growth occurs and an undulating epiphyseal line is the result.

Because of the inability of the capillaries to achieve cartilage breakdown, the epiphyseal plate becames unusually broad and has an undulating surface. The broad zone observed in this area is composed of cartilage and not osteoid tissue as was the case in rickets. The diameter of the bone in the vicinity of the epiphyseal plate is increased because cartilage proliferation has continued at a normal rate while the shaft of the bone has not increased in diameter at a similar rate. The lateral protrusion of the epiphyseal plate as observed in rickets does not occur because compression of the mineralized cartilaginous trabeculae does not take place. The distortion of the osseous trabeculae occurs in the diaphysis or the next to the epiphyseal plate. The osseous trabeculae in this region are thin since suppressed bone formation is present. Some bending, twisting, compressing, and fracturing of the osseous trabeculae in this region may result. When this takes place, some lateral protrusion will be observed.

The periosteal bone growth also shows alterations. The osteoblasts derived from the periosteum are few in number or do not appear and, as a result, little or no osteoid tissue is produced. The osteoid tissue that is formed undergoes ossification and forms osseous tissue. Because of this alteration in osteoblast activity, the normal rate of peripheral enlargement of the shaft of the bone does not occur. As a result, the diameter of the ends of the bones is larger in proportion than is the diameter of the shaft.

The bone marrow shows a marked suppression of hematopoiesis. The space between the bony trabeculae contains a few capillaries, strands of connective tissue, and a few myeloid cells.

Bone lesions resulting from a vitamin A deficiency are seen most frequently in guinea pigs, calves, and pigs. Swine fed grain, such as corn, that has been held in storage for several years may show bone lesions of a vitamin A deficiency if other sources of vitamin A are not provided in the ration. Pelleted feeds may be deficient in vitamin A if the speed and temperature of pelleting are not properly controlled.

### Vitamin C Deficiency

The bone alterations in vitamin C deficiency are very similar to those observed in vitamin A deficiency because these two vitamins complement each other. If a deficiency of vitamin C exists, more vitamin A is required. As a result, when a vitamin C deficiency is present, there will also be a deficiency of vitamin A unless additional amounts of vitamin A are provided.

The basic bone and cartilage alterations are the same as those described in a vitamin A deficiency. The difference is that in a deficiency of vitamin C, hemorrhage occurs in the vicinity of the epiphyseal plate. Capillary fragility is one of the characteristics of scurvy. The bending, twisting, compressing, and fracturing of the cartilaginous and osseous trabeculae adjacent to the epiphyseal plate result in injury and rupture of the capillaries in this region. Since the capillary walls in scurvy are fragile, an unusual amount of vascular injury occurs, resulting in excessive hemorrhage in the area. Hemorrhage along the junction of cartilage and bone is serious, as indicated in the discussion of vitamin A deficiency, because cartilage invasion by capillaries will not occur if the capillaries lose contact with the cartilage.

Extensive hemorrhage also involves the periosteum. Because of the capillary fragility, excessive hemorrhage results when the periosteum is subjected to trauma. These traumatic injuries may be the result of blows from the exterior. They also are the result of the insecure attachment of tendons, ligaments, and muscles to the soft bone. When stress is applied, a separation of these structures from the bone may take place. This separation results in damage to the capillaries in the region.

Most of our domestic animals are capable of synthesizing vitamin C in their digestive tracts. In addition, the nature of the ration is such that vitamin C is usually provided. Hence, a deficiency of vitamin C is of little clinical importance. The disease is observed in the guinea pig when fresh vegetables are not included in the ration.

### Hypoplasia of Bone As the Result of Starvation

Hypoplasia of bone occurs in the starving animal when the constituents necessary for anabolism are not provided in the ration. Protein is one of the most important requirements. The nutritional anemias of swine caused by a deficiency of vitamin B and iron will cause suppression of the rate of bone growth. A well-balanced ration in adequate amounts is necessary if normal bone growth and metabolism are to be accomplished.

### Hypoplasia of Bone As the Result of Specific Infectious Diseases

Hypoplasia of bone occurs in specific infectious diseases as the result of altered metabolism, increased requirements of essential constituents of the ration, or starvation.

Certain infectious diseases are especially likely to produce alterations in bone growth. This is especially true of **hog cholera**. The hog cholera virus damages the endothelial cells. Because of this injury to the endothelial cells, there is a suppression of the rate of cartilage invasion along the epiphyseal plate. The hyperplasia of the capillary endothelium does not take place. The great metabolic activity of the capillaries in this region is not observed. The breakdown of the walls of the cartilaginous lacunae does not take place. The formation of osteoblasts from endothelial cells does not occur, and as a result osteoid tissue is not formed. In addition, the growth rate of the cells of the bone marrow is suppressed. The lesions are very similar to those observed in vitamin A deficiency, and because of this, a broad epiphyseal plate and a hypoplastic bone are observed.

This alteration in bone growth occurs in swine affected with hog cholera or in swine that have been vaccinated for hog cholera. The amount of suppressed bone growth in vaccinated swine depends on the amount of reaction produced by the vaccine and the type of vaccine used. Other infectious diseases of the pig, such as erysipelas, salmonellosis, and swine influenza, may also bring about alterations in the rapidity of bone growth.

Most cases of so-called rickets in the dog are the result of suppressed cartilage breakdown and hypoplasia of the osteoblast associated with certain infectious diseases such as **canine distemper.** This is observed particularly in the larger breeds of dogs where rapid bone growth must take place. The bone lesion most closely resembles the alterations that have been described under vitamin A deficiency.

Since infectious **canine hepatitis** is a disease that injures capillary endothelium, it is quite possible that some of the bone alterations observed in young dogs are also the result of this disease. The debilitating diseases of the dog, such as hookworm anemia, cause a suppressed rate of bone formation.

## INFLAMMATION

### Terminology

**Periostitis** — inflammation of the periosteum.

**Ostitis** — inflammation of the bone.

**Endostitis** — inflammation of the endosteum.

**Osteomyelitis** — inflammation of the bone marrow.

### Acute Periostitis

Acute periostitis usually occurs as a local inflammation of the periosteum. Occasionally all of the periosteum of a small bone may be involved.

**Serous, fibrinous,** and **hemorrhagic** periostitis are usually the result of trauma. They are most frequently observed in the bones of the legs since these extremities are most subject to injury. Lesions of this type may involve the mandible of the horse when severe breaker bits and bridles are used. **Suppurative** periostitis occurs when the periosteum is invaded by pyogenic bacteria. The bacteria may invade the periosteum through wounds that extend into the periosteum from the exterior (knife, bullet, wire cut, and caulk wounds), by extension from suppurative inflammation adjacent to the bone, or carried to the periosteum by way of the blood vascular system. Suppurative periostitis is observed most frequently in the mandible and in the bones of the legs.

### Chronic Periostitis

Chronic periostitis is very common in domesticated animals and is most frequently observed in the leg bones of the horse. It occurs as the result of **injury,** particularly of a traumatic nature (contusions, sprains, luxations, and fractures). **Deficiency diseases** of bone bring about an increased incidence of periostitis since the bone has less strength to withstand traumatic injury. When tension is placed on tendons and ligaments, minute fractures or even a separation of the tissues may take place at the junction of the tendon and ligament with the bone, or the constant tension exerted on the soft bone results in irritation and causes hyperplasia of bone in these areas. A deficiency of phosphorus in the ration often results in a sharp increase in the incidence of chronic periostitis in a group of animals.

Chronic periostitis usually occurs as a **serous** or **suppurative** type of inflammation. Chronic serous periostitis is the most frequent type. Chronic suppurative periostitis occurs when pyogenic bacteria have invaded the periosteum through wounds or compound fractures.

Chronic serous periostitis is characterized by the presence of a serous exudate in the tissues. In addition there is the deposition of connective tissue and osseous tissue in the area. If the new growth is composed primarily of white fibrous connective tissue, it is referred to as **fibrous periostitis**. It appears on the surface of the bone as a raised mass of white fibrous connective tissue which is interwoven with the adjacent tissue and is firmly attached to the underlying bone. **Osseous periostitis** is characterized by the presence of bone in the new growth. The new osseous tissue is firmly attached to the underlying bone. It may occur as a flat plaque, a wartlike mass, or as spicules projecting from the bone. These bony protrusions are called **exostoses**.

Specific terms are used to indicate focal areas of periostitis in the equine. A **spavin** is a term used to describe a focal periostitis of the tarsal bones. A spavin is most frequently observed on the medial side of the hock. The cause is trauma to the tarsal bones when the attachment of ligaments to the tarsal bones has been damaged by sprains or overwork. A **ringbone** is a focal periostitis involving the phalanges. A **splint** is a focal periostitis that occurs as a result of injury to the periosteum at the site of attachment of the interosseous ligament to the splint bones or the metacarpal or metatarsal bones. It is most frequently observed in the front legs and usually involves the attachment of the medial interosseous ligament.

## Ostitis

Both **acute** and **chronic ostitis** are usually the result of extension of a periostitis, an endostitis, or an osteomyelitis into the bone. Bone in the vicinity of inflammation undergoes demineralization. The extent of the demineralization may be focal or diffuse depending on the size of the area of inflammation. This softening and destruction of bone, often showing cavity formation, is termed **rarefying ostitis**.

If bone becomes unusually hard and dense as the result of inflammation, it is said to have undergone **osteosclerosis** or **eburnation**. The protrusion of hyperplastic bone into the marrow cavity as the result of inflammation of the endosteum is designated as **endostosis**.

## Acute Osteomyelitis

**Acute suppurative osteomyelitis** is a diffuse inflammation of the bone marrow. The inflammation may be **serous, fibrinous, hemorrhagic, or suppurative** in type.

**Acute suppurative osteomyelitis** is of most importance because it indicates that pyogenic microorganisms have invaded the bone marrow. The bacteria reach the bone marrow by various routes such as exposure of the bone marrow in compound fractures, perforation by bullet wounds, extension from suppurative inflammation in the vicinity of bone, and by way of the blood vascular system in septicemic diseases such as pullorum disease in chickens.

Hematogenous infections are embolic in nature and result in focal abscesses in the bone marrow. The abscesses are most frequently found in the more vascular spongy portions of the bone. In young growing animals the most vascular portion of the bone marrow is in the diaphysis and the epiphysis near the epiphyseal plate. It is in this region that abscesses are most frequently observed. This can be easily demonstrated if the costochondral junction of the ribs is examined, particularly in the horse with a septicemia as a result of omphalitis. Suppurative inflammation in the vicinity of the epiphyseal plate suppresses or prevents bone growth. Since bone marrow undergoes putrefaction rather late in comparison with the other tissues, uncontaminated bacteriological specimens can often be obtained from the bone marrow of decomposing cadavers.

Suppurative osteomyelitis may occur as

single or multiple abscesses, or the entire bone marrow cavity may be involved in a diffuse suppurative inflammation.

Healing of suppurative osteomyelitis is difficult to accomplish because of the location of the infection within the bone. Suitable drainage cannot be achieved, and in addition, the removal of necrotic tissue by surgical methods is difficult to accomplish.

Suppurative osteomyelitis often results in destruction of the adjacent osseous tissue of the bone shaft. If this destruction is focal, as occurs in the vicinity of abscesses, the cavities that are formed are designated as **caries.**

## Chronic Osteomyelitis

**Chronic osteomyelitis** is the usual termination of the acute form because of the difficulty in obtaining healing. It is usually of the suppurative type and is characterized by irregular hyperplasia of white fibrous connective tissue and osseous tissue and the destruction of normal bone.

Suppurative osteomyelitis can be caused by hematogenous invasion of the bone marrow by Brucella, corynebacteria, staphylococci, streptococci, and other pyogenic microorganisms. It is observed most frequently in swine infected with *Brucella suis* and cattle infected with *Corynebacterium pyogenes.* The most severe lesions are found in the bodies of the lumbar vertebrae, although all bones of the body are involved. The chronic suppurative inflammation results in destruction of the body of the vertebrae. The inflammatory process may extend into the intervertebral articulation or into the vertebral canal. Compression of the spinal cord is of frequent occurrence due to the local hyperplasia resulting from the inflammation. The damaged vertebrae may **fracture** and compress the spinal cord. **Luxation** of the lumbar vertebrae with compression of the spinal cord may occur when the articulation has been damaged. The spinal cord may be compressed by abscesses when the inflammatory process has invaded the vertebral canal.

## ACTINOMYCOSIS

Actinomycosis of bone is caused by *Actinomyces bovis.* It is most frequently observed in cattle but is also encountered in other mammals. Any bone of the body may be involved, but the infection is usually observed in the mandible.

The infection may gain entrance to the bone marrow by hematogenous routes or by direct extension from adjacent abscesses. The higher incidence of the disease in the mandible can be explained by the route of infection. Apparently the organism is brought to an animal on feed contaminated by other animals carrying the organisms in their oral flora. Coarse feed, particularly if it contains barbs and thorns, lacerates the oral mucosa or actually may be inserted into the oral tissues. This is particularly apt to cause infection if the injury occurs around the teeth. Following the introduction of the organism, a focal acute suppurative inflammation occurs. If an acute suppurative alveolar periostitis is the result, the infection can easily be transported by the venous or lymphatic circulation, probably within the cytoplasm of the macrophages, into the bone marrow of the mandible, or it may invade the bone marrow by direct extension. If the microorganisms are not destroyed, a chronic suppurative osteomyelitis of the mandible occurs. This causes an extensive rarefaction of the bone, proliferation of connective tissue, and irregular hyperplasia of osteoid tissue resulting in a greatly enlarged mandible.

As in any chronic suppurative osteomyelitis, numerous **sinus tracts** to the exterior may be present. The pus is greenish yellow in color, has little odor, is thick and tenacious, and contains numerous small yellow granules that resemble grains of sulfur.

The ostitis and osteomyelitis may extend into the adjacent tissues. The teeth may be demineralized and invaded by the infection. Because of the destruction of the alveolus, the teeth may fall out. If bone destruction is great, a fracture of the mandible may occur.

The microscopic appearance of the lesion is that of a chronic focal suppurative inflammation in the center of which is an irregular eosin-staining mass of radiating clublike structures. These eosin-staining masses can also be observed on gross examination of the tissue and appear as firm granules that have a yellow color and vary in size from just visible to 2 millimeters in diameter. Because of their size and appearance they are called **sulfur granules.** If these distinctive structures are stained with the Gram stain, the Gram-positive *Actinomyces bovis* can be demonstrated within them. Immediately adjacent to the sulfur granules there is a dense mass of neutrophils, and both are surrounded by an encapsulating mass of lymphocytes, macrophages, giant cells, and connective tissue.

### TUBERCULOSIS

Tuberculosis of bone, caused by *Mycobacterium tuberculosis,* is most frequently observed as an osteomyelitis. The infection may also involve the periosteum and endosteum. Invasion of the bone proper, particularly that of the shaft of the bone, usually occurs as an extension from the periosteum or the bone marrow.

The acid-fast bacteria usually reach the bone marrow by way of the blood stream, although direct extension from infections in adjacent tissue may occur. Tuberculous osteomyelitis is most frequently observed in chickens, swine, and cattle.

The lesion is usually of the focal or multiple focal type, which indicates an embolic spread from a primary lesion in some other organ. A diffuse involvement of the bone marrow is usually not encountered. The finding of focal lesions in the bone marrow indicates that **generalized tuberculosis** exists.

The basic lesion, in the early stages, consists of a micro-abscess. Later, the central area undergoes caseous necrosis. The necrotic mass becomes surrounded by a zone of macrophages, giant cells, and lymphocytes. This more highly cellular zone is in turn surrounded by an encapsulating zone that consists primarily of lymphocytes, macrophages, and connective tissue. In older lesions the central area of necrosis may become calcified.

The lesions in the bone are frequently miliary in size or may be so small they are not seen on gross examination.

Tuberculosis of bone marrow is usually of the caseo-necrotic or caseo-calcific type, although this will vary with the species of animal concerned. Occasionally a suppurative type of inflammation may be observed.

In the immediate vicinity of the tuberculous inflammation, destruction of the bone occurs. Usually, there is no external distortion of the bone, but at times, particularly with suppurative tuberculous osteomyelitis, extensive rarefaction of bone together with hyperplastic periostitis and endostitis may occur.

About 90 per cent of chickens infected with tuberculosis have tuberculous osteomyelitis. The lesions are most numerous in the long bones of the legs and in the vertebral column.

Malleomyces, blastomyces, histoplasma, toxoplasma, monilia, and aspergilli may also invade bone marrow and produce a chronic osteomyelitis.

### PARASITES

Parasites are seldom found in bone. Occasionally the oncosphere of *Taenia echinococcus* may become located in the bone marrow. As the cyst enlarges, pressure atrophy of the neighboring bone marrow and bone occurs.

### NEOPLASMS OF BONE

Tumors in bone may be primary or secondary. The general discussion on tumors of bone can be found in the chapter on neoplasms.

The **primary tumors** of bone are **fibroma, chondroma, osteoma,** and their malignant type, the **sarcoma.** Neoplasms of the bone marrow are of the **myeloid** and **lymphoid** types. These tumors may cause extensive destruction of the osseous tissue.

**Secondary tumors** of bone marrow are

quite common. Metastatic sarcomas and carcinomas are brought to the bone marrow by the blood stream or they may invade the bone by infiltration when the primary tumor is located in the vicinity of bone. Extensive destruction of bone may result as the tumor grows and invades the osseous tissue.

# Muscular System

The muscular system of the body is extremely important because it is necessary for locomotion. It is also of indirect importance because it provides the most important protein in the ration of the human being, carnivorous animals, and other animal species where meat or meat by-products are used. There is a tendency to overlook the muscular system in routine post-mortem technics, but the evaluation of the lesions within the muscles is exceedingly important and frequently gives an indication as to the cause of death.

## CIRCULATORY DISTURBANCES

### Hyperemia

**Acute general active hyperemia** occurs when hyperemia of the entire body exists as the result of a septicemic disease (erysipelas or salmonellosis). A physiological acute general active hyperemia is observed when the muscles throughout the entire body are undergoing an increased metabolic rate as the result of exercising or fighting.

In packing houses there is a carcass alteration known as the **dark cutter syndrome** or **dark cutting beef** in which the musculature is excessively dark red in color. The pigmentation is found in cattle which are subjected to adverse weather conditions, trauma, excitement, fatigue, and various infectious diseases prior to slaughter. In these animals there is either an acute general active hyperemia or an acute general passive hyperemia. In either case the increased pigmentation of the musculature is due to the increased amount of blood which is contained within the muscle. Because of the dark red color the beef is graded lower in market value and there is an increased difficulty in preserving it since the carcass does not bleed out properly during slaughter. Blood in the vessels aids bacterial growth and putrefaction.

**Acute local active hyperemia** is observed when injury has involved a single muscle or a portion of a muscle. It occurs in the vicinity of local infectious diseases (abscess), in the neighborhood of parasites (trichinae, taeniae, or sarcocysts) which are encysting in muscle, or in areas of traumatic injury.

**Acute general passive hyperemia** occurs throughout the entire body when a lesion is present in the heart or lungs.

**Chronic general passive hyperemia** occurs when a lesion persists in the heart or lungs for a long period of time. Usually connective tissue deposition does not occur to any great extent in the muscles of animals except in the legs or in the more dependent portions of the body where edema occurs and where the impaired circulation is more pronounced because of the influence of gravity.

**Acute local passive hyperemia** occurs when there is a local obstruction to the flow of blood from a muscle. This may be caused by constricting bandages around a limb, or may occur when thrombi are present in the veins draining a particular muscle.

**Chronic local passive hyperemia** occurs when the obstruction to the venous flow persists for a long period of time. It is most frequently observed in the muscles of the legs of horses which are confined in stables and are not allowed to exercise. The influence of gravity causes a hypostatic hyperemia.

## Anemia

General anemia of the musculature occurs when a hemorrhagic, hypochromic, hemolytic, or aplastic anemia exists. General anemia is a prominent lesion in the copper and iron deficiency anemia of swine. Anemia of the musculature is very common in swine that die from gastric hemorrhage. It is commonly observed in puppies with severe hookworm infections, in sheep with stomach worm infections (haemonchus, ostertagia, trichostrongylus), nematodirus infections, or in coccidiosis of chickens, sheep, and cattle. Anemia of the musculature is one of the manifestations of trichloroethylene poisoning in cattle.

**Ischemia** occurs when thrombi or emboli obstruct a major artery of a muscle. This type of injury is not common because the collateral circulation of muscle is so complete that unless very major arteries (femoral or brachial) are involved, a local anemia will not be observed. The most common causes of ischemia are compressing bandages or tourniquets placed around a limb.

**Macroscopic appearance.** The muscle lacks its normal red intense color and has a pink, white or yellow color depending upon the species of animal and the normal color of the muscle. If the ischemia persists, necrosis and gangrene are the result.

**Microscopic appearance.** The blood vessels contain very little blood. Depending upon how long the ischemia has been present, the muscle cells may show degenerative and necrotic changes. The most common alterations as the result of ischemia are fatty degeneration, coagulative necrosis, and gangrene.

## Hemorrhage

Hemorrhage in muscle is usually the result of traumatic injury from whips, clubs, and canes, or the traumatic injuries produced when animals run into objects or receive violent injuries while fighting. This type of bleeding is usually hemorrhage per rhexis.

Hemorrhages per diapedesis or rhexis may occur when local or general infectious diseases are present. When bacteria are introduced into the tissues through gunshot wounds, dog bites, or hypodermic syringe needles, hemorrhage may occur in the vicinity of the injury. Hemorrhage is observed in the musculature in trichloroethylene and bracken poisoning in cattle; salmonellosis, hog cholera, and erysipelas in swine; anthrax, malignant edema, and blackleg in cattle; salmonella, shigella, and streptococcal infections in horses; and hemorrhagic disease, fowl pest, erysipelas, and pasteurellosis in chickens.

Hemorrhages often occur in animals at the time of slaughter and are particularly common in swine and cattle. Hemorrhages of this nature are especially common in well-finished cattle slaughtered by the kosher method. The hemorrhages are most numerous in the muscles of the neck and the longissimus dorsi. In fat beef cattle coagulative necrosis of the muscle is present prior to the time of slaughter, and the necrotic muscle ruptures very easily when the agony of violent death occurs. When rupture of the muscle takes place hemorrhage is the result.

Histologically the hemorrhages are recognized by an abundance of erythrocytes in the area. Whether it is hemorrhage or hemorrhagic inflammation is determined by the proportion of erythrocytes to leukocytes. In inflammation there is an increase in the number of leukocytes.

## Edema

**General edema** of muscle involves the entire body and is caused by general passive hyperemia (as the result of lesions in the heart or lungs), diminished blood protein (extensive hemorrhage, parasitism, or in cachectic animals as is observed in starvation), or increased capillary permeability (as occurs in shock).

**Local edema** occurs when there is an obstruction to the venous or lymphatic circulation from an area. Venous obstruction is usually the result of constricting bandages, rubber bands, or scar tissue which compress the veins, or thrombi which obstruct the venous circulation. Lymphatic obstruction occurs when bandages or constricting devices compress the lymphatics, or when chronic inflammatory diseases (histoplasmosis or blastomycosis) or tumors (lymphosarcoma) invade the regional lymph nodes.

**Macroscopic appearance.** The muscles lack their normal intense red color when lymphatic obstruction is present because the fluid interferes with the flow of blood through the part. The muscles are hyperemic if venous obstruction is present. Most of the edema is located in the interstitial connective tissue and appears as a clear lymphlike fluid between the muscle bundles. When the muscle is incised, fluid flows slowly from the cut surface.

**Microscopic appearance.** The fluid is located for the most part in the interstitial connective tissue. The muscle fibers and connective tissue cells are spread apart by the accumulation of fluid which appears as a faintly granular homogeneous substance that stains slightly pink with eosin.

## DISTURBANCES IN GROWTH

### Atrophy

**Etiology.** A common cause of atrophy is senility. Whether it is observed or not depends upon the age to which the animal is allowed to live. Beef cattle and swine as a rule are slaughtered for food long before atrophy occurs. Dogs, milk cows, horses, and ewes frequently show muscular atrophy because of their longer life span. Starvation atrophy is observed in times of drouth when food is not available or when diseases of the digestive tract prevent the animal from utilizing the food which is available. Muscular atrophy is often observed in chronic debilitating diseases such as tuberculosis, paratuberculosis, and neoplasia. Disuse atrophy often occurs following fractures in the legs of animals. Neurotrophic atrophy is observed when nerves to a group of

muscles are injured. In the horse this is the lesion associated with roaring when the recurrent laryngeal nerve is injured, and in atrophy of the supraspinatus and infraspinatus muscles when the suprascapular nerve is injured. Pressure atrophy may occur when tumors, parasites, hematocysts, saddles, or collars compress muscles. Pressure atrophy is caused by the inadequate nutrition associated with an interference with the circulation to the muscle.

**Macroscopic appearance.** The muscles are pink, white, gray, or yellow in appearance. They do not retain their normal size and they lack normal muscle tone. With atrophy there is often considerable distortion of the animal. If one group of muscles becomes smaller and another does not, the disproportion causes disfiguration. With general atrophy of muscle as occurs in senility or starvation, the osseous skeleton becomes more prominent.

**Microscopic appearance.** The muscle cells are smaller in size when compared with normal muscle cells. Since degenerative and necrotic muscle alterations are brought about by the same group of etiologic factors which produce atrophy, changes such as cloudy swelling, fatty degeneration, and coagulative necrosis may be present in the muscle cells. When replacement fibrosis occurs, there is an increased amount of connective tissue in the area. Metaplasia of connective tissue to adipose tissue may take place and the area may become infiltrated with fat.

### Hypoplasia

**Etiology.** Hypoplasia of muscle is often observed in young animals. It is usually the result of some defect in the blood vessels or nerves in the region. This is frequently observed in the posterior extremities of young animals when embryological defects occur in the spinal cord or the sciatic nerves. A **hypoplastic lipomatosis** is often observed in animals in which the muscles are approximately their normal size but are extensively infiltrated with adipose cells. Only a few muscle strands remain. This is especially common in the longissimus dorsi of cattle and swine. The etiology of this lesion has not been determined.

**Macroscopic appearance.** The muscles are small when compared with those of normal animals and are usually pink, white, gray, or yellow in color. Because the involved muscles or muscle groups are smaller than normal, there is often considerable disfiguration of the animal, and the osseous skeleton may be more prominent than normal.

**Microscopic appearance.** The muscle cells are smaller in size when compared with normal muscle cells. The cells usually lack their angular appearance when viewed in cross section, and Cohnheim's fields are absent or only few in number. Usually there is considerable space between the individual muscle cells, and this space contains a loosely arranged connective tissue, some adipose tissue, and may be slightly edematous.

### Hypertrophy

**Etiology.** Enlargement of muscles as the result of an increase in the size of the individal cells is observed in animals subjected to excessive work or exercise. It is most frequently observed in working dogs, draft horses, saddle horses, and race horses. Hypertrophy of paired muscles is frequently observed when one of the pair is injured. The other pair enlarges as the result of the increased work load placed upon it. This is frequently observed in the legs of animals that are lame.

**Macroscopic appearance.** Hypertrophy of muscle is recognized grossly by an increase in size when compared with the same muscle of a normal animal. The color of the hypertrophic muscle is about that of normal muscle.

**Microscopic appearance.** As a result of the constant stimulation, the muscle cell becomes larger than normal. The angularity of the cells when observed in cross section is retained even though the cell is larger than normal.

### Hyperplasia

General hyperplasia of muscle seldom occurs. There is, however, a condition known as giant calves or giant lambs (doppellender or storkalvern) which is characterized by a great increase in the size of the musculature of the calf or lamb. It is a hereditary congenital hyperplasia of muscle. It affects all of the more important muscles of the trunk and limbs but especially the muscles of the lumbar region, thigh, and shoulder. Because of the increase in the size of the muscle, the young animals are much larger than normal. The condition in lambs is also characterized by a remarkable shortage of subcutaneous, abdominal, and intermuscular as well as intramuscular fat.

Since only certain groups of muscles are involved, the hyperplastic muscles cause a marked distortion of the newborn animal because the involved muscles are out of proportion to the rest of the muscle groups.

**Microscopic appearance.** The enormous increase in volume of the muscle is due to an increase in the number of muscle cells. Other than the increased number of cells and the shortage of fat, the muscles appear normal.

**Local hyperplasia** of muscle is observed in areas of injury when the stimulation of the irritant causes an excessive regeneration of the muscle cells and there is a gross enlargement of the muscle. Histologically it is recognized by an increased number of cells when compared with a normal muscle from an animal of the same size.

### Metaplasia

Metaplasia of muscle to bone is frequently observed in areas of old traumatic injury or in areas where a chronic inflammatory disease has been present in sheep, cattle, dogs, horses, and swine. In swine it is most commonly observed in the abdominal muscles of the flank region where castration injuries have occurred. Bone may appear in the muscles of the back or in the muscles of the neck of horses where the saddle or the harness has pressed. Bone occurs in the muscles of the legs of old turkeys. Bone is observed in the pectoral muscles of cattle as the result of multiple injuries to this region as the animal moves through brush and rocky terrain. It is also observed in the brisket muscles following an infection with *Onchocerca gibsoni*.

**Macroscopic appearance.** The presence of bone in muscle is recognized by its firm, dense consistency and its gritty character when it is incised with a knife. The bone may or may not be preceded by the formation of cartilage. The osseous tissue is deposited in an irregular manner and is of the spongy type.

**Microscopic appearance.** Bone in muscle is recognized by the typical architecture produced by osteoblasts, lacunae, osteoid tissue, and osseous tissue.

## DISTURBANCES IN CELL METABOLISM

### Cloudy Swelling

**Etiology.** Cloudy swelling of muscle is observed after violent physical exercise. It is associated with the toxemia and fever which occur with various infectious diseases. It is the first alteration which takes place in muscles when vitamin E or selenium deficiency is present. This is also the first alteration that occurs in azoturia.

**Macroscopic appearance.** The muscles are enlarged and firm. There may or may not be an alteration in color. The cloudy swelling which follows violent exercise is masked by the hyperemia of the muscle.

**Microscopic appearance.** The individual muscle cells have a greater diameter than normal. They lack their normal angularity when viewed in cross section and become round in shape. Cohnheim's fields are not as sharply delineated as normal and the cells stain more intensely with eosin.

**Significance and result.** Cloudy swelling indicates that a mild irritant or disturbance in metabolism has injured the cell. If the etiologic agent is removed, the part returns to normal with no permanent alteration in the area. If the injurious substance persists or becomes more intense, a more severe type of degeneration occurs.

### Hydropic Degeneration

**Etiology.** The same etiologic factors which produce cloudy swelling will cause hydropic degeneration of muscle. However, they are more intense and persist for a longer period of time. Usually hydropic degeneration is an alteration of epithelium, but it may occur at times in muscle.

**Macroscopic appearance.** There is little variation in appearance from that of cloudy swelling except that the muscles are more moist.

**Microscopic appearance.** The cells in hydropic degeneration are distended to a greater extent than in cloudy swelling, and cell angularity, in cross section, is lost. Cohnheim's fields are indistinct. Multiple droplets of edematous fluid are present within the cytoplasm of the cells which do not stain with fat or glycogen stains.

### Fatty Degeneration

**Etiology.** Fatty degeneration of muscle is most frequently observed with anemia, especially anemia which has persisted for several days or weeks. It is the type of muscle alteration observed in infectious viral equine anemia or hypoferric anemia in swine. Fatty degeneration of muscle may also occur when chemical poisons such as phosphorus have been administered to the animal. It is also observed in metabolic diseases such as diabetes, acetonemia, and pregnancy disease.

**Macroscopic appearance.** The muscles lack their normal intense red color and have a white or yellow tinge depending upon the color of the fat of the species involved. The muscles are greasy in consistency and may or may not be enlarged. The alterations in color and consistency are very prominent in diabetes in the dog.

**Microscopic appearance.** The individual muscle cells are larger than normal and have lost some or all of their angularity. Cohnheim's fields and the muscle columns of Koelliker are indistinct; cross striations are not as prominent as in normal muscle; and the muscle contains numerous fat droplets whose nature can be verified by various fat stains. The size of the fat droplets is an indication of how long the disturbance in cell metabolism has been present. With various infectious diseases or phosphorus poisoning the fat droplets are small. In metabolic diseases such as diabetes the fat droplets are large.

Fatty degeneration should not be confused with fatty infiltration. Fatty infiltration occurs in the adipose and white fibrous connective tissue between the muscle cells. It is the type of alteration which occurs in the muscles of fat animals during the process of fattening them for market.

**Significance and result.** The presence of fatty degeneration indicates that a severe irritant or metabolic disease is present. If the cause can be removed, the muscle will return to normal in a comparatively short period of time.

### Calcification

**Etiology.** Calcification of muscle occurs when degenerative and necrotic alterations have taken place in muscle cells. **General calcification** is observed following coagulative necrosis of muscle as the result of vitamin E or selenium deficiency. It also occurs if excessive amounts of vitamin D are being fed. This is often observed in calves which are fed excessive amounts of cod-liver oil or fish products. General calcification occurs when parathyroid tumors are present with which there is decalcification of the skeleton, a hypercalcemia, and a subsequent precipitation of calcium in muscle.

**Focal calcification** of muscle appears as the result of a local degenerative, necrotic, or inflammatory alteration. Degenerative or necrotic tissue must be present before calcification occurs. Dead parasites (sarcosporidia, trichinae, and tapeworm cysts) within the muscle undergo calcification.

**Macroscopic appearance.** The calcium appears as firm, dense masses or granules which are white, gray, or yellow in color. When incised with a knife they grit against the blade. The size of the area of calcification depends entirely upon the extent of the degenerative or necrotic muscle alteration which preceded it.

**Microscopic appearance.** Masses of calcium staining blue with hematoxylin are found in the degenerating and necrotic muscle. Specific calcium stains (von Kossa's technic) or microincineration may be used to identify the blue material as calcium.

### Pigmentation

The normal color of muscle varies greatly both with the species and age of the animal. Muscle color is dependent upon the concentration of myoglobin, the amount of blood contained within the muscle, and the degenerative or necrotic alterations which may be present. The musculature of cats and chickens is normally pale red when compared with the deep red of equine musculature. The muscles of young animals often have only a slight pink color and at times are almost white. As the animal grows older, myoglobin accumulates and the color becomes more intense. Some animals at birth and even during adult life lack normal muscle color, which suggests inadequate myoglobin formation.

A disease in the Netherlands known as **Enter's disease** of swine is characterized by an exceedingly colorless muscular tissue. The etiology of the disease is not known, but nutritional disturbances are suspected. For the most part no locomotor disturbances are observed in the animals during life. At slaughter the muscles are nearly colorless and are quite edematous. Edematous fluid may drip from the carcass. The nuclei and sarcolemma of the muscle cells show no anatomical abnormalities, but the myofibrils and Cohnheim's fields are not distinct or are absent. Interstitial edema is present between the muscle cells. No inflammatory alterations are observed in the involved muscles.

Myoglobin is very similar chemically to hemoglobin. Iron, copper, protein, and other essential substances are also needed for myoglobin production. As a result, when hypoferric or hypocupric anemia is present the muscles of the cadaver are unusually pale in color because there is an inadequate production of myoglobin as well as hemoglobin. This is especially noticeable in the hypoferric and hypocupric nutritional anemia of swine. The pale musculature in these animals is also due to the cloudy swelling and fatty degeneration which is present because of a deficiency of oxygen.

Muscle also loses its intense red color when degenerative or necrotic alterations are present. Coagulative necrosis associated with vitamin E or selenium deficiency or azoturia results in **pink, yellow, or white** muscles because the pigment containing myoglobin is liberated and diffuses out of the tissue.

When icterus is present the muscles have a **yellow** tinge. Focal areas of a **green** color in muscles are caused by accumulations of eosinophils. The eosinophils accumulate in areas where parasites (sarcocysts, trichinae, or tapeworm cysts) are present or when myeloid tumors composed of eosinophils invade the muscles of mammals.

A **brown** or **black** pigmentation is observed when excessive amounts of melanin are present in muscle. The melanin usually appears in focal areas and is arranged as masses or streaks in the muscle. The pigment is found in the melanophores contained within the intermuscular connective tissue.

A **brown** or **yellow** pigmentation of muscle is often observed in old emaciated animals, especially cattle. The pigmentation is due to fat soluble xanthochromes found in the cytoplasm of the muscle cells. The pigment appears as granules which stain with fat stains (oil red "O"). This pigment is most frequently observed in the heart, diaphragm, tongue, and the muscles of mastication. Because it is most frequently associated with emaciation and senility it is often called wear and tear pigment.

A **chocolate-brown** pigmentation of muscle is observed when a metmyoglobin is present. Nitrate or chlorate poisoning is the most common cause of metmyoglobin.

## NECROSIS

### Coagulative Necrosis

**Etiology.** How many factors are concerned in muscle metabolism and coagulative necrosis is not known. Many experiments on a number of species of animals have clearly demonstrated that vitamin E is of extreme importance in regulating muscle metabolism. When a deficiency of vitamin E is present, coagulative necrosis of muscle occurs.

**Vitamin E** and probably other substances have antioxidant properties and serve as protective mechanisms in controlling muscle metabolism. When vitamin E is absent, the oxygen consumption of muscle increases 200 to 400 per cent, which indicates the increased rate of metabolism taking place in the muscle cell. Actually the rate of cellular metabolism is so great that the cells burn themselves up and coagulation of the sarcoplasm occurs.

Muscle degeneration has been produced experimentally in guinea pigs, rats, mice, hamsters, chickens, and cattle by withholding vitamin E. It has also been shown that cod-liver oil interferes with the utilization of vitamin E, and although the animals are obtaining adequate amounts of vitamin E they are not able to utilize it because the fat-soluble vitamin is eliminated in the feces with the oil or undergoes oxygenation in the intestinal tract.

**Selenium** is much more efficient in controlling muscle metabolism than is vitamin E. Very minute amounts of the element are needed in the ration, but in some areas of the United States even this small amount is not present. In western United States the deficiency is most frequently observed in calves born of cows fed an all-alfalfa ration during the late months of pregnancy. It is also extremely common in lambs from ewes fed rations consisting of ladino clover, chaff, and oats.

Undoubtedly there are a number of other factors that can produce coagulative necrosis of muscle. In domestic mammals it probably occurs most frequently when multiple deficiences, particularly hypovitaminoses, are present. In the Scandinavian countries coagulative necrosis has been observed in the muscles of calves subjected to a deficiency of both **vitamins C and B**$_1$. It has been shown that a deficiency of **thiamine** causes myocardial coagulative necrosis in pigs. Since this will occur in cardiac muscle, it will probably also occur in skeletal muscle.

It would seem that in areas of drouth, necrosis of muscle is due to a combination of multiple deficiences and toxicities and is not due to any single deficiency. Although vitamin A has been frequently suspected as causing muscle necrosis, it has never been shown that it is capable of doing this except perhaps in a secondary role.

It has been shown that abnormal rumen fermentation can be a **stress factor** in the production of muscle necrosis. The rumen often contains a decomposing mass of ingesta, and it is possible that toxic decomposition products are absorbed by the digestive tract and are a stress factor in the production of muscle necrosis. In northern Europe where altered rumen floras are quite common as the result of soil deficiencies such as cobalt, it has been suggested that vitamin B plays a part in the production of coagulative necrosis of muscle. Since there is an alteration in the rumen flora, no or very little vitamin B is synthesized.

**Macroscopic appearance.** In the early stages of the disease the muscles swell and begin to lose the intense red color characteristic of skeletal muscle due to colloidal changes within the sarcoplasm. As the disease progresses and coagulative necrosis of the muscle takes place, myoglobin is liberated. With the liberation of myoglobin the intense red color is lost and the muscle becomes pale pink, yellowish red, gray, or white in color. This color alteration is due to the loss of myo-globin as well as to the change in the protein of the muscle cells. The protein is coagulated and, just as in the coagulation of egg white, it changes its optical characteristics from clear and translucent to white and opaque. The injured muscle is dry, inelastic, and firm in comparison to normal muscle.

After a few days the necrotic muscle, acting as an irritant, causes an inflammatory reaction. If the muscle alteration is not too severe, a remarkable regeneration of the muscle may take place, and after a period of several weeks there may be little or no indication of the necrotic changes which were present. At other times the muscle necrosis is so severe and extensive that the muscle is not able to regenerate, and then the involved muscle becomes infiltrated with connective tissue and fat after the necrotic tissue is removed. When this occurs there is distortion of the animal since the area occupied by the muscles is not filled in to complete normal configuration.

The myoglobin which is liberated is capable of passing through the renal glomerular filter and appears in the urine. The urine may be brown, red, or chocolate brown in color depending upon the amount of myoglobin. Myoglobin is extremely injurious to glomerular and tubular epithelium and, as a result, nephritis (especially in the horse with azoturia) is a frequent complication.

Great care should always be exercised so as not to confuse myoglobinuria with hemoglobinuria. There are many diseases which will cause a red urine. One of the very common errors is to mistake myoglobinuria for hemoglobinuria and to make an erroneous diagnosis of leptospirosis since occasionally in leptospiral infections there is a hemolysis of the erythrocytes and a hemoglobinuria.

Frequently in the coagulative necrosis associated with blackleg and malignant edema there is little hemorrhage, gas, and edema and very few leukocytes are present in the area. Casual examination might overlook an anaerobe infection.

**Microscopic appearance.** The first alteration noticed in muscle undergoing coagulative necrosis is cloudy swelling. The cells swell, the normal angularity of the cells when viewed in cross section is lost, and because of the increased fluid within the cells the sarcolemma becomes distended. As the condition progresses there is coagulation of the protein within the cell and with this, Cohnheim's fields, the muscle columns of Koelliker, and the cross striations disappear. The muscle cell when coagulated appears as a homogeneous mass filling the distended sarcolemma. The muscle cytoplasm stains more intensely pink with eosin than normal. Gomori's trichrome stain is very effective in demonstrating this alteration as the necrotic muscle loses its red staining characteristic and becomes purple or green in color.

If the necrosis is very severe, the nuclei of the cells undergo necrotic alterations. However, if the cytoplasm of the necrotic cells is coagulated but the nuclei of the cells are still viable, the cell may undergo regeneration since the living nuclei are capable of regenerating the muscle cytoplasm. Before this can be accomplished the necrotic cytoplasm must be removed. In some muscle cells the cellular enzymes not destroyed by the alteration that brought about the necrotic change digest the necrotic cytoplasm. Vacuoles and fissures appear in the cytoplasm as disintegration of the coagulated protein takes place. Since coagulated necrotic tissue is not particularly irritating, the appearance of phagocytes is rather slow and they do not appear in the muscle in great numbers for several days.

Neutrophils, macrophages, lymphocytes, and eosinophils are present within the muscle, but it is the macrophages which do most of the removal of the necrotic tissue. If the entire muscle cell is dead, all of the material is phagocytosed. Many of the necrotic cells, however, still have living muscle nuclei, and in this case only the necrotic cytoplasm is removed by the phagocytes. The phagocytes invade the sarcolemma sheath and remove the necrotic cytoplasm. While phagocytosis is going on, muscle nuclei under the sarcolemma are undergoing hyperplasia, multiple nuclei are being formed, and new sarcoplasm and myofibrils are being produced. These hyperplastic muscle nuclei frequently occur in clumps and have the appearance of giant cells. Very frequently regenerating muscle is mistaken for neoplastic tissue, and extreme care should be taken so as not to confuse these proliferating cells with those of rhabdomyosarcomas, giant cell tumors of bone, and osteosarcomas.

After a period of several weeks all of the necrotic muscle will have been removed, the sarcolemma sheaths will again be filled with sarcoplasm and myofibrils, and when regeneration is complete the hyperemia as well as the phagocytes will disappear. Then, except for a small amount of connective tissue and adipose tissue which may have been deposited in the muscle, little or no alteration will be observed.

Calcium and phosphorus are deposited in necrotic muscle and frequently extensive mineralization of the dead muscle occurs. The muscles of calves sometimes contain as much as 20 times more calcium and twice as much phosphorus as normal. The mineral deposition is the result of the necrosis and does not represent a primary muscle alteration.

### STIFF LAMB DISEASE

Coagulative necrosis of the muscle of lambs can be produced experimentally when the ewes are fed a ration composed of alfalfa hay and cull beans during the gestation period, or by feeding a ration composed of alfalfa hay, cull beans, oats, and barley. Both of these rations are deficient in vitamin E. When these rations are supplemented with wheat germ oil, muscle necrosis does not occur. Lambs deficient in vitamin E, if given a preventive dose of 100 mg. of alphatocopherol shortly after birth, do not develop the disease. When stiff lambs are treated with

150 to 300 mg. of alphatocopherol, many of the lambs will recover.

Lambs deficient in vitamin E are normal as long as they are confined in a small enclosure and are not allowed to exercise. If they are turned out into a lot and allowed to run and frolic or if they are driven, the lambs become stiff in a matter of a few minutes or hours and show typical muscle lesions of coagulative necrosis. This shows that exercise is an important factor in the production of the disease. To illustrate this, a weight is tied to the back of a confined animal. In a short time coagulative necrosis of the muscles occurs, indicating that the work factor is of importance in the development of the muscle alteration.

The afflicted animals move slowly, are stiff, and hesitate to jump or step over small objects. The symptoms are usually most pronounced in the hind legs. The animals tend to move their feet close together under their bodies and stand with their backs arched. In the more severe cases there is paralysis of the legs and the animals are unable to stand on their feet. Some animals die suddenly without showing typical stiffness. These usually have extensive cardiac lesions.

The coagulative necrosis involves both skeletal and cardiac muscles. The lesions appear as white or buff opaque foci or streaks in the muscle. The streaks run parallel with the muscle fibers. The lesions are bilaterally symmetrical and are usually most pronounced in the muscles of the legs where the tendon feathers into the muscle. All of the body musculature may be involved in very severe cases, but the muscle alterations are most frequently observed in the legs, then in the rump, loin, and neck muscles, and less commonly in the diaphragm, intercostal muscles, and the tongue. The lesions in the heart muscle are most numerous in the wall of the left ventricle, especially in the large papillary muscle and under the endocardium and epicardium. Animals with cardiac alterations have a general passive hyperemia and frequently have a complicating pneumonia.

## WHITE MUSCLE DISEASE IN CALVES

White muscle disease is observed at any time from birth to 6 months of age, especially in areas where drouth is present or where cows have been on lush alfalfa pasture. It may also occur in stabled animals if the mothers of the calves have been fed inferior roughage and little or no grain during the last 3 to 4 months of pregnancy. The calves are stiff and have difficulty in moving about. Usually the calves will nurse as long as they can follow the cow. Many calves die suddenly due to cardiac involvement. Extensive coagulative necrosis of muscle is observed. The disease can be prevented by feeding the cows good leafy alfalfa hay with grain or by placing them on green pasture. In phosphorus-deficient animals better results are obtained when vitamin E and some source of phosphorus are added to the poor ration of the dam. In herds where the disease is a problem, a preventive dose of 500 mg. of alphatocopherol by mouth at the time of birth, with an additional 300 mg. twice weekly during the critical period when the white muscle disease is likely to occur, will prevent the disease. Stiff calves should receive 500 to 1,000 mg. of alphatocopherol intramuscularly, followed by 200 to 300 mg. every other day until the symptoms disappear.

## MUSCLE NECROSIS IN DROUTH-STRICKEN RANGE CATTLE

Coagulative necrosis of muscle is very common in cattle which are subjected to severe drouth, particularly if the drouth has continued for several years. The course of the disease varies somewhat depending upon the age of the animal and various stress factors which may be present.

**Acute form in calves and older animals.** The acute form of the disease occurs in young animals, particularly in calves under 6 months of age. It is observed in older animals up to 2 years of age and occasionally in elderly cows. Quite commonly the afflicted animals are found dead on pasture. This sudden death is most frequently observed in calves. In those animals that are observed to be ill, the course of the disease is very rapid. They have no fever, are markedly depressed, and develop a pronounced dyspnea associated with a foamy white or sanguineous nasal discharge. Death usually occurs within 6 to 12 hours after the animals are first observed to be ill. Many of the animals are observed to have a red urine as the result of the myoglobin which is being eliminated.

Post-mortem examination reveals extensive necrosis of the skeletal muscles throughout the cadaver. The necrotic alterations are most noticeable in the heavy muscles of the thigh and shoulder. The muscles are white to yellowish white in color and have a cooked or fish-flesh appearance. Calf muscle is normally quite pale, but when it is compared with normal muscle from other calves of the same age the difference is apparent. At times the course of the disease is so rapid that macroscopic lesions do not have time to develop and then microscopic confirmation of the necrosis is necessary. In the more advanced cases there is extensive coagulative necrosis of the myocardium, particularly in the wall of the left ventricle and especially in the papillary muscles. There is an acute edema and congestion of the lungs, and the trachea and bronchi are filled with a white or sanguineous foam.

**Subacute form occurring in calves and older animals.** When these animals are first observed, they do not have a fever. Later there may be a temperature rise which is due to the terminal pneumonia. For several days these calves show a progressive stiffness which usually begins in the posterior extremities. The animals have great difficulty in moving about and appear to be in severe pain. The condition becomes progressively worse; finally the animals are unable to stand, become recumbent, and frequently do not rise again. Cattle on the range are unable to obtain food and water and eventually die from starvation and exposure. At some time during the course of the disease a myo-globinuria is observed. This is usually seen at the time the stiffness first appears or shortly thereafter. It is usually of relatively short duration, and after a day or two the urine returns to its normal color when all of the liberated myoglobin has been eliminated.

The skeletal muscles throughout the cadaver show extensive coagulative necrosis. They are white or yellowish white in color and have a cooked or fish-flesh appearance. The lesions are most extensive in the heavy muscles of the thigh and shoulder. At times the longissimus dorsi, psoas, gastrocnemius, popliteus, semitendinosus, and semimembranosus show very marked alterations. White or yellowish-white foci and streaks of coagulative necrosis are present in the myocardium, especially in the wall of the left ventricle and in the large papillary muscles. The edema and congestion of the lungs and the resulting pneumonia are due to the myocardial failure. In a few animals there is necrosis of the muscles of mastication and the muscles of the tongue. These latter changes interfere with the prehension and mastication of food.

The disease is most commonly observed in animals that have been subjected to some unusual stress factor. Calves recently weaned are very likely to suffer from this disease. Heavily parasitized animals suddenly develop muscle necrosis. Animals consuming toxic plants are frequently involved. Cattle that are driven, castrated, vaccinated, branded, or shipped are very prone to develop this muscular disease. In this way it is similar to stiff lamb disease where exercise is the factor which precipitates the muscle lesion.

A secondary subacute form is observed in animals afflicted with metritis, mastitis, impaction of the rumen, and other diseases. Usually these animals are in very poor condition, and because of their emaciation they do not respond to treatment, become progressively worse, finally become recumbent, and eventually die or are euthanized.

A very serious form of the disease is observed in animals fed a large amount of cottonseed meal. In the drouth areas cottonseed meal is relatively cheap, and during periods of drouth it is often the only feed available. It is capable of producing extensive coagulative necrosis of muscle. Cottonseed meal should not be fed to calves under 4 months of age and should be fed with caution to animals under 6 months of age. It should not even be fed to older animals unless they are given good quality hay or green feed or are on good pasture. In addition, an adequate supply of minerals should be given since cottonseed meal contains an abundance of phosphorus. If excessive amounts of cottonseed meal are fed during periods of drouth when adequate supplementation is not possible, cottonseed meal toxicity along with coagulative necrosis of muscle will occur. It is especially common in range cattle because it is the practice of the rancher to place a mixture of salt and cottonseed meal in bunkers where animals can have it free choice. In periods of drouth when hay, supplemental grains, or pasture are not available, excessive amounts of the meal are consumed to maintain life. The excellent condition of flesh of these animals indicates they are consuming a large amount of cottonseed meal.

### STIFFNESS IN CATTLE ON FULL FEED

Stiffness is often observed in prime and choice beef cattle that are on full feed particularly if the ration contains a large amount of corn and the animals have lush legume (especially alfalfa) pasture available. The stiffness is most frequently observed in the cattle having the highest finish.

The cattle are first observed to be stiff when they attempt to rise and during the first few steps after they have arisen. When the symptoms first appear the stiffness appears to be in the shoulders. The affected animals often have a diarrhea and the feces have a slight sour odor. In many instances nothing more than stiffness is observed. If the concentrate ration is reduced in amount and the ani-

mals are fed some hay prior to being placed upon the lush legume pasture, the stiffness soon disappears. If the full feeding is continued, the disease becomes progressively worse, the animals are unable to move about, and typical lesions of coagulative necrosis are found in the muscles at necropsy.

### STIFFNESS IN CATTLE ON HEAVILY PHOSPHATED LUXURIANT PASTURE

Stiffness in cattle is frequently observed in animals that have been moved from poor range to heavily phosphated luxuriant pasture, especially if it is a legume pasture. The stiffness usually appears 2 to 7 days after the cattle are placed on the luxuriant growth. The severity of the stiffness varies from animal to animal. Some show a slight locomotor disturbance which is not observed unless the animals are allowed to move about undisturbed. In others the stiffness is so severe they refuse to move even when excited by strangers or dogs, and they will not move about to obtain food or water. Some animals show anorexia and have a diarrhea. The cattle usually recover from this stiffness and after a few weeks show no ill effects from the disease except they are not in quite as good condition as the remainder of the herd. This disease should not be confused with arthritis or with founder since joint and hoof involvement is not present.

The condition is apparently associated with abnormal gastrointestinal fermentations resulting from the overloading of the digestive tract with the lush pasture grasses or legumes. It appears that the stress factor of the digestive disturbance brings about the alterations in muscles deficient in vitamin E or some other agent which controls muscle metabolism.

A similar cattle disease has been observed along the Gulf of Bothnia in Finland when young cattle confined to barns are turned out to lush spring pasture. After the animals have been on pasture for several days they become stiff, move with great difficulty, finally are unwilling to move, and then lie down. Coagulative necrosis of the skeletal muscle is observed. Older cows are also affected but the symptoms are not as severe. This disease is also apparently associated with digestive disturbances resulting from placing the animals on the new pasture growth.

### MUSCLE STIFFNESS IN CATTLE IN LATE WINTER

In late winter, cows frequently have difficulty in getting up or have no desire to do so. These animals have a transitory red urine due to the myoglobin passing through the renal system. Post-mortem examination reveals coagulative necrosis of the muscles. The necrotic changes are probably the result of a deficiency disease which developed during the winter when only poor feed was available.

Heifers that have been confined all winter in the barn frequently develop stiffness and red urine a short time after being turned out into the barnyard or pasture. In this respect it is very similar to stiff-lamb disease where the stress of exercise is the factor that precipitates the muscle disease. This disease is frequently erroneously diagnosed as leptospirosis.

### COAGULATIVE NECROSIS OF THE MUSCLES OF HORSES

**Azoturia** is a disease of horses characterized by coagulative necrosis of the heavy muscles of the thigh, back, and shoulder. The etiology of the disease is not known, but recent work in sheep, cattle, poultry, and laboratory rodents indicates it is probably a deficiency of vitamin E, selenium, or some other regulator of muscle metabolism. The exact chemical reaction within the muscle cells of these animals has never been determined since the exact chemistry of muscle cell physiology is unknown.

It is most frequently observed in the spring of the year, especially during the period when animals are worked excessively and particularly in green horses (that is, horses recently broken or not in working condition). It is particularly common on days following periods of rest,

such as weekends or holidays. Usually within 30 minutes to 1 hour after the animal is again put to work he begins to sweat, his gait becomes stiff, and soon he is reluctant to move. The lameness first appears and is usually most severe in the hind legs but may also involve the front legs. As the disease progresses the horse may no longer be able to stand or he may sit on his haunches like a dog. Most horses become very restless, make repeated efforts to rise, and when unable to do so thrash about violently, thus causing additional muscle exertion and thereby bringing about more coagulative necrosis of muscle. Eventually the animal becomes recumbent. The affected muscles are usually those of the loin, gluteal region, and thigh, and are quite readily recognized because they become swollen and firm in appearance and consistency.

Early in the course of the disease the urine becomes red or brown in color due to the large amount of myoglobin which is being passed. This myoglobin passing through the kidneys is extremely injurious to both the glomerular and tubular epithelium and, as a result of this injury, nephritis and uremia appear. In a few days the uremia may bring about the death of the animal.

In a mild case the animal will recover and show little evidence of the disease. In a severe case in which the animal survives, there is frequently extensive atrophy of the involved muscle. Because of the destruction of the muscle the animal may be worthless for work or show.

Post-mortem examination reveals coagulative necrosis of the involved muscle. There are both myoglobinemia and myoglobinuria. If the animal has lived for several days an acute nephritis will be present. In an animal that has recovered, atrophy and fibrosis of the involved muscles will be observed.

Some plants will cause coagulative necrosis of the muscles of horses. This is frequently observed in horses and mules that have grazed on *Pentzias* and *Salsola* shrubs.

## COAGULATIVE NECROSIS IN NURSING FOALS

This disease is observed in the spring of the year and usually appears 2 to 3 days after the mare is turned out to pasture. The foal becomes stiff, has difficulty in following his mother, has a myoglobin-tinged urine, and death frequently occurs. Necropsy reveals extensive coagulative necrosis of the skeletal and cardiac muscles.

## COAGULATIVE NECROSIS IN HORSES CONFINED TO STABLES

All ages of horses are subject to this disease. A red-colored urine is usually the first indication of illness. Later the animals are stiff and unable to stand. Symptoms of cardiac impairment are also observed. Necropsy reveals extensive coagulative necrosis of the skeletal and cardiac muscles.

## NECROSIS OF THE MUSCLES OF MASTICATION IN THE EQUINE

The disease is usually observed in animals that are on dry feed. More than 90 per cent of the cases occur in foals and young horses. In about 30 per cent of the animals the muscles of the extremities are also involved. Hemoglobinuria is observed in about 10 per cent of the horses. It would appear that the disease is the result of a deficiency of a regulator of muscle metabolism such as vitamin E. The reason the muscles of mastication are most frequently involved is probably due to the stress factor which occurs when the animal masticates its food. The muscle involvement is bilaterally symmetrical.

Affected animals are first observed to have eating and swallowing difficulties and later may show locomotor disturbances, especially of the front legs. The muscle involvement interferes with the prehension and mastication of feed. Foals die from starvation because they are unable to nurse. At first the involved muscles of mastication are swollen and later they undergo atrophy. Upon incision they show the typical white cooked appearance of coagulative necrosis.

This necrotic change in the muscles of mastication must not be confused with the *Streptococcus equi* invasion of muscle that occurs in this region of the head in horses with strangles.

## LINGUAL NECROSIS (LINGUAL MYOSITIS) IN HORSES

Lingual necrosis is observed in young horses in the early spring. The tongue swells to a tremendous size, the animals have a high fever, and there is a profuse salivation. The disease apparently begins as a coagulative necrosis of the muscles of the tongue. The myositis is the result of the irritation produced by the necrotic muscle.

## WHITE MUSCLE DISEASE IN SWINE

The highest incidence of coagulative necrosis of the muscles of swine is observed in hogs fed excessive amounts of cottonseed meal. Whenever more than 9 per cent of the ration consists of cottonseed meal, muscle injury can be expected. In many areas farmers are feeding as much as 50 to 60 per cent of the ration as cottonseed meal. When it is fed in this excessive amount without adequate supplemental green pasture, good quality alfalfa, and adequate supplemental grain, coagulative necrosis of muscle can be expected. Quite often the cottonseed meal is fed in self feeders where the hogs can eat all they desire. Since the meal is palatable, they consume excessive amounts.

Clinically, these pigs show edema and congestion of the lungs and muscular stiffness. Eventually they are unable to move about, become recumbent, and die. Necropsy reveals acute edema and congestion of the lungs, bronchopneumonia, hydrothorax, hydroperitoneum, general edema of the entire body, cardiac dilatation, and multiple yellowish and yellowish-white foci and streaks of coagulative necrosis in the myocardium, especially in the wall of the left ventricle. The edema and passive hyperemia of the entire animal and the bronchopneumonia are secondary to the myocardial injury.

There also is extensive coagulative necrosis of the skeletal muscles throughout the cadaver. The lesions are most severe in the heavy muscles of the thigh and shoulder. The etiology of the muscle lesion is not entirely explained. Cotton-seed meal contains practically no vitamin E since it is removed in the process of extracting the oil. How much additional injury the gossypol in the cottonseed meal does is not known.

### COAGULATIVE NECROSIS IN THE CANINE

Coagulative necrosis of muscle is sel-dom observed in carnivorous animals and is quite difficult to produce experimentally.

In the canine a nutritional muscular dystrophy similar to that which has been produced in animals by eliminating vita-min E from the ration is observed in dogs having biliary fistulas and maintained on adequate rations. It is suggested that faulty absorption of vitamin E as the result of the absence of bile in the intes-tine is the cause of the dystrophy.

**Chronic eosinophilic myositis** of the masseter, temporalis, and pterygoid mus-cles is observed quite frequently in the dog in Europe and less commonly in the United States. The etiology of the condi-tion has not been determined but appar-ently is the result of a deficiency of a regulator of muscle metabolism such as vitamin E. At first there is acute swelling and coagulative necrosis of the muscles of mastication, and later this is followed by atrophy. The involvement of the mus-cles is bilaterally symmetrical. The jaws become fixed in a closed position and as a result the animal dies from malnutrition. In the early stages of the disease there is coagulative necrosis of the muscle fol-lowed by infiltration of the muscle with leukocytes, especially eosinophils. The necrotic muscle is removed by the leuko-cytes, and extensive fibrosis and atrophy takes place. A differential leukocyte count reveals an eosinophilia in the circulating blood.

### NUTRITIONAL MUSCULAR DYSTROPHY IN RABBITS

Coagulative necrosis of the psoas mus-cles of rabbits is quite common. It is frequently observed in laboratory rabbits, and it appears that white rabbits are more susceptible than those with pigmented skins. The rabbits may or may not show clinical signs of the psoas muscle involve-ment. At times the muscle damage may be so great that the animal has difficulty in moving about. Because of the inability to use the posterior extremities properly the rabbits are said to be paralyzed. This is an error because it is the muscles and not the nerves that are involved. The etiology of the disease is not known but is probably a deficiency of vitamin E or some other regulator of muscle meta-bolism. Since the psoas muscles in the rabbit are very powerful and are sub-jected to violent contractions when the animal runs or struggles, this work factor explains why this particular muscle shows the necrotic alterations if a deficiency dis-ease exists. Some of the rabbits also have foci of necrosis in the cardiac muscle.

### MUSCULAR DYSTROPHY IN MICE AND RATS

A nutritional muscular dystrophy is observed in mice and young rats fed a ration deficient in vitamin E. It should be remembered that in mice the Coxsackie virus can produce muscular dystrophy which is easily confused with a vitamin E deficiency.

### NUTRITIONAL MYOPATHY IN DUCKLINGS

A nutritional myopathy is observed in ducklings fed a diet of skim milk powder, casein, cornstarch, lard, cod-liver oil, yeast, salt, and paper pulp. The muscle altera-tions are the result of a deficiency of vita-min E and consist of coagulative necrosis followed by an inflammatory reaction when the body attempts to remove the necrotic tissue and repair the muscle.

### Liquefactive Necrosis

Liquefactive necrosis of muscle occurs when large numbers of neutrophils are present in the muscle. The proteolytic enzymes of the neutrophils cause the liquefaction. Bacteria are the most com-mon cause of liquefactive necrosis since they attract large numbers of neutrophils to the muscle. A few drugs such as tur-pentine and various tranquilizers will cause liquefactive necrosis when injected into muscle.

## Caseous Necrosis

Caseous necrosis of muscle is not common since the bacteria which usually produce this alteration are seldom found in muscle. Occasionally *Mycobacterium tuberculosis* invades muscle and then caseous necrosis may be produced.

## Gangrene

Gangrene of muscle is frequently observed in all domestic animals. It is most often seen in the extremities where injury produced by freezing, tight bandages, and rubber bands causes infarction of the part. The infarcted area is invaded by saprophytic bacteria and gangrene is the result. A special form of gangrene, commonly observed in cattle, sheep, and occasionally in other animals, is caused by members of the clostridium group of organisms (*Clostridium chauvoei, welchii*, and *septicum*).

## INFLAMMATION

Inflammation of muscle is known as **myositis**. The classification of myositis follows the terminology used in other organs. It may be acute or chronic, and the type of exudate determines the terminology used. The most common cause of myositis is traumatic injury.

A separation in the continuity of muscle can be caused by the various traumatic factors listed in the chapter on etiology (incisions, lacerations, perforations, and rupture).

The amount and appearance of the injury varies greatly depending upon the type of etiologic agent which produced the injury. Muscles may be completely torn in two, may contain perforations (pitchfork and bullet wounds), or may contain incisions produced with a knife. Muscle rupture is frequently observed in the dog following injuries from an automobile. Muscle rupture also occurs as the result of kicks, horn thrusts, and violent muscular contractions resulting from fighting, playing, or working. Muscle rupture is most frequently observed in the psoas, longissimus dorsi, gastrocnemius, and ventral abdominal muscles.

Hemorrhage occurs in the area of injury, clotting takes place, and with healing the clot is organized. The gap between the muscle fibers is filled in with white fibrous connective tissue. With contraction of the scar and relative approximation of the injured muscle surfaces, the injured muscle may again be able to perform its normal function. If complete rupture of the muscle has occurred, as with the gastrocnemius muscle, the torn ends of the muscle may be so far apart that they cannot be approximated. The muscle may then be so long that it is impossible for it to flex or extend the joint.

## Serous Myositis

**Etiology.** A serous myositis occurs when relatively mild injury to muscle has taken place. It is often caused by overexertion (excessive working or fighting). It may occur when traumatic injury (blows and kicks) of a mild nature has occurred. It is frequently associated with degenerative and necrotic alterations in muscle which occur when a vitamin E or selenium deficiency is present.

**Macroscopic appearance.** The cardinal signs of inflammation are present. The muscle is excessively moist because of the serous exudate.

**Microscopic appearance.** The cellular and vascular alterations characteristic of inflammation are present. Neutrophils are the predominant leukocyte in the area. The intermuscular connective tissue is distended with a homogeneous, finely granular, protein substance which stains slightly with eosin. This homogeneous material between the muscle cells is the serous exudate, and since it is the most prominent constituent of the exudate it is called a serous myositis. The muscle cells show various degenerative alterations (cloudy swelling and fatty degeneration) and may undergo coagulative necrosis.

**Significance and result.** When the cause of the myositis is removed, healing occurs quite rapidly since the serous fluid and the neutrophils are capable of returning quite easily to the general circulation.

## Suppurative Myositis

**Etiology.** Suppurative myositis is usually the result of an infection with pyogenic bacteria when the microorganisms are introduced into the muscle by means of incisions, lacerations, or perforating wounds. Hematogenous infection may occur from primary suppurative lesions (strangle and glanders) in other portions of the animal. It may also occur when drugs such as turpentine or tranquilizers are injected into muscle.

**Macroscopic appearance.** The cardinal signs of inflammation must be present, and the most characteristic alteration in the area is the presence of pus either as a diffuse infiltration (phlegmon) or as a focal accumulation (abscess).

**Microscopic appearance.** The cellular and vascular alterations characteristic of inflammation are present. The predominant constituent of the exudate is the neutrophil. The muscle cells in the area of inflammation show degenerative and necrotic alterations, and because it is a suppurative inflammation the most prominent alteration is liquefactive necrosis.

**Significance and result.** Suppurative inflammation of muscle almost always indicates that pyogenic bacteria are present in the muscle. Healing may occur with organization of the exudate and the formation of a scar. Occasionally a suppurative myositis terminates in a septicemia.

## Eosinophilic Myositis

Eosinophilic myositis is characterized by an abundance of eosinophils in the exudate. It is most frequently observed in the bovine and occasionally in swine. Eosinophilic myositis is frequently confused with a myelosarcoma, but the tumor is also observed in the bone marrow, lymph nodes, and other hematopoietic tissue.

**Etiology.** The muscle reaction is an allergic type. Parasites (sarcosporidia and trichinae) may be found in muscle and yet no eosinophilic reaction is present. At other times an extensive infiltration with eosinophils is found. This would suggest that a previous sensitizing infection which causes an allergic response when subsequent infections occur.

It is quite possible that an animal may become sensitized to muscle protein. If an animal has experienced coagulative necrosis of muscle with liberation of myoglobin, subsequent muscle necrosis with liberation of myoglobin may produce an allergic muscle reaction with an accumulation of eosinophils.

**Macroscopic appearance.** The presence of eosinophils in muscle gives the area of inflammation a green color. The muscle may show a focal or diffuse involvement. A multiple focal distribution of the lesions in the muscle is the type usually observed. Many muscles or only an occasional muscle in the animal may show these alterations. The lesion may be acute or chronic depending upon how long it has been present. When the muscle alteration is observed during the process of meat inspection, the pigmented portion of the carcass is condemned. Massive involvement of muscle may occasionally cause death, especially when there is extensive involvement of the cardiac muscle resulting in acute heart failure.

**Microscopic appearance.** The tissue alterations may be acute or chronic, focal or diffuse. In the majority of instances there are multiple focal areas of extremely acute eosinophilic inflammation. Within these areas of inflammation structural remnants suggesting the remains of parasites may be seen. The involved muscles show extensive cloudy swelling and coagulative necrosis. In the early stages only neutrophils and eosinophils are present, but as the disease progresses, macrophages, lymphocytes, plasma cells, and fibroblasts become numerous. The leukocytes are scattered between the muscle cells. If the myocytes are necrotic, phagocytosis of the muscle takes place. The eosinophils often invade the muscle and appear to be causing lysis of the muscle cells, which suggests they may be secreting lytic enzymes. The involved muscle may regenerate and return to approximately its normal state, or there may be extensive fibrosis of the muscle.

### Hemorrhagic Myositis

**Etiology.** A hemorrhagic myositis is caused by extremely injurious agents. It may follow traumatic injuries when very severe muscle injury has taken place. The most common cause of hemorrhagic myositis is infection with *Clostridium chauvoei, welchii, septicum,* and other clostridia.

**Macroscopic appearance.** The cardinal signs of inflammation are present and they are especially severe. The outstanding feature of the inflammatory reaction is the presence of a large amount of blood in the exudate.

**Microscopic appearance.** The vascular and cellular alterations characteristic of inflammation are present. The predominant constituent of the exudate is blood which infiltrates into the loose connective tissue between the muscle cells. The principle cellular constituent of the exudate is the neutrophil. Macrophages and other leukocytes may be present, but since the inflammation is very severe the animal is usually dead before they appear in the area.

**Significance and result.** A hemorrhagic inflammation always has a very serious prognosis since the etiologic agent is always very severe and usually brings about the death of the animal.

### BLACKLEG

Synonyms for blackleg are symptomatic anthrax, black quarter, and quarter ill. It is an acute infectious disease of cattle, exceptionally of sheep and goats, caused by *Clostridium chauvoei.* In the Middle Western and Western Plains states, *Clostridium chauvoei* is sometimes combined with *Clostridium septicum* and *Clostridium novyi* in the disease in sheep and cattle. Formerly it was considered to be a wound infection disease accompanied by a severe toxemia. Usually, cases are encountered in which no wound at the site of the lesions is apparent.

The mode of entrance of the bacteria in these cases is not clear but it is probably by the digestive tract. The disease is characterized by an emphysematous and edematous swelling of the subcutaneous tissues and muscles. The lesions are usually located upon and extend over the greater part of a hind quarter or shoulder. It seldom occurs in cattle under 6 months or over 2 years of age.

In the West, infection takes place in sheep through shearing wounds, docking, castration, and following lambing.

Spores may enter wounds in company with other microorganisms and foreign bodies (soil, dust, briars, thorns). They germinate, multiply by fission, and produce a serohemorrhagic inflammation, degeneration and necrosis of the musculature, and the formation of gas which has the odor of rancid butter due to the fermentation of carbohydrates. Toxins produced and absorbed disturb the heat-regulating center (fever). The period of incubation is generally 3 days.

In the muscles, affected areas show crepitant swellings above which the skin is stiff, parchment-like, and dark red, almost black. The subcutaneous tissue is red or infiltrated with yellowish gelatinous exudate, at places intermixed with hemorrhages and gas vesicles. The inter- and intramuscular connective tissue is similarly involved. The musculature of the swollen part is dirty brown or dark red and contains a bloody fluid which diminishes in quantity with the increase of gas. The affected muscle has the odor of rancid butter (butyric acid).

Microscopically, the muscle fibers show coagulative necrosis, cloudy swelling, and fatty degeneration. The fibers are separated by gas vesicles, extensive edema, and hemorrhage. Microorganisms are present everywhere in the affected areas. In the center of the affected areas, there is necrosis; at the periphery, leukocytic infiltration.

The regional lymph nodes show a hemorrhagic lymphadenitis and emphysema. The internal organs when involved show similar lesions of hemorrhagic inflammation, especially in the lungs, heart, stomach, and intestine. An acute ulcerative endocarditis is often observed in the heart. The most common location of this lesion is in the left atria. This cardiac lesion is considered pathognomonic for blackleg. Blackleg usually terminates in death in 12 to 36 hours.

### MALIGNANT EDEMA

Malignant edema is an acute wound infection disease of solipeds, sheep, swine, sometimes of cattle, goats, and carnivora, caused by *Clostridium septicum* and characterized by edematous and later crepitating swellings at the place of infection.

The infection enters by way of wounds in the skin, oral cavity, digestive tract (bradsot or braxy of sheep in Europe), vagina and uterus, and castration wounds. Rarely, it is introduced by means of contaminated hypodermic needles or in contaminated material injected into animals. The disease process resembles blackleg, except that hemorrhagic edema is much more conspicuous than emphysema, the location of the lesions is usually different, and the species of susceptible animals are more varied. The basic tissue alteration is necrosis of muscle fibers due to an exotoxin.

## Chronic Myositis

### TUBERCULOSIS

Tuberculosis of muscle is quite uncommon but when observed is usually found in the bovine and porcine. It is most frequently observed in those animals in which there is a diffuse dissemination of the acid-fast organisms throughout the entire body. The infection reaches the muscle by way of the blood stream or extends into the muscle directly from infected organs or lymph nodes. In the muscle the bacteria produce tubercles in the intramuscular connective tissue. The type of reaction varies with the species of animal. In monkeys the alteration is a chronic focal suppurative reaction, while in cattle and swine the lesion is a chronic caseo-calcific type of alteration.

### ACTINOMYCOSIS AND ACTINOBACILLOSIS

These two diseases are most frequently observed in the bovine and are especially common in the muscles of the tongue, cheek, and throat. The lesion produced by these two diseases consists of a chronic multiple focal suppurative myositis. The exudate is extremely thick and tenacious, is pale green in color, and contains numerous yellow granules.

### NODULAR PSEUDOTUBERCULOSIS OF MUSCLE

This is a disease of cattle characterized by a chronic multiple-focal necrotic myositis. The necrotic alterations may be liquefactive or coagulative in type. The etiology is not known. No lesions have been examined in the acute stage. All have been observed in the stage of healing, and this perhaps explains why the etiology has not been determined. The disease has not been transmitted to cattle or experimental animals.

The lesions usually measure from 1 to 7 centimeters in diameter and are usually found intramuscularly, but sometimes similar lesions are observed in the subcutaneous tissue. There is a predilection for the superficial muscles such as the panniculus and the muscles of the tail. The lesions are most prevalent in the legs, trunk, neck, and the ventral musculature of the proximal third of the tail. Necrotic lesions are also frequently observed in the testicle.

The yellowish-gray nodules are firm, round, painless, cold, and do not interfere with the locomotion of the animal. Upon incision they appear dry and homogeneous. They develop rather slowly and frequently are observed for several months before they attain their maximum size. The nodules may disappear after being present for a number of weeks or months. The majority of the nodules are located just below the muscle sheath and bulge into the muscle as well as the surrounding connective tissue. All of the nodules are surrounded by a connective tissue capsule, and the central, yellow, necrotic mass is arranged in concentric rings much like the arrangement of an onion. Some of the nodules have areas of calcification in their centers.

The lesions begin as multiple-focal abscesses which contain an abundance of neutrophils. As the disease progresses, the suppuration becomes less prominent and the area becomes infiltrated with macrophages and lymphocytes and becomes surrounded with a connective tissue capsule. Giant cells are quite frequently observed in the area. Because of the chronicity and appearance of the lesions, they are often confused with those of tuberculosis.

Finally the lesions consist of a central necrotic mass, containing foci of calcification, which are surrounded by concentric rings of necrotic inflammatory tissue. The radiating rings indicate variations in the rapidity of growth of the lesions. At times there is apparently little growth and then at other times there is rapid growth which causes the ringed arrangement.

## PARASITIC DISEASES OF MUSCLE

### Sarcosporidiosis

Sarcosporidiosis is caused by the invasion of muscle with *Sarcocystis meischneriana, muris, blanchardi,* and *tenella.* The life cycle of these parasites is not known. They are extremely common in all animals but are most frequently observed in cattle, sheep, horses, pigs, and ducks.

**Macroscopic appearance.** The lesions are found in skeletal and cardiac muscle and appear as yellowish-gray elliptical masses which measure 0.5 to 4 mm. in length and 0.5 to 3 mm. in width. The long axis of the parasitic cysts is arranged parallel with the direction of the muscle fibers. They are extremely firm, dense masses in the tissue and are frequently calcified. If the meat is eaten, the calcified cysts resemble granules of sand in the muscle. In most instances there is no inflammatory reaction in the vicinity of the encysted parasites nor is there any history of lameness in the animals possessing the parasites. At other times there is a violent inflammatory reaction in the muscle and the

accumulation of large numbers of eosinophils. These masses of eosinophils cause focal green areas to appear within the muscle. Apparently this allergic inflammatory reaction occurs when a previous infection has sensitized the host. Once the living parasite has encysted there is no additional inflammation in the area, but later on when the parasite dies an acute inflammatory reaction occurs in the area.

**Microscopic appearance.** The parasite appears as a cylindrical cyst within the muscle cell. The cyst contains numerous small elliptical sporozoites. Once the parasite has encysted in the muscle there is no inflammatory reaction within the area. When the parasite dies the liberation of the protein of the parasite in a sensitized animal produces a severe inflammatory reaction. The area becomes heavily infiltrated with eosinophils; there is extensive coagulative necrosis of the muscle cells in the area; and as the disease progresses, macrophages, lymphocytes, and fibroblasts become numerous in the vicinity of the parasite. The leukocytes may phagocytose and remove the parasite. At other times the dead parasite and cyst become mineralized.

### Cysticercosis

Tapeworm cysts of various types are found in domestic animals, and the species of the parasite varies with the genus of animal involved.

#### CYSTICERCUS BOVIS

In the bovine the parasite found in the skeletal muscle is *Cysticercus bovis,* the larval stage of *Taenia saginata.* The adult form of *T. saginata* is found in the intestinal tract of the human being. The ova of *T. saginata* are ingested by the bovine and the larvae are liberated in the intestinal tract. They migrate into the wall of the intestine and are then carried by the lymph and blood streams to the body musculature. They are found in muscles throughout the body but are most frequently observed in the tongue, heart, and muscles of mastication. The encysted parasites are found in the interstitial connective tissue of the muscle and vary in size from just visible to the fully developed larval form which measures 1 cm. in diameter. The cysts are oval, pearly white in color, distended with fluid, and contain a yellowish-white scolex which measures 1 to 2 mm. in diameter. An acute inflammatory reaction occurs in the muscles when migration of the larvae is taking place. Once the parasite encysts, the inflammatory reaction disappears.

**Microscopic appearance.** The scolex is enclosed in two walls. One is produced by the larva and the other by the body of the host. When the parasite first invades the muscle there is an acute inflammatory reaction which is soon replaced by a chronic type of inflammation in which lymphocytes and macrophages predominate. The inflammatory reaction is usually slight considering the size of the parasite. When the parasite is migrating, eosinophils are numerous in the area and may become very numerous if the animal is allergic to the protein of the tapeworm. As the cyst enlarges, pressure atrophy of the surrounding musculature occurs. When the parasite dies, the fluid of the cyst becomes cloudy and eventually both the fluid and the parasite become mineralized. At other times the cyst is invaded with macrophages which phagocytose the necrotic parasite as well as the cyst itself, and the area is then filled in with connective tissue.

## CYSTICERCUS CELLULOSAE

*Cysticercus cellulosae* is the larval form of *Taenia solium*. The adult form of the parasite is found in the intestinal tract of man. The tapeworm ova are passed in the feces of man and are usually ingested by swine. The larvae are liberated in the intestinal tract of swine, invade the wall of the intestine, and are carried to the muscles of the body by way of the lymph and blood streams. The parasite is most frequently observed in swine but may invade any mammal (man, dogs, rats, and apes) that ingests the ova.

**Macroscopic appearance.** The fully developed cyst in the muscle appears as a vesicle measuring 1 cm. in diameter and contains a clear fluid in which a yellowish-white scolex which measures 1 to 2 mm. in diameter can be seen. The cysts are found in any muscle of the body but are most frequently observed in the diaphragm, neck, shoulder, and intercostal muscles, tongue, and heart. At times they are observed in other organs such as the brain, spleen, lymph node, lung, liver, and eye. The vesicles are located in the interstitial connective tissue of the muscle. The muscle alterations are similar to those observed when *C. bovis* is present. The number of *C. cellulosae* cysts in muscle is usually much greater than *C. bovis*. Occasionally the invasion of the heart and brain may become so great that death will occur.

## CYSTICERCUS OVIS

The larval form of *Taenia ovis* is frequently observed in sheep. The adult form of the tapeworm is found in carnivora, and the sheep dog guarding the sheep is usually the carrier of the adult parasite. The larvae are most frequently observed in the heart, diaphragm, tongue, and cheek muscles.

## Coenurosis

*Coenurus serialis*, the larval form of *Multiceps serialis*, is observed in the muscles and connective tissue of the rabbit, chinchilla, and other rodents. It is particularly serious in chinchillas where the large subcutaneous cysts disfigure the fur-bearing animal.

## Trichinellosis

Trichinellosis is a disease of muscle caused by *Trichinella spiralis*. The adult form of the parasite is found in the intestinal tract, and the larvae produced by the female are carried to the muscle by the lymph and blood streams where they invade the skeletal muscle cells.

Trichinella are observed in those animals which consume flesh which contains encysted larvae. As a result they are most frequently observed in carnivorous and omnivorous animals. Herbivorous animals may be artificially infected with the parasite. The adult parasites can be found in the intestinal tract of birds, but muscle involvement apparently does not occur. All skeletal muscles of the body may be involved and tremendous numbers of encysted parasites may be present (400 to 2,000 trichinella larvae per gram of tissue). They are most frequently observed in the more active muscles of the body such as the diaphragm, tongue, intercostal, and masticatory muscles which, because of their activity, usually have a low glycogen content.

**Macroscopic appearance.** Usually no alterations are observed in the muscle. In very acute cases where large numbers of parasites are invading the muscle an acute serous myositis may be present. In previously sensitized animals an eosinophilic myositis may occur in which multiple green foci are scattered through the muscle in the vicinity of the invading larvae. When the parasites die and become mineralized they may be seen as small, barely visible foci in the muscle.

**Microscopic appearance.** The parasite invades the muscle cell and produces an acute serous myositis. The muscle cell undergoes cloudy swelling and later coagulative necrosis. At first many neutrophils are present in the vicinity of the involved muscle. Along with the neutrophils the eosinophils appear, and eventually in very sensitized individuals large numbers of eosinophils may accumulate. As the disease progresses, lymphocytes and macrophages appear in the area surrounding the encysted parasite. About 2 months after the muscle cell has been invaded by the parasite it is enclosed in two cyst walls, one produced by the parasite and the second produced by the body. The latter is composed of eosinophils, macrophages, lymphocytes, and connective tissue. After the parasite becomes encysted the leukocytes disappear, the muscle cell itself has disappeared, and the parasite becomes dormant. The cyst is oval in shape and its long axis is arranged parallel with the muscle cells in the area. The cyst contains one or several larvae which in fresh preparations can be seen to move slightly. The larvae persist in the muscle for many years. The cyst wall often becomes mineralized in a few weeks to 2 years. When the parasite dies, the dead parasite as well as the cyst becomes mineralized. At either or both poles of the encysted parasite there are frequently quite a few adipose cells.

## NEOPLASMS

Primary neoplasms in the musculature of domestic animals are occasionally observed. Lipomas, liposarcomas, fibromas, fibrosarcomas, and rhabdomyosarcomas have been described.

Metastatic tumors, both sarcomas and carcinomas, are observed in muscle but not as frequently as would be expected. Apparently muscles are not a suitable medium for tumor transplantation. Lymphosarcomas and myelosarcomas are quite common in the bovine and chicken. The myeloid tumor in the muscle of the bovine is green in color and may have a focal or diffuse arrangement. It is frequently confused with parasitic invasion of muscle, but can be differentiated because the myelosarcoma involves the lymph nodes, bone marrow, spleen, and other hematopoietic structures. The myelosarcoma in the chicken is white in color and is most frequently observed in the intercostal muscles.

# Articular System

## DISTURBANCES OF GROWTH

### Atrophy

Articular changes take place in aging animals. In the young animal the articular cartilages are relatively thick, bluish-white in color, and semitransparent. With age the cartilage becomes thin, yellowish white in color, and opaque. As the articular cartilages undergo atrophy, the bony articular surfaces of the epiphysis of the bones become visible. As the atrophy continues, the articular surface of the joint may consist of bone rather than cartilage. Around the periphery of the articular surface there is hyperplasia of the cartilage with protruding excrescences, giving the border of the articular cartilage a very rough irregular surface. These cartilagenous projections may break off and become foreign bodies within the joint capsule. They are known as **joint mice.** Mineralization of these fragments of cartilage as well as of the menisci may occur.

Degeneration of the articular cartilage is particularly common in old horses, dogs, and cattle. In all of these species it is especially common in the stifle and hip joints. In cattle it is particularly common in the carpal articulations.

**Intervertebral disc protrusion** is seen in all domestic animals and is most common in those species which are allowed to live long enough for senile alterations to take place. As a result they are most frequently observed in dogs and horses. The disease is much more common in the dog than in other species of animals because man has so manipulated the skeleton of some breeds by inbreeding that they are much more prone to skeletal diseases. Disc protrusions are especially common in breeds, such as the dachshund, that have a chondrodystrophic type of skeleton.

Disc protrusion may be the result of violent traumatic injury in which the soft intervertebral disc is compressed between the osseous bodies of the vertebrae. This causes the softer structure to protrude in a peripheral direction. The protrusion may be into the vertebral canal or may be lateral or ventral to the body of the vertebrae.

The most common cause of disc protrusion is senility. With senility there is degeneration of the fibrocartilage and elastic tissue of the annulus fibrosus, and with this it loses its ability to contain the softer central nucleus pulposus. The nucleus pulposus also undergoes senile alterations, changing from a soft mucoid structure to a drier mass which may contain calcium salts. If compression is placed upon the disc by the adjacent osseous vertebrae, the degenerate annulus fibrosus is no longer able to withstand this pressure; it ruptures, and the semisolid nucleus pulposus herniates through the rent in the annulus fibrosus. The direction of herniation depends entirely upon the location of the rent in the annulus fibrosus. This tendency to herniate through the weakest point is well shown by the fact that herniation is usually observed in the cervical, terminal thoracic, or lumbar portions of the vertebral column and is seldom observed in the thoracic region. The reason for this is that in the vertebral canal of the thoracic portion of the spinal column there is a reinforcing ligament on the floor of the vertebral canal. This reinforcement tends to prevent herniation in this region. In addition, the discs in the thoracic region are very thin and therefore are less likely to herniate.

Following herniation there is an acute inflammatory reaction which, after 1 to 2 weeks, changes into a chronic type of inflammation. Since degenerating and necrotic tissue is present both in the annulus fibrosus and the protruding nucleus pulposus, mineralization of the tissue altered by senility and trauma occurs. The inflammatory reaction which follows the protrusion of the nucleus pulposus aggravates the initial injury because of the swelling associated with inflammation. The disease is particularly serious when the herniated mass protrudes into the vertebral canal because the mass, as well as the swelling associated with the inflammatory reaction, causes a compression of the spinal cord. The degree of injury of the cord depends entirely upon the pressure. Mild pressure causes a slight to moderate impairment of function. When the pressure is great, atrophy of the spinal cord takes place and eventually the cord may completely disappear in the area.

### Hypoplasia

Congenital defects in the formation of joints are quite common in all animals. Any joint may be involved but it is most frequently observed in the coxofemoral, stifle, shoulder, and elbow articulations. The disorder is especially common in the toy breeds of dogs where manipulation of body conformity by selective breeding has resulted in marked alterations in skeletal and articular development. The involved bones are usually shorter and more slender than normal and the articular surfaces are smaller than normal and may have an abnormal angularity. The alteration in the size of the bones is frequently difficult to appreciate unless other dogs of the same age, size, and breed are available for comparison. If the articular defect is unilateral, the bones of one limb can be compared with those of the opposite limb.

**Hypoplasia of the coxofemoral articulation** is frequently observed in domestic animals. It is most common in dogs and is especially prevalent in the German shepherd breed. Both hip articulations are usually involved. Symptoms of the disease become apparent when the dogs are about 3 months of age. Dogs with this defect should be spayed or castrated since it is a hereditary disease.

This defect is primarily a disturbance in the growth of the acetabulum which is small and shallow. Because of this formation it does not contain and hold the head of the femur, and luxation of the hip joint is very common unless the surrounding musculature and connective tissue are able to hold the head of the femur in place. The disproportion in the size of the acetabulum and the head of the femur causes abnormal articular pressure and excessive wear of the articular surfaces. This is especially prominent in the head of the femur. As the result of the irritation there is hyperplasia of bone around the periphery of the acetabulum and the head of the femur.

**Hypoplasia of the stifle** occurs in all animals but is most frequently seen in dogs, especially in the toy breeds (Chihuahua, Pekingese, and Pomeranian). It is also observed in foals and calves. There is imperfect development of the articular surfaces and periarticular tissues, and as

the result of this the patella undergoes dislocation. The dislocation is usually to the medial side of the articulation. The disease may involve one or both stifles.

## INFLAMMATION

Inflammation of an articulation is called **arthritis** and may involve one joint or a number of joints. When several joints are involved it is designated as **polyarthritis.** The inflammation may be acute or chronic, and the type of reaction is classified according to the exudate (serous, fibrinous, suppurative, hemorrhagic, and gangrenous) produced.

Various traumatic injuries may cause dislocation and inflammation of an articulation. This frequently occurs when animals are run over by automobiles, when running animals collide with objects, or when injuries are received during fighting. When the supporting structures of the joint are torn and the articular surfaces are no longer in their normal approximation, the joint alteration is known as a **luxation.** When the periarticular supporting structures and joint capsule which hold the joint together have been stretched or torn slightly but the articular surfaces are still in their normal approximation, the condition is known as a **strain** or **sprain.** As a result of the injury there is hemorrhage into the joint cavity, joint capsule, and the surrounding periarticular tissue. The tearing and stretching of the tissues as well as the hemorrhage causes inflammation. Quite frequently following healing there is restricted movement or no movement of the joint as the result of improper approximation of the articular surfaces, union of the articular surfaces by connective tissue, and immobility caused by the connective tissue deposited around the joint. These factors cause abnormal bending and positioning of the joint which is known as **ankylosis.**

**Gout,** the deposition of sodium and calcium urate in joints, is frequently observed in birds, poultry, and reptiles, especially alligators. It is of no importance in domestic animals. The crystals of urate are deposited in the joint capsule, the periarticular tissue, and within the joint cavity. The crystals are irritating and a chronic inflammation is produced with the deposition of large amounts of connective tissue. Because of the proliferative type of reaction, there is impairment in the movement of the joint.

### Serous Arthritis

**Etiology.** Serous arthritis is caused by very mild irritants which are ordinarily of a traumatic nature. For the most part only one joint is involved and usually follows over-extension. Serous arthritis may occur when there has been excessive use of the joint as in the case of the horse that stands for long periods of time in the stable or is forced to trot or gallop for long periods of time on concrete or cobblestones.

**Macroscopic appearance.** The cardinal signs of inflammation are present. The joint capsule is distended with an excessive amount of synovial fluid, is hyperemic as the result of inflammation, and may contain a few petechial hemorrhages.

**Microscopic appearance.** The joint capsule shows the typical vascular and cellular alterations associated with inflammation. A few leukocytes are present and, for the most part, they are neutrophils.

### Fibrinous Arthritis

**Etiology.** Fibrinous arthritis occurs when a more severe irritant, usually of a traumatic nature, is applied to an articulation.

**Macroscopic appearance.** The alterations are similar to those of serous arthritis except that the joint fluid contains yellow or white strands of fibrin. The masses of fibrin are usually compressed into flattened, elongated structures and float free in the joint fluid. These structures are commonly known as **joint mice.**

**Microscopic appearance.** The cellular changes are very similar to those of serous arthritis except that the inflammatory reaction is more severe. The principal constituent of the exudate is fibrin, and neutrophils are quite numerous both in the joint capsule and in the joint fluid.

### Suppurative Arthritis

**Etiology.** Suppurative arthritis is caused by various infectious agents (streptococci, staphylococci, corynebacteria, erysipelothrix, and pleuropneumonia-like organisms) which enter the joint. The bacteria may gain entrance to the joint through wounds. The bacteria may also invade the joint from periarticular suppurative processes in the skin, the subcutaneous connective tissue, or in the epiphysis of the bone below the articular cartilage. The bacteria may also invade the joint when a septicemia is present since the organisms are brought to the joint capsule by the circulating blood stream. A polyarthritis indicates a septicemia has been present.

One of the most common causes of suppurative arthritis is an umbilical infection at the time of birth. Following the umbilical infection there is a septicemia and the microorganisms are carried throughout the body. Some of the bacteria invade the joints. Umbilical infection is usually characterized by a polyarthritis, although the involvement of a single joint may occur (Fig. 21.2). Suppurative arthritis is also associated with metritis, mastitis, traumatic gastritis, pneumonia, endocarditis, and other bacterial diseases which produce a septicemia. Salmonella, particularly *Salmonella typhimurium*, causes a polyarthritis, and this is most frequently observed in pigeons. In swine *Erysipelothrix rhusiopathiae* may cause an arthritis. *Brucella abortus* and *suis* may also invade joints and are most frequently observed in swine. Sporadic bovine encephalomyelitis is characterized by a polyarthritis which is particularly noticeable in the legs. Infections with pleuropneumonia-like organisms in swine are also characterized by a polyarthritis. They are the most common cause of arthritis in swine.

Once bacteria gain entrance into a joint it is extremely difficult for the body defenses to cope with the infection. The reason for this is that the bacteria within the joint cavity are so far removed from the blood vessels in the joint capsule that the complicated vascular and cellular reaction necessary for the removal of the bacteria cannot reach the microorganisms. In addition, the synovial fluid is an ideal medium for bacterial growth. Because of its fluid nature the organisms are spread throughout the entire joint cavity quite quickly.

**Macroscopic appearance.** The cardinal signs of inflammation must be present. The joint is swollen, and because of the pain of the arthritis and the swelling, impairment of movement of the articulation is usually present. The most characteristic alteration in this type of arthritis is the white, yellow, or green mass of pus which distends the joint capsule. The pus is thin and watery in consistency and nearly colorless in PPLO infections. It is white or yellow in color and thin, creamy, or thick in consistency in streptococcic or staphylococcic infections. The exudate is green in color and rather thick and tenacious when corynebacteria are present. When the inflammatory process has been there for a considerable period of time, an abundance of connective tissue is deposited in the joint capsule and periarticular tissue. Whether the arthritis is acute or chronic is indicated by the deposition of connective tissue.

With a suppurative arthritis there is usually considerable destruction of the cartilage of the articular surfaces, particularly in chronic suppurative arthritis of long standing. Nearly all of the articular surface may be destroyed. The inflammatory process may extend into the underlying epiphysis of the bone and may also extend into the surrounding periarticular tissue. Quite often the suppurative process will cause destruction of the periarticular tissue, and a sinus to the exterior of the body is formed through which the pus may drain. Joint mice which are composed of masses of exudate as well as fragments of disintegrating cartilage and bone are very common.

**Microscopic appearance.** The typical vascular and cellular alterations associated

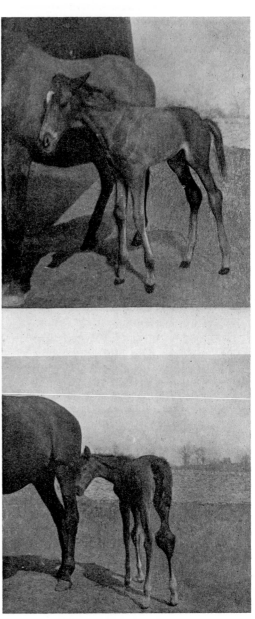

Fig. 21.2 — Suppurative arthritis in a foal. (Hardenbergh, Jour. A.V.M.A.)

with inflammation are present. Neutrophils are the primary constituent of the exudate.

**Significance and result.** The presence of a suppurative arthritis indicates that bacteria are present. The prognosis is always unfavorable because healing of the arthritis is difficult to obtain. If healing is accomplished, there is frequently a union of the articular surfaces which prevents movement of the joint, or the abundance of connective tissue deposited in the joint capsule and the periarticular tissue restricts the movement of the joint.

### Hemorrhagic Arthritis

**Etiology.** Hemorrhagic arthritis may be caused by severe traumatic injury as is observed in sprains and luxations of the joint. The most common cause of a hemorrhagic arthritis produced by bacteria is observed in the bovine when an infection with *Clostridium chauvoei* or *septicum* extends into the articulation.

**Macroscopic appearance.** The cardinal signs of inflammation are present and are particularly prominent. The principal constituent of the exudate is blood.

**Microscopic appearance.** The vascular and cellular reactions characteristic of inflammation are present. There is an abundance of erythrocytes in the exudate. It is differentiated from hemorrhage by the presence of large numbers of leukocytes.

### Gangrenous Arthritis

Gangrenous arthritis occurs when gangrene of an extremity is present as the result of embolism, thrombosis, freezing, or ergot poisoning. Gangrene may occur in an articulation if saprophytic bacteria are introduced into the joint through wounds. These bacteria grow in the necrotic tissue and cause putrefaction.

# CHAPTER 22

# Cutaneous System

The skin is the largest and one of the most important organs of the body. Since the skin occupies such a critical position in the body, it is particularly subject to trauma, chemical irritation, radiation injury, extremes of heat and cold, infections, or parasitic diseases. Because of this vulnerable and yet protective position, the alterations in the skin of animals are of extreme importance to the veterinarian.

In addition to its mechanical protective purpose, the skin is also of extreme importance in the heat-regulating mechanism of the body. The sweat glands serve to cool the individual by means of the evaporation of the sweat that is poured out on the skin. The accessory skin structures (hair, fur, or feathers) serve as insulation, protecting the individual from extreme heat or cold.

## DISTURBANCES OF CIRCULATION

The circulatory disturbances of the skin of domestic animals are rather difficult to observe because of the hair, feathers, or wool that covers the individual. As a result, in most species of animals the skin can only be observed on the ventral surface of the abdomen, the inguinal or axillary region, the inner surface of the ear, or in any area where the hair, feathers, or wool has been removed by shaving, clipping, or traumatic injury. The skin altera-

tions are best studied in the white pig where the skin is readily visible over the entire body.

### Hyperemia

**Acute general active hyperemia** involves the skin of the entire cutaneous surface of the individual. It is observed in acute infectious diseases where acute general active hyperemia exists. The lesions of acute general active hyperemia are best observed in the white pig during winter. The stimulation of the cold causes the entire cutaneous surface of the pig to be pink or red. The color of the skin is caused by an abundance of oxyhemoglobin contained within the erythrocytes in the dilated capillaries of the skin.

**Acute local active hyperemia** involves a portion of the cutaneous surface of an individual. It is usually observed in an area where traumatic injury or chemical irritation has occurred. The area is pink or red in color depending on the intensity of the hyperemia.

**Acute general passive hyperemia** involves the skin of the entire cutaneous surface of the individual and occurs when an acute general passive hyperemia exists within the individual as a result of cardiac or pulmonary disease of short duration. The skin will have a cyanotic color because poorly oxygenated blood is present in the circulatory system. The lesions of general passive hyperemia are best observed in the white pig, where it will be noted that the color alteration in the skin is most pronounced in the ventral abdominal and thoracic wall, the legs, and the dependent portions of the ears.

**Acute local passive hyperemia** involves the skin of a portion of the individual such as a leg, the tail, or an ear. The color of the skin is cyanotic as the result of poorly oxygenated blood in the affected portion of the skin. It indicates a recent local obstruction to the flow of venous blood from the part in the form of a ligature, bandage, or other constricting device, or it may be the result of a thrombus within a vein.

**Chronic general passive hyperemia** occurs when the obstruction in the heart or lungs persists for a long period of time. The skin will be cyanotic in color and, in addition, will be thicker and more inelastic than normal because of edema and connective tissue deposition. The lesions are most pronounced in the legs, ventral underline, the dependent portions of the ears and tail, and in the ventral neck and mandibular regions due to the influence of gravity on the circulatory system.

**Chronic local passive hyperemia** involves only a portion of the skin such as the tail, ear, or leg. It is the result of a persisting obstruction to the venous flow from the area. Quite frequently it results from a bandage, ligature, or a rubber band placed around the ear, tail, or the leg. These objects may exert enough pressure to restrict the venous flow of blood from the area without obstructing the arterial blood supply. The skin in the area is thicker than normal as the result of edema and the deposition of white fibrous connective tissue.

### Hemorrhage

Hemorrhages within the skin are extremely common since the cutaneous surface is so vulnerable to traumatic injury. They are associated with septicemic diseases (hog cholera, leptospirosis, strangles, erysipelas) or any other infectious disease in which there is injury to endothelium or alterations in the bleeding and clotting time of the blood. Hemorrhages in the skin are frequently associated with various toxemias (ingestion of dicoumarol either in the form of rat poison or sweet clover, the excessive administration of sulfa drugs, the feeding of cattle for long periods of time on trichloroethylene-extracted soybean oil meal). Hemorrhages occur in the vicinity of insect bites where the mouth parts of the insect have penetrated into the skin.

The hemorrhage may be confined to a local area of the individual or may be scattered through the entire cutaneous surface. Hemorrhage as the result of trauma is localized, occurring in and around the site of injury. Those hemorrhages associated with the infectious diseases involve all portions of the skin of the individual if a septicemia is present. Multiple hemorrhages throughout the entire integument may occur in a toxemia when the bleeding or clotting time is prolonged.

The size of the hemorrhage varies with the amount of injury and the size of the vessels that have been damaged. Petechial hemorrhages are found in infectious or septicemic diseases since the injury is to the capillaries and only a small amount of blood escapes (hog cholera). Petechial and ecchymotic hemorrhages, suffusions, and hematocysts are observed when a toxemia is present that has caused an alteration in the bleeding and clotting time of the blood (sweet-clover poisoning). Local hemorrhages or hematocysts are usually the result of traumatic injury in which many vessels in a local area are injured or in which the larger veins and arteries in the skin have ruptured.

### Edema

Edema of the skin occurs when there is an increased amount of lymph in the connective tissue of the dermis and in the subcutaneous tissue. Edema of the skin may be local or general.

Local edema occurs when there is a local passive hyperemia or when a lymphatic obstruction to a local area of the skin is present. In those animals, especially in the horse, in which the circulation becomes sluggish as the result of inactivity, the local edema is most pronounced in the legs.

General edema of the skin occurs when there is a general passive hyperemia or a hypoproteinemia. The edema will be most pronounced in the skin of the ventral underline, the legs, and in the skin ventral to the mandible — in other words, in the dependent portions of the body where the edematous fluid accumulates due to the influence of gravity. General edema is observed in newborn pigs when the sows have been immunized against hog cholera during pregnancy. Edematous piglets, lambs, and foals are observed as the result of erythrocyte destruction by iso-antibodies. General edema of the skin is observed in individuals that have a deficiency of iodine.

**Macroscopic appearance.** The skin is thicker than normal, tense and turgid in consistency, cuts with ease, and has a transudate flowing from the cut surface. On examination of the cut surface, it will be noted that the prominent structures of the skin are separated from each other by clear fluid. Pitting on pressure occurs, and the part is cold as compared with the remainder of the body as the result of the sluggish circulation. If the edema persists, the skin becomes firm, inelastic, and does not return to normal if the cause of the edema can be removed. This is the result of the deposition of connective tissue in the area since connective tissue proliferates in areas of impaired circulation.

**Microscopic appearance.** The histological structures of the skin are separated by a faintly granular, eosin-staining material which is lymph. If the edema remains for a considerable period of time, the fibroblasts are stimulated by the reduced oxygen tension in the area, the stretching of the tissue, and the accumulation of waste materials; and then fibroblasts and collagen appear in the dermis and the subcutaneous tissue.

**Result.** The skin will return to normal if the cause of the edema can be corrected in a comparatively short period of time. If the cause of the edema cannot be removed, and the transudate persists, then white fibrous connective tissue is deposited and permanent distortion of the part is the result. This is the reason for the thick skin of the legs of horses that are confined to barns or small lots where they cannot obtain sufficient exercise.

## DISTURBANCES OF GROWTH

### Aplasia

Areas of skin may fail to develop. This condition is known as **epitheliogenesis imperfecta.** It is most commonly observed in the Holstein-Friesian breed of cattle and is a heritable factor (lethal gene). Since the skin is absent, these individuals are invaded with bacteria, and death from septicemia is the result.

A similar sex-linked epithelial defect is observed in newborn male Berkshire swine in which the epithelium and hair follicles fail to develop.

### Hypoplasia

Incomplete development of the skin is known as hypoplasia. The hypoplasia may involve the epithelium, the hair and hair follicles, and the sweat or sebaceous glands. The most common alteration is congenital alopecia in which the hair is imperfectly developed and the animal is bald. It is most commonly observed in Jersey calves. Alopecia may be the result of an iodine deficiency in the newborn.

Hypoplasia of the antlers of deer and moose is observed. It is apparently associated with hormone disturbances and cryptorchidism. The antlers do not extend in a dorsal direction in their normal position but remain close to the head. As they proliferate they cover the dorsal surface of the cranium, giving the animal the appearance of wearing a wig.

## Atrophy

Atrophy of the skin occurs in old age. As the result of senile changes, there is a reduction in the amount of hair, the number of sweat and sebaceous glands, and the intensity of pigmentation. Atrophy of the skin may occur when there is a circulatory disturbance in the part in which the nutritional requirements of the skin are not supplied. When this occurs, all structures of the skin decrease in size.

## Hypertrophy

The cells of the skin may be larger than normal when there is stimulation of the skin as the result of irritation. Hypertrophy of the sweat glands and sebaceous glands is observed when the skin is stimulated into activity by a need for sweat or oil on the skin. The glands of the skin become larger during the summer and decrease in size during the winter.

## Hyperplasia

Hyperplasia of the skin occurs when the skin is stimulated by some irritating factor. One of the more common examples of hyperplasia is the callus that occurs on the posterior surface of the elbow and on the lateral surface of the stifle of the dog. These parts are stimulated as they are pressed against the ground or floor when the animal is in a recumbent position. The epithelium becomes much thicker than normal, and large amounts of keratinized epithelium are present on the surface of the skin. At the same time there is hyperplasia of the skin glands, and epidermal inclusion cysts and sebaceous cysts are commonly found in the hyperplastic skin. As a result of the chronic irritation, white fibrous connective tissue is deposited in the dermis and the subcutaneous tissue. A similar hyperplasia is observed on the anterior surface of the knees of cattle. A general hyperplasia of the skin of calves is known as **ichthyosis**. It is a congenital disease in which there is general hyperkeratosis of the cutaneous surface. The entire skin is covered with a thick layer of keratinized epithelium divided by clefts and furrows that are formed as the result of the movement of the individual. Along with the hyperkeratosis there is usually an increased amount of hair.

Hyperkeratosis of the skin associated with an increased pigmentation is known as **acanthosis nigricans**. It is most frequently observed in the dog. The alterations in the skin are most pronounced in the axilla, ventral thoracic and abdominal wall, and the inguinal region. The skin is thicker than normal, quite inelastic, and forms prominent folds. Usually there is a decreased amount of hair. Along with these alterations there is also an increase in the pigment content of the skin, and as a result the skin becomes gray or black in color. The disease is most frequently associated with sustentacular-cell tumors of the testicle and with hypoplasia of the pituitary gland. Microscopic examination of the skin reveals hyperkeratosis, and the basal cells of the skin contain an abundance of melanin.

Focal hyperplasia of hair may occur in swine. Kernkamp has described **hypertrichosis partialis** in localized areas on the snout, nostrils, lips, and chin in five out of a litter of seven pigs. The hair was as much as 5 inches in length.

Hyperplasia of the skin structures also occurs when the skin is subjected to various bacterial and parasitic diseases (mange, ringworm, and pox).

**Hyperplasia of the scrotum** of old dogs is quite common. There is a thickening of the dermis and epidermis and a marked hyperkeratosis. The etiology of the condition has not been determined, but it probably represents the reaction to irritation and trauma over a long period of time.

**Hyperplasia of the ears of swine** is quite common as the result of an infection with various bacteria (streptococci, stapyhlococci, corynebacteria, and actinobacilli). The bacteria usually gain entrance to the ear through wounds received from fighting or through the epithelial defects produced by sunburn. The chronic inflammation causes a great increase in the amount of connective tissue in the dermis and subcutaneous tissue as well as hyperplasia of the skin glands and the epithelium. Usually, only one ear is involved. As the result of the chronic inflammation and the contraction of connective tissue, the ear acquires a cauliflower appearance. A somewhat similar hyperplasia of the ear may occur when various vascular disturbances resulting from erysipelas or constricting devices, such as rubber bands placed around the ear, are present.

Hyperplasia of the skin structures is observed along the ventral underline from the premaxilla to the perineum, the legs, and occasionally the distal end of the tail in animals in which there is a local or general passive hyperemia and edema. The thickening of the skin is due primarily to hyperplasia of white fibrous connective tissue.

**Hyperkeratosis of cattle.** A disease known as hyperkeratosis occurs in cattle. It occurs primarily in young animals 6 to 12 months old. The skin of the neck, back, and rump becomes thick and crusty (Fig. 22.1). Later this dermal thickening extends down the sides. Wartlike growths on the oral mucosa make mastication difficult.

Lacrimation is often prominent. Other symptoms are loss of weight, diarrhea, and polyuria. Hyperkeratosis is the name given to the condition because it is the most prominent lesion.

Hyperkeratosis has been reproduced by subjecting animals (cattle and laboratory animals), either by contact or by feeding, to substances suspected of containing the causative agent. In this manner the condition has been produced by feeding suspected hay, a processed wheat concentrate, pelleted dehydrated alfalfa containing dicalcium phosphate, and a ration containing machine lubricants in which highly **chlorinated naphthalenes** were present. It has also been produced by confining calves to pens, the boards of which had been treated with a wood preservative containing a naphthalene.

The causative agent is excreted in the cow's milk so that nursing calves develop the same condition. It is also absorbed through the skin. Insecticides containing naphthalenes, when applied to the skin, and machine lubricants which become incorporated into processed cattle feeds may be the chief sources of the agent.

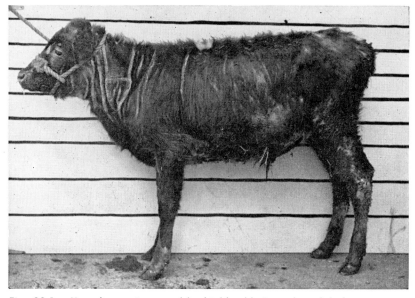

Fig. 22.1 — Hyperkeratosis caused by highly chlorinated naphthalenes present in lubricating oils and wood preservatives. (Department of Veterinary Pathology, Michigan State University.)

It is postulated that the causative agents of hyperkeratosis have an antivitamin-A effect, perhaps by interfering with the conversion of carotene to vitamin A.

## DISTURBANCES IN CELL METABOLISM

### Hydropic Degeneration

Hydropic degeneration is very common in the skin of domestic animals as the result of irritation of a rubbing nature with various chemical or blistering agents (croton oil, red iodide of mercury), from extreme heat or cold (sunburn or frostbite), and various infectious diseases (pox, foot-and-mouth disease, and contagious ecthyma).

**Macroscopic appearance.** Hydropic degeneration appears as a local swelling in the skin at the site of injury. The epidermis contains a blister or vesicle which, when incised, appears as a cystic structure containing a thin lymphlike fluid. The superficial surface of the blister is composed of the cornified layer of the stratified squamous epithelium. The basal layer of the blister consists of the basal cells of the skin.

**Microscopic appearance.** The histological appearance of hydropic degeneration is an intracellular edema in which the cells swell and burst when the cell wall can no longer contain the increased cell volume. Hydropic degeneration usually involves the prickle cell layer of the skin, but when severe irritation is present, the stratum germinativum may also be involved. The stratum corneum does not show this alteration since it is a dead structure and cannot undergo a disturbance in cell metabolism. As adjacent cells rupture, large masses of fluid accumulate in the epithelium, forming a vesicle.

### Fatty Degeneration

Fatty degeneration is of no concern in in the skin. It does not involve the stratified squamous epithelium. The sebaceous glands normally contain an abundance of fat. The sweat glands seldom show this alteration. Fat does accumulate in the dermis and subcutaneous adipose connective tissue. This is actually fatty infiltration and not a degenerative process.

### Glycogen Infiltration

Glycogen infiltration of the skin is of no concern in domestic animals. There are no diseases of animals associated with its deposition in the skin in excessive amounts.

### Amyloid Infiltration

Amyloid infiltration of the skin is most commonly observed in the equine. It is seldom observed in the United States but is quite common in Sweden. The disease appears as multiple nodules and masses in the skin of the head, neck, shoulders, and chest. The amyloid is deposited around the capillaries of the dermis and appears as a homogeneous material staining red with eosin and Congo red. The location of the lesion in the anterior portion of the individuals suggests that it is a contact allergic manifestation that occurs when the animals come in contact with a sensitizing substance in the process of feeding.

### Disturbances in Pigment Metabolism

MELANIN

A deficiency of pigment in the skin is known as **hypopigmentation**. The pigment defect is a hereditary transmissible disturbance. Total or partial **albinism** is observed in horses, cattle, dogs, and cats. Frequently it is associated with deafness. The skin lacks melanoblasts necessary for the production of pigment. Focal areas of hypopigmentation follow injury to the skin when there has been imperfect regeneration in the healing of cutaneous injury. The more specialized structures of the skin, such as the melanoblasts, do not regenerate, and the area of injury appears as a white spot. It is particularly noticeable in black horses in areas where saddle, collar, or harness injuries have occurred. It may also be observed in areas where ulcers have been present in the skin of horses affected with dourine. A deficiency of pigment is not as serious in domestic animals as it is in man because most of our domestic animals have sufficient amount of hair to protect the skin from the sun's rays. In swine, especially the Chester White and Landrace, considerable solar injury in the form of sunburn may occur because of the inadequate pigmentation that is characteristic for the breed. This is particularly true if the hogs are consuming photosensitizing vegetation.

**Hyperpigmentation** is observed in the skin of the inguinal, axillary, ventral thoracic, and abdominal regions in dogs affected with sustentacular-cell tumors of the testicle and in acanthosis nigricans. Focal areas of hyperpigmentation known as **melanosis maculosa** are frequently observed in the skin of swine and sheep. These represent areas where there is an abundance of melanoblasts. Many of these areas disappear with maturity of the individual. Hyperpigmentation is particularly common in Duroc hogs.

Depending upon the breed, type, and the normal color markings, there is considerable variation in the pigmentation of the individual. Jersey and Guernsey cattle have a **yellow** or **orange**-colored skin as the result of the high lipochrome and xanthochrome content of the tissue. Alterations in the color of the skin may be associated with the ingestion of various pigments such as carmine, which imparts a pink color to the skin. The application or the use of silver salts results in a **gray** skin color. Various **blue, green,** and **red** colors are observed when dyes of various types are administered to animals for therapeutic reasons. The skin of the cadaver is often **gray, green,** or even **black** as the result of putrefactive alterations. The skin of the cadaver may also be **red** or **pink** when imbibition with blood is present.

### Disturbances in Mineral Metabolism

Calcification of the skin is quite common in domestic animals when degenerative or necrotic alterations have occurred. Calcium salts are deposited in the altered tissue.

### PRESTERNAL CALCIFICATION

This lesion is most commonly observed in the chicken, cow, and sheep. The basic skin alteration is traumatic injury as the result of pressure when the animal is recumbent on its sternum. In cattle, injury from brush and thorns may also result in calcification of the sternal region. Calcification of the skin occurs in the degenerating or necrotic tissue in the area. The alterations are most extensive in the subcutaneous connective tissue and consist of multiple white or gray nodules varying from 1 millimeter or less to as much as 5 to 6 centimeters in diameter. The mass is chalky in consistency and is surrounded with a dense zone of white fibrous connective tissue. Microscopic examination of the area reveals a chronic inflammation, which may or may not be suppurative in nature, and masses of calcium in the form of calcospheres that are deposited on or infiltrating the necrotic or degenerating tissue.

### CALCIFICATION OF THE FOOT PADS

This lesion is quite common in older dogs. It is sometimes called calcium gout, but this is a misnomer because the term gout should be reserved for the deposition of sodium and calcium urate. The accumulation of calcium salts in the elastic and white fibrous connective tissue of the foot pads causes extreme pain, and the animal has difficulty in moving about. The etiology of the condition has not been established, but it is apparently associated with degeneration of elastic and white fibrous connective tissue. No association has been established between this calcification and renal disease in the dog. The incidence of the condition appears to vary from community to community.

**Macroscopic appearance.** When the foot pad is incised, masses of white, semisolid, chalky material are found. These are arranged in multiple foci that vary from 1 millimeter or less to as much as 10 millimeters in diameter. When the white chalky content is exposed to air, it dries, leaving a crumbly mass that resembles chalk.

**Microscopic appearance.** The histological appearance of the area varies considerably with the age of the lesion. The disease first appears as a deposition of calcospheres on and in the white fibrous and elastic tissue of the pad of the foot. As the condition advances, more and more calcium salts are deposited in the area. The salts act as a foreign body, especially when the animal moves about, and produce a chronic inflammation. The cellular exudate consists primarily of macrophages, lymphocytes, and giant cells. The areas of calcification and inflammation become encapsulated with white fibrous connective tissue.

### CALCIFICATION OF THE SKIN

This alteration occurs in various infectious and noninfectious diseases. Foreign bodies such as thorns and splinters inserted into the skin may become calcified, or the degenerating and necrotic tissue in the vicinity of the foreign body may be calcified. Following traumatic injury in which fat necrosis occurs, calcium salts are deposited in the necrotic fat. In tuberculosis the degenerating and necrotic tissue in the area becomes calcified.

## NECROSIS

### Coagulative Necrosis

Coagulative necrosis of the skin may be seen shortly after the application of phenol to the skin, or when the surface of the skin has been coagulated with heat in the form of actual cautery. Coagulative necrosis is also observed when *Spherophorus necrophorus* invades the skin. In coagulative necrosis of the skin the architecture remains but the cellular detail is lost. Uncomplicated coagulative necrosis of the skin is usually not observed because of the presence of bacteria in and on the skin.

### Liquefactive Necrosis

Liquefactive necrosis of the skin is very common because of the presence of pyogenic bacteria in and on the skin. The characteristic features of liquefactive necrosis are the absence of architectural and cellular detail and the presence of large numbers of neutrophils in the area. When bacteria are able to invade the skin following traumatic injury, infectious diseases (pox), and thermal injury (burns and freezing), the presence of bacteria attracts the neutrophil to the area, and the powerful proteolytic enzymes of the neutrophil liquefy the dead or injured tissue. The result is the presence of liquefactive necrosis and pus.

### Caseous Necrosis

Caseous necrosis is present when no cellular or architectural detail is present. The area contains relatively few neutrophils, and the necrotic tissue is dry, homogeneous, and surrounded with a connective tissue capsule. It is most frequently observed in skin tuberculosis or in tuberculoid infections of the skin.

### Fat Necrosis

Fat necrosis of the skin appears as a mass of opaque, white or gray material in the dermis or subcutaneous connective tissue. It occurs as the result of injury in which the circulation to an area of skin has been damaged. As a result of this injury, necrosis of the fat in the region occurs. It is usually the result of crushing traumatic injury as might occur following heavy blows from a club, or at the site of a bite wound where the skin has been traumatized by the blow from the teeth and jaws.

Necrotic fat in the skin is a chronic irritant and, in response to this irritation, considerable local inflammation is produced. These areas of fat necrosis and the resulting inflammatory reaction are often mistaken for wound infection, but it is soon observed that they do not respond to the usual treatment and surgical methods. Healing does not occur until all of the necrotic fat has been removed by surgery or phagocytosis.

In the area of fat necrosis there is a chronic inflammation characterized by the presence of an abundance of white fibrous connective tissue, lymphocytes, macrophages, and giant cells. These areas of fat necrosis frequently become invaded with bacteria, and then a complicating suppurative inflammation is present. Fat necrosis in the dog is particularly apt to be observed in the legs, back, and sacral region. The injury to the back and sacrum apparently occurs when the dog is retreating after being defeated in a dog fight, or when the dog has been stared down in the game of bluff and makes a hurried retreat and the victorious dog hastens his departure with a crushing bite in the dorsoposterior portion of the body.

### Gangrene

Gangrene of the skin is characterized by the disappearance of cellular and architectural detail and the invasion of the area with saprophytic microorganisms. Before gangrene will occur in an area there must first be necrosis, and secondly there must be invasion of the area with saprophytic bacteria of a putrefactive type.

Gangrene of the skin occurs when there is interference with the blood supply of a part. The cause of the gangrene is of two types: (1) gangrene as the result of pressure on the skin that compresses the capillaries (pressure necrosis or decubital gangrene), and (2) gangrene as the result of stenosis of the arteries or veins in the area.

Gangrene may be found in any area of the skin, but its usual site is in those areas where collateral circulation is inadequate to maintain the life of the part if the blood vascular system to an area of the skin is injured. It usually involves the ears, tail, legs, comb or wattles, or those areas in close proximity to the osseous skeleton (the skin over the wing of the ileum or over the zygomatic arch of the skull).

Pressure necrosis of the skin is very common in those animals that are unable to maintain an upright position when they are ill. As the animal lies in a recumbent position, portions of the skin are pressed against the bedding, floor, or the ground. This pressure prevents the blood from entering the capillaries of a portion of the skin and, if continued for a long period of time, death occurs in the area. Following death, the area is invaded with saprophytic organisms from the surface of the skin, and an area of gangrene is the result. It is most commonly observed over the bony body protuberances such as the wing of the ileum, spine of the scapula, the lateral surface of the hock and stifle joints, and the zygomatic arch of the skull. Frequent turning of the animal together with skin massage is necessary if this type of gangrene is to be prevented.

Gangrene as the result of stenosis of an artery or a vein occurs when ligatures, bandages, rubber bands, and other objects are placed around the ear, tail, or leg. The constant pressure hinders the venous and arterial blood supply, and the circulation to the extremity is impaired. Gangrene may also occur when vascular spasms (primarily arterial) associated with the ingestion of ergot occur. The ergot causes vasoconstriction, and the blood supply to an extremity is so reduced that death and necrosis occur. A fungus similar to classical ergot is present in fescue grass and causes vasoconstriction and gangrene of the feet, tail, and ears of cattle.

Gangrene may occur when bacterial or viral diseases damage an artery to an area of skin, thus causing thrombosis and interference with the arterial blood supply. This is frequently observed in erysipelas in swine.

Hemorrhage in the skin, especially if it is ecchymotic in size or larger, may so interfere with the circulation in an area by causing pressure stenosis of the blood vessels that life cannot be maintained and a focal area of skin undergoes necrosis.

Bacterial, parasitic, tumor, fibrin, and platelet emboli may lodge in an artery supplying an area of skin and cause infarction and necrosis of the skin in a focal area.

# DERMATITIS

**Definition.** Dermatitis is an inflammation of the skin. **Eczema** is a general term used to indicate any inflammation of the skin. Because of its nonspecific character and because more specific terms can be given to the skin lesions, the term should not be used. It is much more preferable to use the term dermatitis and indicate whether it is serous, papular, suppurative, necrotic, or parasitic, thus giving a much more specific description of the skin alteration.

Dermatitis is classified according to the type of exudate present, and a discussion of each of these types is presented below.

## Serous Dermatitis

Serous dermatitis of the skin occurs when the irritant is mild. A very good example is sunburn in its early stages when there is hyperemia of the skin and before blister formation has occurred. It may also follow mild friction from harnesses, collars, or ropes, mild irritating chemicals or drugs, or the application of heat or cold to the skin.

**Macroscopic appearance.** The cardinal signs of inflammation are present, and the exudate consists primarily of serous fluid. Usually there is hypersecretion of oil and sweat, and a small amount of serous fluid may be present on the skin surface. Frequently, the involved skin has a granular or raised appearance that is sometimes referred to as a **papular dermatitis.** This results from a characteristic of the skin architecture in which some of the papular areas of the dermis show more reaction than others, giving the skin a rough granular surface.

**Microscopic appearance.** Hyperemia, edema, and a few leukocytes, particularly neutrophils, are present in the area. The tissue reaction is mild, and cell destruction is not present.

**Result.** The skin recovers quickly when the cause of the dermatitis is removed. There is no permanent injury or scarring in the area. If the irritant persists or becomes more acute, a more severe type of dermatitis develops.

### VIRAL PAPULAR DERMATITIS OF HORSES

A mild papular dermatitis has been described in the equine. It is a highly contagious skin disease that tends to involve the entire skin surface of thoroughbred horses.

**Macroscopic appearance.** The lesion appears as small, raised, papular nodules that do not show the typical vesicle formation of pox. The papule becomes covered with a crust of dry exudate, and when this mass of encrusted hair falls away a small circumscribed area of alopecia remains.

## Hydropic Dermatitis

Hydropic or vesicular dermatitis occurs when the edematous fluid in the dermis and epidermis becomes excessive and microscopic or macroscopic accumulations of fluid, commonly known as blisters, appear.

**Etiology.** The cause of hydropic dermatitis is an irritant more severe than that which produces serous inflammation and resulting in a greater alteration in cell protoplasm. The best example of this type of alteration is the second-degree injury that results from sunburn or the application of other forms of heat (hot water or hot metal). This type of inflammation may occur with specific infectious diseases such as pox. It may be a manifestation of photosensitization in which the individual becomes sensitized to light as the result of the presence of various porphyrin compounds within the skin. It may represent an antigen-antibody reaction.

**Macroscopic appearance.** The cardinal signs of inflammation are present. In addition, the dermis is infiltrated with a large amount of edematous fluid. As a result, it is greatly thickened, and fluid will flow from the cut surface. In the epidermis there will be a raised bladder-like structure in the skin known as a blister or vesicle. This fluid accumulates in the middle layers of the epidermis, and the superficial stratum corneum is tense and taut because of the fluid pressure in the area. If the vesicle is incised, a clear lymphlike fluid spurts from the blister, and the underlying body surface in the base of the blister is pink or red as the result of hyperemia.

**Microscopic appearance.** Hydropic degeneration of the dermis is characterized by hyperemia and the accumulation of an edematous fluid in the tissues. The dermal structures are separated by a material that is granular and stains pink with eosin, which is the edematous fluid. Varying numbers of leukocytes are present, and of these, the neutrophils predominate. Hydropic degeneration of the epidermis begins as an accumulation of intracellular fluid in the prickle-cell layer. As the fluid accumulates in these stratified squamous cells, they become larger and larger, and soon the cell membranes are no longer able to contain the fluid and the cell bursts. As adjacent cells undergo a similar change, a large amount of fluid accumulates in the epidermis, and the stratum corneum is pushed to the exterior. This results in a raised swelling in the skin that is recognized as a vesicle or blister. Since the superficial layer of the skin, stratum corneum, is a dead structure, it cannot undergo hydropic degeneration. The dead stratum corneum contains the fluid, thus protecting the underlying structures and, in addition, it serves as a membrane preventing the entrance of bacteria into the fluid of the vesicle. Eventually, due to increasing pressure or as the result of trauma, the stratum corneum of the blister ruptures and the fluid escapes. Unless the irritation to the skin is very severe, the basal-cell layers, stratum germinativum, of the skin are not damaged to any great extent and are able to regenerate and form new stratified squamous epithelium. Usually by the time the vesicle ruptures, sufficient regeneration of the epithelium has occurred so that an effective barrier against the entrance of bacteria is present. The newly formed epithelial cells are hyperchromatic and have large nuclei. The more superficial cells begin to undergo keratinization, eventually cornify, and in

a relatively short period of time the skin has returned to normal, leaving no permanent injury or scar in the area.

While these changes are taking place in the epithelium, leukocytes are coming into the area, and the neutrophil will be found in the dermis and infiltrating into the epidermis and even into the fluid of the vesicle. However, since the most characteristic and outstanding feature of the lesion in the area is the vesicle, the term hydropic dermatitis is used to describe the alteration.

**Result.** No permanent injury to skin occurs. Regeneration of both dermis and epidermis is complete. If the irritant becomes more severe, or if bacteria invade the area of inflammation, a more severe type of skin alteration may result.

### MAMMALIAN POX

Pox, or variola, is an acute, infectious disease which usually runs a typical course and is characterized by a skin eruption consisting first of papules, then vesicles, next pustules, and finally scabs. Pox may affect any of the farm quadrupeds, but in this country it apparently occurs most frequently in cattle (cowpox) and hogs (swine pox). The causative virus, *Borreliota variolae*, will pass through only relatively coarse filters and is present in the vesicles.

The virus has an affinity for the epithelial layers of the skin and mucous membranes. At the points of localization of the virus, the epithelial cells proliferate at first (**papule** formation) but soon undergo a hydropic degeneration (**vesicle** formation) (Fig. 9.6). Cells resisting the degenerative changes are drawn out into thin threads which form a loose network in the vesicles. Migration of leukocytes into the contents of the vesicles changes the contents from a serous to a purulent exudate (**pustule** formation). The center of the pustule becomes depressed. Next, the pustule dries, forming a **scab** with regeneration of the epithelium underneath. If the inflammatory process penetrates the dermis and persists, a chronic inflammation is the result. As the newly formed connective tissue in the dermis contracts with age, a **pit** (scar) remains. The period of incubation of cowpox is 4 to 7 days; of swine pox, 6 to 16 days.

In **cowpox (*Variola vaccina*)** in cattle the characteristic pox lesions occur on the teats and udder. Pea-sized nodules in a day or two give way to bean-sized vesicles. The vesicles vary in color (reddish or bluish or yellowish white). Their shape is round on the udder, but on the teats they are slightly elongated dorsoventrally. They are surrounded by a hyperemic zone. Soon the vesicles become pustules. At the end of a week or 10 days the center becomes depressed, and a little later the pustule gives way to a scab which dries, drops off, and leaves behind a depressed white cicatrix (pit). Usually, there is a succession of vesicles which seldom number more than 15 to 20.

**Cowpox (*Variola vaccina*) in swine.** The majority of outbreaks of pox in swine are caused by the vaccinia virus. The disease is somewhat milder than the true swine pox. Vaccinia does not prevent an infection with the true swine pox, indicating that they are immunologically distinct viruses. Vaccinia and true swine pox (*Variola suilla*) can only be differentiated by cross-immunity tests in susceptible animals.

**Swine pox.** In the Corn Belt the disease occurs rather frequently and is caused by *Borreliota suis*. Pox infections in swine are most frequently spread by the hog louse (*Haematopinus suis*). The virus may also be transmitted by flies or by direct contact between animals. The characteristic pox lesions occur on the skin of the abdomen and inner surfaces of the legs (Fig. 22.2). When extensive, they appear also on the sides of the body, sometimes also along the back and on the face and ears. Central depression of the vesicle is not always present. The scab resulting from a pustule usually stands out above the general level of the skin. A scar or pit seldom results.

**Horse pox** is often known as contagious pustular stomatitis, coital vesicular exanthema, sore heel, or scratches. The virus of horse pox is very similar, if not identical, to cow pox (vaccinia). It spreads by direct contact between horses and is often introduced into a group of horses when cows infected with vaccinia are introduced into the herd or when human beings recently vaccinated with vaccinia come in contact with horses. The incubation period is usually about 10 days, although in severe epidemics this period may be greatly reduced.

Lesions are most frequently observed and most numerous on the nose and in the mouth of the horse. For this reason it is often known as contagious pustular stomatitis. The lesion in the mouth begins as a catarrhal stomatitis. Soon small elevated areas known as papules develop in the mucous membrane of the mouth or in the skin of the lips and nose. The papules soon undergo hydropic degeneration, and vesicles are then present. Later these vesicles become invaded with bacteria, and pustules are found in the area. When the vesicles and pustules rupture, ulcers are the result. In very severe cases a diffuse necrotic stomatitis may be present and the infection may extend into the nasal mucous membrane, the larynx, pharynx, esophagus, and conjunctiva. At times similar lesions will be observed on the external genital organs. It is possible that flies carry the virus from the mouth to the genital organs. When the infection becomes established in the genital organs it may be transmitted from animal to animal by coitus (coital vesicular exanthema).

The virus of horse pox may also contaminate wounds. This is particularly common in the legs of horses in the region of the fetlock (scratches). It is frequently a complication of the dermatitis associated with poor cleanliness of the feather and fetlock region of the horse such as when the area is macerated with mud. It may also invade wounds produced by wire cuts. The initial infection of the fetlock region produces papules and vesicles as were observed in the mouth. Once the initial infection is accomplished, bacteria in the area are able to invade, and a complicating bacterial dermatitis develops. As a

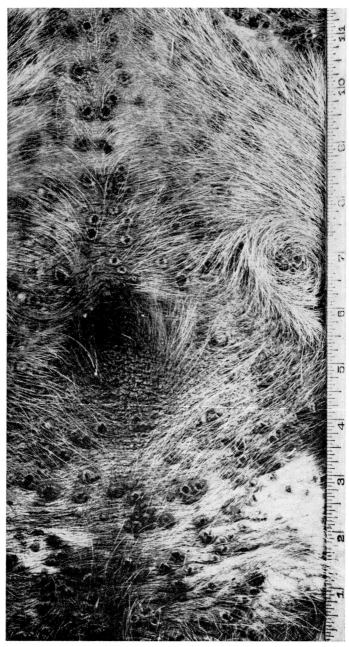

Fig. 22.2 — Swine pox lesions on skin of abdomen. (McNutt, Murray, and Purwin; Jour. A.V.M.A.)

result of the bacterial and viral stimulation, large masses of connective tissue (excessive granulation tissue) appear in the area.

## FOWL POX

Contagious epithelioma, sore head, avian diphtheria, and chicken pox canker are other names applied to fowl pox. It is an acute viral disease of birds caused by *Borreliota avium* and is characterized by wartlike nodules on the external surface of the head (Fig. 22.3) and by the formation of ulcers in the mouth. The period of incubation is 6 to 12 days.

**Pathogenesis.** The virus is contained within the nodules occurring on the comb, wattles, ear lobes, and face of the affected birds. It is transmitted to healthy birds through breaks in the continuity of the skin of the head. At certain seasons and in certain localities this occurs by means of mosquitoes (*Culex pipiens*). Mosquitoes have carried the infection 58 days and may possibly carry it during the entire course of their lives. At the site of infection the virus causes a hyperplasia of the epithelium. Within the epithelial cells are inclusions known as **Bollinger bodies** which contain numerous smaller inclusions (**Borrell bodies**). The latter can be

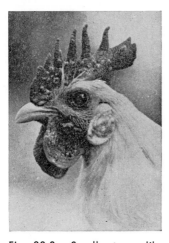

Fig. 22.3 — Small, tumor-like nodules in the epithelium of the comb, wattles, and ear lobes in fowl pox.

agglutinated by homologous immune serum. Centrally, these nodules first show hydropic degeneration of their cells, later, necrosis. Nodules having a similar histogenesis in their earlier stages may appear in the epithelium of the mouth, esophagus, and crop. Secondary infection with saprophytes, however, alters the manner in which they develop in later stages.

**Lesions.** External lesions have the appearance of **wartlike nodules** on the skin of the head. In size they are an eighth to a fourth of an inch in diameter. They first appear as small whitish foci which rapidly increase in size. They reach their maximum size in 4 to 6 days and become yellowish in color as they develop (**pustules**). Later they become dark brown or black (**scabs**). After a week or 10 days the scabs drop off leaving white scars (**pits**). In the mouth, sometimes also in the esophagus and crop, grayish-red, raised, diphtheritic patches develop. They appear dry and cheesy, and when removed leave behind bleeding erosions. Histologically, they consist of areas of fibrinonecrotic inflammation (**fowl pox canker**) containing superficially numerous colonies of bacteria (secondary invaders). This form of the disease is called **avian diphtheria.** The inflammatory process may extend from the mouth into the sinuses, particularly the infraorbital sinus, resulting in a tumor-like swelling as large as a hazelnut anterior to the eye. The contents of the swollen sinus is a grayish-yellow, dry, caseous material. Histologically, this disease can be differentiated from similar lesions in laryngotracheitis and nutritional and bacillary roup by the presence of Borrell bodies.

## CONTAGIOUS ECTHYMA

Contagious ecthyma, also called infectious pustular dermatitis and soremouth, is an acute viral disease of sheep and goats on the range and in feed lots. It also affects nursing lambs and kids. It is characterized by the formation of rather typical pox lesions on the lips, and sometimes on woolless or hairless areas of the skin. The cause is an epitheliotropic virus, *Borreliota ecthymatis,* which will pass through a Berkefeld V but not through a Mandler normal filter.

The lesions of contagious ecthyma are frequently confused with those of sheep pox and blue tongue. As a matter of differentiation, sheep pox does not occur in the United States. Blue tongue differs from contagious ecthyma in that the ulcerative lesions of the lips are not present and hyperplasia of the epithelium does not occur.

The lesion develops most typically on woolless or hairless parts of the skin such as the face, eyelids, inside the ears, under the base of the tail, on the mammary gland, and on the inside of the thighs. In its complete development it resembles the lesion of pox. It begins as a papule, a sharply defined nodule resulting from epithelial cell proliferation in the Malpighian layer of the epidermis. The cells in the papule soon undergo hydropic degeneration, swell, burst, and a vesicle is the result. When bacteria invade the vesicle, leukocytes infiltrate the lymph of the vesicle and it is converted into a pustule. The pustule ruptures and the exudate dries, forming a crust or scab. Large numbers of these lesions in close proximity cause the skin in the affected area to become greatly thickened and covered with dry hard crusts which become cracked, scale off, and leave a raw, bleeding surface or one covered with newly formed epithelium. The virus also stimulates the epithelium and hyperplasia occurs. As the result of this hyperplasia, large wartlike masses of tissue are present on the lips. Often, the middle stages (vesicle and pustule) may seem to be absent and the lesion appears to progress directly from the papule to the scab. Typically, there is a succession of lesions; they do not all form at once. As a consequence, the disease may last 3 or 4 weeks or longer.

In the mouth the lesion cannot develop the same as it does on the skin because the oral mucosa is moist. Furthermore, the lesions are subjected to constant trauma. As a result, there is no scab formation. Instead, on the highly reddened oral mucosa there are circumscribed, somewhat elevated areas covered with a creamy, whitish-yellow, spongy, membranous deposit. These ulcers bleed easily. On the lips, where desiccation can occur, scabs form. The lips become greatly thickened. It is easy for *Spherophorus necrophorus* or pyogenic bacteria to invade the primary lesion and cause a severe necrotic cheilitis (Fig. 22.4) or necrotic stomatitis (Fig. 17.5). Recovery may also be delayed by screwworm infestation.

Any epithelial surface of the body may be involved. Usually the portions of skin covered by wool are not affected because the wool protects the skin from trauma; and likewise, it is more difficult for the viral agent to reach any wound that may be present. In some cases the virus produces lesions in the mouth involving the cheeks, tongue, and palate; and when this occurs, the larynx, esophagus, rumen, reticulum, omasum, and abomasum may also be involved. In these organs where the surface is constantly bathed with saliva or fluids, diffuse necrotic inflammation of the epithelium may occur. Infections of the vulva, sheath, penis, coronet, and soles of the feet are also observed.

When the infection involves nursing lambs, the disease may be transmitted to the udder of the ewe. The udder may become so painful that the ewe will not allow the lamb to nurse. The infection may invade the mammary gland, resulting in a severe mastitis.

**Termination.** Unless complications arise from pyogenic infection or screwworm infestation, there is usually little mortality. It is easy for complications to occur, however, and as a result, the mortality has been reported to be as high as 50 per cent. In uncomplicated cases inability of adult animals to eat or of the young to nurse results in emaciation. Ewes with infected udders may not allow the lambs to nurse or may even disclaim their lambs. Mastitis from retained milk may result.

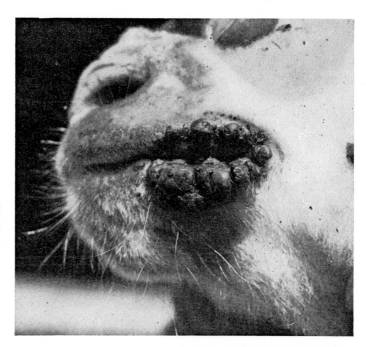

Fig. 22.4 — Necrotic cheilitis in a lamb due to the virus of contagious ecthyma a n d **Spherophorus necrophorus.** (Marsh and Tunnicliff, Jour. A.V.M.A.)

## ULCERATIVE DERMATITIS OF SHEEP

Tunnicliff has described an ulcerative dermatitis of sheep that he considers distinct from contagious ecthyma. It is caused by a viral agent that does not invade the mucous membrane of the mouth. The disease is transmitted by the bucks during breeding, but other methods of contact will also spread the disease. It affects primarily the skin of the lips, legs, and genital organs of both male and female sheep. The lesions on the lip are usually located between the nasal orifice and the margin of the upper lip, the pastern above the coronet, the interdigital pouch, the interdigital space, the lips of the vulva, the prepuce, and the glans penis. The infection is particularly serious in rams because swelling of the prepuce may be so great that the preputial opening is closed and urine accumulates within the prepuce. Lesions of the vulva usually do not extend into the vagina, cervix, or uterus.

The basic lesion is a necrotic dermatitis in which there is extensive ulceration of the involved skin surface. The area is usu-ally relatively free of the usual contaminating bacteria found in skin lesions. This is in contrast to the lesions of contagious ecthyma where secondary infection with staphylococcus, streptococcus, corynebacterium, and spherophorus organisms usually occurs.

## VESICULAR DERMATITIS IN CHICKENS

Vesicular dermatitis in chickens (sod disease) is observed in chickens placed on sod, especially prairie sod. It is primarily a disease of young birds and occurs during the early summer months. The etiology of the disease has never been entirely explained. It may be similar to the dermatitis and itching observed in the human who comes in contact with peat moss.

**Macroscopic appearance.** The disease usually involves the unfeathered portions of the feet, shanks, head, wattles, comb, and vent. The course of the disease is usually 2 to 3 weeks, and the mortality may be as much as 90 per cent. The lesion is first observed as small papules in the skin, particularly between the toes. Later a vesicle develops and bacterial invasion of the vesicle or the site of the vesicle after rupture results in a focal suppurative dermatitis. The masses of exudate on the eyelids cause the lids to adhere to each other. In the more severe cases, gangrene of the toes may occur.

**Prognosis.** The prognosis depends upon the rapidity with which the birds are removed from the sod and the amount of secondary bacterial infection of the skin. The mortality usually ranges from 20 to 90 per cent of the affected birds.

### Suppurative Dermatitis

Suppurative inflammation of the skin occurs when the principal constituent of the exudate is pus.

**Etiology.** Almost without exception, a suppurative inflammation indicates that bacteria are present in the skin. The injection of certain chemicals (turpentine) into the dermis will result in a sterile suppurative inflammation. The usual source of bacteria that invade the skin is the flora on the skin surface. These bacteria are primarily staphylococci, streptococci, and corynebacteria. They enter the skin through lacerations, incisions, or through minor skin alterations that occur when the defense mechanism of the body is impaired by malnutrition, chronic debilitating diseases, or vascular disturbances (anemia or passive hyperemia). A suppurative dermatitis may also result when a septicemia exists and bacteria are brought to the skin by way of the blood vascular system. A suppurative dermatitis is frequently a complication of vesicular dermatitis when bacteria invade the blister and produce a pustule (pox or foot-and-mouth disease).

Dermatitis is observed ventral to wounds or body openings when the skin is moistened by exudate, secretion, or excretion. The discharge from wounds causes a maceration of the skin, and the organisms in the skin or exudate are able to invade the skin surface and produce a suppurative dermatitis. Dermatitis of the face ventral to the eye is frequently observed with pink-eye or rickettsial conjunctivitis.

Dermatitis of the tail, perineum, and the medial surface of the thighs and legs occurs in animals that have a diarrhea. It is especially serious in sheep since the wool holds the mass of feces against the skin, causing maceration and thus lowering the resistance of the skin to bacterial invasion.

Dermatitis of sheep, particularly involving the backs of lambs, is observed when sharp awns and burrs from plants fall into the breaks in the fleece and come in contact with the skin, producing traumatic irritation.

A suppurative dermatitis in dogs is associated with chronic thallium sulfate poisoning. The dermatitis may be serous or suppurative, and the lesions that occur in the skin in the vicinity of the eye and nose of dogs may be confused with the suppurative blepharitis and rhinitis observed in canine distemper.

**Macroscopic appearance.** Suppurative inflammation of the skin may be diffuse or focal, depending on the extent of the invasion with bacteria. Diffuse inflammation of the skin is usually the result of wound infection and the rapid spread of the microorganisms through the dermis and the subcutaneous tissue. This diffuse spread through the tissues is known as a **phlegmon.** It is characterized by the rapid spread of the infection through the tissues in the direction of the heart, the cardinal signs of inflammation, and the accumulation of pus in the skin where the inflammation is present.

A focal suppurative inflammation of the skin occurs when wounds are invaded with pyogenic bacteria and the infection is contained within the immediate vicinity of the wound.

A circumscribed focal suppurative inflammation of the skin is an **abscess.** According to its size and location, specific terms are often given to it. If the focal area of suppurative inflammation is confined and contained within the epidermis, it is called a **pustule.** Pustules are frequently observed in the horse, particularly in the summer, in areas where the skin becomes macerated with sweat (under the saddle or harness). Pustules are common in the skin of the dorsal surface of the nose of the dog. Pustules are observed in areas of skin that become macerated with water (the back of sheep when the wool becomes soaked with rain, the legs of horses that stand in water or mud for long periods of time, or the tail of cattle when it drags in water, urine, or feces). It is a common complication of canine distemper in which multiple pustules are observed in the skin of the inguinal region and the auricula and the external auditory canal of the ear of the dog.

If the focal area of suppurative inflammation involves the hair follicles, sweat glands, or sebaceous glands, it is known as a **furuncle** or **boil**. The furuncle measures from a millimeter to a centimeter in diameter. A larger focal area of suppurative inflammation of the skin which extends into the subcutaneous connective tissue is called an abscess, or in the human being it is referred to as a **carbuncle**.

**Microscopic appearance.** Basically, the tissue alteration is the same whether the suppurative inflammation is focal or diffuse. The cardinal signs of inflammation are present. There is hyperemia and exudation into the area, and the most characteristic alterations are the extensive liquefactive necrosis and the presence of pus in the area. The phlegmon progresses so rapidly that connective tissue does not proliferate in the area. The pustule which involves only the epithelial layer does not stimulate the production of connective tissue. The furuncle, which involves both the epidermis and the dermis and persists for a period of time, causes the proliferation of connective tissue. A similar situation occurs with the abscess or the carbuncle that extends into the subcutaneous connective tissue. The mass of exudate contained within the abscess, particularly when it is inspissated, is referred to as the **core**. The path by which the exudate discharges to the skin surface is known as the **sinus tract**.

## SEBORRHEA

Seborrhea is a functional disturbance of the sebaceous glands in which excessive amounts of sebum pour out on the skin. The condition is associated with a dermatitis.

**Etiology.** The etiology of seborrhea is unknown, but it occurs in those individuals and in those areas of the body in which there is an abundance of skin secretion. It is occasionally observed in the skin of the shoulder, front legs, and flank region of the horse.

**Macroscopic appearance.** The cardinal signs of inflammation are present, and the surface of the skin is covered with dandruff or with oily masses of desquamated epithelium. The amount of oil in the exudate determines whether it is a dry or moist seborrhea. The inflammation usually exists as multiple papular areas where the reaction is unusually acute. The scales and accumulations of exudate on the skin cause itching, and the scratching and rubbing of the skin results in abrasions.

**Microscopic appearance.** Hyperkeratosis of the skin is present along with hyperplasia and hypertrophy of the sweat and sebaceous glands. As a result of the skin alterations and the lacerations or abrasions that may be present, the area is often infiltrated with staphylococci, streptococci, and corynebacteria that produce a complicating suppurative inflammation.

## OTITIS EXTERNA

Otitis externa is an inflammation of the auricula and the external auditory canal of the ear. It is especially common in old dogs with long pendulous ears that contain excessive amounts of hair.

The otitis externa is often initiated by an infection with *Otodectes canis* (ear mite), excessive amounts of water in the ear (from bathing or swimming), the accumulation of wax, epithelial debris and hair, or canine distemper.

The inflammation may be acute or chronic, serous, suppurative, ulcerative, or even gangrenous in type. Once inflammation of the ear is initiated, the abundance of secretion and excretion in the area provides excessively moist surroundings in which various pyogenic and saprophytic organisms multiply. These are capable of invading the macerated skin surface. Quite often the treatment for otitis externa is so irritating that it favors the spread of the inflammation rather than affecting healing.

### PODODERMATITIS AND CORONITIS

Pododermatitis is an inflammation of that portion of the skin which continues down within the horn capsule of the hoof of an animal. Coronitis is inflammation of the skin in the area where the skin joins the coronary border of the hoof.

A pododermatitis and coronitis occurring as a herd problem in domestic animals, whether on the range or in the feed lot, particularly in hogs, cattle, and sheep, is almost without exception an indication of a viral infection (mammalian pox, vesicular exanthema, foot-and-mouth disease, blue tongue, contagious ecthyma, ulcerative dermatitis in sheep, and lumpy skin disease in cattle). This is particularly true when lesions are also observed on the muzzle, in the mouth, on the teats, and around the base of the horns. The lesions, typical of a viral infection, usually appear as papules, become vesicles, later develop into pustules, and then become ulcers.

Some years ago the terms mycotic pododermatitis, coronitis, and stomatitis were introduced into the literature. This was exceedingly unfortunate because the lesions do not represent a primary fungus infection. If fungi are present, it is an indication of a secondary complicating fungus infection. The terms mycotic pododermatitis, coronitis, and stomatitis should never be used since no specific fungus capable of producing a sudden herd outbreak in domestic animals has ever been described.

Occasional outbreaks of pododermatitis and coronitis appear as a herd or flock problem when the hoof and the skin of the legs have been macerated in water or mud. The maceration lowers the resistance of the skin to bacterial invasion (*Spherophorus necrophorus*, corynebacteria, staphylococci, streptococci, and saprophytic bacteria), and a suppurative dermatitis is the result.

The penetration of the larvae of *Strongyloides papillosus* through the skin of the legs of sheep is an important factor in the introduction of the organisms that cause foot rot.

Individual cases of pododermatitis and coronitis are usually the result of traumatic injury (calk wounds, barbed wire lacerations, and brush or rock injury).

### LUMPY WOOL DISEASE

Lumpy wool disease is a suppurative dermatitis that occurs in heavily wooled sheep (confined almost entirely to Merino sheep) in areas in which there is an abundance of rainfall, where mists are common and the humidity is high. Mason and Bekker have isolated *Actinomyces dermatonomus* from the lesions and have reproduced similar lesions in experimental animals. This constantly wet mass of wool macerates the skin, and under these conditions the organism invades the skin and produces a dermatitis.

The organism is probably a normal inhabitant of the wool and skin, and only invades the skin and produces lesions when the wool has been wet for a long period of time. Because the wet mass of wool must be present to produce the lesion, it is in the heavier wooled breeds (Merino) that the disease has been observed. Lambs are particularly susceptible. Experimental skin infections can be reproduced in rabbits, guinea pigs, mice, calves, and cattle.

**Macroscopic appearance.** At first, there is a hyperemia of the skin. Later, papules and pustules, which later enlarge and coalesce, appear in the involved area. The pustules rupture and the pus is discharged into the wool. In addition, considerable serum and plasma exudes from the involved area. The serum, plasma, and pus cause a matting of the wool, resulting in lumps in the fleece. These lumps of matted wool have given the disease the name lumpy wool. Considerable pain is experienced by the animal when it attempts to move and, as a result, the animal walks with a very stiff gait.

**Microscopic appearance.** Histological examination reveals a serous, suppurative, or ulcerative dermatitis.

**Result.** Shearing of the wet wool and the contained exudate results in rapid healing and recovery. If the wet wool and exudate are allowed to remain in the area, the infection persists for months and a chronic dermatitis is the result. Blowflies may deposit eggs in the matted wool, and the resulting blowfly larvae may cause considerable injury and even death of the individual.

### LUMPY SKIN DISEASE IN SWINE

Lumpy skin disease in swine is characterized by an uneven skin surface of the back, shoulder, and thighs of swine. The cutaneous protruberances of the skin are separated by depressions that resemble scars or dimples. To the casual onlooker these areas resemble the raised, diamond-shaped lesions occurring in swine with erysipelas. Closer examination reveals no acute inflammation in the area, and the hyperemia associated with erysipelas is not present.

The disease has been described by Penny in England, and Bohmker (personal communication) reports similar cases in South Dakota. Penny observed the disease in the Large White breed of hogs in England, but the hogs involved in Iowa and South Dakota have been black or almost black in color. Usually the pigs are not ill. There is no anorexia, fever, or diarrhea. Occasionally, a herd in which the disease appears had a history of illness when the pigs were young, but, for the most part, no early specific skin disease has been associated with the condition. The etiology has not been explained. Although many or all litters on a premises may be involved, no hereditary defect has been demonstrated; nor has it been possible to associate the disease with any nutritional deficiency.

**Macroscopic appearance.** Cross section of the skin through the involved area reveals the lumps to be from 3 to 6 centimeters in diameter. These areas of fat appear to be somewhat thicker than the normal back-fat thickness of pigs of a similar age. The depressions between the raised lumps of fat are about half the thickness of the lump, and they contain more connective tissue than is usually found in the skin and the subcutaneous tissue. The cardinal signs of inflammation are not present.

Although the clinical appearance of the pigs suggests that the alterations are found in the skin, the lesion is actually in the subcutaneous tissue.

Although the general appearance of the hogs is quite disturbing as far as the lumps and depressions in the back and legs are concerned, the animals show little evidence of illness. In general it can be said that they are not quite as thrifty or as well developed as unaffected animals. An occasional herd is observed in which the scarring and dimpling of the posterior legs becomes so extensive that difficulty in locomotion is the result, and some animals eventually are unable to rise or move about. The majority of the animals will pass federal meat inspection; and if the lumps and scars in the skin are large and numerous, the involved areas are trimmed out by the inspector.

**Microscopic appearance.** Histological examination reveals that the raised lumps of fat consist entirely of normal-appearing adipose cells. The depressions or dimples between the lumps of fat contain considerably more connective tissue than do the lumps, and a few macrophages and lymphocytes are present in the area. Apparently the dimpling of the skin is the result of the local destruction of fat and the contraction of the scar tissue that is present.

The shape of the depression and the

presence of scar tissue, lymphocytes, and macrophages suggests that these dimples are the site of an old area of infarction as might occur with an erysipelas or a streptococcic infection. However, in the herds that have been observed, a history of erysipelas or streptococcosis has not been obtained.

### LUMPY SKIN DISEASE IN CATTLE

Lumpy skin disease is an acute viral infection of African cattle that is characterized by multiple focal areas of dermatitis, acute lymphadenitis, edema of the legs, and lameness.

**Etiology.** The etiology of lumpy skin disease is a virus that is easily cultivated in eggs. The embryos are stunted in growth, lack feathers (except along the crest), and their skin is very hyperemic.

**Macroscopic appearance.** A focal nodular dermatitis is observed involving the entire cutaneous surface. These areas vary from 0.5 to 3 centimeters in diameter but occasionally are as much as 5 centimeters. In severe cases, the nodules coalesce to form larger masses. As the condition progresses, the center of the nodule under-goes necrosis and an ulcer is the result. In especially severe cases, lesions are observed in the conjunctiva and in the mucous membrane of the mouth and nasal passages. The teats and udder may also be involved. There is a general lymphadenitis. Edema of the legs, brisket, and ventral portions of the neck is present in severe cases.

A few animals have a pododermatitis and coronitis that may extend above the fetlocks and cause severe lameness. In some cattle, multiple circular areas of necrosis are observed in the skin from the hoof to the shoulder.

**Microscopic appearance.** The lesion first appears as a focal serous dermatitis and is primarily a perivasculitis involving the smaller blood vessels (arterioles, venules, and capillaries) of the skin. Extensive edema is present, and later, neutrophils and eosinophils appear in the area. Thrombosis of the small vessels is common. As the result of thrombosis, necrosis occurs and an ulcerative dermatitis is produced. The ulcer is invaded with bacteria found on the surface of the skin, causing a complicating suppurative dermatitis.

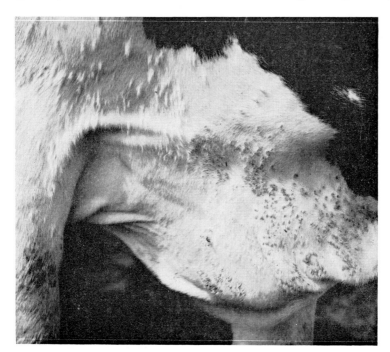

Fig. 22.5 — Lumpy skin disease in Iowa cattle. Brisket region.

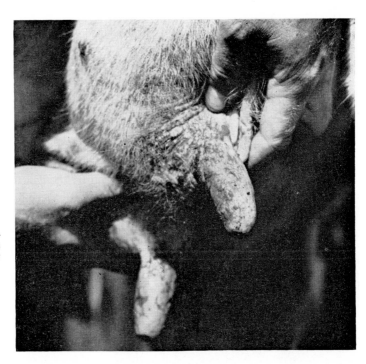

Fig. 22.6 — Lumpy skin disease in Iowa cattle. Dermatitis of the skin of the mammary gland.

One of the microscopic characteristics of the disease is the proliferation of macrophages and fibroblasts in the area of dermatitis. Numerous intracytoplasmic inclusion bodies, that stain pink with eosin, are found in the macrophages, fibroblasts, and epithelial cells. The inclusion bodies are frequently as large as the cell nuclei.

**Prognosis.** The disease is extremely contagious and spreads rapidly through the herd. Great care should be taken so as not to carry the infection to other cattle on other premises. The morbidity is from 50 to 100 per cent of the herd, and the mortality is 0.5 to 1 per cent. Calves and animals in poor condition are more severely affected. The skin lesions heal after 2 or 3 weeks. In the more severe cases, when extensive ulceration is present, healing may be delayed several weeks or months, and incomplete repair with small focal areas of alopecia may remain.

## LUMPY SKIN DISEASE IN IOWA CATTLE

A papular, and later pustular and ulcerative, dermatitis (Fig. 22.5), involving entire herds of cattle, is observed in Iowa during the month of August. The entire surface of the body is affected, and the disease is particularly serious when it involves the udder and teats. When mammary gland lesions are present, considerable difficulty is experienced in milking the animal (Fig. 22.6).

**Etiology.** The etiology of the disease has not been determined. It seems to be more prevalent in low-lying pastures along streams. The condition has not been associated with biting arthropods or toxic vegetation. Whether the disease is the same or similar to lumpy skin disease in Africa has not been determined. Preliminary investigations indicate that it is probably the same disease.

**Macroscopic appearance.** The lesions are found on the pigmented and unpigmented portions of the skin. Itching is not a prominent symptom; in fact it is surprising how little pruritus is present considering the amount of skin area involved. Careful examination of the herds indicates that the morbidity is almost 100 per cent. No deaths have occurred in affected herds. Healing occurs after several weeks, but lesions may persist in particularly severe cases for as long as 4 to 6 months.

The lesions begin as a papule, developing into a pustule that ruptures to form an ulcer. The pus, serum, and plasma cause a scab to form in the hair over the area of ulceration. In some animals extensive ulceration of the legs below the shouder and hock occurs (Fig. 22.7).

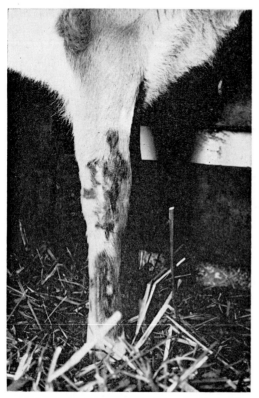

Fig. 22.7 — Lumpy skin disease in Iowa cattle. Ulcers in the skin of the legs.

**Microscopic appearance.** Histological examination reveals a focal suppurative or necrotic dermatitis.

### FACIAL DERMATITIS IN BABY PIGS

A suppurative and later ulcerative dermatitis is frequently observed in the skin of the face of baby pigs as the result of injury from the tusks of other baby pigs of the litter while fighting or nursing. The suppurative inflammation spreads over the face following the initial infection of the tusk wounds. Crusts of exudate cover the skin surface. Considerable mortality may occur as the result of toxemia, shock, and septicemia.

### GREASY PIG DISEASE

**Definition.** Greasy pig disease is an acute dermatitis involving the entire surface of the body of baby pigs. It is characterized by a wet greasy skin covered with crusts of exudate.

**Predisposing factors.** No predisposing factors have been found. The disease is observed throughout the entire year but is most frequently encountered during the spring because more baby pigs are present at that time. There is no evidence to indicate that breed, sex, color, size of litter, housing, chilling, bedding, sanitation, dry lot, pasture, or heredity are concerned with the appearance of the disease. Pigs of the first, second, or third litter are equally affected.

**Etiology.** The etiology of the disease is unknown. Most of the information about the disease has been contributed by Jones. In Europe, staphylococci have been suspected of causing the lesions, but difficulty has been experienced in reproducing the clinical disease. The importance of heredity, nutrition, viral agents, and toxic substances have been studied, but no association with the appearance of the disease has been demonstrated.

**Incidence.** The disease was first reported by Spinola in 1842. In the United States the cutaneous alterations were described in California in 1911. Today, it is apparently found wherever swine are raised, and reports of its presence have appeared from all parts of the world. Evidence seems to indicate that the disease is becoming more prevalent.

The disease affects young pigs between 5 and 35 days of age, with an average of 21 days. The younger the pigs, the lower is the resistance, the shorter is the course, and the higher are the morbidity and mortality. One or more litters on a farm are affected. Usually, if the disease appears in a litter, the entire litter becomes affected. The mortality varies considerably from 5 to 100 per cent, with an average of 68 per cent.

**Macroscopic appearance.** At the onset of the disease the pigs show listlessness, drooping of the ears and tail, and a dull hair coat. A little dandruff is observed.

On the second or third day the attitude varies from dejection and apathy to restlessness and anxiety. Anorexia and thirst are present. The skin is slightly thickened, damp, and oily. Small brown spots appear around the hair follicles and at the mouths of the sweat glands.

As the disease progresses, the depression and anorexia become more marked. Usually the animals are constipated. Fever is not present. The hair is not damaged. Itching and pain are not observed. Soon the entire body is covered with a moist, sticky, greasy exudate composed of sebum, sweat, and serum. This exudate dries on the surface of the skin, forming scabs or crusts. Due to the movement of the animal, these crusts develop fissures. If the scabs are removed, a very hyperemic skin with a very sour or rancid odor is observed. The feet are almost constantly involved in the more severe forms of the disease. Cracking, separation, and peeling of the skin of the digital bulbs and plantar and volar surfaces of the feet are observed.

**Microscopic appearance.** A serous dermatitis is present in the early stages of the disease. Later, a suppurative dermatitis appears as the result of the invasion of the skin with bacteria (primarily staphylococci). Along with the dermatitis there are marked hyperplasia, hypertrophy, and hypersecretion of the skin glands.

Since considerable confusion exists between greasy pig disease and parakeratosis, Table 22.1 is presented.

## TUBERCULOSIS

Tuberculosis of the skin of the bovine, caused by *Mycobacterium tuberculosis*, is a chronic productive inflammation that produces raised areas in the skin measuring a few millimeters to several centimeters in diameter. On cross section, a chronic inflammatory reaction is quite apparent with considerable deposition of white fibrous connective tissue in the area. Throughout the white fibrous connective tissue there are numerous focal areas of caseous necrosis that measure 1 millimeter to 2 centimeters in diameter.

Tuberculosis of the skin of domestic animals in the United States is extremely uncommon at the present time because of the extensive eradication of tuberculosis in this country. Even when tuberculosis was quite prevalent, the incidence of skin tuberculosis was not great.

Tuberculosis of the cow is most frequently observed in the skin of the vulva, and when present, there is a chronic vulvitis that contains multiple areas of necrosis. Sinus tracts may extend from the areas of necrosis to the exterior. Vulvar tuberculosis is the result of a tuberculous metritis or vaginitis in which the exudate pours over the surface of the vulva and macerates the skin, lowering the resistance of the cutaneous tissue so that the bacilli may enter the skin.

Tuberculosis of the skin of the horse shows more connective tissue deposition and less caseation than the lesion does in

TABLE 22.1
DIFFERENTIATION BETWEEN PARAKERATOSIS AND GREASY PIG DISEASE

|  | Parakeratosis | Greasy Pig Disease |
|---|---|---|
| Age | 10 to 12 weeks | 5 to 35 days |
| Season | winter | spring |
| Lesions | dry, thick crusts of exudate | moist, greasy crusts of exudate, sour or rancid odor |
| Mortality | low, usually recover | high |
| Etiology | calcium, phosphorus, zinc ratio | unknown (staphylococci) |
| Pasture | recover quickly | no effect |

the bovine. Skin tuberculosis is quite common in swine, occurring as a caseous dermatitis with calcification of the necrotic tissue. The lesions are usually located in the fat of the subcutaneous tissue. Ulceration of the epithelium above the lesion may occur. Skin tuberculosis is quite frequently observed in the cat, involving the head and especially the dorsal surface of the nose. The involved area shows multiple ulcers in the skin. Tuberculosis of the skin of the bird is occasionally observed and is of the caseous type. Tuberculosis of the pigeon and parrot usually involves the head, especially the eyelids. Hyperkeratosis is particularly prominent in the parrot.

**Microscopic appearance.** Histological examination reveals a chronic caseous dermatitis in which there are numerous macrophages and giant cells. If the tissue is stained with Ziehl-Neelsen's acid-fast stain, the acid-fast organisms can be demonstrated in the lesions.

### TUBERCULOID DERMATITIS OF THE SKIN OF CATTLE

In the United States, acid-fast organisms, probably soil forms, invade the skin of cattle and produce a chronic inflammatory reaction. The lesion is very similar to the alterations produced by *Mycobacterium tuberculosis*. These lesions are of particular importance to the regulatory official because the organisms contained within the focal areas sensitize the individual so that when tuberculin is injected into the animal, a positive skin reaction for tuberculosis occurs.

The alterations are most frequently observed in the skin of the fetlock, pastern, shoulder, knee, and the ventral abdominal wall. The lesion is primarily a chronic caseous dermatitis, and the surface of the lesion may show ulceration. Acid-fast organisms can be demonstrated in the lesion. Calcification of the necrotic tissue occurs.

### GLANDERS

Glanders, caused by *Malleomyces mallei,* involves the skin of the horse where it produces nodules and ulcers. Glanders has been eradicated from the United States. The lesion first appears as a nodule of varying size in the skin, and later the superficial surface undergoes necrosis and an ulcer is the result. When the ulcer heals, an unpigmented scar remains in the area.

**Microscopic appearance.** The histological appearance is a typical chronic suppurative inflammation characterized by the presence of connective tissue, neutrophils, lymphocytes, macrophages, and giant cells.

### STAPHYLOCOCCOSIS

Staphylococcosis is a chronic suppurative skin inflammation caused by *Staphylococcus aureus*. The skin lesion consists of multiple focal areas of suppuration in which there are small yellow granules that may be confused with the sulfur granule of actinobacillosis. When the lesion is stained with the Gram stain, Gram-positive cocci that are morphologically identical with staphylococci are observed in the small yellow granules.

Chronic staphylococcosis is most frequently observed in the horse. In the dog it produces a chronic suppurative inflammation of the tail.

### ACTINOBACILLOSIS

Actinobacillosis of the skin is caused by *Actinobacillus lignieresi* which produces a chronic suppurative inflammation. Within the area of inflammation there are multiple yellow foci that consist of masses of neutrophils within which there is a yellow sulfur granule. When this granule is stained with the Gram stain, it is found that the granule contains numerous Gram-negative rods.

### CRYPTOCOCCOSIS

Cryptococcosis of the skin is occasionally observed in domestic animals, particularly the horse, and is caused by *Cryptococcus neoformans*. It is a chronic suppurative skin inflammation that produces nodules, abscesses, and ulcers. The lesions are circular in shape and have raised borders and depressed centers.

**Microscopic appearance.** Histological examination reveals a chronic suppurative inflammation. Numerous cryptococci can be seen in the multiple suppurative foci. The organism, a budding yeast, can be demonstrated in direct smears when suspended in physiological saline solution. In histological preparations the organisms appear as budding yeasts surrounded by a zone which has the tinctorial properties of glycogen. Numerous lymphocytes, macrophages, and giant cells are present in the area, and the macrophages and giant cells contain phagocytosed cryptococci. Neutrophils are numerous in the active areas where parasites are found.

### BLASTOMYCOSIS

Blastomycosis is caused by a fungus, *Blastomyces dermatitidis*, that occurs in the tissue as a budding yeast and exhibits mycelia when grown on suitable artificial media.

The disease appears as a chronic focal suppurative and ulcerative dermatitis, and tends to spread through the skin, eventually involving a considerable cutaneous area. The disease spreads to the regional lymph nodes by way of the lymphatics and from there may involve the internal organs.

**Microscopic appearance.** Histological examination reveals the budding yeasts in small foci of neutrophils or within the cytoplasm of macrophages and giant cells. The organism has a thin, clear, sharply defined cell wall, and the cell is not surrounded with a clear zone of mucin. Fresh smears of the lesion, suspended in physiological saline solution and examined with the microscope, will reveal the yeasts. In the more chronic lesions the organism may be difficult to demonstrate, being few in number.

### EPIZOOTIC LYMPHANGITIS

Epizootic lymphangitis is a chronic suppurative infection of horses, mules, and donkeys caused by the fungus *Zymonema farciminosum*. The disease is found in Europe, Africa, and Asia. It probably does not occur in the United States.

The infection gains entrance through skin wounds of various types. Following the initial invasion of the skin, the organism spreads by way of the lymphatics to the regional lymph nodes, and in the more advanced cases involves the internal organs.

Epizootic lymphangitis is most common in the anterior legs, the chest wall, and the neck. In severe cases the skin of the entire body may be involved. The lymph vessels in the skin are greatly enlarged and stand out as tortuous cords extending from the lesion to the regional lymph nodes.

Small yeastlike organisms, morphologically similar to histoplasma in some respects, are observed in the exudate and within the leukocytes. Mycelia are occasionally observed in tissue but are usually found only in culture.

### SPOROTRICHOSIS

Sporotrichosis is a chronic suppurative infectious disease caused by *Sporotrichum schencki*. The disease is transmitted to individuals through injuries produced by thorns, awns, and splinters. Sporotrichosis occurs only sporadically, is seldom observed in the United States, and is seen most frequently in horses, mules, dogs, and cattle.

The organism, a short rod-shaped yeast that measures 2 to 3 microns in width and 3 to 5 microns in length, is difficult to demonstrate within the lesion. It is readily cultured on artificial media and there produces hyphae.

The lesion begins as a focal suppurative inflammation of the skin. The foci are usually small, measuring 1 to 2 centimeters in diameter. As the disease progresses, the superficial layers of the skin undergo necrosis, and an ulcer is the result. Although multiple isolated nodules may be found in the skin, this disease usually follows the course of the lymphatics, resulting in multiple nodules along the lymphatics from the primary site of invasion to the regional lymph nodes. Involvement of the bones, joints, and internal organs may occur.

## FAVUS

Favus in dogs, cats, and horses is caused by *Trichophyton schonleinii*. Favus usually involves the head of the dog and cat. Ear infection is particularly common in the cat. The organism produces a dense mat of hyphae and conidia on the surface of the skin, giving a white or gray color to the surface of the lesion. The underlying dermis shows a severe hyperemia and an abundance of leukocytes. The disease probably does not occur in the United States.

Favus in the chicken is caused by *Trichophyton* (Achorion) *gallinae*. It appears on the comb and wattles as white mold-like plaques that may become confluent and cover the entire comb and wattle. The disease probably does not occur in the United States.

## DERMATOMYCOSIS (RINGWORM)

Dermatomycosis in domestic animals is caused by *Trichophyton faviforme* in cattle and horses, *Microsporum canis* in the dog, *Microsporum felineum* in the cat, and *Microsporum equinum* in the horse.

Ringworm is most commonly observed in cattle and cats, and usually involves young animals. It is primarily a disease of the winter months when the animals are crowded together in stables.

The lesions begin as small focal areas that spread peripherally in a circular manner. The most active inflammatory reaction is in the periphery of the lesion where the organism is invading the skin.

## DERMATOMYCOSIS IN CATTLE

Dermatomycosis, caused by *Trichophyton faviforme*, is very common in cattle during the winter months. The disease is most prevalent in calves. The lesions are usually found on the head and neck but may spread over the entire body.

The lesions consist of focal areas of inflammation that vary in appearance from those that show excessive scaliness and partial loss of hair to large asbestos-like plaques that are covered with thick crusts of exudate and desquamated epithelium. Deep skin scrapings suspended in NaOH or KOH solution reveal numerous spores that measure 4 to 6.5 microns in diameter, which are arranged as sheaths around the hairs, and form distinct chains. In addition to the spores, hyphae are found in the skin. Spores and hyphae are also found within the hair shaft.

## DERMATOMYCOSIS IN HORSES

Dermatomycosis in horses is caused by *Trichophyton faviforme* and *Microsporum equinum*. It is most frequently observed in the skin of the neck and back.

The lesion of *Trichophyton faviforme* is somewhat larger and has a thicker scab than does the *Microsporum equinum* lesion. Scrapings of the area reveal hyphae and spores arranged in chains. The spores are large, measuring 4 to 6.5 microns in diameter, and occur in definite chains that can be distinguished even when an entire sheath of spores is present around the hair. The fungus invades the bulbous portion of the hair, which is usually not the case with the *Microsporum*. Fluorescence with filtered ultraviolet light is not observed. The fluorescence sometimes reported is due to the fluorescence of the drugs used in treating the skin disease.

The lesions of *Microsporum equinum* appear on the skin as circular areas that measure 1 to 3 centimeters in diameter. The hair in the area tends to stand rather erect, is sparse in amount, and much of it is broken off just above the surface of the skin. The surface of the skin lesion is dry, and an excessive number of epidermal scales are present. Sheaths of small spores are found around the infected hairs, and a few hyphae may be observed in the lesion. The spores measure 2.5 microns in diameter, thus readily differentiating them from those of *Trichophyton faviforme*. Fluorescence with filtered ultraviolet light is not observed.

## DERMATOMYCOSIS IN DOGS AND CATS

Dermatomycosis in dogs and cats is caused by *Microsporum canis*. It is most commonly observed in young kittens and puppies but may occur in older animals. The lesions in dogs are most commonly found on the neck, withers, dorsal surface of the back, and the legs. In cats the infection is most frequently observed on the face and paws.

The disease appears as a typical ringworm lesion that is circular in shape and measures as much as 2 to 3 centimeters in diameter. The lesion is covered with stumps of broken hair that protrude slightly above the skin surface. The area is covered with excessive numbers of epidermal scales. When the hairs in the lesion are pulled out, they appear dull and lusterless, and are enclosed in a gray sheath that is a mass of spores. Itching is slight or absent.

In the dog a few fluorescent hairs are observed under filtered ultraviolet light. Care should be taken so as not to confuse the fluorescence of medicaments with that of the fungus. Fluorescence of infected hairs is commonly observed in the cat and is of considerable aid in diagnosis. However, a definite diagnosis can only be made when the typical spores and hyphae are demonstrated in or on the hairs, in the skin, and are grown on artificial media and show typical morphology.

Deep scrapings of the involved area and the suspension of the material in KOH or NaOH for clearing purposes will reveal numerous spores located as a spore sheath around the hair and measuring 2.5 microns in diameter. The small size of the spore readily identifies the fungus as a microsporum. Hyphae may also be observed in the hair and in the skin. Histological preparations, suitably stained with fungus stains, reveal the organism in the hairs and in the epidermis.

## DERMATOMYCOSIS IN SWINE

Ringworm has occasionally been described in swine in the inguinal region, the ventral surface of the abdomen, and in the axillary region. The lesions described are circular with raised borders signifying active inflammation in the periphery of the area, and centers that are somewhat depressed and covered with dry crusts and scales. The lesions apparently do not cause great discomfort to the pig. Itching is minimal and alopecia is not present. Difficulty has been experienced in demonstrating a specific fungus. Until a specific organism that will reproduce the disease is described, considerable doubt will exist as to whether ringworm occurs in swine.

## Hemorrhagic Dermatitis

Hemorrhagic dermatitis occurs when very severe irritants are applied to the skin. It is observed when *Bacillus anthracis* or clostridium organisms of various types (malignant edema and blackleg) are introduced into the skin through various wounds (abrasions, lacerations, castration wounds, and insect bites). Because of the violence of the inflammatory reaction that takes place when this occurs, a great amount of edema and hemorrhage appears at the site of infection. When this occurs, an acute hemorrhagic inflammation is present. The infection extends into the underlying subcutaneous tissue, and then a septicemia may result.

**Microscopic appearance.** The histological appearance of the lesion is an acute hemorrhagic inflammation in which extensive hemorrhage, edema, and necrosis are present. Neutrophils are quite numerous in the area. When the site of inflammation is stained with a Gram stain, numerous organisms can be seen.

## Necrotic Dermatitis

Necrotic dermatitis is observed in erysipelas infections in swine. The lesions occur in the skin of the ears, snout, back, and tail, and vary as to size and number. The focal lesions on the back and sides have a square or diamond shape that corresponds to the vascular distribution of a single arterial system. In the more diffuse involvement of the skin, the entire ear or tail or the skin of the entire back and sides may undergo necrosis and slough.

The skin lesions are apparently an allergic manifestation of a local invasion with *Erysipelothrix rhusiopathiae*. Experimentally, similar skin lesions can be produced in sensitized animals when the organism is inoculated into the skin by scarification. In the area of allergic inflammation there is extensive acute active hyperemia and stasis of the blood flow through the area. The erythrocytes within the capillaries show hemoagglutination. As the condition continues, hemorrhage is observed in the area. The reaction extends through the skin and deep into the underlying fat. The area shows the typical appearance of a cutaneous infarct with vascular stasis and death of tissue within the area. Since it is an allergic manifestation and not a local infection of the skin, the erysipelas organism is usually not isolated from the skin lesions.

Necrotic inflammation of the skin of the dog is observed in vitamin B deficiencies. Ulceration of the skin occurs on the anterior and posterior surfaces of the tarsal and carpal articulations.

Blue ointment, when placed on stanchions to control lice in cattle, may produce a very severe necrotic dermatitis. The blue ointment rubs off on the individual and is worked well into the skin of the neck. Extensive sloughing of the skin occurs in the area.

## Gangrenous Dermatitis

Gangrenous inflammation exists when a necrotic portion of skin is invaded with saprophytic microorganisms. A specific type of gangrene is observed when black-leg-malignant edema organisms are introduced through abrasions and incisions in the skin. This is most frequently observed in sheep where it occurs as a wound infection that involves the entire flock following vaccination, shearing, castration, docking, parturition, or wounds received from fighting. This is a very serious problem on certain farms where a particularly malignant type of organism is present in the soil.

**Macroscopic appearance.** There is an intense wound infection with a rapidly spreading inflammation into the surrounding tissue. The area is extremely edematous, and the skin has a cyanotic color with extensive imbibition with blood. A blood-stained exudate frequently flows from the wound. Gas may or may not be present in the area, depending on the type of organism present. This is particularly true with malignant edema. If the animal

recovers, extensive sloughing and ulceration occur in the area.

### FOWL CHOLERA

Acute or chronic inflammation of the wattles is observed in chickens with fowl cholera. The disease appears as an acute serous or suppurative inflammation with extensive edema. As the condition progresses, the wattle becomes necrotic, is invaded with saprophytic bacteria that cause gangrene, and sloughing of the entire wattle may occur.

There is some confusion as to the pathogenesis of this lesion in the wattle. Some maintain it is an allergic reaction, others state it is the result of edema from vascular disturbances, while still others claim there is a local infection within the wattle.

## Contact Dermatitis

Contact dermatitis is a term used to describe an inflammation of the skin caused by chemicals or other irritating agents applied to the cutaneous surface.

A necrotic dermatitis is observed in turkey poults when the tar residue dripping from the stovepipes of brooder stoves heated with gas briquettes is rubbed off on the heads and backs of the poults. The inflammation usually involves the head, face, neck, back, and dorsal surface of the wings when the area is not protected with feathers. Frequently, so many birds are involved that the condition is thought to be an infectious disease. The lesion resembles a burn since there is extensive coagulative necrosis of the skin. The lesion appears 24 to 48 hours after the residue comes in contact with the skin. The reaction is intensified when the poults are exposed to sunlight.

Similar injuries occur in chickens and turkeys when kerosene or fuel oil from brooders come in contact with the skin. It is usually observed on the heads of the birds where the residue has rubbed off the fuel line.

## Sunburn

In general the domestic animals do not suffer from sunburn. They are usually covered with hair, feathers, or wool which screens out the sun's rays, and in addition, most animals have rather heavily pigmented skins. An occasional albino is observed or an occasional individual is found in which focal areas lacking pigmentation are present. In these individuals, local burning may occur. When this is present, the local injury may result in the appearance of hyperkeratosis or tumors (vulva of Ayrshire cattle). Sheep that have been recently shorn or dogs that have been recently clipped may experience sunburn when the protective hair or wool has been removed.

When individuals show an unusual reaction to the sun's rays, the process is called photosensitization. Photosensitization, with its resulting serous, vesicular, suppurative, or necrotic dermatitis, is extremely common in domestic animals and is a serious economic problem.

PHOTOSENSITIZATION

There are several substances called fluorescent or photodynamic agents which, when present in the body with their inherent capability of absorbing certain wave lengths in sunlight, produce the characteristic necrosis and edema of exposed tissues in all species of domestic animals and man. The condition is usually an acquired one, but may be congenital and sometimes familial.

Photosensitization most commonly first involves the ears, eyelids, face, lips, and coronets in sheep and the teats, udder, ears, and eyelids in cows. Lightly pigmented areas of the skin are most sus-

ceptible to the action of sunlight, and open-fleeced and recently shorn sheep may burn badly on the general body surfaces (Fig. 22.8). The details of the photosensitization reactions are as yet somewhat speculative. It is known that sunburn is a reaction of unprotected skin produced by ultraviolet radiation of wave lengths shorter than 320 m$\mu$. The wave lengths involved in photosensitization usually lie in the range of 540 to 600 m$\mu$. Since these longer light waves readily pass through ordinary window glass, sensitized animals may develop characteristic lesions if exposed to sunlight naturally or even through glass.

In past years photosensitization has been of major importance in the United States only in the South and West. It is unfortunate that many outbreaks produced by the ingestion of plants have passed unrecognized or have been diagnosed as eczema or dermatitis. In other parts of the world such as North and South Africa, New Zealand, and Australia, as in the United States, it is most commonly seen in the large grazing areas. Clare of New Zealand has carefully studied photosensitization and classified the resulting diseases into three main types, taking as a basis the origin of the photodynamic agent or the means by which it may reach the peripheral circulation:

Type I     Primary photosensitivity.

Type II    Photosensitivity due to aberrant pigment synthesis.

Type III   Hepatogenous photosensitivity.

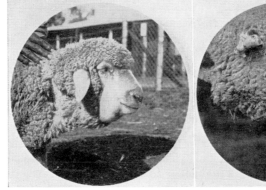
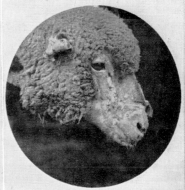

Fig. 22.8 — Photosensitization. These sheep were made sensitive to light by administering hemato-porphyrin. Note edema of the face, throat, and ears of the sheep on the left and the later necrosis and sloughing of the skin of the face and ears of the one on the right. (Quin, Veterinary Services, Union of South Africa.)

Other photosensitivities remain unclassified due to limited and incomplete investigations of the mechanism of the origin of the photodynamic agent involved. These include the clovers, alfalfa, cereal grasses, rape, and vetch. It is discouraging that the most widely seen photosensitization syndromes involving these common forages are of a very sporadic and transient occurrence. As might be expected, conclusive studies have not been attempted to date on many of these reported outbreaks.

**Type I (Primary photosensitivity)** is the group that can strictly be termed photosensitivity diseases in the sense that all the pathologic changes result from photodynamic action on exposed body surface. In other types the photosensitivity is secondary to a disturbance of metabolism or function in one of the internal organs, and is often only an incidental manifestation of minor importance in the disease. One excellent example of a primary photosensitization is St.-John's-wort poisoning (hypericism), and it is related to the presence of a red fluorescent pigment that is absorbed directly from the digestive tract. The other classical example of a primary photosensitization is fagopyrism (**buckwheat sensitivity**) which is also related to a red fluorescent pigment that is absorbed directly. Phenothiazine photosensitivity is an unusual primary photosensitization due to the conversion of phenothiazine in the digestive tract into a sulfoxide. When the sulfoxide is absorbed in large quantities, the liver is unable to convert all of it into a harmless phenothiazine derivative and it accumulates in the tissues. Its accumulation in the tissue spaces of the eye results in a characteristic keratitis in calves and birds. Clare has proven quite conclusively that the sulfoxide was present in the aqueous humor and tears and directly related to the photosensitivity. Claims that phenothiazine produces a hepatogenous photosensitization have never been proven and do not appear to be true. Quin showed that fluorescein dyes including eosin, erythrosin, rose bengal, acriflavin, and methylene blue will induce clinical photosensitization in goats. One should be aware of the hazards of using rose bengal for liver function tests and methylene blue as a therapeutic agent.

**Type II (Aberrant pigment synthesis).** Congenital and acquired porphyria in man have been studied for many years. The origins of many of the porphyrias in man are not understood, and clinical cases do not completely resemble those produced by the injection of porphyrins. In cattle, a congenital porphyria (pink tooth) was first reported by Fourie in 1936 in South Africa and has now been recognized in several herds in the United States. Two porphyrins, uroporphyrins and coproporphyrins, apparently are produced in excessive amounts, and both appear in appreciable amounts in the urine, giving it a reddish-brown color. The uroporphyrin is also deposited in the bones and teeth and causes a discoloration of these tissues.

**Type III (Hepatogenous photosensitivity).** In this type, which is the most common and most important economically, animals are sensitized by the accumulation of phylloerythrin, a product of chlorophyll digestion, in the peripheral circulation. Phylloerythrin is normally excreted into the bile by the liver, but in certain types of diffuse liver damage most commonly associated with a variety of plant, bacterial, and chemical hepatoxins, it is gradually absorbed by the circulatory system until levels are reached that will produce photosensitivity. Quin proved that ligation of the common bile duct also produced hepatogenous photosensitization. The mechanism always seems associated with an almost complete or complete stoppage of the flow of bile in the liver. In the classical facial eczema seen in sheep in New Zealand and associated with the ingestion of an unstable toxin produced by fungi growing on new lush rye pastures, the damage is primarily to the small bile ducts. In the severe outbreak in 1957–58 in Eastern Oklahoma and adjacent areas of Arkansas, Texas, Missouri, and Kansas, a stable hepatoxin for cattle was present in water-damaged hay and acted directly on the liver cells and small bile duct cells, causing them to swell and occlude bile passages. The hay was grown in many of the creek and river bottoms in the involved area.

In South Africa a hepatogenous photosensitization in sheep, Geeldikkop (Tribulosis) is associated with the plants named *Tribulus terrestris* and *Lippia sp.* The *Panicum sp.* are responsible for a similar disease in Australia and New Zealand, and the leaves of a tree, Ngaio (*Myoporum laetum*), were incriminated in New Zealand. *Lantana camara* and *Tetradymia sp.* have produced hepatogenous photosensitization in cattle and sheep in the United States and many foreign countries. The stage of growth and season of the year often play important roles in the incidence of photosensitivities of plant origin.

Extensive liver damage associated with carbon tetrachloride and phosphorus poisoning and with Rift Valley fever are reported to have resulted in a hepatogenous photosensitization.

Elevated blood levels of bilirubin and phylloerythrin are indicative of a hepatogenous origin, and an associated icterus and lowered urobilinogen excretion further substantiate a diagnosis. Liver biopsies are helpful in studying the diseases. It should be remembered that the primary liver disease is often more important in reference to the possible recovery of the animal than the photosensitization.

## Allergic Dermatitis

Allergic dermatitis occurs in those individuals that have become sensitized to certain substances, particularly protein. When the skin comes in contact with these antigens, an allergic type of inflammation occurs at the site. The most commonly observed types of allergic inflammation are those that result from the injection of tuberculin or johnin into the skin of domestic animals. The severity and extent as well as the systemic reaction of the individual depends upon the degree of sensitization present.

Allergic inflammation occurs as single or multiple-focal lesions. The diffuse swelling of the individual that occurs with certain allergic manifestations usually does not represent an inflammation of the skin. It is a general vascular reaction of the individual in which edema of the skin is present.

The focal reaction in the skin where the allergin is applied may be a serous, hydropic, suppurative, or necrotic inflammation. The size of the lesion depends upon the intensity of the reaction. It may be barely visible or it may be 15 to 20 centimeters in diameter with extensive necrosis and ulceration of the skin.

Allergic inflammation is used by the veterinarian in detecting tuberculosis in cattle. The tuberculin is injected into the caudal fold and, after a specified interval of time following injection, the area is examined for allergic inflammation. If no inflammation is present, the animal usually does not have tuberculosis. If an allergic inflammation is present, it is an indication that the animal has been infected with tuberculosis. A somewhat similar reaction may occur in the necks of cattle when johnin is injected into the skin and subcutaneous connective tissue.

A sudden appearing acute dermatitis is frequently observed in dogs, especially during the summer. Many of these skin alterations are the result of an allergic reaction to some sensitizing substance in the food or the environment of the individual. Intradermal injections of various allergins (wheat, salmon, alfalfa, and rice) produce cutaneous reaction indicating that sensitivity is present.

The term allergic dermatitis must be used with considerable caution. For the term to be used properly, the allergin must be identified. Careful examination of the individual as to the location of the lesions, constituents of the ration, and the possibility of contact with agents capable of producing sensitivity will influence the accuracy of the diagnosis. Since the majority of the objects in the environment, the food consumed, and the drugs used are potentially capable of acting as allergins, extremely critical sensitivity tests must be performed if a correct diagnosis is to be accomplished.

## Urticaria

Urticaria (hives) is characterized by the sudden appearance of smooth, slightly elevated, flat areas in the skin that are associated with considerable pruritis. The onset of the disease is sudden, and likewise, it disappears as suddenly, existing for only a few hours or at most a few days. The lesions may appear in one portion of the skin, disappear, and then reappear in another portion of the individual.

Urticaria is observed in all domestic animals but is most frequently found in the horse and dog.

The cause of urticaria is the presence of a specific allergin to which the individual is sensitive. This may be in the form of a vaccine, serum, foreign protein of various types, or drug sensitivity.

**Macroscopic appearance.** R a i s e d , rounded, smooth elevations are present in the skin in local areas, or involving the skin of the entire individual. The lesions may shift from one portion of the skin to another. The size of the focal lesions varies with the individual. They may measure 1 to 2 centimeters in diameter or may consist of large plaques as much as 8 to 10 centimeters in width. At times, adjacent areas join together to form very large raised areas in the skin.

Palpation of the lesions reveals they are tense, rather firm swellings that are, at most, only slightly warmer than the surrounding skin surface.

**Microscopic appearance.** Histological examination reveals the basic lesion is an edema and hyperemia of the dermis. No alterations are observed in the epidermis unless extensive biting or scratching of the area takes place as the result of the itching. The cellular reaction in the area is slight; at most only a few lymphocytes are present. If repeated attacks of urticaria occur, or if the cause of it persists, such as the administration of drugs to which the individual is sensitive, then a chronic dermatitis with hyperkeratosis develops.

## Deficiency Diseases

Skin lesions as the result of deficiency diseases are common. The skin lesions are not sufficiently distinctive to enable one to determine the type of deficiency that is present. Usually, the deficiency as observed in clinical cases is a multiple deficiency and not a deficiency of one single ingredient in the ration. Because of this, specific diagnoses are extremely difficult to make. The skin of animals with deficiency diseases lacks its normal tone and lustre and is untidy and covered with scales. Frequently, a partial or total alopecia is present and the hair is coarse in texture. Bacterial invasion of the devitalized skin is common.

The skin lesions in swine with a nutritional deficiency are of special concern to the veterinarian engaged in a swine practice. A **vitamin A** deficiency produces a hyperkeratosis of the epithelium and keratinization of the accessory skin glands. **Pantothenic acid** deficiency causes the hair coat to be thin and rough, especially over the rump and the center of the back. Eventually, there is a patchy alopecia. The skin is redder than normal due to hyperemia. An excessive number of scales is present on the surface of the skin. **Nicotinic acid** deficiency produces a dermatitis that is particularly severe around the ears. In addition, the skin is scurfy. A **riboflavin** deficiency causes the hair coat to be thin, rough, and dry. A papular, suppurative, or ulcerative dermatitis is present and is most severe on the snout, behind the ears, along the mid-line of the back, in the inguinal region, and over the abdomen. An ulcerative pododermatitis and coronitis may be present, and when this occurs the hoof wall shows ridging and thickening. A **pyridoxine** deficiency causes the hair to be untidy and curled. An **iodine** deficiency causes an alopecia in newborn pigs. The skin is smooth, shiny, thick, and edematous. The hoofs are short and brittle. When there is a deficiency of **iron,** the skin is rough, scaly, and greasy. The skin contains many folds and wrinkles because of emaciation and because of the edema of the dermis and subcutaneous tissue. The hair coat is dry and coarse in texture. When **biotin** is deficient in the ration, an alopecia occurs. Numerous cracks may be present in the soles of the hoofs. A deficiency of zinc produces a disease known as parakeratosis.

## PARAKERATOSIS

**Definition.** Parakeratosis is a skin disease of swine that is characterized by cutaneous hyperplasia. It affects any part of the surface of the body, especially the epidermis of the abdomen and legs.

**Etiology.** A deficiency of zinc in rats will produce dermatitis resembling, in some respects, the lesions observed in swine. This observation resulted in establishing the importance of zinc in the rations of swine. When the role of zinc in swine nutrition was studied, it was found that an imbalance of the calcium-phosphorus-zinc ratio would produce the disease. Pigs should have a minimum of 5 milligrams of zinc per pound of ration fed. Apparently an abundance of calcium or phosphorus interferes with zinc metabolism, and as a result, the amount of calcium in the ration should be adjusted so as not to exceed 0.6 per cent. The practice of force-feeding limestone to limit feed consumption should be discouraged, as this results in a large amount of calcium in the ration. The use of excessively mineralized supplements should be avoided, as a high calcium content of the ration is apt to result.

The disease is widely distributed throughout the United States but is apparently more common in some states than in others. As many as 75 per cent of the individuals in some herds are affected.

The disease has been recognized for at least 30 years. It has been most frequently observed in the well-managed herds such as purebred herds, experiment station herds, and institutional herds, in other words, in those herds where considerable attention has been directed toward balanced rations and good housing.

Parakeratosis is a disease of winter months. It appears in November and December and disappears in March or April. It is seldom seen during the summer months. Recovery is rapid if the pigs are placed on pasture. In some areas an occasional case is observed in swine on pasture. It is most frequently observed in pigs that are 10 to 12 weeks of age. Males and females are equally affected, and apparently all breeds are susceptible.

**Symptoms.** Affected animals show considerable retardation in growth. Although the animals show a remarkable recovery, this retardation is never entirely overcome.

There may or may not be a rise in body temperature. A diarrhea is sometimes observed, and vomiting may occur. Most pigs show some degree of anorexia. At least part of this anorexia is due to oral tenderness. The pigs have difficulty in eating, and buccal ulcers are present. Usually, a period of 12 to 13 days is required for the lesions to develop. The course of the disease varies from 6 to 8 weeks. The morbidity is usually less than 50 per cent of the individuals in the herd, but occasionally it may be as high as 80 per cent. The mortality is very low. Most pigs recover spontaneously after a few weeks. Recovery is much more rapid if the hogs are placed on pasture.

**Macroscopic appearance.** Bilaterally symmetrical lesions involve the skin surface of any part of the body but are especially prominent on legs, inguinal region, perineum, ears, eyelids, shoulders, and thighs.

The skin lesions are first observed as papules and pustules. Later, the skin is covered with crusts of cornified epithelium and exudate that are firmly attached to the underlying tissue. These crusts may measure as much as 5 to 7 millimeters in thickness. Due to the movement of the animal and desiccation, cracks or crevices appear in the crusts. A brown exudate may be present in these crevices due to secondary bacterial invasion of the skin. The involved skin is thicker than normal and hangs in large folds.

There is no permanent skin damage other than an alteration in the color of the hair of the Duroc breed of swine. In this breed the hair coat changes to a strawberry roan or light tan color.

**Microscopic appearance.** Histological examination of the skin reveals it to be covered with a thick layer of cornified epithelium that contains many nuclei and kerato-hyaline granules. There is a marked increase in all epidermal elements except the stratum lucidum.

### Parasitic Dermatitis

Parasitic dermatitis as the result of insect bites is extremely common in domestic animals. The animals have little protection against the insect world and often are stabled, housed, or forced to feed in areas where biting and sucking insects are numerous.

The amount and type of cutaneous reaction to the bites of arthropods vary with the species of arthropod, the species bitten, and the allergic state of the individual.

All insect bites have, in general, the same basic lesion, which consists of a wound in the skin where the epithelium is broken and an acute or chronic inflammatory reaction. Shortly after the bite, extensive edema may appear in the area, particularly if a toxin or proteolytic substance is injected into the skin. Soon leukocytes, primarily neutrophils and eosinophils, appear in the area. The eosinophils become more numerous than they do in the ordinary wound infection. As the condition progresses, necrosis may occur in the area if toxins or other injurious substances are injected. If healing does not take place in a short period of time, a chronic dermatitis occurs and plasma cells, macrophages, and proliferating fibroblasts appear in the area. The chronic inflammation is particularly apt to occur if portions of the mouth parts or sucking tubes (sucking tube of the chigger) remain in the wound. Inflammation at the site of an arthropod bite may persist for months and even years. The tissue reaction may be confused with a lymphosarcoma, histiocytoma, eosinophilic granuloma, or even squamous-cell carcinoma.

Parasitic dermatitis is particularly serious in the dog and the horse in very allergic individuals. The flea is of primary concern in the dog, and biting flies are usually the cause of the skin disorder in the horse. Certain individuals have a persistent dermatitis each summer when the biting arthropods are numerous. During the winter when these parasites are not present, or are greatly reduced in number, healing of the skin lesions occurs.

#### PROTOZOIASIS

Protozoa are of little concern in the skin of domestic animals in the United States. Species of *Globidia* may invade the skin of cattle and horses. The genus *Besnoiti* is found in rodents.

#### APISINATION

Inflammation of the skin is quite common in all domestic animals as the result of bee stings. The intensity of the reaction depends upon the type of bee that is involved and the allergic response of the individual that is stung. Immediately after the bee stings, an inflammation of the skin characterized by massive accumulations of serous exudate in the area is present. The purpose of this vascular response is to dilute the irritant and prevent extensive damage. Shortly thereafter, neutrophils and eosinophils begin to appear in the area. The number of eosinophils depends upon the allergic response of the individual. Sensitized individuals have many eosinophils in the area. If considerable toxin is placed in the skin, as is usually the case, coagulative necrosis occurs at the site. The area is usually microscopic in size, but in extremely sensitive or allergic individuals a macroscopic area of necrosis may be visible. When necrosis occurs, the area becomes surrounded with leukocytes and connective tissue, and an ulcerative dermatitis may develop.

#### SIMULIASIS

Parasitic dermatitis as the result of *Simulium* (black flies) bites is observed. The *Simulium* have biting mouth parts, and extensive laceration is observed in the skin of the head and the ventral abdominal wall of the host.

#### HYPODERMYIASIS

*Hypoderma lineatum* and *Hypoderma bovis*, the cause of hypodermyiasis, are extremely common in the skin of the backs of cattle.

A small wound is produced in the skin

of the legs of cattle where the fly lays her eggs. The wound is produced by the migrating larva that hatched from the egg attached to the hairs of the skin. After the larva of the parasite wanders through the body, it eventually reaches the subcutaneous tissue of the back. As the parasite enlarges in the subcutaneous tissue of the back, a raised nodule appears in the skin that varies in size from just visible to 3 centimeters in diameter. In the center of this raised nodule there is an opening through the skin from the encysted larva in the subcutaneous tissue to the exterior. This opening is needed to supply the oxygen requirements of the parasite. When the larva is mature, this opening is enlarged and the parasite escapes to the exterior.

A chronic inflammation of the subcutaneous tissue is present. If the encysted parasite in the backs of cattle is ruptured by a blow on the back, a very severe allergic reaction may occur with extensive hemorrhage and edema in the area.

### GASTEROPHILOMYIASIS

An edema and dermatitis of the face of the horse from the corner of the mouth to the eye is observed as the result of the wandering of *Gasterophilus* l a r v a e through the skin. The *Gasterophilus* larvae hatched from the eggs deposited on the hairs of the horse come in contact with the mouth, penetrate into the skin of the lips, and then wander in a posterior direction through the skin towards the visceral portions of the body.

The serous or suppurative inflammation of the skin appears as lines or streaks covered with crusts of exudate that extend in a general direction from the corners of the mouth to the region of the eye. The intensity of the inflammatory reaction varies with the individual and probably depends upon the allergic sensitivity of the host.

### TROMBICULIASIS

*Trombicula* mites (harvest mites or chiggers) invade the skin of all domestic animals. The incidence of infection varies with the species of animal as well as with the species of mite concerned.

**Macroscopic appearance.** Clusters of mites are observed in the ears, behind the ears, in the perineal region, or around the vent of animals. The mites may also occur in the skin of any portion of the individual. Some individuals show considerable inflammatory reaction to the presence of the mites, and papular, nodular, or ulcerative lesions occur. Examination of these lesions with the hand lens may reveal the presence of the mites if they have not finished feeding and detached.

**Microscopic appearance.** Histological examination of the involved skin areas reveals the mites attached to the skin. Cleared specimens of unstained skin at the site of attachment of the mite will reveal the long sucking tubes of the parasite inserted into the underlying skin. When the mite detaches, these sucking tubes remain in the skin, and since they are foreign to the individual, a chronic inflammation results and an ulcer persists for some time at the site of attachment. The local inflammation causes itching, and considerable trauma from scratching may occur. At times, secondary bacterial infection of the site of attachment of the mite occurs, and very disagreeable wound infection is the result.

### GAMASOIDIASIS

*Dermanyssus gallinarum*, *Ornithonyssus sylviarum*, and *Ornithonyssus bursa* produce multiple focal areas of inflammation in the skin of birds and mammals at the site where blood is extracted. Mammals placed in areas occupied by chickens develop extensive dermatitis of the legs and feet. This is especially common in the horse.

### ACARIASIS

Acariasis is produced by sarcoptic, demodectic, otodectic, notoedric, cnemidocoptic, psoroptic, and chorioptic mites. The type of lesion produced and the location of the lesion differ somewhat depending on the species of animal infected and the species of parasite involved.

**Sarcoptic mange** is caused by *Sarcoptes scabiei* var. *equi, bovis, ovis, suis,* and *canis.* The female mite is found in the deeper layers of the stratum corneum where she tunnels through the epidermis by means of her cutting mouth parts and the cutting hooks located on the last segment of the first two pairs of legs. The males, larvae, and nymphs leave the tunnels, following hatching, and are found on the skin surface. The males re-enter the epidermis only to fertilize the females. The tunnels vary in length from a few millimeters to several centimeters. The mites feed on the tissue fluids of the host and probably consume some of the cells of the stratum corneum.

The lesion begins as a serous or papular dermatitis. The first invasion of the mite produces little inflammation, but this initial invasion sensitizes the individual, and subsequent invasion causes a severe allergic dermatitis. As the result of the burrowing of the mite through the epidermis, a mild irritation occurs which produces a hyperkeratosis. Most of the cutaneous injury is the result of scratching and rubbing in response to the pruritus. The infection usually begins on the head and neck and then spreads over the entire body.

In the dog and pig the lesions usually first appear on the head and then extend over the entire body. As the result of the chronic skin irritation, the skin becomes thickened, wrinkled, and creased. Partial alopecia is present. The dermatitis is most severe on the ventral surfaces of the animal (abdomen, inguinal region, and axillary region).

Sarcoptic mange in sheep involves primarily the non-wooled areas of the body and therefore is found on the skin of the head and legs. In goats the infection is particularly serious, and considerable mortality may be experienced. It usually spreads over the entire body.

The mite invades the skin of the head and neck of the horse. In cattle, the mites are found in the skin of the head, neck, brisket, medial surface of the thighs, and the sacral region.

The histological alterations in the skin vary with the severity of the infection and the length of time the mange has been present. Numerous tunnels containing females, eggs and newly hatched larvae are observed in the external two-thirds of the epidermis. The type of inflammation is an acute or chronic, serous, papular, vesicular, suppurative, or ulcerative dermatitis with considerable hyperkeratosis. Neutrophils, eosinophils, and macrophages infiltrate the epidermis and dermis. When the skin infection has persisted for a long period of time and has extended into the dermis, a proliferation of fibroblasts in the dermis occurs. When bacteria invade the devitalized skin, a severe suppurative inflammation results.

**Cnemidocoptic mange** is a poultry disease caused by *Cnemidocoptes gallinae* and *Cnemidocoptes mutans*.

*Cnemidocoptes gallinae* is known as the depluming mite because of the alopecia it produces. The mites burrow into the shaft of the feathers and into the skin around the feather follicle and cause focal areas of dermatitis with severe pruritus. Because of the itching and because the feathers break off easily, the birds deplume themselves. This frequently introduces the vice of feather eating into a flock. It is primarily a disease of the spring and summer months and tends to disappear during the autumn and winter, thus differing from other types of mange.

The feathers of the vent region are usually involved first. Later the infection spreads to the thighs, back, and abdomen. The large feathers of the tail and wings are usually not involved. An infected rooster may spread the infection through the flock during copulation.

*Cnemidocoptes mutans* causes the disease scaly-leg in the domestic fowl. The parasite invades beneath the scales of the metatarsus and phalanges. The scales of the legs become raised as the result of a powdery material and exudate that accumulates. As the condition progresses, the legs become greatly enlarged in diameter, distorted, and covered with crusts of exudate. The skin of the comb, wattles, and neck may also be involved. Because of the itching, the bird will peck at the crusts on the legs. When bacteria invade the lesion, a tendovaginitis or arthritis may occur.

**Psoroptic mange** is caused by *Psoroptes equi* var. *ovis, caprae, cunniculi,* and *bovis.*

Psoroptic mange differs from sarcoptic mange in that the mites are found on the surface of the skin in the exudate and desquamated epithelium. The mites pierce the skin with their mouth parts, causing a focal traumatic dermatitis. Apparently the mites need lymph or tissue fluids for their nutritive requirements.

In goats and rabbits the mite is found primarily in the ears and causes an otitis externa. Few rabbit hutches are free of this infection. The accumulation of desquamated epithelium, lymph, serum, and plasma in the auricula and external auditory canal, together with a complicating bacterial infection, results in a serious suppurative otitis externa that may extend into the internal ear and on into the cranial cavity, causing a suppurative meningitis and encephalitis. The lesions in cattle appear on the withers, on the top of the neck, or at the root of the tail; and from these points they spread over the entire surface of the body. Psoroptic mange in the horse is found in the skin of the more protected areas such as beneath the forelock and mane, the root of the tail, along the ventral surface of the body, and in the auricula and external auditory canal of the ear.

It is the most common type of mange encountered in sheep and occurs in the skin of the thickly wooled parts of the skin. Mange can be detected early in a band of sheep when a local area of clean wool appears on an animal as the result of the biting and chewing of the wool by the animal in response to the pruritus. As the biting and chewing continues, the wool is pulled out and an area of alopecia is present.

**Chorioptic mange** is caused by *Chorioptes bovis* var. *equi, caprae, ovis,* and *cunniculi.* It is quite similar to psoroptic mange except the lesions are usually restricted to the feet, perineum, and the base of the tail.

Chorioptic mites feed on the scales of the epidermis. As a result, they are found on the skin surface and do not penetrate into the skin. Because of their feeding habits they produce little skin damage other than that caused by the traumatic injury produced by the host as the result of itching.

Chorioptic mange in the horse usually involves the feet in the fetlock region. It is especially common in those horses that have considerable feather. It rarely extends above the hock or the knee. Because it is localized to the feet and legs, it is often called foot or leg mange. In cattle the infection involves the legs and tail.

**Otodectic mange** is caused by *Otodectes cynotis.* The mite invades the skin of the ears of dogs, cats, rats, and foxes, producing an otitis externa. The lesions and feeding habits of the parasite are very similar to those of the psoroptic mites. The mites insert their mouth parts into the skin of the host and suck the tissue fluids.

Otodectic mange is exceedingly common in the ears of dogs. The parasitic infection is complicated by the maceration of the skin with secretion and excretion. The position and shape of the auricula and the external auditory canal prevent the exudate and secretion from leaving the ear. As a result, bacterial invasion of the macerated skin occurs, and a serious acute or chronic suppurative dermatitis of the auricula and the external auditory canal develops. Otodectic mange is the most common cause of the traumatic injury (scratching to relieve itching) to the ear of the cat.

**Demodectic mange** is caused by *Demodex folliculorum* var. *bovis, ovis, caprae, suis,* and *canis* depending on the species of animal infected. The disease is of particular importance in the dog where it is known as red mange. The term red mange results from the intense hyperemia of the skin.

Demodectic mange mites are found in

the hair follicles, sebaceous glands, and sweat glands. As they grow and multiply, the hair follicles and skin glands become distended with the parasites and desquamated epithelium. Usually the mite is arranged in the lesion so that the head faces the exterior. Due to bacterial infection, a multiple focal suppurative inflammation is present. There is some question as to just how much damage in the skin is due to allergic manifestations and bacterial infection and how much is due to the mites. If a suppurative inflammation, indicating the presence of bacteria, is not present, it is surprising how little reaction is actually found within the skin.

Because the infection usually persists over a long period of time, the skin becomes thickened due to hyperplasia of epithelium and connective tissue. The skin becomes wrinkled and hangs in folds. The folds are the result of hyperplasia, the swelling associated with inflammation, emaciation, and the cutaneous and subcutaneous edema. Because of the involvement of the hair follicles, together with the constant scratching and rubbing, a partial alopecia is present.

The mite is carried to the regional lymph nodes by the lymphatics and produces a chronic serous lymphadenitis.

The disease in pigs involves primarily the thin skin of the ventral underline, extending from the snout along the ventral cervical, thoracic, and abdominal regions, to the flanks and medial surface of the thighs. The lesion usually appears as a pustular dermatitis that must be differentiated from ringworm and pox. In cattle the mites produce a focal pustular dermatitis that is found most prevalent around the ears, shoulders, and back. Demodectic mange in dogs is particularly common in short-haired animals (bulldogs, fox terriers, and Dalmatians). It is most commonly observed in young dogs. The infection first appears on the head (nose, lips, and forehead), then spreads to the feet, and finally extends to other parts of the body.

**Notoedric mange** is caused by *Notoedres cati*. It is a disease of cats that is usually restricted to the head, neck, and paws. The paws of the cat become infected when he scratches or washes his face. Occasionally, the external genital organs of the cat are involved. The mites cause a severe diffuse chronic suppurative dermatitis with considerable hyperplasia and thickening of the skin.

**Laminosioptes cysticola.** Although *Laminosioptes cysticola* is not located in the skin proper, it is observed in the subcutaneous tissue when the skin is removed, and because of this, it is often regarded as a skin parasite.

The parasite is particularly common in wild birds (especially ducks). In some areas of the tropics the majority of older birds have these parasites. It is occasionally observed in the domestic fowl. The mites within the subcutaneous connective tissue produce little tissue reaction. When the mite dies, it undergoes calcification and becomes enclosed in a connective tissue capsule. Calcified mites appear in the subcutaneous tissues as white or yellow elliptical masses that vary in size from 0.5 to 1 millimeter in width to 1 to 3 millimeters in length.

### TREMATODIASIS

For the most part, trematodes do not cause injury to the skin. Certain trematodes (schistosomes) invade the host through the skin as do some nematode larvae (hookworms). The cercariae of the schistosomes penetrate the skin and produce a minute traumatic lesion at the site of invasion. In certain individuals, probably those sensitized by previous infections, a severe focal papular, vesicular, suppurative or ulcerative dermatitis may occur.

The only adult trematode found in the skin of domestic animals in the United States is *Collyriclum faba*, which infects the domestic fowl. This parasite is found in the subcutaneous tissue of chickens and turkeys in cysts that protrude above the surrounding skin surface. These cysts probably represent an invaded feather follicle. The parasite is apparently confined to the state of Minnesota. The cysts measure 4 to 6 millimeters in diameter. Each cyst contains two flukes suspended in a black fluid. The character of the black fluid resembles the melanin found in the feather follicles of certain breeds of birds. An opening is present in the external surface of the cyst through which the ova of the fluke are discharged to the exterior. The encysted flukes are found primarily around the vent and the skin of the ventral abdominal wall.

## NEMATODIASIS

A parasitic dermatitis is frequently observed in domestic animals, particularly the horse, when larvae or microfilaria are found in the skin.

**Habronemiasis.** The larvae of *Habronema majus*, *Habronema muscae*, and *Draschia megastoma*, stomach worms of the horse, produce areas of ulceration of varying size in the skin. They are particularly common in the skin of the sheath and inguinal region, probably because flies are quite numerous in this area and because of the rather moist nature of the skin. The larvae may also invade the canthi of the eye and the conjunctiva. The areas of ulceration vary in size from 1 to 6 centimeters in diameter. They are frequently confused with various nonparasitic inflammations of the skin or with squamous-cell carcinoma.

The ova of the adult parasite are passed in the feces of the horse. On the ground the ova embryonate, hatch, and larvae are liberated. The larvae attach themselves to flies that are present in the feces. When the flies feed on exudate from wounds in the skin of the horse, the larvae leave the flies and invade the wound. It must be remembered that habronemiasis is a wound infection and does not occur if the skin is not broken. This is of importance in differentiating the lesions from microfilariasis. The presence of the larvae in the skin causes a chronic inflammation, and wound healing is retarded. Because of the prolonged course of the disease, the difficulty in effecting healing unless surgical methods are used, and because the wounds are numerous in the summer, the lesions are called summer sores.

An area of ulceration is present in the skin that may or may not be covered with crusts of exudate. The ulcer is usually white or yellow in color. If the ulcer is incised and the cut surface is examined, multiple yellow foci 1 millimeter in diameter are observed.

If the surface of the ulcer is scraped and the scrapings suspended in a small amount of warm physiological saline solution and examined with a microscope, the larvae may be observed. Histological examination of the ulcer reveals an area of chronic suppurative inflammation in which many eosinophils are found in the exudate. The yellow necrotic foci observed on gross examination are found to contain larvae surrounded with many leukocytes. The parasites may or may not have been alive at the time the tissue was fixed. The dead larvae stain with eosin and show little cellular detail. The larvae that were alive at the time of fixation show hematoxylin-stained internal structure that aids in recognizing the type of parasite present.

Healing of the area occurs readily if the ulcer is removed by surgical methods and is then protected from flies. It is extremely important to examine skin wounds of horses, particularly those of the sheath, for the presence of these parasites. All too frequently a clinical diagnosis of squamous-cell carcinoma of the sheath is made and radical surgery is performed, when actually the skin lesion was not serious.

**Strongyloidiasis.** A papular or pustular dermatitis is frequently observed in dogs as the result of the invasion of the skin with the larvae of *Strongyloides stercoralis* and *Rhabditis strongyloides*. These lesions may appear on all parts of the skin and have been reported to be most frequent in the skin of the posterior legs. At times the surface of one side of the dog's body will show the dermatitis, indicating that probably the dog was recumbent on that side, perhaps lying on a manure pile or on an area where feces had been deposited. An acute or chronic parasitic dermatitis is present, and the parasites can be observed on microscopic examination of the involved skin area. The larvae are also found in the regional lymph nodes.

Although invasion of the skin by **hookworm larvae** is of considerable concern in the human being, this type of dermatitis does not appear to be of great importance in the dog because he is the definitive host of the dog hookworm. However, it is quite probable that in heavy infestations with hookworm larvae a dermatitis will result following the invasion with these parasites.

**Microfilariasis.** Microfilaria are found in skin lesions of domestic animals. It is thought that these microfilaria are those of *Onchocerca cervicalis, Onchocerca gutturosa, Onchocerca reticulata, Onchocerca gibsoni, Parafilaria multipapillosa, Parafilaria bovicola,* and *Dirofilaria immitis.* The disease is most frequently observed in the tropics or in the warmer areas of the world, and has been reported to be particularly common in the Philippines.

The lesions are quite variable in appearance depending upon the duration of infection, the number of microfilaria present, and the amount of traumatic injury inflicted by the animal. The dermatitis may appear as multiple papules in the skin or as large ulcerated areas that result from the injury inflicted by the animal. Pruritis is present, and because of this the animal bites or scratches the involved area or rubs against objects in an attempt to relieve the itching. The lesions are most common on the ears, crest, withers, shoulders, breast, ventral neck region, abdomen, sheath, inguinal region, and legs. It is frequently diagnosed as eczema when no attempt is made to demonstrate the microfilaria. The lesions may be acute or chronic, depending upon the length of time they have persisted. They may be confined to a small area or may involve multiple areas and considerable surface of the body. The lesions tend to be smaller and more papular in nature in the thin-skinned regions of the body, while in the thicker-skinned areas the nodules are larger, more irregular in shape, and tend to show a more proliferative type of reaction. The microfilaria are most easily demonstrated in the more active areas of acute inflammation. In those wounds that have been present for a considerable period of time and in which the inflammation is chronic in type, the microfilaria are much more difficult to demonstrate. The lesions involve the epidermis and the superficial portions of the dermis. The microfilaria can be seen within the capillaries of the papillary bodies of the dermis just below the epithelium.

Considerable confusion exists between the lesions of microfilariasis and the lesions of habronemiasis, in the equine commonly called summer sores. Habronema larvae gain entrance to the skin through a wound; in other words it is a wound infection. The larvae of the Habronema are carried to the wound by flies, and while the fly is feeding on the area, the larvae escape into the wound. The Habronema larvae are large, while the microfilaria are small. The Habronema larvae have an immature digestive tract, while the microfilaria do not possess a digestive tract. The microfilaria gain entrance to the skin by way of the blood vascular system when liberated into the circulatory system by the adult parasites and are not brought to the skin by flies.

Although a parasitic dermatitis has been reported as being due to the microfilaria of *Dirofilaria immitis,* some question does exist concerning whether the parasites found in these skin lesions are actually the microfilaria of *D. immitis* or some other parasite. At least in the Midwest, filarial parasitic dermatitis is seldom observed even though *Dirofilaria immitis* is found in adult dogs.

**Stephanofilariasis.** *Stephanofilaria stilesi* invasion of the skin is extremely common in cattle. The majority of old or aged cattle in the Midwest have the skin lesions of this parasite. They are seldom observed in calves.

The lesions are found in the skin of the ventral surface of the abdomen and the sheath. They appear as circular, dry, raised areas that measure from 2 to 15 centimeters in diameter and 0.5 to 2 centimeters in thickness. The surface of the lesion may show hyperkeratosis and be covered with scales; or in the more active lesions, blood and serum, which dries and forms crusts, may be present on the surface.

The histological examination of the skin reveals a chronic suppurative parasitic dermatitis. Both adults and larvae are found throughout the lesion, and neutrophils and eosinophils are present in the immediate vicinity of the parasite. Hyperplasia of the epithelium is present. If the area is scraped with a sharp knife and the material is suspended in warm physiological saline solution and examined with a microscope, the adult parasites and their larvae can be demonstrated. It must be remembered that parasites are easily found in the more active lesions, while they are more difficult to find in the old chronic lesions. It is imperative that deep scrapings be made. One of the most common reasons why the parasites are not demonstrated is that the skin scrapings are too superficial.

This lesion must not be confused with the acute or chronic dermatitis that occurs in recumbent animals in those portions of the abdomen and thorax that are pressed against the floor or bedding.

**Elaeophoriasis.** *Elaeophora schneideri* is the cause of a filarid dermatitis of sheep that has been reported in the western United States. The adult filarid is found in the major arteries throughout the animal (aorta, carotid, and iliac arteries). The microfilaria of this parasite cause a dermatitis of the thinly wooled portions of the head, beginning at the poll and extending forward over the face to the nostrils and lips. In about 25 per cent of the sheep, the hind foot used to scratch the head is similarly involved; and in 10 per cent of the animals, lesions are found on the abdomen where the skin comes in contact with the infected hind foot. A papular, suppurative, or ulcerative dermatitis is present. The severity of the dermatitis depends upon the number of microfilaria, the traumatic injury produced as the result of the

pruritus, and the amount of bacterial infection in the area.

Histological examination reveals an acute or chronic, papular, suppurative, or ulcerative inflammation. The microfilaria are observed in the capillaries of the papillae of the dermis just below the epithelium. Numerous neutrophils and eosinophils are found in the lesion. If deep scrapings of the area are made and the material obtained is suspended in warm physiological saline solution and examined with the microscope, the microfilaria may be observed.

## ALOPECIA

Loss of hair frequently occurs in animals with various skin diseases and is especially common in housed animals during the winter months. These animals show an intense pruritus and rub against objects, scratch their body with their legs, and lick themselves. The hair is probably removed by the constant friction of the area in the attempt to relieve the itching. It is often the result of a fungous infection or an infestation with lice, fleas, or mites.

There are cases of alopecia in which none of the more common infectious etiologic agents can be found. Many of these animals show evidence of poor management, feeding, and care. Their hair coats are filthy from the accumulation of dirt and manure. Often their backs are covered with hay and chaff. This is especially common in bulls that throw bedding on their backs as they paw with their forefeet when irritated. Proper grooming and brushing of these animals together with an improvement in the general cleanliness and the ration fed will often bring about relief from the pruritus. When trauma to the area is no longer present, the hair returns.

Alopecia, resulting from dermatitis, occurs in dogs with chronic thallium sulfate poisoning. The hair can be pulled out with comparative ease, and when the dog is handled there is excessive falling of the hair.

Alopecia may occur as a result of an infectious disease. Following an acute or chronic infectious disease, the hair falls out, and partial or complete baldness occurs. This is especially common in sheep that have recovered from blue tongue.

Feeding on certain plants such as *Chrysodoma tenurisolia, Tamarindus indica, Senecio,* and *Astragulus* results in alopecia, especially in sheep and goats, but may also occur in horses, mules, and cattle.

Hutt and Saunders describe **viable genetic hypotrichosis** transmitted as a simple autosomal, recessive character in Guernsey cattle. The calf most severely affected lacked hair at 8 weeks except on the end of the tail, inner surface of the ear, eyelids, lips, dewlap, and umbilicus. At maturity the heifer had hair in these areas, also on the extremities of the legs, between the toes, and in lesser amounts elsewhere. Histological examination revealed that the hair follicles lacked papillae, the cells were not differentiated as in normal follicles, and sweat glands were cystic.

**Hypotrichosis congenita** (lethal hairless) has been described by Mohr and Wriedt. Homozygous calves are born alive at full term but die within a few minutes after birth. Hair is found only on the muzzle, eyelids, ears, tail, and pastern. The teeth and hoofs are normal, the sweat glands are cystic, the hair follicles are arrested in development, and fat is lacking in the subcutaneous tissue.

**Semihairlessness.** This simple, recessive, autosomal mutation is observed in Oklahoma and California in polled Herefords. The animals have coarse wiry hair that is never present in its normal amount. The hair coat is patchy, and the hair on the legs and back is longer and thicker than in other portions of the body.

**Hypotrichiosis with anodontia** is apparently a sex-linked recessive defect involving males. Calves are completely hairless and toothless at birth; sweat glands are cystic and hair follicles are rudimentary.

## HOOFS

Excessive wear of the hoof causes sore-footed swine, cattle, sheep, goats, and horses when the animal moves on gravel, rock, or concrete. It is particularly common in the animals in a feed lot paved with concrete. As the result of the excessive wear, the walls of the hoof are worn away and all of the weight of the animal is placed on the sole of the foot. These animals are reluctant to move, and if forced to move, they experience considerable pain.

It is often confused with the sore-footedness associated with vesicular exanthema in swine or foot-and-mouth disease in cattle. Examination of the coronet readily differentiates these diseases. The excessive wear of the hoof wall in the horse, and the sore-footedness associated with it, may be confused with the symptoms of founder.

Dogs or cats, although not having hoofs, experience similar wear and pain of their digital pads when they travel for long distances over rocky soil or over crusted snow or granular ice.

The shoeing of horses and oxen with rubber or metal shoes prevents hoof wear. The feet of sled dogs are frequently enclosed in moccasins to prevent foot injury.

The hoof of the domestic animals is particularly subject to trauma. Frequently nails and other objects, especially in the horse, penetrate the sole of the hoof and allow bacteria to enter into the interior of the hoof where a suppurative inflammation is produced.

Injuries to the coronary band, improper shoeing, nutritional and metabolic diseases, as well as hereditary hoof defects, result in cracks, ridges, and irregular hoof growth. The defects in the hoof wall allow bacteria to invade the internal structures of the hoof, causing a suppurative inflammation.

### Laminitis

Anyone interested in laminitis (founder) should consult the excellent work of Nils Obel. He has pointed out that the previous conception of the lesions in the hoof of the horse afflicted with this locomotor disease are probably in error.

Contrary to popular belief, horses affected with the so-called acute laminitis do not show edema, hemorrhage, and inflammation in the laminar corium. Likewise, histological examination does not reveal the vascular and inflammatory alterations in the sensitive laminae of the hoof that have been previously described. As Obel points out, "It is difficult to understand how serious injury to vessels could exist in the hoof while symptoms are generally lacking of a similar disturbance in other parts of the organism." He further points out that edema of the legs (a vascular reaction) is only occasionally observed in alimentary laminitis or postparturient laminitis, and yet edema of the limbs that is not accompanied by laminitis is often observed in the horse, which would indicate that the alterations in the hoof are probably not associated with vascular disease.

Obel has shown that all severe cases examined by him displayed a disturbance of the process of cornification in the various epidermal parts of the foot.

"This disturbance was evident as a disappearance of the 'keratogenic' structures characteristic of the basal part of the zone of cornification in the various epidermal regions, i.e. the onychogenic substance occurring in the form of comparatively coarse fibrils in the secondary epidermal laminae and in the matrix of the wall, sole and frog, disappeared, as did the keratohyalin occurring as basophilic granules in the matrix of the periople . . . . With regard to the papillary parts the process led to the denudation of a network of extremely fine fibrils passing radially from the cell centre and with distinctly outlined bridge corpuscles. However, in the lamellar region the corresponding epidermal layer was in the main free from fibrillary structures and, moreover, the secondary laminae were greatly deformed through stretching, so that in many places they consisted of a single cell layer. The epidermal part of the laminar layer also displayed . . . horn-like bodies or strings in the middle layer of the secondary laminae, necrobiotic processes in various stages, enlarged nucleoles, coarse meshed

chromatin network and numerous mitoses.

"The changes in the papillary parts of the corium of the foot were, apart from the bending of the coronary papillae, limited to more or less serious hyperemia, which did not always appear. . . . In the laminar part of the foot, however, there proved to be, in addition to hyperemia, fairly considerable changes in the vascular tissues, such as leukocytic infiltration, swelling and dislocation of the secondary sensitive laminae, and in a couple of cases, a serous exudation in the outer part of the laminar layer. It is remarkable that the injuries characteristic of the sensitive laminae only occurred in regions with very severe epidermal changes.

"The peculiar course of the process of cornification in the heavily loaded laminar layer . . . renders it probable that the onychogenic substance possesses the property of increasing the strength of the epithelial fibrils. On this assumption, . . . it is possible to explain the stretching of the secondary epidermal laminae as the result of a discrepancy between the body weight and the strength of the secondary laminae due to the disappearance of the onychogenic substance. As a rule the epithelial fibrils in the laminar layer undergo complete destruction. . . . This difference is probably connected with the deformation of the secondary laminae which may cause mechanical tearing of the fibrillar network.

"Some of the other epidermal changes typical of the laminar layer, the occurrence of numerous mitoses and the partial necrosis of the secondary laminae, are probably also the result of a purely mechanical irritation.

"The changes demonstrated in the laminar corium may without difficulty be explained as secondary to the weakening of the epidermal laminae. The infiltration of leukocytes may be occasioned by the epidermal necroses or by the injuries caused by the overstretching of the connective tissue, appearing in conjunction with the collapse of the basal epidermal laminae."

It is quite possible that the laminitis-causing factor may inactivate some substance that is essential for the normal metabolism in the zone of cornification. The work of Obel indicates that the entire problem of laminitis deals with biochemical alterations in which the process of cornification is not complete. It indicates that there must be a disruption of cell enzyme systems necessary for the production of keratohyalin.

The sinking of the pedal bone and its rotation are brought about by the disturbance in the process of cornification which decreases the strength of the epithelium. In consequence, the body weight gives rise to a stretching of the secondary epidermal laminae and a dislocation of the os pedis. As the os pedis rotates and sinks, the anteroventral border perforates the sole, allowing bacteria to invade the internal structures of the hoof and resulting in a suppurative inflammation (Fig. 22.9).

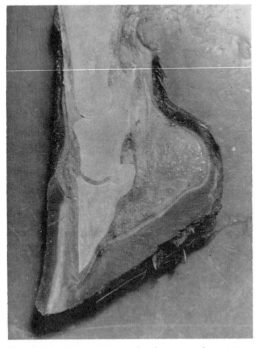

Fig. 22.9 — Laminitis in the horse with rotation of the os pedis. (Photograph retouched to demonstrate the position of the os pedis.)

## NEOPLASMS

For the general discussion of tumors consult the chapter on neoplasms. In the **chicken** the most common tumor of the skin is the lymphosarcoma of the leukosis complex. Hemartia are also quite common in the skin of Leghorn chickens, and fatal hemorrhage from these hemartia may occur. In the **dog** the most commonly encountered tumors are the fibroma, mastocytoma, histiocytoma, melanosarcoma, lymphosarcoma, fibrosarcoma, papilloma, squamous-cell carcinoma, sweat-gland adenoma and adenocarcinoma, sebaceous-gland adenoma and adenocarcinoma, and basal-cell carcinoma. In the **horse** the melanoma, melanosarcoma, fibroma, fibrosarcoma, papilloma, squamous-cell carcinoma, and sarcoid are commonly observed tumors. The **equine sarcoid** resembles a sarcoma and is composed of white fibrous connective tissue. Even though the tumor mass becomes quite large, it does not metastasize to the regional lymph nodes or other organs. It is usually found in the skin of the head and neck. The cause has not been determined, but apparently some of these tumors could be the result of viral infections (bovine wart virus and horse pox). Papillomas are present in the auricula and the external auditory canal of about 15 per cent of older horses. In some areas of the United States papillomas are very common in the skin of the nose of the horse in the vicinity of the external nares and the lips. Cook and Olson have shown that the papilloma of the nose of the horse may be transmitted from one equine to another.

In the **bovine**, fibroma, fibrosarcoma, papilloma, and squamous-cell carcinoma are the most commonly encountered tumors. The melanoma and melanosarcoma are most frequently observed in **swine**.

**Epidermal inclusion cysts** are quite common in all animals and involve the sebaceous glands, sweat glands, or the hair follicles. The epidermal inclusion cysts are quite common in swine, where they appear as bluish-green vesicles in the skin of the back and vary in size from just visible to 1 centimeter in diameter. They are often very numerous but do not represent an infectious process. They are apparently a disturbance of growth in which the hair follicle does not develop properly. The vesicle consists of a mass of hair suspended in a reddish-brown fluid. The condition in swine is often called **hypotrichosis cystica.**

Epidermal inclusion cysts are exceedingly common along the dorsal mid-line of the lumbosacral region of the Rhodesian ridgeback dog. These cysts are similar to pilonoidal cysts in man.

Epidermal inclusion cysts are found in the domestic fowl. They vary in size from 1 millimeter to 2 centimeters in diameter. The cysts are comparable to those observed in mammals except that rudimentary feathers are found within the cyst.

## REFERENCES

Clare, N. T.: 1952. Photosensitization in diseases of domesticated animals. Review Series No. 3, Commonwealth Bur. Anim. Health, Farnham, Royal Bucks, England.

———, Whitten, L. K., and Filmer, D. B.: 1947. Photosensitized keratitis in young calves following the use of phenothiazine as an anthelminthic. III. Identification of the photosensitizing agent. Austral. Vet. Jour., 23:344.

Cook, R., and Olson, C.: 1951. Experimental transmission of cutaneous papilloma of the horse. Amer. Jour. Path., 27:1087.

Davis, C., and Kemper, H.: 1951. The histopathologic diagnosis of filarial dermatosis in sheep. Jour. A.V.M.A., 118:103.

Fourie, P. J. J.: 1936. The occurrence of congenital porphyrinuria (pink tooth) in cattle in South Africa (Swaziland). Onderstepoort Jour. Vet. Sci. and Anim. Ind., 7:535.

Hutt, F. B., and Saunders, L. Z.: 1953. Viable genetic hypotrichosis in Guernsey cattle. Jour. Hered., 44:97.

Jones, L. D.: 1956. Exudative epidermitis in pigs. Master's Degree Thesis, Iowa State University.

Kernkamp, H. C. H.: 1933. Five cases of hypertrichosis partialis in swine. Cornell Vet., 23:74.

McIntyre, R.: 1949. Virus papular dermatitis of the horse. Amer. Jour. Vet. Res., 10:229.

Mason, J., and Bekker, J.: 1934. Further notes on lumpy wool in South Africa. Onderstepoort Jour. V.S.A.I., 3:211.

Mohr, O. L., and Wriedt, C.: 1928. Hairless, a new recessive lethal in cattle. Jour. Genet., 19:315.

Obel, N.: 1948. Studies on the histopathology of acute laminitis. Almqvist and Wiksells Boktryckeri AB, Uppsala, Sweden.

Penny, R. H. C.: 1957. An unusual skin condition in the pig. Vet. Rec., 69:1957.

Quin, J. I.: 1933. Studies on the photosensitization of animals in South Africa. I. The action of various fluorescent dye stuffs. Onderstepoort Jour. Vet. Sci. and Anim. Ind., 1:459.

———: 1933. Studies on the photosensitization of animals in South Africa. VI. The effect of surgical obstruction of the normal bile flow. Onderstepoort Jour. Vet. Sci. and Anim. Ind., 1:505.

Tunnicliff, E. A.: 1949. Ulcerative dermatosis of sheep. Amer. Jour. Vet. Res., 10:240.

# Technic for Post-Mortem Examinations

## Horse

### PREPARATION FOR EVISCERATION

1. Place the horse on the right side.

2. Make a median, ventral, cutaneous incision from the chin to the anus. Make the incision dorsolaterally around the mammary gland, or prepuce and penis.

3. Skin as much as possible of the left side of the neck and the left side of the thorax and abdomen. Most rendering plants insist that the hide be removed in good condition.

4. Raise the left forelimb while cutting the pectoral and serratus muscles, and tip the leg over the body in the direction of the withers. Cut the thoracic muscles close to the ribs.

5. Raise the left hindlimb while cutting the inner thigh muscles from the external angle of the ilium to the coxofemoral joint and thence to the anus, keeping laterally around the tuberosity of the ischium. Tip the leg over the body while severing the remainder of the thigh muscles.

6. Finish skinning the thorax and abdomen to the tops of the spinous processes of the vertebrae.

7. From the vertebral end of the last rib to the vertebral end of the first rib make an incision through what remains of the thoracic muscles. Posteriorly this incision will follow the ventral border of the longissimus dorsi muscle. This incision marks the places at which the ribs are to be cut with an ax. Stick a knife in the severed brachial artery and cut through it and the sternocephalicus muscle so as to let any uncoagulated blood escape from the large vessels of the anterior thorax. From the sternal end of the first rib to the xyphoid cartilage make an incision through the unremoved parts of the pectoral muscles. This marks the place for cutting the ribs and costal cartilages with an ax.

8. Open the abdominal cavity by making a xyphoid-pubic incision and a pubic-lumbar incision through the abdominal wall. Cut a handhold in the abdominal muscles at the pubic angle of the severed abdominal wall.

9. Pull upward and forward the large flap of abdominal wall and cut the diaphragm dorsoventrally close to its attachment to the ribs and remove the whole left side of the animal. This can be used for a clean place on which to examine organs in the field.

### EVISCERATION

#### Abdominal Cavity

1. Pick up the pelvic flexure of the great colon and pull the organ, together with the cecum, out of the abdominal cavity. Extend them at right angles to the long axis of the body.

2. Remove the spleen, left kidney, and left adrenal.

3. Pick up the small colon and lay it over the back of the animal in the lumbar region. Sever it at the rectum and at the duodenal-colic fold. Finish removing the small colon by cutting its mesentery.

4. Sever the small intestine at the duodenal-colic fold and remove it by cutting its mesentery close to the intestine attachment

along the whole length of the organ. Sever the small intestine again about six inches from the ileocecal valve.

5. Remove the stomach and duodenum.

6. With scissors open the posterior aorta from a few inches anterior to the crura of the diaphragm to the bifurcation of the iliac arteries. Open the stump of the coeliac artery. Open the root of the anterior mesenteric artery and its three branches.

7. Remove the great colon and cecum.

8. Remove the right adrenal, right kidney, and ureter.

9. Cut the ligamentous attachment of the liver to the diaphragm and remove the liver.

10. With an ax cut the symphysis of the pubis. Saw through the shaft of the ileum above the coxofemoral joint. Remove the resulting detached portion of the pelvic girdle and then the internal genital organs, the rectum, and the bladder.

### Thoracic Cavity

1. Open the pericardial sac from the apex to the base of the heart and inspect the contents of the sac.

2. Cut off the posterior aorta at the crura of the diaphragm and then cut anteriorly between the aorta and the spinal column. Continue cutting forward until the trachea and esophagus are reached. Sever them together with the large vessels and nerves of the anterior thorax. Cut posteriorly along the floor of the thoracic cavity, freeing the heart and cutting the right half of the diaphragm close to its rib attachment. With the left hand grasp the large vessels at the base of the heart and remove the thoracic organs.

### Neck and Mouth Organs

1. Grasp the trachea at the thoracic entrance and remove it together with the esophagus, the cervical blood vessels, and muscles of the ventral cervical region by dissecting toward the head.

2. Without severing the above structures, continue the dissection around the larynx. Cut the omohyoideus and mylohyoideus muscles close to the rami of the mandible. Separate the hyoid bone at the middle cornua where it is easy to cut through the cartilaginous attachments. Pull the neck organs forward and continue dissecting until the tongue flips around posteriorly. Then, while continuing to pull the neck organs forward, lay the knife with the cutting edge to the rear on the rami of the mandible and finish cutting the omohyoideus muscles.

### Brain

1. Remove the head at the occipitoatloid joint.

2. With the head in the normal position and with the nose pointing toward the prosector, run a dorsal median cutaneous incision from the nose up over the poll.

3. Skin each side of the head lateroventrally from this incision down below the ear and eye.

4. With a saw make a transverse cut through the calvarium into the cranial cavity along a line just posterior to the supraorbital processes of the frontal bones.

5. With a saw connect each end of this incision with the foramen magnum. The incision on each side should extend from the notch dorsal to the occipital condyle toward the eye.

6. Remove the detached calvarium.

7. Remove the brain by slipping the handle of a scalpel down in front of the olfactory lobes and then working the lobes back. Slip the index finger of the left hand down in front of the cerebral hemispheres and lift the brain up, exposing the optic chiasm. Sever it, and then continue to work the brain back, exposing next the pituitary body and then the pons. Slip the left index finger down under the pons and medulla and roll the brain upward and backward.

## Ruminants

### PREPARATION FOR EVISCERATION

Proceed as with the horse except: 1. Place the ruminant on the left side. 2. Reverse the median, ventral, cutaneous incision. Make it from the anus to the chin because it is awkward to make it from the chin to the anus. 3. Reverse the xyphoid-pubic incision.

### EVISCERATION

### Abdominal Cavity

1. Palpate between the reticulum and diaphragm for evidences of foreign body penetration in cattle.

2. Remove the omentum by cutting dorsally and also at the right laterally along the omental attachment to the duodenum. Also, cut its two attachments to the rumen.

3. Remove both kidneys and the ureters.

4. Sever the rectum and the duodenum. The duodenum is cut in two places — six inches on either side of the place where the

gall bladder lies over it. Remove the intestine by then cutting its mesentery.

5. While the assistant exerts traction on the stomachs, cut their attachments and the esophagus, and pull them out.

6. Remove the liver and the pelvic organs as in the horse.

(The remainder of the procedure in the ruminant is the same as in the horse.)

## Dog and Cat

### PREPARATION FOR EVISCERATION

1. Make a median, ventral, cutaneous incision from the chin to the anus. In the male make this incision as far as the penis and prepuce. From there to the anus run double parallel incisions so that the penis may be reflected to the ischial arch. Do not detach the organ.

2. Beginning at the brisket, skin the thorax, removing the thoracic muscles with the skin and separating, but not completely detaching, the forelimbs from the thorax. Finish skinning both sides of the dog, and open the coxofemoral joint so that the hind-limbs lie flat on the table.

3. Examine the superficial lymph nodes and the thyroids.

4. Open the thorax and abdomen by cutting the costochondral junctions and removing a strip of abdominal wall from the sternum to the pubis.

### EVISCERATION

#### Abdominal Cavity

1. Working at the side of the carcass with the animal's head to the prosector's left, pick up and remove the omentum.

2. Sever the colon near the bladder and the duodenum at the posterior end of the pancreas. While pulling on the intestine, cut the mesentery and remove the organ.

3. With the index and second fingers of the left hand, straddle the hepatic vein, posterior vena cava, and the esophagus and sever these three structures. Lift out the five organs just detached — stomach, duodenum, liver, spleen, and pancreas.

4. Remove both adrenals, both kidneys, and the ureters.

5. Cut the symphysis of the pubis with a knife or saw, and spread the pelvis so that the bladder, internal genitals, rectum, and anus can be removed intact.

#### Thoracic Cavity

1. Cut the diaphragm close to its attachment.

2. With the first two fingers of the left hand straddle the trachea and adjacent structures and pull the chest organs back. With a long-bladed knife cut down between the first and second ribs on each side simultaneously, severing all the structures at the thoracic entrance. Pull the thoracic organs posteriorly, stripping them loose from their attachment along the spinal column. Cut the posterior aorta at the crura of the diaphragm.

(Remove the neck and mouth organs as in the horse.)

## Swine

The technic for swine is similar to that for the dog except that: (1) Often the intestine is not severed from the stomach at the time of removal, and (2) the urinary bladder is usually removed without splitting the pelvis.

## METHODS FOR EXAMINING ORGANS

### Brain

1. Place the brain on the table with the brain-stem below and the medulla towards the prosector.

2. Inspect the outer surface of the various parts.

3. Beginning medially on each cerebral hemisphere, cut ventrolaterally into each lateral ventricle.

4. Medially cut down through the cerebellum in an anteroposterior direction into the fourth ventricle.

5. Follow the aqueduct of Sylvius into the third ventricle. Inspect all ventricles especially for edema.

6. Beginning at the olfactory lobes and proceeding posteriorly, make rather thin transverse, vertical incisions completely through the brain and inspect for symmetry of form of corresponding structures, for tumors, foci of softening, abscesses, parasitic cysts, hemorrhages, and for increased prominence and numbers of bleeding points.

### Mouth and Neck Organs

1. Inspect the tongue.

2. With an enterotome open the pharynx and esophagus.

3. With the enterotome open the larynx and trachea.

**Thoracic Organs**

1. Place the thoracic organs on the table with the heart nearest the prosector and with the apex pointing to his right. This places the heart in the position in which it would lie in an animal facing the prosector.

2. With an enterotome open the esophagus.

3. Examine the bronchial and mediastinal lymph nodes.

4. Examine the lungs — the three lobes of the left lung first and then the four of the right.

5. Open the pericardial sac of small animals. It has already been opened in large animals.

6. Inspect the outside of the heart and open it in the following manner:

a. Beginning ventrally in the right ventricle, make an incision in an upward direction parallel and close to the left longitudinal groove through the pulmonary semilunar valve into the pulmonary artery.

b. Rotate the heart to the right and continue the incision from the point of beginning in the right ventricle laterally to the left almost to the right longitudinal groove, then dorsally along the groove through the tricuspid into the right atrium.

c. Place the heart in the original position. Stick a knife into the apex of the left ventricle and cut dorsally parallel and close to the left longitudinal groove through the mitral valve into the left atrium.

d. With an enterotome open the aortic semilunar valve and continue the incision along the aorta.

**Abdominal Organs**

1. The stomach, duodenum, pancreas, liver, and spleen are placed in front of the prosector in this manner: (1) liver at the right with gall bladder up, (2) stomach at the left with duodenum and pancreas toward the prosector, (3) spleen at end of stomach farthest removed from the prosector. Examine the spleen, the liver, the gall bladder, the cystic, hepatic and common bile ducts, and the pancreas. Then open the duodenum and stomach, keeping to the left side of the latter in order to follow the greater curvature. (This technic is for these organs in small animals.)

2. Cut the mesentery close to the intestine and open the organ with an enterotome.

3. Make an incision through the cortex of each kidney and inspect for swelling. Then finish the incision to the pelvis. Remove the capsule if possible.

4. The pelvic organs are placed with the bladder uppermost and with its vertex toward the prosector. Open the bladder at the vertex and carry the incision toward the urethra and then down the latter. Reverse the position of these organs. In the female open the vagina, cervix, and uterus. Open the rectum and, in dogs, examine the anal glands.

## MATERIAL FOR LABORATORY EXAMINATION

In selecting material for bacteriological examination, prevent as far as possible outside contamination. If a septicemia of any kind is suspected, tie off the vessels of the heart and send the intact organ. With it send the spleen and some of the affected lymph nodes. Place the organs in a small container *without* a preservative, and place this container in a second but much larger one. Pack enough chopped ice in sawdust in this larger container to insure the arrival of the organs at the laboratory in an undecomposed state. Heads of rabies suspects should also be sent in this manner. Blood for serological tests need not be sent in this way if the samples are collected in sterile containers under good conditions.

Material for sectioning and parasites for identification should be sent in a 10 per cent solution of ordinary commercial formaldehyde solution.

Regardless of the nature of the material sent, a complete history and description of the case should accompany the specimens. It is much more satisfactory to include this information with the specimens than to send it in a letter which may not reach the laboratory until after the specimens. In most instances it is better to address material to a laboratory rather than to an individual in a laboratory.

## POST-MORTEM CHANGES

As an aid to making a differentiation between alterations that occur in the body before death and those which take place after death the following descriptions of postmortem changes are given. The changes are given only for parts of the body where they most often occur and where they are most likely to lead to confusion.

**Heart**

At death the heart is in diastole. Within the first hour rigor mortis develops, beginning with the left ventricle. As a consequence, the left ventricle becomes almost empty and the right ventricle only about half full. If the myocardium is degenerated, rigor mortis may not appear. Under usual conditions rigor mortis disappears in 20 to 30 hours (1 to 1½ days). Necropsy at this time shows a flabby heart with an empty left ventricle. However, if at this time the heart is flabby and the left ventricle is filled with coagulated blood, it is an indication that there is myocardial degeneration, and rigor mortis did not occur at all or only slightly. On the other hand, if the heart is flabby and filled with uncoagulated blood, rigor mortis may have occurred, but the fluid blood returned to the ventricle (asphyxia, hemolysis). Usual post-mortem coagulation occurs slowly with separation of the clot into two portions, upper "chicken fat" clot, lower "currant jelly" clot. Predominance of the former indicates slow death. Post-mortem granular coagulation of the sarcoplasm of the cardiac muscle cells resembles cloudy swelling in color. The endocardium is frequently blood-stained (imbibition of blood). Occasionally gas vesicles appear in the myocardium as a result of post-mortem decomposition.

## Forestomachs of Ruminants

Post-mortem **tympany** is produced by continued fermentation after death. It is differentiated from ante-mortem tympany by lack of passive hyperemia of the thoracic and abdominal organs and absence of ecchymoses in the serous membranes. Extreme distension may cause **rupture** of the rumen or diaphragm. This can be differentiated from ante-mortem rupture by the absence of hemorrhagic infiltration and swelling of the border of the rupture. Another change which is frequently noted by veterinarians is loosening of the epithelium by **maceration**. It occurs within a few hours after death and is noticed particularly in the omasum.

## Stomach

**Hypostatic congestion.** The lowermost portions of the mucosa and serosa have a bluish-red color, and the blood vessels are injected. There is a perivascular diffusion of hemoglobin (**imbibition of blood**). By the formation of sulfmethemoglobin and iron sulfide, the color becomes grayish-blue or grayish-green (**pseudomelanosis**). Intravital hemorrhages undergo the same change. **Imbibition of bile.**

There is a yellowish discoloration of the mucosa. A faded yellow or green discoloration can be seen also on the serous coat in the vicinity of the gall bladder. **Autolysis.** The degree of self digestion depends upon the digestion period at the time of death, upon the stomach contents, and the rapidity with which the carcass cools. It is not dependent upon putrefactive changes. It begins with swelling of the mucosa, which becomes soft, transparent and glassy, and strips off easily leaving the submucosa bare. The process begins at the tops of the folds and rarely affects the muscular coats and serosa. When it does, post-mortem rupture may occur. **Putrefactive emphysema.** The dirty, grayish-red mucous membrane becomes raised into blisters by gas. **Tympany.** Fermentative and decomposition changes after death produce gas which distends the stomach and may produce rupture of the stomach and diaphragm. Like ante-mortem rupture it occurs on the greater curvature. It must be differentiated from ante-mortem rupture.

## Intestine

Post-mortem changes in the intestine are quite similar to those of the stomach. To the list must be added post-mortem displacements such as torsion and invagination. Absence of hyperemia, edema, and hemorrhage in the displaced intestines marks the difference between post-mortem and ante-mortem displacements.

## Liver

**Hemolysis and imbibition of hemoglobin** are observed first perivascularly. The color may be dark green or bluish-black due to the formation of sulfmethemoglobin and iron sulfide. **Emphysema** may occur soon after death. It is common in sheep and hogs. As a result of **autolysis** the organ becomes a soft, pulpy mass. Microscopically, the nuclei disappear, and the plasma shows granular disintegration. **Imbibition of bile** is manifested by a pale yellow or greenish discoloration in the area where the gall bladder is in contact with the liver. **Post-mortem bacterial emboli** may be differentiated from ante-mortem emboli by the absence of accompanying tissue changes.

# Index

[ 719 ]